Research Advances in

# Alcohol and Drug Problems

Volume 10

# Research Advances in Alcohol and Drug Problems

## Volume 10

Edited by

Lynn T. Kozlowski, Helen M. Annis, Howard D. Cappell,
Frederick B. Glaser, Michael S. Goodstadt, Yedi Israel,
Harold Kalant, Edward M. Sellers, and Evelyn R. Vingilis

Addiction Research Foundation and
University of Toronto
Toronto, Ontario, Canada

Springer Science+Business Media, LLC

The Library of Congress cataloged the first volume of this title as follows:

Research advances in alcohol & drug problems. v. 1 -

New York [etc.] J. Wiley, 1974-
v. 24 cm. annual.
"A Wiley biomedical health publication."
ISSN 0093-9714

1. Alcoholism—Periodicals. 2. Narcotic habit—Periodicals.
RC565.R37 616.8′6′005 73-18088

ISBN 978-1-4899-1671-6 ISBN 978-1-4899-1669-3 (eBook)

DOI 10.1007/978-1-4899-1669-3



Originally published by Plenum Press, New York in 1990
Softcover reprint of the hardcover 1st edition 1990

# Contributors

ZALMAN AMIT, Centre for Studies in Behavioural Neurobiology, Department of Psychology, Concordia University, Montreal, Quebec, Canada

PATRICIA G. ERICKSON, Drug Policy Research Program, Prevention Studies Department, Addiction Research Foundation, Toronto, Ontario, Canada

KAYE MIDDLETON FILLMORE, Institute for Health and Aging, Department of Social and Behavioral Sciences, University of California–San Francisco, San Francisco, California

EDITH S. LISANSKY GOMBERG, School of Social Work, and Alcohol Research Center, Department of Psychiatry, School of Medicine, University of Michigan, Ann Arbor, Michigan

NEIL E. GRUNBERG, Medical Psychology Department, Uniformed Services University of the Health Sciences, Bethesda, Maryland

DOROTHY HATSUKAMI, Departments of Psychiatry and Psychology, University of Minnesota, Minneapolis, Minnesota

STEPHEN T. HIGGINS, Departments of Psychiatry, Psychology, and Family Practice, University of Vermont, Burlington, Vermont

JOHN R. HUGHES, Departments of Psychiatry, Psychology, and Family Practice, University of Vermont, Burlington, Vermont

MARK KELLER, Rutgers University, Piscataway, New Jersey

JIM ORFORD, Department of Psychology, University of Exeter, Washington Singer Laboratories, Exeter, and Department of Clinical and Community Psychology, Exeter Health Authority, Larkby, Exeter, United Kingdom

ROBIN ROOM, Alcohol Research Group, Institute of Epidemiology and Behavioral Medicine, Medical Research Institute of San Francisco, Berkeley, California

BRIAN R. SMITH, Centre for Studies in Behavioural Neurobiology, Department of Psychology, Concordia University, Montreal, Quebec, Canada

KAREN J. SPIVAK, Addiction Research Foundation, Toronto, Ontario, Canada

VALERIE A. WATSON, Drug Policy Research Program, Prevention Studies Department, Addiction Research Foundation, Toronto, Ontario, Canada

THOMAS ASHBY WILLS, Department of Epidemiology and Social Medicine, Albert Einstein College of Medicine, Bronx, New York

# Preface

This is the tenth volume in the *Research Advances* series and the seventh published by Plenum Press. Volume 10 is another omnibus volume, providing specialized and advanced reviews in a number of areas related to the use of alcohol, illicit drugs, and tobacco. We include also a brief history of the Center for Alcohol Studies that gives Mark Keller's unique perspective on this noted institution. Two of the chapters are decidedly longer than the others—very long chapters have appeared occasionally in the past, and we think that it is one of the strengths of the series that we are able to accommodate such reviews.

Again the editorial board has changed. After several years of service, Reginald G. Smart has stepped down. New to the board are Helen M. Annis, Michael S. Goodstadt, Lynn T. Kozlowski, and Evelyn R. Vingilis. This is likely to be the sole volume for which Goodstadt is on the board, since before completion of this volume he moved from the Addiction Research Foundation to the Center for Alcohol Studies, Rutgers University.

The Editors

*Toronto*

# Contents

# 1

# Does Acetaldehyde Play a Role in Alcoholism?

## Behavioral versus Biochemical Analysis

BRIAN R. SMITH, KAREN J. SPIVAK, and ZALMAN AMIT

## 1. INTRODUCTION

The issue whether acetaldehyde plays a functional role in the actions of alcohol remains a controversial area following more than two decades of investigation. The publication of several extensive reviews (Lindros, 1978; Amir et al., 1980; von Wartburg, 1980; Brien and Loomis, 1983, Amit and Smith, 1989) have left little doubt that the first metabolic product of alcohol oxidation is an important contributor to some of the consequences of exposure to ethanol. Unfortunately, despite the massive literature that accumulated during this period, there is, as yet, little consensus concerning which actions of alcohol (if any) are a function of the formation of acetaldehyde.

This chapter therefore reviews and evaluates the behavioral and psychopharmacological data on the possible role of acetaldehyde in the actions of alcohol. Furthermore, we have based the argument on the contention that the positive reinforcing properties of alcohol are the primary variables underlying the development of dependence on alcohol. It follows logically that any suggestion that acetaldehyde may play a role in alcoholism must incorporate within its framework evidence supporting the involvement of acetaldehyde in those reinforcing and dependence-producing properties of alcohol. This chapter was written as an attempt to do so. Finally, we have attempted to evaluate the relevance of primarily negative biochemical data and contrast it with the significance of a growing body of behavioral data supportive of this notion.

BRIAN R. SMITH and ZALMAN AMIT • Centre for Studies in Behavioural Neurobiology, Department of Psychology, Concordia University, Montreal, Quebec H3G 1M8, Canada. KAREN J. SPIVAK • Addiction Research Foundation, Toronto, Ontario M5S 2S1, Canada.

## 2. ACETALDEHYDE AS A TOXIC SUBSTANCE

Traditionally, acetaldehyde has been viewed as a toxic by-product of ethanol metabolism (Hald and Jacobsen, 1948; Jacobsen, 1952). It is known, for example, that prolonged ethanol exposure may disrupt liver function (Hasumura et al., 1975). It was perhaps because of these earlier observations that acetaldehyde's aversive effects have initially drawn the greatest attention. The apparent toxicity of peripheral accumulation of acetaldehyde has in fact served as the basis of a treatment model for alcoholism (Ritchie, 1970; Sellers et al., 1981). This presumably toxic elevation in blood concentration of acetaldehyde was brought about through the use of pharmacological agents that are capable of inhibiting hepatic aldehyde dehydrogenase (ALDH). Two such agents widely used in the treatment of alcoholism are disulfiram (Antabuse) and the cyanamide derivative calcium carbimide (Temposil) (Ritchie, 1970; Sellers et al., 1981). In the presence of alcohol, these agents induce a reaction known as the disulfiram–alcohol reaction. Manifestations of this interaction include vasodilatation, tachycardia, decreased blood pressure, dizziness, nausea, and vomiting (Kitson, 1977; Truitt and Walsh, 1971). In more severe cases, respiratory depression, cardiovascular collapse, and death may occur (Jacobsen, 1952).

It had long been thought that the elevation of acetaldehyde levels via the use of these agents served to limit alcohol drinking (Eriksson, 1980*a*; Lindros et al., 1975; Schlesinger et al., 1966; Sellers et al., 1981). It was demonstrated in both humans as well as laboratory animals (although exceptions were, in fact, reported) that administration of disulfiram or cyanamide reduced voluntary consumption of ethanol (see Lindros, 1978). This notion has been supported by investigations of the innate alcohol sensitivity observed in some Orientals (Goedde et al., 1979; Mizoi et al., 1983; Wolff, 1972). These studies revealed that approximately 50% of Japanese lack the hepatic mitochondrial low $K_m$ isozyme of ALDH (Harada et al., 1980; Mizoi et al., 1983). Ingestion of low to moderate doses of alcohol in these individuals results in much higher blood acetaldehyde levels than that found in Caucasians after ingestion of similar amounts of alcohol. Because of the inability to metabolize acetaldehyde quickly and efficiently, these Orientals have a heightened sensitivity to alcohol and experience dysphoric reactions (Goedde et al., 1979; Mizoi et al., 1979). This reaction is similar to that observed in alcoholics who consume alcohol while receiving disulfiram or calcium carbimide (Brien and Loomis, 1983; Tottmar et al., 1977). In a study conducted by Harada et al. (1983), approximately 40% of healthy Japanese males sampled displayed a deficiency in the low $K_m$ isozyme of ALDH; however, only 2.3% of Japanese alcoholics were in this group, suggesting that the deficiency of this isozyme of ALDH in Orientals may be a genetic factor protecting this subpopulation from excessive alcohol intake and the subsequent development of alcoholism.

## 3. ACETALDEHYDE AS A REWARDING AGENT

The foregoing seems to support the view that the effects of acetaldehyde were primarily aversive in nature; however, clinical evidence and more recent experimental data suggest that this may not be the case in every instance. There can be no question that high concentrations of acetaldehyde circulating in blood have aversive consequences (Kitson, 1977); however, there are increasing data to suggest that lower levels may in fact be "euphoric." There are now several reports in the literature which indicate that not only do individuals continue to drink despite receiving disulfiram (Chevens, 1953; Minto and Roberts, 1960) but that the perceived effects of the disulfiram–alcohol interaction are reported to be pleasurable (Chevens, 1953; Minto and Roberts, 1960; Peachey et al., 1980; Brown et al., 1983). Further support for this notion was provided by a report in which alcohol-induced increase in "positive" mood (i.e., talking easy and feeling good) was found to be positively correlated with blood acetaldehyde levels (Behar et al., 1983).

Animal research appears to support this notion as well. Sinclair and Lindros (1981) demonstrated that prevention of the accumulation of peripheral acetaldehyde by concurrent treatment with cyanamide and the alcohol dehydrogenase inhibitor 4-methylpyrazole still resulted in the suppression of alcohol drinking in rats. Despite the fact that a suppression in ethanol intake was observed, the authors concluded that acetaldehyde accumulation in the periphery was not responsible for this effect, but rather was the result of some central regulating mechanism related to brain ALDH activity (Sinclair and Lindros, 1981). In addition, several studies have been reported in which the administration of cyanamide failed to reduce ethanol consumption in rats and at least one case produced a transient increase (Amit et al., 1976*b*, 1980). In a recent study, the prior administration of cyanamide was found to increase ethanol consumption when the latter was presented following termination of the drug treatment (Sinclair and Gribble, 1985). Finally, in a recent series of studies Spivak and Amit (1987), using a paradigm similar to that used by Sinclair and Lindros (1981), demonstrated a complex interaction between the various manupulations of brain ALDH and voluntary ethanol consumption. These data supported the notion that these changes in ethanol intake were not merely a function of changes in enzyme activity (e.g., brain ALDH), but were possibly related to the resultant fluctuations in brain acetaldehyde concentration and its capacity to mediate ethanol's positive reinforcing properties.

It appears, therefore, that acetaldehyde accumulation may result in either aversive or, in many instances, positive effects and that the occurrence of each of these effects seems to be related to either peripheral or central concentration levels of this substance. The indication that some level of accumulation of acetaldehyde may not be aversive in nature led to the suggestion that acetaldehyde may possess psychopharmacological effects which are actually opposite in nature (i.e., positive or reinforcing effects). The first indication in support of this notion came from a series of studies by Amir (1977, 1978*a,b*; Amir and Stern, 1978). It was reported that ALDH activity in liver and brain was positively correlated with previous ethanol intake in rats given free acces to ethanol (Amir, 1977). Although significant correlations were obtained with liver ALDH activity and ethanol intake, brain ALDH was relatively more important in predicting ethanol consumption (Amir, 1977). These findings led Amir (1977) to suggest that some interaction of acetaldehyde with brain mechanisms may dictate the effects of ethanol and that brain ALDH activity could ultimately be responsible for differences in the behavioral response to ethanol. Recent studies have supported these initial reports, as ethanol consumption correlated better with levels of brain rather than liver aldehyde-oxidizing capacity in three different strains of rats (Socaransky et al., 1984, 1985). Furthermore, brain ALDH activity did not differ as a function of exposure to ethanol, in contrast to the higher ALDH levels in liver measured in ethanol-drinking animals (Socaransky et al., 1984).

The relationship of acetaldehyde-metabolizing enzymes and ethanol intake provided indirect support for the notion that the pharmacological properties of acetaldehyde may be important in the mediation of ethanol consumption. This, in turn, led to a direct investigation of the possible psychopharmacological properties of acetaldehyde. It was reported that naive rats would self-administer acetaldehyde into the cerebral ventricles but would not perform the operant task when ethanol infusions were used as the reinforcer (Brown et al., 1979). These same authors also reported that the propensity to self-administer acetaldehyde intraventricularly was positively correlated with subsequent ethanol preference in the same animals (Brown et al., 1980). It was suggested that acetaldehyde not only possessed positive reinforcing properties, but that these psychopharmacological effects may mediate, at least in part, voluntary ethanol intake in rats (Brown et al., 1980).

These studies, taken together, provided a strong suggestion that the presence of acetaldehyde in brain may be reinforcing. Moreover, more recent research has provided evidence that this may also be the case in the periphery. Consistent with the central self-administration studies, several laboratories reported that animals would learn to self-administer acetaldehyde intravenously (Myers et al., 1982, 1984*a,b*; Takayama and Uyeno, 1985). These results support the previously described clinical evidence indicating that low peripheral concentrations of acetaldehyde may have reinforcing properties. Once again, in agreement with the central studies described earlier, it was also shown that animals with a prior history of acetaldehyde self-administration subsequently consumed more ethanol when they were later presented with a free choice of increasing concentrations of ethanol and water, indicating that prior exposure to acetaldehyde may facilitate subsequent acquisition of ethanol intake or, even more interestingly, that the two are related (Myers et al., 1984*a,b*). Furthermore, it has been reported that naïve rats self-administered intravenous acetaldehyde at higher rates compared to animals lever-pressing for infusions of ethanol, suggesting that acetaldehyde may be a more potent reinforcer than ethanol (Takayama and Uyeno, 1985).

Studies using the behavioral paradigm known as place conditioning have demonstrated that conditioned place preferences occur to a variety of self-administered drugs, such as morphine (Mucha et al., 1982; Katz and Gormezano, 1979; Blander et al., 1984), heroin (Bozarth and Wise, 1981*a*; Schenk et al., 1983), and cocaine (Mucha et al., 1982; Spyraki et al., 1982). Consistent with these findings, Smith et al. (1984) demonstrated that multiple intracerebroventricular infusions of acetaldehyde were capable of inducing a conditioned place preference in rats and that its magnitude was similar to that observed with other self-administered drugs. These experiments, then, utilizing two routes of administration (central and intravenous), as well as two distinctly different paradigms which are considered at present to be the most suitable instruments for detecting the reinforcing properties of abused drugs, indicate that acetaldehyde can support operant responses and appears, therefore, to possess positive reinforcing properties.

## 4. THE MEASUREMENT OF ACETALDEHYDE *IN VIVO*

Despite the consistency of the clinical observations and the behavioral experiments described earlier, there has been a "consistent" reluctance to accept the notion that acetaldehyde has positive reinforcing properties or that these psychopharmacological properties play a mediational role in alcohol intake (i.e., Deitrich, 1987; Erikkson, 1983). Much of this objection stems not from theoretical considerations, but rather from the apparent limitations (particularly in view of the strength of the behavioral data) of the current state of analytical technology and its inability to measure acetaldehyde either in the periphery or directly in brain. There seems to be a consensus that most of the acetaldehyde formed following consumption of moderate quantities of ethanol is rapidly oxidized and only minute amounts can be detected in the peripheral circulation (Eriksson, 1977; Eriksson and Sippel, 1977). When larger doses of ethanol (>2 g/kg) were administered, elevated peripheral acetaldehyde concentrations were measured, indicating that the rate of ethanol oxidation may have exceeded the rate of hepatic acetaldehyde elimination capacity (Lindros et al., 1972; Raskin and Sokoloff, 1972; Weiner, 1979). However, it has been argued that these elevated concentrations of acetaldehyde may be related to confounds in assay technique alone and, therefore, are artifactual (Eriksson, 1980*b*, 1983; Lindros, 1983). Using controlled assay procedures, Eriksson et al. (1984) have reported that following a challenge dose of 3 g/kg ethanol in mice, no acetaldehyde could be detected in blood.

The attempt to determine the presence of acetaldehyde in brain following alcohol exposure has yielded equally ambiguous results. It has frequently been reported that ethanol can diffuse through body tissues and can be readily detected in brain tissue (Ritchie, 1970; Sunahara et al., 1978). Acetaldehyde has a high lipid affinity and, therefore, can also diffuse through various organs including brain tissue (Akabane, 1970; Lindros, 1978). Earlier studies reported the presence of acetaldehyde in brains of ethanol-treated animals at concentrations equal to or greater than acetaldehyde levels measured in cerebral blood (Duritz and Truitt, 1966; Kiessling, 1962; Majchrowicz, 1973). However, as with the early studies examining peripheral blood levels of acetaldehyde, the reports of brain concentrations of acetaldehyde were later questioned on the grounds of technical and methodological difficulties (Eriksson, 1980*b*, 1983; Eriksson et al., 1984; Lindros, 1983). As with blood, the major difficulty here appeared to be the nonenzymatic formation of acetaldehyde during sample preparation (Sippel, 1972; Truitt, 1970). When this nonenzymatic formation was inhibited through the use of thiourea in the assay methodology, acetaldehyde levels were extremely low or undetectable in brain tissue following ethanol administration at doses as high as 3 g/kg (Eriksson and Sippel, 1977; Sippel, 1974). With appropriate (albeit current) assay techniques, acetaldehyde appears to be measurable in brain tissue only if blood levels are artifically elevated with pretreatment of ALDH inhibitors (Eriksson and Sippel, 1977; Westcott et al., 1980).

## 5. DOES PERIPHERAL ACETALDEHYDE ENTER THE BRAIN?

The inability to detect appreciable quantities of acetaldehyde in brain has led to the proposal that there may be an enzymatic blood–brain barrier which limits the entry of circulating acetaldehyde to the brain (Erikkson and Sippel, 1977; Kiianmaa and Virtanen, 1978; Sippel, 1974; Tabakoff et al., 1976). However, other studies have indicated that acetaldehyde may, in fact, cross the blood–brain barrier, as acetaldehyde has been measured in cerebrospinal fluid (CSF) of rats injected with ethanol (Hillbom et al.,

1981; Kiianmaa and Virtanen, 1978; Petersson and Kiessling, 1977; Westcott et al., 1980). The concentrations of acetaldehyde detected in CSF were in the nanomolar range even though the dose of ethanol administered can be considered to be very high (4.5 g/kg) (Westcott et al., 1980).

The foregoing seems to suggest that while acetaldehyde cannot, at present, be detected in brain tissue, it is possible that acetaldehyde may exist in the interstitial fluid of brain following ethanol exposure. However, it seems unlikely to reach the brain from the periphery (Deitrich, 1987; Eriksson and Sippel, 1977; Sippel, 1974) as hepatic ALDH is extremely efficient in its elimination of acetaldehyde (Lindros, 1978) and metabolism can also occur in extrahepatic tissues, including kidney and muscle (Deitrich, 1966). The presence of acetaldehyde in the interstitial fluid of brain, together with the strength of the behavioral data supporting its presence, despite the unlikely event of its originating from the peripheral circulation, leads to the notion that acetaldehyde may be formed directly in brain itself (Cohen et al., 1980). However, research has indicated that alcohol dehydrogenase, the principal route of metabolism of ethanol in the liver, while present in various areas of brain (Buhler et al., 1983), is essentially unreactive (Raskin and Sokoloff, 1970; Tabakoff and von Wartburg, 1975).

This lack of direct evidence of a mechanism for ethanol metabolism in brain has been another major stumbling block in the acceptance of a possible mediational role for acetaldehyde in alcohol's psychopharmacological actions. Despite these difficulties, however, there is now a growing body of behavioral evidence, both clinical and experimental, which indicates that acetaldehyde may indeed be endowed with psychopharmacological properties which exert their effects during alcohol ingestion and which are central in origin. In contrast, and as mentioned earlier, there are some negative findings from biochemical studies which fail to support this notion. It is important to remember that this failure is not theoretical in nature but seems exclusively related to the inability to detect acetaldehyde in brain or to identify a process by which it may arrive from the periphery.

## 6. BEHAVIORAL VERSUS BIOCHEMICAL STUDIES: THE ISSUE OF PARSIMONY

As described earlier, there are many technological difficulties which remain in the biochemical measurement of acetaldehyde and its various routes of formation (Eriksson, 1980*a*, 1983; Eriksson et al., 1984; Lindros, 1983). Consequently, the attempts to obtain a quantitative measure of the presence of acetaldehyde following ethanol exposure have to date yielded results that have been far from consistent. On the other hand, the behavioral data that have been accumulating are in fact very consistent and highly replicable. Given that alcoholism and particularly voluntary consumption are behavioral phenomena by definition and given that the behavioral data are reliable and replicable, it would seem logical and parsimonious that the behavioral findings should take precedence in an attempt to draw conclusions concerning the functional role of acetaldehyde in brain. The failure to secure positive biochemical data, therefore, should be taken merely as technological difficulties yet to be resolved, rather than an indication that the behavioral results are artifactual or irrelevant.

Several examples of recent research suggest that this conclusion may be accurate. First, recent studies have indicated that the brain may, in fact, possess the enzymatic capability to metabolize ethanol. It has been reported that cultured neural tissue was extremely efficient in metabolizing ethanol to acetate (Wickramsinghe, 1987). Moreover, ethanol metabolism in this preparation was significantly reduced in the presence of an inibitor of the enzyme catalase (Wickramsinghe, 1987). Various biochemical and histochemical methods have verified that catalase is present in brain (Brannan et al., 1981; Gaunt and DeDuve, 1976; McKenna et al., 1976). Cohen et al. (1980) have presented evidence that ethanol oxidation can occur *in vivo* in brain via the peroxidatic activity of brain catalase. In addition, and once again drawing on data generated from behavioral studies, a significant positive correlation was observed between brain catalase activity and voluntary ethanol consumption in rats (Aragon et al., 1985*c*). No differences in mean brain catalase activity between water- and forced-ethanol-drinking animals were detected, suggesting that inherent differences in brain catalase may be one of the factors determining an animal's propensity to voluntarily consume ethanol (Aragon et al., 1985*c*).

An examination of the involvement of catalase in the mediation of some of the psychopharmacological effects of ethanol seems to support and greatly strengthen the latter notion. Pretreatment with the catalase inhibitor 3-amino-1,2,4-triazole (AT) was reported to attenute an ethanol-induced conditioned taste aversion (CTA) (Aragon et al., 1985*a*). This effect of AT appeared to be specific to the effects of ethanol, as CTAs to morphine and lithium chloride were unaffected by AT pretreatment (Aragon et al., 1985*a*). In addition, pretreatment with AT was also shown to attenuate ethanol-induced locomotor depression in rats (Aragon et al., 1985*b*). These findings support the notion that acetaldehyde may be formed centrally via the peroxidatic activity of brain catalase and that this centrally formed acetaldehyde is functionally active. While the effect of catalase inhibition appears to affect several actions of ethanol, however, it has been reported to be ineffective in altering the hypothermic response to injected ethanol (Aragon and Amit, 1985). This negative finding may not represent an inconsistency, as it has been suggested that the mechanisms mediating ethanol-induced hypothermia may not be related to voluntary intake (Cunningham and Bischoff, 1987). Furthermore, the contention that acetaldehyde may mediate many of ethanol's behavioral effects does not in any way preclude a role for ethanol itself in affecting behavior. Taken together, these findings are consistent with the previously described behavioral data indicating that acetaldehyde's presence in brain may play an important role in the psychopharmacological actions of ethanol.

It is interesting to note in this context that despite earlier notions that peripherally formed acetaldehyde is incapable of arriving in brain and highlighting the inconsistency of the biochemical literature, it has been proposed that acetaldehyde is capable of binding reversibly to various proteins (von Wartburg and Ris, 1979; Summers et al., 1980; Nomura and Lieber, 1981; Donohue et al., 1983; Tuma et al., 1984), hemoglobin (Eriksson et al., 1977; Nguyen and Peterson, 1984), and, in particular, erythrocytes (Baraona et al., 1987; DiPadova et al., 1986). It has been suggested that the low levels of acetaldehyde previously reported may be attributed to those assay techniques which focused only on unbound acetaldehyde and that significantly higher concentrations can be detected when bound acetaldehyde is also measured (DiPadova et al., 1986). Furthermore, an active transport of acetaldehyde bound in erythrocytes was suggested by these authors (DiPadova et al., 1986). Thus, it seems amply clear from these studies that even if future research unequivocally demonstrates that the proposed central formation of acetaldehyde is inaccurate, these latter findings indicate that acetaldehyde may still be capable of reaching the brain via its capacity to reversibly bind to some proteins.

## 7. THE THRESHOLD OF BEHAVIORAL SENSITIVITY TO ACETALDEHYDE

It is clear that whatever the source of brain acetaldehyde, the amounts of unbound acetaldehyde generated following voluntary ethanol intake are at present at the limits of detection (Deitrich, 1987; Eriksson and Sippel, 1977; Sippel, 1974). However, it is at present unclear what concentration of acetaldehyde is necessary in order to trigger a behavioral response. In order to maintain some perspective, it is important to remember that the initial self-administration studies using the opiate morphine suggested that milligram quantites of this drug would be necessary to support operant behavior (Collins et al., 1984); however, it is now clear that doses in the microgram range can maintain operant responding (Amit et al., 1976*a*; Bozarth and Wise, 1981*b*; Collins et al., 1984). Similarly, it was long thought that animals voluntarily consuming ethanol did not generate sufficient blood ethanol levels and that this consumption, therefore, was not pharmacologically meaningful (Cicero, 1980; Lester and Freed, 1973). Recent studies, however, have indicated not only that animals will voluntarily consume ethanol to produce significant blood ethanol concentrations (Gill et al., 1986; Grant and Samson, 1985; Samson, 1986), but that the concentrations detected are behaviorally relevant (Gill et al., 1986). These examples seem to argue quite strongly that arbitrary judgments as to what constitutes a sufficient concentration to trigger a response should be determined by behavioral observations.

Alcoholism, like all other consummatory behaviors, is a motivated and regulated behavioral phenomenon. As such, alcohol dependence is mediated primarily via ethanol's positive reinforcing properties. The emerging clinical and experimental data indicate that acetaldehyde may be the most likely and most parsimonious candidate to mediate these positive psychopharmacological effects. The neural mechanisms that interact with acetaldehyde to produce these central effects remain to be elucidated. However, the data on acetaldehyde and the central enzymology related to its possible formation are already enabling behavioral researchers to understand the rudiments of a motivational regulatory system mediating the intake of alcohol.

The ongoing disagreement concerning the role of acetaldehyde in the above-mentioned motivational regulatory system probably stems primarily from different conceptions about "levels of explanation." Following the same logic as pursued by the "failure to detect" argument, one would have to argue that schizophrenia is an artifactual and irrelevent phenomenon since, to date, all attempts to measure a reliable central substrate have failed. However, both schizophrenia and alcoholism are "real" disorders whose substrates are central in origin. What remains is a combined neurochemical and neurobehavioral effort to identify them.

## REFERENCES

Akabane, J., 1970, Aldehydes and related compounds, *Int. Encycl. Pharmacol. Ther.* **2**:523–560.

Amir, S., 1977, Brain and liver aldehyde dehydrogenase: Relations to ethanol consumption in Wistar rats, *Neuropharmacology* **16**:781–784.

Amir, S., 1978*a*, Brain aldehyde dehydrogenase: Adaptive increase following prolonged ethanol administration in rats, *Neuropharmacology* **17**:463–467.

Amir, S., 1978*b*, Brain and liver aldehyde dehydrogenase activity and voluntary ethanol consumption by rats: Relations to strain, sex and age, *Psychopharmacology* **57**:97–102.

Amir, S., and Stern, M. H., 1978, Electrical stimulation and lesions of the medial forebrain bundle of the rat: Changes in voluntary ethanol consumption and brain aldehyde dehydrogenase activity. *Psychopharmacology* **57**:167–174.

Amir, S., Brown, Z. W., and Amit, Z., 1980, The role of acetaldehyde in the psychopharmacological effects of ethanol, in: *Alcohol Tolerance, Dependence and Addiction* (H. Rigter and J. C. Crabbe, (eds.), pp. 317–337, Elsevier/North Holland, Amsterdam.

Amit, Z., and Smith, B. R., 1989, The role of acetaldehyde in alcohol addiction, in: *Human Metabolism of Alcohol, Vol. II* (K. E. Crow and R. D. Batt, eds.), pp. 193–200, CRC Press, Boca Raton, FL.

Amit, Z., Brown, Z. W., and Sklar, L. S., 1976*a*, Intraventricular self-administration of morphine in naïve laboratory rats, *Psychopharmacology* **48**:291–294.

Amit, Z., Levitan, D. E., and Lindros, K. O., 1976*b*, Suppression of ethanol intake following administration of dopamine-beta-hydroxylase inhibitors in rats, *Arch. Int. Pharmacodyn. Ther.* **223**:114–119.

Amit, Z., Brown, Z. W., Amir, S., Smith, B., and Sutherland, E. A., 1980, Behavioral assessment of the role of acetaldehyde in the mediation of alcohol intake in animals and humans, in: *Animal Models in Alcohol Research* (K. Eriksson, J. D. Sinclair, and K. Kiianmaa, eds.), pp. 159–165, Academic Press, New York.

Aragon, C. M. G., and Amit, Z., 1985, Ethanol-induced hypothermia may not be mediated by catalase produced brain acetaldehyde. Paper presented at the Research Society on Alcoholism, Isle of Palms, SC.

Aragon, C. M. G., Spivak, K., and Amit, Z., 1985*a*, Behavioral evidence for the role of brain catalase in the mediation of acetaldehyde related actions of ethanol, *Alcoholism: Clin. Exp. Res.* **9**:209.

Aragon, C. M. G., Spivak, K., and Amit, Z., 1985*b*, Blockade of ethanol-induced conditioned taste aversion by 3-amino-1,2,4-tryazole: Evidence for catalase-mediated synthesis of acetaldehyde in rat brain, *Life Sci.* **37**:2077–2084.

Aragon, C. M. G., Sternklar, G., and Amit, Z., 1985*c*, A correlation between voluntary ethanol consumption and brain catalase activity in the rat, *Alcohol* **2**:353–356.

Baraona, E., DiPadova, C., Tabasco, J., and Lieber, C. S., 1987, Red blood cells: A new major modality for acetaldehyde transport from liver to other tissues, *Life Sci.* **40**:253–258.

Behar, D., Berg, C. J., Rapoport, J. L., Nelson, W., Linnoila, M., Cohen, M., Bozevich, C., and Marshall, T., 1983, Behavioral and physiological effects of ethanol in high risk and control children: A pilot study, *Alcoholism: Clin. Exp. Res.* **7**:404–410.

Blander, A., Hunt, T., Blair, R., and Amit, Z., 1984, Conditioned place preference: An evaluation of morphine's positive reinforcing properties, *Psychopharmacology* **84**:124–127.

Bozarth, M. A., and Wise, R. A., 1981*a*, Heroin reward is dependent on a dopaminergic substrate, *Life Sci.* **29**:1881–1886.

Bozarth, M. A., and Wise, R. A., 1981*b*, Intracranial self-administration of morphine into ventral tegmental area in rats, *Life Sci.* **28**:551–555.

Brannan, T. S., Maker, H. S., and Raes, I. P., 1981, Regional distribution of catalase in rat brain, *J. Neurochem.* **86**:307–309.

Brien, J. F., and Loomis, C. W., 1983, Pharmacology of acetaldehyde, *Can. J. Physiol. Pharmacol.* **61**: 1–22.

Brown, Z. W., Amit, Z., and Rockman, G. E., 1979, Intraventricular self-administration of acetaldehyde but not ethanol in naïve laboratory rats, *Psychopharmacology* **64:**271–276.

Brown, Z. W., Amit, Z., and Smith, B. R., 1980, Intraventricular self-administration of acetaldehyde and voluntary consumption of ethanol in rats, *Behav. Neur. Biol.* **28:**150–155.

Brown, Z. W., Amit, Z., Smith, B. R., Sutherland, E. A., and Selvaggi, N., 1983, Alcohol-induced euphoria enhanced by disulfiram and calcium carbimide, *Alcoholism: Clin. Exp. Res.* **7:**276–278.

Buhler, R., Pestalozzi, D., Hess, M., and von Wartburg, J. P., 1983, Immunohistochemical localization of alcohol dehydrogenase in human kidney, endocrine organs and brain, *Pharmacol. Biochem. Behav.* **18**(Suppl. 1)**:**55–59.

Chevens, L. C. F., 1953, Antabuse addiction, *Br. J. Med.* **1:**1450–1451.

Cicero, T. J., 1980, Animal models of alcoholism, in: *Animal Models of Alcohol Research* (K. Eriksson, J. D. Sinclair, and K. Kiianmaa, eds.), pp. 99–117, Academic Press, New York.

Cohen, G., Sinet, P. M., and Heikkila, R., 1980, Ethanol oxidation by rat brain *in vivo, Alcoholism: Clin. Exp. Res.* **4:**366–370.

Collins, R. J., Weeks, J. R., Cooper, M. M., Good, P. I., and Russell, R. R., 1984, Prediction of abuse liability of drugs using IV self-administration in rats, *Psychopharmacology* **82:**6–13.

Cunningham, C., and Bischoff, L., 1987, Tolerance to ethanol hypothermia does not alter oral self-administration. Paper presented at the Research Society on Alcoholism, Philadelphia, PA.

Deitrich, R. A., 1966, Tissue and subcellular distribution of mammalian aldehyde-oxidizing capacity, *Biochem. Pharmacol.* **15:**1911–1922.

Deitrich, R. A., 1987, Specificity of the action of ethanol in the central nervous system: Behavioral effects, in: *Advances in Biomedical Alcohol Research* (K. O. Lindros, R. Ylikahri, and K. Kiianmaa, eds.), pp. 133–138, Pergamon Press, Oxford.

DiPadova, C., Alderman, J., and Lieber, C. S., 1986, Improved methods for the measurement of acetaldehyde concentrations in plasma and red blood cells, *Alcoholism: Clin. Exp. Res.* **10:**86–89.

Donohue, T. M., Tuma, D. J., and Sorrell, M. F., 1983, Acetaldehyde adducts with proteins: Binding of [14C] acetaldehyde to serum albumin, *Arch. Biochem. Biophys.* **220:**239–246.

Duritz, G., and Truitt, E. B., 1966, Importance of acetaldehyde in the action of ethanol on brain norepinephrine and 5-hydroxytryptamine, *Biochem. Pharmacol.* **15:**711–721.

Eriksson, C. J. P., 1977, The distribution and metabolism of acetaldehyde in rats during ethanol oxidation. II. Regulation of the hepatic acetaldehyde levels, *Biochem. Pharmacol.* **26:**249–252.

Eriksson, C. J. P., 1980*a*, Problems and pitfalls in acetaldehyde determinations, *Alcoholism: Clin. Exp. Res.* **4:**22–29.

Eriksson, C. J. P., 1980*b*, The aversive effect of acetaldehyde on alcohol drinking behavior in the rat, *Alcoholism: Clin. Exp. Res.* **4:**107–111.

Eriksson, C. J. P., 1983, Human blood acetaldehyde concentrations during ethanol oxidation (update 1982), *Pharmacol. Biochem. Behav.* **18:**141–150.

Eriksson, C. J. P., and Sippel, H. W., 1977, The distribution and metabolism of acetaldehyde in rats during ethanol oxidation. I. The distribution of acetaldehyde in liver, brain, blood and breath, *Biochem. Pharmacol.* **26:**241–247.

Eriksson, C. J. P., Sippel, H. W., and Forsander, O. A., 1977, The occurrence of acetaldehyde binding in the rat blood but not human blood, *FEBS Lett.* **75:**205–208.

Eriksson, C. J. P., Atkinson, N., Petersen, D., and Deitrich, R. A., 1984, Blood and liver acetaldehyde concentrations during ethanol oxidation in C57 and DBA mice, *Biochem. Pharmacol.* **33:**2213–2216.

Gaunt, G. L., and DeDuve, C., 1976, Subcellular distribution of D-amino acid oxidase and catalase in rat brain, *J. Neurochem.* **26:**749–759.

Gill, K., Frances, C., and Amit, Z., 1986, Voluntary ethanol consumption in rats: An examination of blood/brain ethanol levels and behavior, *Alcoholism: Clin. Exp. Res.* **10:**457–462.

Goedde, H. W., Harada, S., and Agarwal, D. P., 1979, Racial differences in alcohol sensitivity: A new hypothesis, *Hum. Genet.* **51:**331–334.

Grant, K. A., and Samson, H. H., 1985, Induction and maintenance of ethanol self-administration without food deprivation in the rat, *Psychopharmacology* **86**:475–479.

Hald, J., and Jacobsen, E., 1948, A drug sensitizing the organism to ethyl alcohol, *Lancet* **2**:1001–1004.

Harada, S., Misawa, S., Agarwal, D. P., and Goedde, H. W., 1980, Liver alcohol dehydrogenase and aldehyde dehydrogenase in the Japanese: Isozyme variation and its possible role in alcohol intoxication, *Am. J. Hum. Genet.* **32**:8–15.

Harada, S., Agarwal, D. P., Goedde, H. W., and Ishikawa, B., 1983, Aldehyde dehydrogenase ioenzyme variation and alcoholism in Japanese, *Pharmacol. Biochem. Behav.* **18**(Suppl. 1):151–153.

Hasumura, Y., Teschke, R., and Lieber, C. S., 1975, Acetaldehyde oxidation by hepatic mitochondria: Its decrease after chronic ethanol consumption, *Science* **189**:727–728.

Hillbom, M. E., Lindros, K. O., and Larsen, A., 1981, The calcium carbimide–ethanol interaction: Lack of relation between electroencephalographic response and cerebrospinal fluid acetaldehyde, *Toxicol. Lett.* **9**:113.

Jacobsen, E., 1952, Deaths of alcoholic patients treated with disulfiram (tetraethylthiuram disulfide) in Denmark, *Q. J. Stud. Alcohol* **13**:16–26.

Katz, R. J., and Gormezano, G., 1979, A rapid inexpensive technique for assessing the reinforcing effects of opiate drugs, *Pharmacol. Biochem. Behav.* **11**:231–253.

Kiessling, K-H., 1962, The effect of acetaldehyde on rat brain mitochondria and its occurrence in brain after ethanol injection, *Exp. Cell. Res.* **26**:432–434.

Kiianmaa, K., and Virtanen, P., 1978, Ethanol and acetaldehyde levels in cerebrospinal fluid during ethanol oxidation in the rat, *Neurosci. Lett.* **10**:181–186.

Kitson, T. M., 1977, The disulfiram–ethanol reaction, *J. Stud. Alcohol* **38**:96–113.

Lester, D., and Freed, E. X., 1973, Criteria for an animal model of alcoholism, *Pharmacol. Biochem. Behav.* **1**:103–107.

Lindros, K. O., 1978, Acetaldehyde: Its metabolism and role in the actions of alcohol, in: *Research Advances in Alcohol and Drug Problems, Vol. 4* (Y. Israel, F. B. Glaser, H. Kalant, et al., eds.), pp. 111–176, Plenum Press, New York.

Lindros, K. O., 1983, Human blood acetaldehyde levels: With improved methods, a clearer picture emerges, *Alcoholism: Clin. Exp. Res.* **7**:70–75.

Lindros, K. O., Vihma, R., and Forsander, O. A., 1972, Utilization and metabolic effects of acetaldehyde and ethanol in perfused rat liver, *Biochem. J.* **126**:945–952.

Lindros, K. O., Koivula, T., and Eriksson, C. J. P., 1975, Acetaldehyde levels during ethanol oxidation: A diet-induced change and its relation to liver aldehyde dehydrogenases and redox states, *Life Sci.* **17**:1589–1598.

Majchrowicz, E., 1973, The concentration of ethanol and acetaldehyde in blood and brain of alcohol-dependent rats, *Proc. Am. Soc. Neurochem.* **4**:113.

McKenna, O., Arnold, G., and Holtzman, E., 1976, Microperoxisome distribution in the central nervous system, *Brain Res.* **117**:181–194.

Minto, A., and Roberts, F. J., 1960, "Temposil" a new drug in the treatment of alcoholism, *J. Ment. Sci.* **106**:288–295.

Mizoi, Y., Ijiri, Y., Tatsuno, T., Kijima, T., Fujiwara, S., Adachi, J., and Hishida, S., 1979, Relationship between facial flushing and blood acetaldehyde levels after alcohol intake, *Pharmacol. Biochem. Behav.* **10**:303–311.

Mizoi, Y., Tatsuno, Y., Adachi, J., Kogame, M., Fukunaga, T., Fujiwara, S., Hishida, S., and Ijiri, I., 1983, Alcohol sensitivity related to polymorphism of alcohol-metabolizing enzymes in Japanese, *Pharmacol. Biochem. Behav.* **18**(Suppl. 1):127–133.

Mucha, R. J., van der Kooy, D., O'Shaughnessy, M., and Bucenieks, P., 1982, Drug reinforcement studies by the use of place conditioning in the rat, *Brain Res.* **243**:91–105.

Myers, W. D., Ng, K. T., and Singer, G., 1982, Intravenous self-administration of acetaldehyde in the rat as a function of schedule, food deprivation and photoperiod, *Pharmacol. Biochem. Behav.* **17**: 807–811.

Myers, W. D., Ng, K. T., Marzuki, S., Myers, R. D., and Singer, G., 1984*a*, Alterations of alcohol drinking in the rat by peripherally self-administered acetaldehyde, *Alcohol* **1**:229–236.

Myers, W. D., Ng, K. T., and Singer, G., 1984*b*, Ethanol preference in rats with a prior history of acetaldehyde self-administration, *Experientia* **40**:1008–1010.

Nguyen, L. B., and Peterson, C. M., 1984, The effect of acetaldehyde concentrations on the relative rates of formation of acetaldehyde-modified hemoglobins, *Proc. Soc. Exp. Biol. Med.* **177**:226–233.

Nomura, F., and Lieber, C. S., 1981, Binding of acetaldehyde to rat liver microsomes: Enhancement after chronic alcohol consumption, *Biochem. Biophys. Res. Commun.* **100**:131–137.

Peachey, J. E., Brien, J. F., Loommis, C. W., and Rogers, B. J., 1980, A study of the calcium carbimide-ethanol interaction in man: Symptom responses, *Alcoholism: Clin. Exp. Res.* **4**:322–329.

Petersson, H., and Kiessling, K-H., 1977, Acetaldehyde occurrence in CSF during ethanol oxidation in rats and its dependence on the blood level and on dietary factors, *Biochem. Pharmacol.* **26**:237–240.

Raskin, N. H., and Sokoloff, L., 1970, Alcohol dehydrogenase activity in rat brain and liver, *J. Neurochem.* **17**:1677–1687.

Raskin, N. H., and Sokoloff, L., 1972, Enzymes catalyzing ethanol metabolism in neural and somatic tissues of the rat, *J. Neurochem.* **19**:273–282.

Ritchie, J. M., 1970, The aliphatic alcohols, in: *The Pharmacological Basis of Therapeutics* (L. S. Goodman and A. Gilman, eds.), pp. 135–150, Macmillan, New York.

Samson, H. H., 1986, Initiation of ethanol reinforcement using a sucrose-substitution procedure in food and water-sated rats, *Alcoholism: Clin. Exp. Res.* **10**:436–442.

Schenk, S., Hunt, T., Colle, L., and Amit, Z., 1983, Isolation versus grouped housing in rats: differential effects of low doses of heroin in the place preference paradigm, *Life Sci.* **32**:1129–1134.

Schlesinger, K., Kakihana, R., and Bennet, E. L., 1966, Effects of tetraethylthiuram disulfide (Antabuse) on the metabolism and consumption of ethanol in mice, *Psychosom Med.* **28**:514–520.

Sellers, E. M., Naranjo, C. A., and Peachey, J. E., 1981, Drugs to decrease alcohol consumption, *N. Engl. J. Med.* **305**:1255–1262.

Sinclair, J. D., and Gribble, P. A., 1985, Cyanamide injections during alcohol deprivation increase alcohol drinking, *Alcohol* **2**:627–630.

Sinclair, J. D., and Lindros, K. O., 1981, Suppression of alcohol drinking with brain aldehyde dehydrogenase inhibition, *Pharmacol. Biochem. Behav.* **14**:377–383.

Sippel, H. W., 1972, Thiourea, an effective inhibitor of the non-enzymatic ethanol oxidation in biological extracts, *Acta Chem. Scand.* **24**:541–550.

Sippel, H. W., 1974, The acetaldehyde content in rat brain during ethanol metabolism, *J. Neurochem.* **23**:451–452.

Smith, B. R., Amit, Z., and Splawinsky, J., 1984, Conditioned place preference induced by intraventricular infusions of acetaldehyde, *Alcohol* **1**:193–195.

Socaransky, S. M., Aragon, C. M. G., Amit, Z., and Blander, A., 1984, Higher correlations of ethanol consumption with brain than liver aldehyde dehydrogenase in three strains of rats, *Psychopharmacology* **84**:250–253.

Socaransky, S. M., Aragon, C. M. G., and Amit, Z., 1985, Brain ALDH as a possible modulator of ethanol intake, *Alcohol* **2**:361–365.

Spival, K. J., and Amit, Z., 1987, The role of acetaldehyde-metabolizing enzymes in the mediation of ethanol consumption: An investigation using a simulated drinking bout, in: *Advances in Biomedical Alcohol Research* (K. O. Lindros, R. Ylikahri, and K. Kiianmaa, eds.) pp. 361–365, Pergamon Press, Oxford.

Spyracki, C., Fibiger, H. C., and Phillips, A. G., 1982, Cocaine-induced place preference conditioning: Lack of effects of neuroleptics and 6-hydroxydopamine lesions, *Brain Res.* **253**:195–203.

Summers, M. C., Gidley, M. J., and Sanders, J. K., 1980, Acetaldehyde-enkephalins: Elucidation of the structure of the acetaldehyde adducts of methione-enkephalin and leucine-enkephalin, *FEBS Lett.* **111**:307–310.

Sunahara, G. I., Kalant, H., Schofield, M., and Grupp, L., 1978, Regional distribution of ethanol in the rat brain, *Can. J. Physiol. Pharmacol.* **56**:988–992.

Tabakoff, B., and von Wartburg, J. P., 1975, Separation of aldehyde reductases and alcohol dehydrogenase from brain by affinity chromatography: Metabolism of succinic semialdehyde amd ethanol, *Biochem. Biophys. Res. Commun.* **63**:957–966.

Tabakoff, B., Anderson, R. A., and Ritzmann, R. F., 1986, Brain acetaldehyde after ethanol administration, *Biochem. Pharmacol.* **25**:1305–1309.

Takayama, S., and Uyeno, E. T., 1985, Intravenous self-administration of ethanol and acetaldehyde by rats, *Jpn. J. Psychopharmacol.* **5**:329–334.

Tottmar, O., Marchner, H., and Lindberg, P., 1977, Inhibition of rat liver aldehyde dehydrogenases *in vitro* and *in vivo* by disulfiram, cyanamide and the alcohol sensitizing compound coprine, in: *Alcohol and Aldehyde Metabolizing Systems, Vol. II* (R. G. Thurman, J. R. Williams, et al., ed.), pp. 203–212, Academic Press, New York.

Truitt, E. B., 1970, Ethanol-induced release of acetaldehyde from blood and its effects on the determination of acetaldehyde, *Q. J. Alcohol* **31**:1–12.

Truitt, E. B., and Walsh, M. J., 1971, The role of acetaldehyde in the actions of ethanol, in: *The Biology of Alcoholism, Vol. I* (H. Kissin and H. Begleiter, eds.), pp. 161–195, Plenum Press, New York.

Tuma, D. J., Donohue, T. M., Medina, V. A., and Sorrell, M. E., 1984, Enhancement of acetaldehyde-protein adduct formation by L-ascorbate, *Arch. Biochem. Biophys.* **234**:377–381.

von Wartburg, J-P., 1980, Acetaldehyde, in *Psychopharmacology of Alcohol* (M. E. Sandler, ed.), pp. 137–147, Raven Press, New York.

von Wartburg, J-P., and Ris, M. M., 1979, Determination of acetaldehyde in human blood, *Experientia* **35**:1682–1683.

Weiner, H., 1979, Aldehyde dehydrogenase. Mechanism of action and possible physiological role, in: *Biochemistry and Pharmacology of Ethanol, Vol. I* (E. Majchrowicz and E. P. Noble, eds.), pp. 107–123, Plenum Press, New York.

Westcott, J. Y., Weiner, H., Shultz, J., and Myers, R. D., 1980, *In vivo* acetaldehyde in the brain of the rat treated with ethanol, *Biochem. Pharmacol.* **29**:411–417.

Wickramsinghe, S. N., 1987, Neuroglial and neuroblastoma cell lines are capable of metabolizing ethanol via an alcohol–dehydrogenase independent pathway, *Alcoholism: Clin. Exp. Res.* **11**:234–237.

Wolff, P. H., 1972, Ethnic differences in alcohol sensitivity, *Science* **175**:449–450.

# 2

# Critical Explanations—Biological, Psychological, and Social—of Drinking Patterns and Problems from the Alcohol-Related Longitudinal Literature

## Critiques and Strategies for Future Analyses on Behalf of the World Health Organization

KAYE MIDDLETON FILLMORE

## 1. INTRODUCTION

Generalization of scientific findings is contingent on replication of results. This is particularly critical for research concerning the correlates and prediction of human behavior where cultural and temporal factors may alter findings. Alcohol-related longitudinal research is rich and bountiful; it permits exploration of the degree to which replication of findings has taken place, particularly replication across differing cultural and temporal frames, and the development of research strategies that might provide tests of replication.

The longitudinal research design, itself, is a persuasive technique for examining a number of research questions with regard to human behavior in general and alcohol-related behavior in particular. This design can (1) determine the antecedents of particular behaviors, (2) assess and describe the incidence and chronicity/remission of behaviors and their correlates, and (3) differentiate in the timing of antecedents and correlates of behaviors (Clausen, 1978). Longitudinal research designs using normal representative populations are ideal for shedding light on the understudied and little-understood issues of incidence, chronicity, and remission of given drinking patterns and alcohol problems over the life course and their correlates and antecedents, for assessing social change as it

---

KAYE MIDDLETON FILLMORE • Institute for Health and Aging, Department of Social and Behavioral Sciences, University of California–San Francisco, San Francisco, California 94133.

influences individual lives, for assessing the relationship of alcohol use to morbidity and mortality, and for disentangling biological, social, and personality factors (and their possible interactions) as they contribute to the incidence, chronicity, and remission of drinking patterns and problems.

This chapter deals with three major research findings emerging from the alcohol-related longitudinal literature, which has used, for the most part, general population samples. The three general research findings are: (1) an antecedent to serious alcohol problems is youthful antisocial behavior (conduct disorder); (2) an antecedent to serious alcohol problems is a genetic predisposition to them; (3) environmental change on the aggregate level can govern the incidence, chronicity, and remission of serious alcohol problems on the individual level.

This chapter considers the degree to which these findings have actually been replicated across existing studies, the degree to which the studies suffer from methodological weaknesses, and the degree to which the subjects in these studies represent culturally and historically distinct groups of people, thereby contributing to stronger statements regarding generalization. Further, the chapter not only is oriented toward a critical appraisal of the research findings as they now exist, but also proposes new research strategies which would systematically replicate findings and correct methodological weaknesses.

## 2. RESEARCH FINDING 1: AN ANTECEDENT TO SERIOUS ALCOHOL PROBLEMS IS YOUTHFUL ANTISOCIAL BEHAVIOR (CONDUCT DISORDER)

A tradition of studies from the 1950s sought to locate behaviors in childhood and youth that would ultimately predict alcohol-related adult behaviors. Although not all of them focused on "deviant" youth, many did. For instance, Robins utilized a longitudinal design of white, child-guidance-clinic patients (Robins, 1966); the McCords used delinquency-prone boys (McCord and McCord, 1962); Vaillant used a sample of Harvard students and also a sample of inner-city boys (Vaillant, 1983); and Monnelly and his colleagues used a sample of boys in residential treatment for youth with behavioral problems (Monnelly et al., 1983). On the other hand, Jones's sample (1968, 1971) was white and middle class, while Amundsen's sample consisted of all 19-year-old boys screened for the military in Norway (Amundsen, 1982).

The ages of measurement for these studies differed as well: Robins measured males between ages 13 and 46; the McCords measured boys between a mean age of 8 until they reached their 30s; Vaillant's college students were measured first at age 18 and then at age 59 and his inner-city boys at 16 and 47; Monnelly et al.'s boys were under age 16 at Time 1 and over 60 at Time 2; Jones's sample was 10 years old at first measurement and 43 at last measurement; Amundsen's universe of boys was first measured at age 19 and last measured at age 50.

Taken together, these studies suggest that boys exhibiting antisocial behavior at first measurement tend to become alcoholic more often than boys who do not. Further, they tend to experience other problems in adulthood (see Robins, 1984, for a review of these findings). Antisocial behavior, roughly speaking, is defined as a collectivity of behaviors:

> These predictive behaviors for early childhood were not limited to illegal acts, but involved a set of signs of resistance toward authority, hostility to peers and adults, impulsiveness, and precocious assumption of behaviors reserved for adults: drinking, sexual relations, running away from the parental home, and leaving home. (Robins, 1984, p. 1)

The results from these studies suggest that this is a sex-linked finding. Since it seems to hold up only for males (see Robins, 1984), we exclude findings on females from this discussion. The evidence as it stands is summarized as follows.

The McCords found that more aggressive or more sadistic boys were likely to become alcoholic. Amundsen found truancy to predict those men who were later hospitalized for alcoholism (through examination of records). Robins found antisocial behavior and lower social status, among other variables, to predict adult alcohol problems. Monnelly and his colleagues, while not defining alcoholism, found body build, namely gynemorphy, to be a strong predictor, but found assertive masculine behavior to predict alcoholism as well. Jones found that assertive, independent, less considerate, rebellious boys were more likely to become alcoholic. Zucker and Gomberg (1984), recasting Vaillant's data on inner-city boys, found boys who were later alcohol-dependent to have more school behavioral problems, truancy, and dropout.

At first glance these findings seem persuasive; however, they may be problematic. The majority of the studies used nonrepresentative samples, concentrating on children or adolescents in the most disadvantaged segments of society where the combination of disadvantage and early problems would seem to exacerbate later maladjustment among adults (at least from the white, middle-class point of view).

Unlike most of the studies from that era is the Amundsen study, which is not a sample but an actual universe of 19-year-old boys in Norway. While the analysis in this study is only in its initial phases, it is instructive to note those demographic variables at or before age 19 which were associated with alcoholism (measured by institutional records) before age 50. Living in an urban environment and marital change in parents during primary school were the best predictors after a multiple discriminant analysis had been performed; the second group of predictors indicate low intelligence, low education, and low social status to be related to later alcoholism. In the group of neurotic inventory items, truancy and sometimes drinking to get away from trouble/worries are the best predictors. This study indicates that lower socioeconomic status and maladjustment in primary school are interacting to predict later alcoholism. This suggests (in concert with Robins's work) that the antisocial personality findings may derive from differences in socioeconomic status.

Robins (1984) reports that longitudinal studies of representative general population samples find that conduct disorder in childhood is predictive of antisocial behavior (alcohol problems included in these definitions) in adulthood but that cross-sectional studies find higher rates of conduct disorder in lower-class urban areas. In these respects, we may tentatively conclude that alcohol problems among lower-class men may be linked to the continuation of "bad boy" life styles. If adult alcohol problems are, in effect, class-linked, then it may be suggested by extrapolation that the etiologies of alcohol problems are multicausal and are contingent on group membership. In other words, early antisocial behavior accounts for alcohol problems only among lower-class men.

Four recent studies spanning the adolescent to adult years contain samples including the middle class, which should provide some clarification of whether the antisocial behavior phenomenon can be generalized to other social groups. Furthermore, these studies began in a later historical period (the 1960s and 1970s), bringing with them differing assumptions regarding the dependent variable. The newer assumptions included the concept that disaggregated alcohol problems rested on a continuum rather than use of a dichotomous variable, alcoholism, implying a distinct entity. In addition, there was a shift to measures of consumption and differing sampling techniques (e.g., age-specific, general-population samples as opposed to samples almost solely confined to "deviant youth").

Loper et al. (1973) and Hoffmann et al. (1974) studied the MMPIs of students attending a midwestern university, comparing those who would later become institutionalized for alcoholism with those who would not. They found no evidence of gross maladjustment among the students who would become alcoholic:

> As a group, the prealcoholics appeared more gregarious, impulsive and less conforming than their peers. The lack of differences on most of the MMPI empirical scales combined with the low scores on the maladjustment scale suggest that few signs of gross maladjustment appear at this age. (Loper et al., 1973)

Using a dependent variable of alcoholism (derived from existing records), this study clearly suggests that among a middle-class sample, early antisocial behavior does not predict adult alcoholism.

The Jessors and colleagues' studies (Jessor, 1983; Donovan et al., 1983) measured respondents from their adolescent/college years to young adulthood using probability sampling in schools and a problem-drinking-dependent variable. They found considerable discontinuity between problem drinking over this period, confirming other longitudinal epidemiological research findings (Fillmore, 1985, 1987*a,b*) that this period in the life course is characterized by *both* high rates of high incidence and remission. However, their measures of "psychosocial proneness to problem behaviors" in adolescent/college significantly discriminated between those who would exhibit continuity of problems over time and, to a lesser degree, discriminated between nonproblem drinkers in youth who would and would not report alcohol problems in young adulthood. Those adolescents who had "greater involvement in 'other' problem behavior, such as general deviant behavior and involvement with marihuana, and less involvement with the conventional situations of the church and school" were more likely to be problem drinkers in young adulthood (Donovan et al., 1983).

On the surface, the Jessors' work appears to support the antisocial behavior theory; however, Zucker (1979) points out that "it is difficult to fully evaluate whether it is the engagement in transgressive or antisocial behavior that is critical, or whether it is *the involvement in behaviors that are productive of independence from family and established institutions*" (emphasis added). Since the Jessors find that the nonconventional behaviors adopted during the adolescent years change toward conventionality with age, it is suspected that the antisocial behavior studied by the earlier researchers is somewhat different than the type studied here. Rather the trends found are more "normal" than "abnormal." Furthermore, the Jessors and colleagues fail to control for social class. Nonetheless, in this predominantly middle-class sample some sort of personality variables measured in adolescence may be promoting later alcohol problems. Whether these may be classified as "conduct disorder" is open to question.

A 12-wave study of a sample of boys in the general population studied between ages 18 and 31 (50% middle class; 74% living in small cities or towns) by Temple and Fillmore (1985*a*) used a framework similar to the Jessors' research. Like the Jessors, they found a discontinuity or remission of "problem drinking" (in this case, the frequency of drinking to the point of "feeling high") over time. Measures of family social class, family support, school success, successful self-concept, and positive and negative peer networks were good cross-sectional predictors of "problem drinking" at age 18. However, the predictive value of these variables measured at age 18 dropped by at least half by a year later and by the mid-20s vanished altogether. But, as in the Jessors' research, measures of antisocial behavior were not directly assessed.

Recently, Temple and Fillmore (1985*b*) found that a measure of delinquency is strongly related to the frequency of getting high when both are measured at age 18. However, by age 31, even controlling for the drinking measure at age 18, the relationship between youthful delinquency and drinking to get high did not hold in the sample as a whole. Remarkably, delinquency in youth did *not* predict the drinking measure among the lower class but among the middle and upper classes, almost twice as many as those who were delinquent in youth were likely to drink regularly to get high at age 31 as those who were not delinquent in youth. These findings contradict results supporting the antisocial hypothesis in lower-class samples and, instead, argue that delinquency among the more privileged classes (itself a rare demographic phenomenon) is linked to later "alcohol problems." This study confuses the issue even more than before by finding no one-to-one link between delinquency (measured as at least one arrest) and later drinking behavior and, moreover, finding no special link among the more economically disadvantaged.

The last study we have found to have implications for the antisocial hypothesis is important because it contains a large group of highly deviant children and a large group of "normal" children across a spectrum of social classes. Kandel et al. (1984) studied a high-school sample and a sample of absentees from the same schools in New York State; this very large sample was followed up in their mid-20s. Both truancy and dropping out of school, among a number of other variables, were used as independent variables to predict alcohol use. Among the males, neither frequency of use (four or more times in the last week) nor quantity–frequency (5+ drinks per day in the last month) at last measurement point could be differentiated using absenteeism or school dropout measured earlier. However, school dropout and absenteeism held severe consequences regarding employment, divorce or separation, and cigarette smoking for men. Noteworthy is that absentees were more likely to be black, to drop out of school, and to have been more delinquent during the high-school years. This study, on a much more representative and larger sample than any cited heretofore, raises substantial doubts about the antisocial behavior hypothesis.

Overall, these diverse findings indicate strongly that the antisocial behavior hypothesis needs reexamination. Not only have the majority of these studies shown that antisocial behavior is not predictive of adult alcohol problems, many have also illustrated that having alcohol problems in youth is also not predictive of adult alcohol problems. Together, these findings suggest that both may be transient behaviors of youth. The differences in findings regarding the antisocial behavior hypothesis may be attributed to at least three sources. First, the operational definitions differed by historical epoch of study such that after the 1960s, researchers adopted a "problem drinking" approach, thereby "liberalizing" the definition to include alcohol-related problems that are not necessarily "alcoholic" or do not necessarily come to the attention of the societal authorities. Also, measures of consumption were introduced. If the source of difference is attributable to differential operational definitions, a reanalysis of the more recent longitudinal studies should, where possible, recode the dependent variables to make them more consistent across studies. Second, the independent variables utilized used in more recent studies may have been too different from those used in earlier research. Again, this problem can be addressed through use of consistent operational definitions when trying to replicate. Third, even with more consistent operational definitions, it may be that the results from the earlier studies cannot be generalized to the later studies because the samples from which the earlier results were derived were not representative of the general population.

In the future, every effort should be made to collectively reanalyze data sets to determine the degree to which and under what conditions youthful antisocial behavior in particular and youthful problematic behavior in general predict adult drinking practices and problems (measures of alcoholism included). A pragmatic and compelling reason to do so is that antisocial behavior (now called "conduct disorder") has been accepted in the *Diagnostic and Statistical Manual* of the American Psychiatric Association as a predisposing factor for alcoholism, among other "adult antisocial behaviors." This has rather far-reaching implications for institutions charged with either the prevention or treatment of alcohol problems, among them the possibility that "false positives" may be identified and subjected to intervention measures based on faulty evidence.

A research strategy that seeks to simultaneously replicate multiple studies, representing different age cohorts, cultures, and historical periods, has numerous advantages. Because different studies took measures at different ages (with a particularly wide range in the adult years), one could examine at which ages, if any, the hypothesis is relevant. In addition, the nature of the relationship under variable cultural conditions could be examined. A project of this kind would be important given the hypothesis that the chronicity (or enduringness) of drinking problems differs according to age (see Fillmore, 1985, 1987*a,b*). (For instance, it has been found that alcohol problems, while highly prevalent in youth, are transient, but while less prevalent in middle age, are more chronic.) Because recent longitudinal studies have made clear that drinking practices and problems are age-related within certain cultural groups—contrary to much research in the alcohol field, where the assumption has been that alcohol problems, once attained, persist in the adult years—the relationship between antisocial behavior and drinking problems needs to be explored in light of when incidence, chronicity, and remission are highest. Other analyses in a systematic replication effort should try to find out (1) just what elements of the antisocial behavior hypothesis, alone or in concert, may be contributing to alcohol problems in adulthood and (2) the degree to which the relationship holds up under differing socioeconomic and racial/ethnic contexts.

The existing data on the antisocial behavior hypothesis are limited to the 20th century and to North American and northern European cultures. To determine the cross-cultural generality of the degree to which behavioral characteristics in youth predict behavioral characteristics in adulthood, a wider frame of cultures is crucial.

## 3. RESEARCH FINDING 2: AN ANTECEDENT TO SERIOUS ALCOHOL PROBLEMS IS A GENETIC PREDISPOSITION TO THEM

In the 1970s a group of adoptee studies were used to explain the origins of drinking problems (from Denmark: Goodwin et al., 1973, 1977; from Sweden: Bohman, 1978; Bohman et al., 1981; Cloninger et al., 1981; from the United States: Cadoret and Gath, 1978; Cadoret et al., n.d., 1980). These studies tested the premise that a genetic factor promotes the development of alcoholism. This interest represents a reemergence of a dominant scientific theme from the turn of the century when heredity was thought to be a cause of many mental disorders, alcoholism included.

At the end of the 19th and the beginning of the 20th centuries, the notion of a hereditary link between alcoholism in parents and problems in their children was popular in medical, psychiatric, and social thinking (Bynum, 1984). Theories regarding alcoholism (or dipsomania) were embedded in larger theories of mental disorders in general. The "degeneration" theory of alcoholism was strongly supported during this period:

> Between 1860 and 1910 almost all the accumulated data seemed to support the general conclusions of the degenerationists. Although it was occasionally pointed out that much of the scientific work on alcohol was produced by those already active in temperance movements, and accepting some version of a degenerationist position, there is no doubt that the bulk of the medical literature of the period implicitly or explicitly embodied many of the causal assumptions of alcoholic degeneration. (Bynum, 1984, p. 63)

The influence and popularity of these theories diminished with the work of Pearson and Elderton (1910) and with the growing influence of the Freudian movement. In 1926, Pearl addressed what he regarded as the two divisions in the study of the biology of alcohol: "the racial or hereditary effect of alcohol" and "the effect of alcohol upon the duration of life of the individual" (p. 16). On the first issue, he summarized animal studies that used experimental design and concluded that "the prevalent notion that parental alcoholism tends to cause the production of weak, defective, or monstrous progeny is not supported by the extensive body of experimental work which has been done on the problem" (p. 229). In Pearl's view, the introduction of experimental design in the laboratory and the use of statistics in human populations advanced knowledge in the field on these questions by critically reevaluating older assumptions and theoretical perspectives.

There are parallels between the science postulating hereditary links in alcoholism at the turn of the century and today. In both periods, the existing data on the matter was assumed to prove the thesis; at neither time did a "critical experiment" emerge to demonstrate beyond a shadow of a doubt that a biological basis for alcoholism exists. In contemporary times, the adoptee studies (and, to a lesser degree, twin and half-sibling studies) have laid the groundwork for an explosion of U.S. studies seeking to locate the "biological marker or markers" that might point to this genetic factor. The following statement issued from the U.S. National Institute of Alcohol Abuse and Alcoholism testifies to the importance of this research agenda.

> The realization that genetically transmitted determinants and varieties or stages of dependence both play important roles in the disease process of alcoholism has continued to spur the development of research to identify the differences between individuals predisposed to problems with alcohol and those who are not. This body of research has the potential to greatly increase our ability to effectively prevent, diagnose, and treat alcohol abuse and alcoholism, and the Institute continued this year to focus research attention on the heritability of alcoholism. (NIAAA, 1986)

Almost 80 years have passed since the hereditary theories were last in vogue. They have returned and are beginning to dominate scientific thought on the origins of alcoholism. The importance of the contemporary reemergence of this scientific trend, both for scientific explanation and for social consequences, directs us to more closely scrutinize the scientific material in the longitudinal area on which these explanations are based. Noteworthy is that these genetic hypotheses are often treated as "facts" with the emergence of studies seeking to "find" the "marker" implied by the adoption and twin studies.

Schuckit (1984) outlines criticisms of the adoptee studies in the context of genetic research in general. According to him, the findings may be compromised by unknown illness in second-degree relatives and through assortative mating. In the latter case, adults with problems (psychiatric or behavioral) are not likely to mate randomly. El-Guebaly and Offord (1977) conclude also that the nature-vs.-nurture argument is not yet resolved. Although the genetic studies have become more sophisticated, early environmental stress may increase the probability of alcoholism; later alcohol problems may be influenced by "sensory deprivation in childhood, parental separation or rejection, or more subtle disturbances of the parent-child relationship" (p. 363).

I advance these further criticisms. It is assumed that adoptee studies are interested in something called chronic alcoholism or, put more simply, alcohol problems that occur over many years. Chronic alcohol problems, both in clinical studies and in the general population (Armor et al., 1978; Fillmore and Midanik, 1984), are normally found among men in the late 30s and 40s. Interestingly, the ages chosen for follow-up in adoptee studies are usually not the ages at risk for *chronic* problems, but are the ages at which the incidence, prevalence, and remission of problems are highest. Over 75% of the adoptive men Goodwin follows up are under 34 at Time 2; Cadoret and his colleagues study adoptees between 18 and 31; Bohman and his colleagues measure adoptees between ages 23 and 43. Not all of these studies match for age and, importantly, the *chronicity* of problems does not seem to be the issue, rather some measure of "ever alcoholic" or "current alcoholic." This suggests that some of the "alcoholism" picked up by these studies may be transient age-related alcohol problems, not a collectivity of problems or a "syndrome" lasting for many years. This criticism, of course, is applicable to many other studies, including longitudinal studies. However, many studies from the psychosocial framework have explored the transience of alcohol problems in adulthood.

But while the ages studied in this research are certainly not those when chronic alcohol problems are likely to appear either in clinics or in the general population, the point is clear that the probands report or are found to have a higher rate of alcohol problems than the controls. Unfortunately, most of these studies present extremely limited information regarding the life course of the subjects under study, leaving the interested reader with little or no information on the lives of these people between birth and measurement in adulthood. Even with this paucity of information, potential non-genetic explanations may be found for the differences between the probands and the controls. A description and critique of each of the adoption studies are detailed below.

Goodwin (1984) drew samples from 5483 nonfamilial adoptees originally studied by Kety et al. (1968) in a large schizophrenia study in Denmark. Three phases were employed in this study: (1) In the first phase 55 men with an alcoholic biological parent were age-matched to 78 controls. Alcoholism in biological parents was determined by examination of central registries maintained in Denmark for alcoholic hospitalization. Alcoholism in sons was determined by psychiatric interview. Sons of alcoholics were four times more likely to be diagnosed as alcoholic as sons of nonalcoholics. (2) In the second phase the adoptive probands were compared with brothers who had been raised by the biological parents. These brothers, like their adopted siblings, had a higher rate of alcoholism than controls. The severity of alcoholism in the biological parents was related to the alcoholism in both groups. (3) In the third phase daughters of alcoholics raised by foster parents and by alcoholic biological parents and controls were compared. The female samples were small (49 adopted-out daughters of alcoholics and 48 controls). There was no relationship between alcoholism in parents and alcoholism in female offspring, although it was found that depression and drug abuse were higher among daughters raised by an alcoholic parent.

This series of studies has been criticized on a number of important dimensions. The sex of biological parent with alcoholism was not always stated, sample loss was above 20% at follow-up, and, for the men, two control groups (one whose biological parents had been hospitalized for psychiatric conditions and one whose biological parents had not) were combined (Murray et al., 1983). Perhaps the most serious criticism has been directed toward the means by which alcoholism was diagnosed in the adoptees. The criteria for a diagnosis of alcoholism included relatively infrequent drinking, reports of parental disapproval of drinking, and a single traffic arrest for drinking.

> These criteria do not appear very strict but nevertheless produce a curious anomaly. If the cut-off point for abnormality is widened to include not just alcoholism but also problem drinking, then evidence for any genetic predisposition vanishes. Indeed, the control adoptees were more frequently categorized as heavy or problem drinkers than the index adoptees. This finding contradicts the evidence of Kaij's twin study and Clonginger's adoption study . . . that not only alcoholism but also milder alcoholic abuse is under some degree of genetic influence. Furthermore, this finding runs counter to all the evidence that heavy drinking and alcoholism are closely related (Bruun, K., Edwards, G., Lumio, M. et al, 1975; Royal College of Psychiatrists, 1979). Could it be that Goodwin's findings are simply an artifact produced by the threshold for alcoholism accidentally dividing heavy drinkers in the index and control groups unevenly? (Murray et al., 1983, p. 42)

At the time when these children were adopted, the Mother's Aid in Denmark followed a procedure in which children were matched by social class of biological and adopted father (Jacobsen and Schulsinger, 1981). Other factors taken into consideration for matching were intelligence, educational background, and physical appearance. It is posited here that (1) if there is variation in both the biological and adoptive parents' social class and ethnoreligious groups, (2) if matching of adoptions occurs on the basis of social class or ethnoreligious groups, and (3) if alcoholism is more likely to occur in particular class and ethnoreligious groups (Armor et al., 1978; Cahalan, 1970), then (4) adopted children from alcoholic biological parents are more likely themselves to be alcoholic, not necessarily as a function of the biological parents' alcoholism, but as a function of the matching of social categories at adoption.

The distinct possibility of a major selection bias can be indirectly examined in this study. As mentioned earlier, two control groups were combined for the analysis of the males—one a group whose biological parent(s) were hospitalized for schizophrenia (which is most likely to occur in the lower classes, at least in the United States—see Hollingshead and Redlich, 1958), the other a group with no evidence of psychiatric illness or alcoholism. However, in the analysis of the female sample, a control group of schizophrenic biological parents was not used. Eighteen percent of the female probands had adoptive parents with "below average" economic status compared to 6% of the controls, but there were no economic status differences in the male sample. We posit here that the combined use of the schizophrenic (reflective of lower-class biological parents) and nonschizophrenic control groups in the male study disguised the social class differences in light of the fact that clear nonrandom adoption matching took place among the females.

Put another way, I argue that the female children of alcoholic biological parents (who have a higher probability of being lower class) were matched in the adoption process with lower-class adoptive parents, and female children of nonalcoholic/non-schizophrenic parents (who have a higher probability of not being lower class) were matched in the adoption process with like adoptive parents. This is tentatively confirmed by the economic differences for adoptive parents who fostered female children of alcoholics as compared to those who fostered female children of nonalcoholics/non-schizophrenics. Had the male control group *not* included the children of schizophrenics, then a clear social class difference would have been found, with lower-class adoptive parents being overrepresented among the probands and middle-class adoptive parents being overrepresented among controls. Consequently, I hypothesize that the differences in alcoholism between probands and controls would have reflected social class differences rather than biological ones. Had the male control group *not* included the children of nonschizophrenics, then no social class difference would have been found between the adoptive parents of probands and controls. Consequently, I hypothesize that no differences in drinking would have been found. In this respect, the results of the male study may be related more to differences in social class than to differences in genetic makeup. Careful matching of probands and controls by social class of adoptive parents would address this issue. Otherwise, we are left with the question posed by Murray and colleagues with regard to the combination of the two control groups for the male sample: "Could this have been to increase the likelihood of finding significant differences?" (1983, p. 41).

Other evidence suggests that the male probands and controls were different with respect to important variables often related to drinking patterns. In the male sample, 38% of the probands were never married or divorced, compared to 26% of the controls. While the Danish study provides no temporal order of marital status and alcohol problems, epidemiological evidence has repeatedly shown a relationship between alcohol problems and marital status, with the maritally unattached being highly likely to experience problems (e.g., Cahalan, 1970). Further analyses of these data, either controlling for marital status or establishing temporal order of alcohol problems and divorce, would address this problem.

Two major adoptee studies performed by Bohman and colleagues in Sweden are summarized below. The first study did not find differences in the measure of alcohol abuse among children with biological parent(s) with and without alcohol problems. This study utilized a sample of children who were candidates for adoption in 1956–1957; 93 children were adopted, 118 were raised by the biological mother, and 118 were placed with foster parents (Bohman, 1971). A control group was selected from classmates when the children were measured at age 11. Later follow-ups were at ages 15, 18 (males only), and 23. The aims of the study were twofold: (1) to examine genetic factors in criminality and alcohol abuse and (2) to examine the social processes regarding adoption.

Indicators of alcohol abuse and alcoholism among both biological parents and children were collected from the criminal register and the excise board register for offenses against the Temperance Act. Family type was an important predictor of alcohol problems in the children. Those children adopted and those raised by the biological mother did not differ from controls with regard to alcohol abuse at age 23. However, children raised by foster parents were highly likely to be recorded by the excise board register. The analysts note that there was no relationship between parental alcoholism and alcohol problems in offspring for each of the family types:

> Cross-tabulation of alcohol abuse among boys and their biological parents did not show a significant correlation in any of the three groups [adopted. raised by biological mother, placed in foster homes]. As alcohol abuse and criminality was common among the parents in all three groups, it is obvious that the boys in foster homes have reacted differently and much more negatively in their social outcome. (Bohman and Sigvardsson, 1985, p. 153)

The second study supportive of the genetic hypothesis consisted of a sample of children born in Stockholm between 1930 and 1949 ($N = 2324$) who were placed for adoption before the age of three (Bohman, 1978). At follow-up (the early 1970s), the children ranged between 23 and 43 years of age. The results showed that male offspring of biological parents who had been registered by the temperance boards for alcohol abuse were themselves more likely to be registered. Further refinement of this study matched by age a limited number of male adoptees whose biological fathers were repeatedly registered with the temperance boards with those whose biological fathers were not (Cloninger et al., 1981). Twenty percent of the probands showed a history of alcohol problems in contrast to 6% of the controls.

Limited information on adoptive parents has enabled these analysts to examine the potential interaction between hereditary and environmental factors, finding that a subset of the children display alcohol abuse associated with both alcohol abuse and criminality in biological fathers, while environmental factors (e.g., occupational status of adopted father) play a stronger role in a larger group.

Murray et al. (1983) have criticized this study for its reliance on temperance board data—data used as the sole source on the extent of alcohol abuse in both biological parents and children. Notably, whether those registered by the temperance boards are actually representative of alcohol abusers in the general population is in question. Kaij (1972) found, for example, that alcohol abusers coming to the attention of the temperance boards were more likely to be psychopathic than alcohol abusers known in the general population who had not come to the boards' attention.

The findings of the Swedish adoptee study indicated that lower occupational status of adoptive fathers was related to severe forms of alcohol abuse in their adoptive sons. Possibly the subculture in which the adoptee was placed is *reflecting* the subculture of the biological father, by virtue of the adoptee selection process, rather than *interacting* with the genetic makeup of the biological fathers.

Children placed for adoption by the Lutheran Social Services in the State of Iowa between 1938 and 1962 were studied (Cadoret and Gath, 1978). The sample, however, was not drawn with an alcoholism study in mind. A total of 190 adoptees who had been separated from biological parents at birth with one or more parents exhibiting psychiatric symptoms were matched to 194 adoptee controls who had no evidence of psychiatric symptoms in the biological family. Matching took place on the basis of age, sex, age of biological mother, and time in foster care. To examine alcoholism's heritability among adopted adults, only 173 of the adoptee pool were age 18 or older at time of examination in 1982. The age at follow-up was a mean of 25.4 for males and 24.8 for females (the range for both sexes was 18–40). Sample loss was further increased by nonlocation of 10% of this subsample and by 40% of the adoptive parents refusing interview. The resulting sample consisted of 127 men and 87 women.

Both first-degree and second-degree biological relatives were appraised in this study. A "definite" alcohol problem in a biological relative was defined as one recorded by the adoption agency as a "heavy drinker with one or more social, police, work, or medical problems due to drinking, or the individual had been hospitalized for treatment of alcoholism"; a "possible" alcohol problem was defined as a person being a heavy drinker or "as drinking too much for her/his own good" (Cadoret et al., n.d., p. 5). The adoptees' alcohol problems were appraised by interviews with adoptive parents and in roughly half the cases through a telephone interview with the adoptees themselves. School records and treatment records, when relevant, were requested from those adoptees consenting to interview. Definite and possible alcoholism was diagnosed by the Feighner criteria; primary and secondary alcoholism was also specified (Robins and Guze, 1972).

Significant relationships were found between evidence of alcoholism in biological parents and evidence of alcoholism in their offspring for both males and females. Like the Swedish study, the U.S. study examined environmental variables to the extent possible. Antisocial behavior in the adoptive family was unrelated to alcohol problems among adoptees, while alcohol problems in the adoptive family were. Adoptees raised in a rural environment were more likely to have higher rates of alcoholism if there was alcoholism in the adopted family.

This study has been criticized on the bases of possibly impressionistic alcoholism diagnosis by the personnel of the adoption agency, the small sample, sample loss, use of parents' interviews to diagnose alcoholism, and use of the distinction between secondary and primary alcoholism (Murray et al., 1983). The analysts themselves realized that the sample is young and that selective placement can take place in the adoption process. With regard to the latter, they state the following:

> In most adoption settings, some matching of adoptee to adoptive family occurs. The most obvious is the attempt to match on physical features as hair and eye color. Other matching also occurs but is less clearly defined and often involves a match based on the "child's potential." Possible IQ and social background of the adoptee seem to be elements in this match and determine in part whether a child is placed into an upper social class home with high achievement expectation or a different kind of adoptive home. Such a matching process likely operated in this sample of adoptees yet it is difficult to find evidence for it. (Cadoret et al., n.d., p. 18)

It is common knowledge that in the United States the adoption process has been traditionally nonrandom. In some parts of the United States, adoptions could not be across religious or ethnic lines. Hair and eye color may be regarded as surrogate variables for ethnic and religious groups, both demographic variables that have been found to be highly related to drinking patterns. As with the Danish study, these variables may be confounding the results.

A more serious problem may be related to the ages of not only the children, but their parents. The mean age of biological mothers was roughly 21; we may assume that the biological fathers were 1 or 2 years older. As the analysts point out, the likelihood of chronic alcoholism being solidly evident at these ages is relatively low. This may mean, then, that the control group's biological parents consisted of a number of false negatives, a problem this group of analysts cannot address with their limited data. Furthermore, the fact that the biological parents were in their early 20s from the late 1930s to the early 1960s warrants attention. During this period the definition of alcohol problems in U.S. society was in a state of flux, as was treatment for alcohol problems. (For instance, Mulford, 1965, notes significant changes in alcoholism commitments to Iowa State institutions between 1934 and 1965 as well as a major increase in per capita consumption.) Younger birth cohorts of biological mothers and fathers may have had a higher likelihood of being described as alcoholic by the adoption agency than older birth cohorts. These potential confounding factors suggest that future research using this data set should match for age of biological parents in an effort to control for differential definitions in alcoholism across time.

The potential confounding factors in these studies suggest the need for caution in interpretation and care in reanalysis. Noteworthy is the lack of integration of other theoretical perspectives and important findings in the contemporary alcohol field in this body of work. These studies tend to ignore or only pay lip service to the many studies of powerful environmental variables in the development of alcohol problems—for instance, childhood acquisition of deviant drinking and subsequent deviant drinking (Jessor and Jessor, 1977; Donovan et al., 1983), the relative impact of availability of alcohol on individuals' drinking (Wish et al., 1979), the relationship between per capita consumption and alcohol problems in societies as a whole (Bruun et al., 1975), the effects of economics in reducing alcohol problems on the individual and aggregate levels (Kendell et al., 1983). Because some of the advocates of the hereditary argument see alcoholism as an "either/or" concept, the notions of a continuum of alcohol problems and alcohol problems as nonstatic behaviors tend to be dismissed (e.g., the findings of

Cahalan and Room, 1974, on the continuum of alcohol problems in the general population; the findings of Fillmore et al., 1979, and Roizen et al., 1978, on the sporadic character of drinking problems in the general population; the findings of Polich et al., 1981, on the sporadic character of drinking problems among treated alcoholics).

On the other hand, however, few longitudinal studies with a psychosocial framework have examined the biological question of the inheritance of drinking practices. A number of these studies do include information on parental drinking and they may be used for comparative analyses. At least two studies demonstrate the importance of assessing parental drinking. Robins et al. (1962) found that parental problem drinking was one of a constellation of other parental antisocial behaviors that antedated alcoholism among former patients of a child guidance clinic. In this respect, the inadequacy of parental roles may be of more importance than the way in which the roles are fulfilled (e.g., the presence of parents). Fillmore et al. (1979) found that the frequency of parental drinking, as well as parental attitudes toward drinking, contributed far more to the prediction of drinking status of respondents in middle age than did parental drinking problems. This result was even more pronounced when the drinking status of the respondents in youth was controlled. These analysts concluded that the general milieu of alcohol use in the family had an independent effect on the likelihood of respondents exhibiting alcohol problems several decades after they left home.

Because both psychosocial and adoptee studies tend not to test competing hypotheses, it is recommended here that both types of studies could benefit from analysis plans developed by teams representative of each group working together. The objectives of such an enterprise would include examining the possibility of self-selection bias in the adoptee studies and examining the independent and interactive effects of parental drinking and other early measures on alcohol problems in offspring in the general population. This joint effort, using two distinct longitudinal designs, should better describe the independent impact of parental drinking in general (alcoholism included) on children. The critical importance of such an effort is outlined below.

There is a contemporary explosion of studies aiming to locate the biological "marker" or "markers" implied by the findings of the adoptee and other studies. These studies have been criticized (Peele, 1986) on the basis that a persuasive genetic mechanism has not yet been proposed to account for what is known about social variations in the development of alcohol problems and, further, because the genetic models to date oversimplify explanations of human drinking behavior, which is exceedingly complex.

Apart from issues of scientific validity and issues of integrating "facts" from other theoretical perspectives into this body of literature, it is also important to consider the implications of these studies within the broader frameworks of social policy, treatment, and prevention of alcohol problems.

In the United States, the genetic research has been used to support the disease model in which biological predispositions are implicated in etiology. Popular notions of the nature of alcohol problems support the conclusion that the genetic hypothesis fills out the theoretical frame offered by Jellinek (1952), where the loss of control over drinking among only a minority of drinkers pointed toward a "predisposing X factor."

The current assertions of the "genetic model" also give credibility to the popularity of the Alcoholics Anonymous ideology, where the response to alcohol is predestined among those who become alcoholic and "once an alcoholic, always an alcoholic.'' Thus, a genetic predisposition emphasizes the role of victim of a disease, relieving the victim of responsibility for his or her condition. Peele states:

> Popular writing and thinking about alcoholism have not assimilated the trend in genetic research and theory away from the search for an inherited mechanism that makes the alcoholic innately incapable of controlling his or her drinking. Rather, popular conceptions are marked by the assumption that any discovery of a genetic contribution to the development of alcoholism inevitably supports classic disease-type notions about the malady. For example, Milan and Ketcham (1983) and Pearson and Shaw (1983) both argue vehemently in favor of a total biological model of alcoholism, one that eliminates any contribution from individual volition, values or social setting (any more than takes place, according to Pearson and Shaw, with a disease like gout). As Milan and Ketcham repeatedly drive home, ''the alcoholic's drinking is controlled by physiological factors which cannot be altered through psychological methods such as counselling, threats, punishment, or reward. In other words, the alcoholic is powerless to control his reaction to alcohol'' (p. 42). (1986, p. 69).

If genetic findings are pointing the way to asserting a condition that is not amenable to treatment, then what will the treatment consist of? Chemical means have been suggested (see Peele, 1986). But, notwithstanding scientific discoveries of a workable medical intervention, it is not far-fetched to consider other avenues of intervention.

Diseases or conditions with hypothesized genetic origins—as opposed to those which are ''communicable''—may occupy a special place in treatment philosophies under differing social and political conditions. An excursion into the last century points to a time when it was suggested by Reid (as quoted by Edwards, 1984) that alcoholics might refrain from marriage. Likewise, Bynum reports of that period: ''The only way to abolish habitual drunkenness would be to prevent alcoholics from having children, for a child could inherit an 'alcoholic diathesis', i.e., a constitution which made deep and repeated indulgence pleasurable'' (1984, p. 67). And, it was only 40-odd years ago when a ''genetic hypothesis'' pointed the way to sterilization or liquidation for alcoholics, as was the case in Nazi Germany (Fahrenkrug, 1984). As Bynum comments in his work on the degenerationist theories at the turn of the century: ''Inevitably, we look at degenerationism through lenses the curvature of which is affected not simply by DNA or the 'central dogma', but also by Nazism and concentration camps'' (p. 69).

The prevention of alcohol problems under the genetic rubric might take a different form from that which we know today. As mentioned earlier, a simple, but effective means would be to prevent alcoholics from having children in the first place. But should this control mechanism not be employed, children of alcoholics might be seen to deserve special consideration in the society such that labeling would take place at an early age and abstinence would be required of them. Needless to say, the emphasis on the genetic approach would deflect attention away from consideration of such factors as the availability of alcohol, so that, as Edwards (1984) so aptly put it, it ''would be a convenient message for those wanting no meddlesome tampering with the liquor supply.''

Much thoughtful work directed toward the social consequences of the disease concept has been generated among the community of scholars interested in alcohol problems (e.g., Gusfield, 1984; Room, 1983; Conrad and Schneider, 1980), but only a few have began to think about the social implications of a genetic origin of alcoholism. Because this hypothesis and the scientific findings implied by it hold strong potential for supporting racism and determinism in some social and political settings, it is the obligation of the scientific community not only to carefully scrutinize the studies from which these findings emerge, but to ensure that they are reanalyzed so that all confounding factors are taken into account.

## 4. RESEARCH FINDING 3: ENVIRONMENTAL CHANGE ON THE AGGREGATE LEVEL CAN GOVERN THE INCIDENCE, CHRONICITY, AND REMISSION OF SERIOUS ALCOHOL PROBLEMS ON THE INDIVIDUAL LEVEL

A relatively new tradition of longitudinal research began in the 1970s which sought to address changes in the environment hypothesized to affect drinking practices. These longitudinal studies contribute to a larger literature—sometimes called the public health perspective. The theoretical framework specifically relevant to the alcohol field on which much of this research rests emphasizes situational factors influencing drinking patterns and problems, above and beyond psychological or biological factors, which until the 1960s and 1970s had dominated the field (see Lemert, 1967; Bruun, 1971; Makela, 1978). It is postulated that the social control system and the contexts and situations of drinking may be used to explain much drinking behavior. The complicated question being addressed, then, is to what degree can drinking patterns and problems change—on either the individual or aggregate level—if the environment is manipulated or, if there is a manipulation, as such, as a result of the individual(s) being exposed to one or another naturally occurring environment?

These considerations are ultimately relevant to cross-cultural research. For instance, examination of environmental factors can address the question of the degree to which industrialization and the emergence of modern complex societies increase or decrease social and psychiatric problems. Voorhees-Rosen and Rosen (1981) summarize this larger question in the context of psychiatric epidemiology and generally conclude that the evidence is not yet in on the degree to which rapid social change affects these problems. They point out that the question is an exceptionally complex one in which social change is potentially interacting with psychosocial and genetic variables with regard to vulnerability.

There have been a number of critiques of the public health perspective literature in general, particularly on the grounds that the conclusions reached are based on scanty evidence, particularly with regard to the relationship of per capita consumption and the number of heavy drinkers in a given society (Duffy, 1977; Pittman, 1980; Tuck, 1980). Among the problems, this literature has relied on aggregate statistics—a problem that can potentially be corrected by using longitudinal data. However, as will be shown below, the longitudinal studies relevant to this broader literature carry with them their own problems, making conclusions regarding environmental effects less than certain.

Seven longitudinal studies were located that assess environmental change. A pronounced difficulty in all of these studies is either the absence of control groups or their inadequacy due to "self-selection" bias.

The Robins' study (Robins, 1973) of heroin use in U.S. Vietnam veterans is instructive for alcohol use as well. Among other findings, the decreased availability of alcohol in Vietnam and the youth of the subjects could account for a drop in alcohol problems during that time:

> In Vietnam, narcotics were of excellent quality and readily, if illegally, accessible. Legal access to alcohol use was restricted both because many of the enlisted men were under legal drinking age and because Army policy limited liquor purchases by lower ranking enlisted men to beer. By the time of return to the United States, men were over 21 years of age and all types of alcohol were much cheaper and more plentiful than narcotics. Even ignoring the psychological effects of being at war in a strange country, it should not be surprising that the relative popularity of narcotics and alcohol should be reversed under these vastly different conditions of supply. (Wish et al., 1979, p. 256)

Once the veterans returned to the United States, their alcohol problems increased at the time of discharge and tended to stabilize at that level, in comparison to a control group who had not entered the armed forces. The analysts were interested not only in the Vietnam experience, but in ascertaining the degree to which the "self-selection" process of entering the military was related to the higher rate of problems among this group. In this regard, they selected a sample matched on the bases of place of residence, education, eligibility for the draft, and age. However, even with these matching procedure, the veterans reported higher rates of alcohol problems and antisocial behavior prior to induction as compared to controls who retrospectively reported this information.

The problem of adequate control groups is reflected as well in Plant's study (1979), which compared newly recruited manual workers to the brewing industry to controls recruited to a nonbrewing industry. In this case, the recruits to the drink trade were both younger and heavier drinkers than the controls prior to their employment. While the exposure to the drink trade did increase alcohol problems among this group—which was interpreted on evidence of greater availability and increased peer pressure—the self-selection problem is again a concern.

A Shetland Island study may have been the least affected by this problem, although information is too limited in the reports to adequately evaluate possible differences. Two regions geographically distinct from one another were studied. The target region was directly affected by the impact of the rapidly developing oil industry. Increases in mean alcohol consumption were noted in both regions, but particularly in the target zone and particularly among subjects under age 30. Availability of alcohol and a rise in income were interpreted to contribute to the increase in consumption (the increase in consumption being attributable to increases in frequency of drinking, rather than quantity per occasion) (Caetano et al., 1983). Nonetheless, generalization from this study is tentative in that there are few assurances that the communities were evenly matched with respect to a multitude of characteristics prior to the social change.

A fourth study evaluated the effects of an increase in the price of alcohol in an area in Scotland (Kendell et al., 1983). Although this study reported decreases in consumption and adverse consequences among all drinkers, it did not include a control group. Apart from the methodological flaws, the study addresses the criticisms of the per capita consumption argument—that is, the thesis that alcohol problems in the aggregate tend to follow the rise and fall of per capita consumption (Bruun et al., 1975). The criticism has been that even with social controls exerted on a population, those controls (such as price) would affect only "social" drinkers, not heavy or problematic drinkers (Nathan,

1983). This study observed a decrease in consumption and problems even among heavy and problematic drinkers.

A fifth study attempted to evaluate an alcohol abuse prevention program using a naturalistic longitudinal design in a U.S. college setting (Greenfield and Duncan, 1984). Levels of exposure to the multicomponent program were confounded by self-selection into various living groups (e.g., fraternities vs. dormitories) with widely differing drinking norms, potentially biasing estimates of program impact. These analysts faced up to their complex self-selection bias by modeling the way individual characteristics determine choice of living groups and then using these selection results to adjust the equations for estimating program effects. The analysts regard their findings as most tentative and classify them as a methodological pilot study. However, one finding has relevance to the debate on the extent of environmental influences. They found that an agglomeration of like individuals, rather than direct peer influence, accounted for the substantial differences in living-group drinking patterns.

A sixth study evaluated the impact of roadside random breath tests in one city in New South Wales (Homel, 1986). While the deterrence model was supported in this research, there was no control community.

Finally, a quasiexperimental design study of two Ontario communities is currently in the field where an education program introduced in one community will be evaluated (Giesbrecht and McKensie, 1983). Although matching occurred across communities (i.e., on the bases of population distribution by age, low population change, predominantly English speaking, low unemployment, and alcohol sales), the Time 1 results report differences in mean alcohol consumption.

The inadequacy of control groups (or their nonexistence) only increases the complexity and difficulty of the questions this research seeks to address. Often the self-selection and control group problems are unavoidable in this kind of research. These studies do not necessarily reflect poor planning—rather they are inadequate because many of them study social forces that are rarely under the researchers' control.

This research suffers from at least two additional difficulties. First, the time between measurement points is inadequate to evaluate the long-term effects of the environmental change. Most of these studies have used a 3-year period between baseline and follow-up. The more important question to be addressed is the long-term influence of social change on a population.

While accumulation of social and medical statistics over the long term can partially evaluate this issue and while the intervention can get lost in other historical changes, the importance of observing new cohorts "born into" the already existing historical change must be addressed. In other words, it is one thing to conclude that, at least in the short term, heavy drinkers are decreasing or increasing their consumption, but it is another to suggest that the social change will influence the same persons over the long term or will influence new generations. For instance, younger middle-class birth cohorts during the "Roaring Twenties" in the United States were in blatant opposition to alcohol controls (Warner, 1970). In this respect, multiple follow-ups over longer periods of time, as well as incorporation of new birth cohorts into these follow-ups, should yield designs that more specifically address the long-term effects of social controls and social change.

Assessment of long-term effects has immediate practical significance in terms of contemporary prevention frameworks which seek to curtail the availability or access to alcohol. If only short-term effects can be demonstrated, as has been true for a number of interventions—such as harsher Driving While Intoxicated (DWI) laws where enforcement was less than fully practicable—these policies must be subject to renewed consideration.

Second, these studies are in the position to integrate variables from other disciplinary frameworks which might include psychiatric or genetic "vulnerability." Although this information would most likely be retrospective in nature (e.g., the presence of a family history of alcohol problems), it might add to an understanding, above and beyond demographic characteristics, of who is more likely to be affected by social change or environmental manipulation. While Robins's study did include such questioning, the analysis regarding drinking change as a "function" of the hypothesized predisposing factors was not performed (Goodwin et al., 1975).

Regardless of these problems, the accumulation of this type of research should enable the interested scholarly community to begin to disentangle the effects of social change on drinking behavior. Toward this end, scholars engaged in "natural experiment" or quasiexperimental longitudinal research should develop some common instruments so that results across studies can be used for comparisons. The same recommendation would, of course, be applicable to repeated sampling designs concerned with environmental questions. It is also recommended that the burgeoning econometric literature on the ways of handling selectivity problems be consulted (Barrow et al., 1980; Maddala, 1983; Muthen and Joreskog, 1983).

However, the major recommendation we have regarding the potential contribution of longitudinal studies to this literature is not confined to only those studies which were designed to evaluate social change or natural experiments. If the weaknesses of the trend or repeated measurement studies and the weaknesses of the longitudinal studies that have been used to assess the public health perspective hypotheses are taken into account, it is obvious that the recommendations above are *not* sufficient to adequately generalize from this body of research for many years to come. We propose an analytical scheme that will more clearly, albeit not perfectly, address the impact of cultural, historical, and economic conditions that hypothetically change the nature of drinking patterns in the general population on both the aggregate and individual levels.

It would be possible to make use of many of the longitudinal studies at hand for purposes for which they were not originally designed. Because we know that the prevalence of heavy drinking and alcohol problems varies historically and cross-culturally and because it is hypothesized that this variation is at least partially a function of differing social and economic conditions, it would be possible to reconstruct the social and economic conditions of the periods in which many of the existing longitudinal studies were performed (a number now approaching 100—see Fillmore, 1988). Doing that, studies could be used as "controls" for each other (e.g., where price remained constant but income varied across studies).

While this analytical scheme would not be one where causality is implied, it would serve as a descriptive step toward more systematically delineating the conditions under which incidence and chronicity of levels of consumption and alcohol problems are likely to change. In turn, the analyses would provide a set of guidelines for future data collection where environmental and social factors, are hypothesized to influence drinking patterns.

Finally, the scheme would integrate two quite disparate bodies of research—research traditions that have often been used in "critique" of each other. By considering "maturational hypotheses" and cultural, economic, and political hypotheses within the same research framework, the relative power of the two explanatory frameworks could be assessed in a competitive manner.

The "natural experiment" studies are in their infancy; major problems impair generalizing their results. Nevertheless, they sharply remind longitudinal researchers of the importance of history as a component that may change the direction of the drinking practices of a population. Rarely are traditional longitudinal studies even couched in a discussion of the social changes taking place in their subjects' environment as a whole, not to mention social, economic, or political trends in the period under measurement. At the very least, future longitudinal research should document the history of social change which may have affected selected cohorts or the entire population of those under study.

Clear social consequences are implied by the studies performed under the public health rubric. Because they suggest prevention in the form of manipulating the environment by reducing the availability of alcohol or increasing the cost of alcohol (among other efforts), they may run the risk of interfering with the civil rights of the populace. In this sense, it is important to more carefully assess both the short-term and long-term effects of environmental manipulation in replicated research designs.

## 5. CONCLUSION

Three themes of findings from the alcohol-related longitudinal literature are examined in depth, each representing distinct explanatory frameworks of drinking patterns and problems. All have methodological weaknesses, self-selection problems, and control group problems. But of greater importance, each of the explanatory frameworks has given little attention to testing competing hypotheses, and none of them has attempted to systematically test findings cross-historically, cross-culturally, or across birth cohorts. By trying both to test competing hypotheses and to systematically replicate findings, the potential gain from longitudinal research—a design that most closely can deal with issues of causality—will be met.

To this end, the work represented in this chapter, which was drawn from a larger report (Fillmore, 1988), laid the foundation for an ongoing project which brings together longitudinal collaborators worldwide to perform a coordinated and systematic analysis of their respective data so that replication of results can be tested in the light of historical and cultural differences (Fillmore et al., 1987).

### Acknowledgments

Support for the preparation of the report (Fillmore, 1986) from which this paper derived came from the World Health Organization (WHO) and from a National Institute of Alcohol Abuse and Alcoholism Research Scientist Development Award (1 KO1 AA 00073) to the author. Portions of this paper have been reported elsewhere (Fillmore,

1987c; Fillmore, 1988). My deepest appreciation is extended to M. Grant of WHO who entrusted me with this project, and for his support in work resulting from it, to A. Jablensky, formerly of WHO, who contacted scholars worldwide in search of alcohol-related longitudinal research and to NIAAA for providing me the time and support to engage in such a project.

## REFERENCES

Amundsen, A., 1982, Who became patients in institutions for alcoholics? Paper presented at the ICAA Epidemiology Section Meetings, Helsinki, Finland.

Armor, D., Polich, J. M., and Stambul, H. B., 1978, *Alcoholism and Treatment,* Wiley, New York.

Barrow, B. S., Cain, G. G., and Goldburger, A. S., 1980, Issues in the analysis of selectivity bias, in: *Evaluation Studies Review Annual, Vol. 5* (E. W. Stromsdorfer and G. Farkas, eds.), pp. 43–59, Sage, Beverly Hills, CA.

Bohman, M., 1971, A comparative study of adopted children, foster children and children in their biological environment born after undesired pregnancies, *Acta Paediatr. Scand.* (Suppl. 221).

Bohman, M., 1978, Some genetic aspects of alcoholism and criminality, *Arch. Gen. Psychiatry* **35:**269.

Bohman, M., and Sigvardsson, S., 1985, A prospective longitudinal study of adoption, in: *Longitudinal Studies in Child Psychology and Psychiatry* (A. R. Nicol, ed.), pp. 137–154, Wiley, New York.

Bohman, M., Sigvardsson, S., and Clonigner, C. R., 1981, Maternal inheritance of alcohol abuse. Cross-fostering analysis of adopted women, *Arch. Gen. Psychiatry* **38:**965.

Bruun, K., 1971, Implications of legislation relating to alcoholism and drug dependence, in: *International Congress on Alcoholism and Drug Dependence* (L. G. Kiloh and D. S. Bell, eds.), Butterworths, Sydney.

Bruun, K., Edwards, G., Lumio, M., Makela, K., Pan, L., Popham, R. E., Room, R., Schmidt, W., Skog, O. J., Sulkinen, P., and Osterberg, E., 1975, *Alcohol Control Policies in Public Health Perspective,* Finnish Foundation for Alcohol Studies, Helsinki, Finland.

Bynum, W. F., 1984, Alcoholism and degeneration in 19th century European medicine and psychiatry, *Br. J. Addiction* **79:**59.

Cadoret, R. J., and Gath, A., 1978, Inheritance of alcoholism in adoptees, *Br. J. Psychiatry* **132:**252–258.

Cadoret, R. J., O'Gorman, T. W., Troughton, E., and Heywood, E., n.d., Alcoholism and antisocial personality: Interrelationships, genetic and environmental factors, Dept. of Psychiatry, University of Iowa College of Medicine, Ames.

Cadoret, R. J., Cain, C. A., and Grove, W. M., 1980, Development of alcoholism in adoptees raised apart from their alcoholic biologic relatives, *Arch. Gen. Psychiatry* **37:**561.

Caetano, R., Suzman, R. M., Rosen, D. H., and Voorhees-Rosen, D. J., 1983, The Shetland Islands: Longitudinal changes in alcohol consumption in a changing environment, *Br. J. Addiction* **78:**21.

Cahalan, D., 1970, *Problem Drinkers,* Jossey-Bass, San Francisco.

Cahalan, D., and Room, R., 1974, *Problem Drinking among American Men,* Publications Division, Rutgers Center of Alcohol Studies, New Brunswick, NJ.

Clausen, J. A., 1978, Longitudinal studies of drug use in the high school: Substantive and theoretical issues, in: *Longitudinal Research on Drug Use: Empirical Findings and Methodological Issues* (D. B. Kandel, ed.), Hemisphere (Halstead/Wiley), Washington, DC.

Cloninger, C. R., Bohman, M. and Sigvardsson, S., 1981, Inheritance of alcohol abuse, *Arch. Gen. Psychiatry* **38:**861.

Conrad, P., and Schneider, J., 1980, *Deviance and Medicalization: From Badness to Sickness,* Mosby, St. Louis.

Donovan, J. E., Jessor, R., and Jessor, L., 1983, Problem drinking in adolescence and young adulthood: A follow-up study, *J. Stud. Alcohol* **44:**109.

Duffy, J. C., 1977, Estimating the proportion of heavy drinkers, in: *Alcohol Education Centre: The Ledermann Curve,* Alcohol Education Centre, London.

Edwards, G., 1984, Alcoholism, genetics and society, *Br. J. Addiction* **79:**353.

El-Guebaly, N., and Offord, D., 1977, The offspring of alcoholics: A critical review, *Am. J. Psychiatry* **134:**357.

Fahrenkrug, W. H., 1984, Conceptualization and management of alcohol-related problems in Nazi Germany, 1933–45, Paper presented at the Social History of Alcohol: Drinking and Culture in Modern Society Conference, Berkeley, CA.

Fillmore, K. M., 1985, A meta-analysis of the epidemiological results of existing alcohol-related longitudinal studies by age and sex: Implications for intervention and prevention of alcohol problems, in: *Alcohol, Drugs, and Tobacco: An International Perspective—Past, Present and Future, Vol. 2,* pp. 310–313, Alberta Alcohol and Drug Abuse Commission, Edmonton.

Fillmore, K. M., 1988, *Alcohol Use across the Life Course: A Critical Review of 70 years of International Longitudinal Research,* Addiction Research Foundation, Toronto.

Fillmore, K. M., 1987*a*, Prevalence, incidence and chronicity of drinking patterns and problems among men as a function of age: A longitudinal and cohort analysis, *Br. J. Addiction* **82:**77.

Fillmore, K. M., 1987*b*, Women's drinking across the adult life course as compared to men's: A longitudinal and cohort analysis, *Br. J. of Addiction* **82:**801–811.

Fillmore, K. M., Grant, M., Hartka, E., Johnstone, B. M., Sawyer, S. M., Speiglman, R., and Temple, M. 1988, Collaborative longitudinal research on alcohol problems, *Br. J. Addiction* **83:** 441–444.

Fillmore, K. M. and Midanik, L., 1984, Chronicity of drinking problems among men: A longitudinal study, *Journal of Studies on Alcohol.* **45:**228–236.

Fillmore, K. M., Bacon, S. D. and Hyman, M., 1979, The 27 year longitudinal panel study of drinking by students in college, 1949–1976, Final report to the National Institute on Alcohol Abuse and Alcoholism under Contract No. (ADM)281-76-0015, Social Research Group, University of California at Berkeley, Berkeley.

Giesbrecht, N., and McKenzie, D., 1983, Alcohol consumption and responses to a secondary prevention programme: A survey and intervention in a small Ontario community, Paper presented at the epidemiology section of the ICAA, Padova, Italy.

Goodwin, D. W., 1984, Studies of familial alcoholism: A growth industry, in: *Longitudinal Research in Alcoholism* (D. W. Goodwin, K. T. Van Dusen, and S. A. Mednick, eds.), Kluwer-Niojhoff, Boston.

Goodwin, D. W., Schulsinger, F., Hermansen, L., Guze, S. B., and Winokur, G., 1973, Alcohol problems in adoptees raised apart from alcoholic biological parents, *Arch. Gen. Psychiatry* **28:**238.

Goodwin, D. W., Davis, D. H., and Robins, L. N., 1975, Drinking amid abundant illicit drugs, *Arch. Gen. Psychiatry* **32:**230.

Goodwin, D. W., Schulsinger, F., Knop, J., Mednick, S., and Guze, S., 1977, Alcoholism and depression in adopted-out daughters of alcoholics, *Arch. Gen. Psychiatry* **34:**751.

Greenfield, T. K., and Duncan, G. M., 1984, Evaluation of an alcohol abuse prevention program correcting for self-selection, Paper presented at the 92nd Annual Convention of the American Psychological Association, Toronto, Canada.

Gusfield, J. R., 1984, On the side: Practical action and social constructivism in social problems theory, in: *Studies in the Sociology of Social Problems* (J. Schneider and J. I. Kitsuse, eds.), pp. 31–51, Ablex Publishing, Norwood, NJ.

Hoffmann, H., Loper, R. G., and Kammeier, M. L., 1974, Identifying future alcoholics with MMPI alcoholism scales, *Q. J. Stud. Alcohol* **35:**490.

Hollingshead, A. B., and Redlich, F. C., 1958, *Social Class and Mental Illness: A Community Study,* Wiley, New York.

Homel, R., 1986, Policing the drinking driver: Random breath testing and the process of deterrence, 1986, Department of Transportation, Federal Office of Road Safety. Report No. CR42, New South Wales, Austrialia.

Jacobsen, B., and Schulsinger, F., 1981, The Dannish adoption register, in: *Prospective Longitudinal*

*Research: An Empirical Basis for the Primary Prevention of Psychosocial Disorders* (S. A. Mednick and A. E. Baert, eds.), pp. 225–230, Oxford University Press, Oxford.

Jellinek, E. M., 1952, Phases of alcohol addiction, *Q. J. Stud. Alcohol* **13**:673.

Jessor, R., 1983, The stability of change: Psychosocial development from adolescence to adulthood, in: *Human Development: An Interactional Perspective,* Academic Press, New York.

Jessor, R., and Jessor, S. L., 1977, *Problem Behavior and Psychosocial Development: A Longitudinal Study of Youth,* Academic Press, New York.

Jones, M. C., 1968, Personality correlates and antecedents of drinking patterns in adult males, *J. Consult. Clin. Psychol.* **32**:2.

Jones, M. C., 1971, Personality antecedents and correlates of drinking patterns in women, *J. Consult. Clin. Psychol.* **36**:61.

Kaij, L., 1972, Definitions of alcoholism and genetic research, *Ann. NY Acad. Sci.* **197**:110.

Kandel, D. B., Raveis, V. H., and Kandel, P. I., 1984, Continuity in discontinuities: Adjustment in young adulthood of former school absentees, *Youth and Society* **15**:325.

Kendell, R. E., de Roumanie, M., and Ritson, E. B., 1983, Effect of economic changes on Scottish drinking habits 1978–82, *Br. J. Addiction* **78**:365.

Kety, S. S., Rosenthal, D., and Wender, P. H., 1968, The types and prevalence of mental illness in the biological and adoptive families of adopted schizophrenics, in: *The Transmission of Schizophrenia* (D. Rosenthal and S. S. Kety, eds.), pp. 345–362, Pergamon Press, Oxford.

Lemert, E. M., 1967, *Human Deviance, Social Problems and Social Control,* Prentice-Hall, Englewood Cliffs, NJ.

Loper, R. G., Kammeier, M. L., and Hoffmann, H., 1973, MMPI characteristics of college freshman males who later became alcoholics, *J. Abnorm. Psychol.* **82**:159.

Maddala, G. S., 1983, *Limited-Dependent and Qualitative Variables in Econometrics,* Cambridge University Press, Cambridge.

Makela, K., 1978, Levels of consumption and social consequences of drinking, in: *Research Advances in Alcohol and Drug Problems. Vol. 4* (Y. Israel et al., eds.), pp. 303–348, Plenum Press, New York.

McCord, W., and McCord, J., 1962, A longitudinal study of the personality of alcoholics, in: *Society, Culture and Drinking Patterns* (D. J. Pittman and C. R. Snyder, eds.), pp. 413–430, Wiley, New York.

Milan, J. R., and Ketcham, K., 1983, *Under the Influence: A Guide to the Myths and Realities of Alcoholism,* Bantam Books, New York.

Monnelly, E. P., Hartl, E. M., and Elderkin, R., 1983, Constitutional factors predictive of alcoholism in a follow-up of delinquent boys, *J. Stud. Alcohol* **44**:530.

Mulford, H. A., 1965, *Alcohol and Alcoholics in Iowa, 1965,* The University of Iowa, Iowa City.

Murray, R. M., Clifford, C. A., and Gurling, H. M. D., 1983, Twin and adoption studies: How good is the evidence for a genetic role? in: *Recent Developments in Alcoholism. Vol. 1. Genetics, Behavioral Treatment, Social Mediators and Prevention, Current Concepts in Diagnosis* (M. Galanter, ed.), pp. 25–48, Plenum Press, New York.

Muthen, B., and Joreskog, K. G., 1983, Selectivity problems in quasi-experimental studies, *Evaluation Rev.* **7**:139.

Nathan, P. E., 1983, Failures in prevention: Why we can't prevent the devastating effects of alcoholism and drug abuse, *Am. Psychologist* 459.

NIAAA, 1986, *Official Highlight of Activities,* National Institute of Alcohol Abuse and Alcoholism, Washington, D.C.

Pearl, R., 1926, *Alcohol and Longevity,* Knopf, New York.

Pearson, D., and Shaw, S., 1983, *Life Extension,* Warner, New York.

Pearson, K., and Elderton, E. M., 1910, *A Second Study . . . Being a Reply to Certain Medical Critics of the First Memoir and an Examination of the Rebutting Evidence Cited by Them,* Eugenics Laboratory Memoirs, No. 13, London.

Plant, M., 1979, Drinking Careers: Occupation, Drinking Habits, and Drinking Problems, Tavistock, London.

Peele, S., 1986, The implications and limitations of genetic models of alcoholism and other addictions, *J. Stud. Alcohol* **47**:63.

Pittman, D. J., 1980, Primary prevention of alcohol abuse and alcoholism: An evaluation of the control of consumption policy, Social Science Institute, Washington University, St. Louis.

Polich, J. M., Armor, D. J., and Braiker, H. B., 1981, *The Course of Alcoholism: Four Years after Treatment,* Wiley, New York.

Robins, E., and Guze, S., 1972, Classification of affective disorders: The primary–secondary, the endogenous–reaction and the neurotic psychotic concepts, in: *Recent Advances in the Psychobiology of the Depressive Illnesses* (M. M. Katz and J. Shield, eds.), pp. 288–298, U.S. Government Printing Office, Washington, DC.

Robins, L. N., 1966, *Deviant Children Grown Up,* Williams & Wilkins, Baltimore.

Robins, L. N., 1973, The Vietnam drug user returns, Final report to the Special Action Office for Drug Abuse Prevention, Contract No. HSM-42-72-75.

Robins, L. N., 1984, Changes in conduct disorders over time, in: *Risk in Intellectual and Psychosocial Development* (D. C. Farran and J. D. McKinney, eds.) Academic Press, New York.

Robins, L. N., Bates, W. M., and O'Neal, P., 1962, Adult drinking patterns of former problem children, in: *Society, Culture and Drinking Patterns* (D. Pittman and C. R. Snyder, eds.), Wiley, New York.

Roizen, R., Cahalan, D., and Shanks, P., 1978, "Spontaneous remission" among untreated problem drinkers, in: *Longitudinal Research on Drug Use* (D. B. Kandel, ed.), pp. 197–224, Hemisphere (Halstead/Wiley), Washington, DC.

Room, R., 1983, Sociology and the disease concept of alcoholism, in: *Research Advances in Alcohol and Drug Problems, Vol. 7,* pp. 47–91, Plenum Press, New York.

Royal College of Psychiatrists, 1979, *Alcohol and Alcoholism,* Travistock, London.

Schuckit, M. A., 1985, Studies of populations at high risk for alcoholism, *J. Psychiatr. Dev.,* **3.**

Temple, M., and Fillmore, K. M., 1985*a*, The variability of drinking patterns and problems among young men, age 16–31: A longitudinal study, *Int. J. Addictions* **20**:1595.

Temple, M., and Fillmore, K. M., 1985*b*, Delinquency in youth and drinking in adulthood. Working paper, Alcohol Research Group, Berkeley, CA.

Tuck, M., 1980, Alcoholism and social policy: Are we on the right lines? Home Office Research Study No. 65, H.M.S.O., London.

Vaillant, G. E., 1983, *The Natural History of Alcoholism,* Harvard Unversity Press, Cambridge, MA.

Voorhees-Rosen, D. J., and Rosen, D., 1981, Shetland: The effects of rapid change on mental health (Scotland), in: *Prospective Longitudinal Research: An Empirical Basis for the Primary Prevention of Psychosocial Disorders* (S. A. Mednick and A. E. Baert, eds.), pp. 178–189, Oxford University Press, Oxford.

Warner, H. S., 1970, Alcohol trends in college life: Historical perspectives, in *The Domesticated Drug* (G. L. Maddox, ed.), pp. 45–88, College and University Press, New Haven, CT.

Wish, E. D., Robins, L. N., Hesselbrock, M., and Helzer, J. E., 1979, The course of alcohol problems in Vietnam veterans, in: *Currents in Alcoholism* Vol. 6 (M. Galanter, ed.), Grune and Stratton, New York.

Zucker, R. A., 1979, Developmental aspects of drinking through the young adult years, in: *Youth, Alcohol and Social Policy* (H. T. Blane and M. E. Chafetz, eds.), pp. 91–140, Plenum, New York.

Zucker, R. A. and Gomberg, E. S. L., 1984, *The horse and the cart: The case for a biopsychosocial process in the etiology of alcoholism,* Michigan State University Press, Lansing, MI

3

# Measuring Alcohol Consumption in the United States

## Methods and Rationales

ROBIN ROOM

## 1. INTRODUCTION

This chapter lays out the methods of measuring alcohol consumption that have been used in survey studies of the general population of the United States and discusses their development and rationales. As was already clear by 1970 (Room, 1970*b*), there are two major strategies for asking respondents about their current pattern of drinking: (1) asking them to list all recent drinking occasions; and (2) asking them to summarize their current patterns. In general terms, British and Scandinavian researchers have followed the first strategy, while North American researchers have followed the second (see Room, 1977, and Auth and Warheit, 1982/83, on U.S. traditions). Recently, some European researchers have challenged U.S. traditions of measuring drinking patterns, arguing in favor of the "recent occasions" approach (Duffy, 1982, 1984; Alanko, 1984). On the other hand, a recent empirical analysis of Finnish data concluded that "for most descriptive purposes" on a population level, "the choice of measurement procedure is irrelevant," and furthermore that an approach in the U.S. tradition may least underestimate consumption among the heaviest drinkers (Simpura, 1987). These discussions and analyses, along with recent discussions by U.S. researchers (e.g., Greenfield, 1986; Knupfer, 1987*a*, 1987*b*), do remind us of "the extremely complicated structure of the concept of alcohol consumption" (Alanko, 1984, p. 209) and of the need for new developmental work taking account of the different national traditions. As Alanko concludes, our "awareness of the problems" in existing approaches "should stimulate further research leading to improved methodology" (p. 224).

In sketching the history and development of measurements of the amount of drinking in North American surveys, this chapter focuses on surveys of the general adult

ROBIN ROOM • Alcohol Research Group, Institute of Epidemiology and Behavioral Medicine, Medical Research Institute of San Francisco, Berkeley, California 94709.

population, although, as noted below, two other quantititative research traditions—studies of teenage drinking and studies of amount of drinking among clinical alcoholics—have intersected with the tradition of adult drinking practices surveys. Our attention is on the logic and procedures of measurement and of aggregation for reporting; readers are referred elsewhere for general reviews on the validity of measures of alcohol consumption (Pernanen, 1974, Midanik, 1982).

## 2. NORTH AMERICAN APPROACHES TO MEASURING AMOUNT OF DRINKING

Methodological discussions of the best way to measure drinking patterns and problems date back at least to Pearl's discussion (1926, pp. 69–92) of the importance of separating steady daily drinkers from occasional heavy drinkers. Until the 1950s, however, surveys of the general population confined themselves to simple distinctions between drinking and abstaining (e.g., Gallup, 1972; Billings, 1903) or by frequency of drinking (Riley and Marden, 1947). The crucial step in moving to a fuller measurement of alcohol consumption was to start asking also about amount of drinking on an occasion or in a given period of time.

In this sense, the modern North American tradition of questions on amount of drinking starts with Straus and Bacon's path-breaking study (1953) of *Drinking in College*. Straus and Bacon's approach to measuring patterns of drinking was to ask, for each type of beverage (wine, beer, and spirits), the frequency of drinking and the average amount ordinarily consumed at a sitting (see Fig. 1). A similar method was adopted in the Iowa general-population studies of Mulford and associates, starting in the late 1950s (Fitzgerald and Mulford, 1982; their 1979 survey specified the time period covered to the last 30 days). Variations on this method have been widely used (Fig. 2).

Meanwhile, a separate tradition, starting with the San Francisco Bay Area studies of the California Drinking Practices Study in the early 1960s (Knupfer et al., 1963; Knupfer and Room, 1964), asked, for each beverage type, the frequency of drinking and then the proportion of drinking occasions on which one or two drinks, three or four

Now I'd like to ask you about your use of alcoholic beverages in just *the past month.*

About how often did you drink any wine in the past month?

More often than every day/every day/5 or 6 days a week/3 or 4 days a week/1 or 2 days a week/less often than weekly/did not drink any/can't remember.

(If at all in last month): Think of all the times you had wine in the past month. When you drank wine, how much did you usually have *at one time, on the average,* during this past month? ____ glasses (PROBE IF NECESSARY: If you're not sure, just your best guess will do)/can't remember.

(Same question sequence repeated for "beer" and for "gin, whiskey, vodka, mixed drinks, things like that" — then abbreviated to "liquor.")

Figure 1. The Straus and Bacon "usual quantity" questions: 1986 National 6 version. This version, like many versions coming in the wake of NIAAA's treatment evaluation studies (Polich and Orvis, 1979; Armor and Polich, 1982), uses a 1-month time base. The original Straus and Bacon and Mulford and Miller studies used an implicit 1-year time base.

drinks, and five or more drinks were consumed (Fig. 3). This series of questions was carried over to the national drinking surveys of Cahalan and associates (1969) and to studies by Jessor and associates (1968, pp. 483–486). They have also been used in a number of other surveys (see Fig. 4). To maintain comparability with the 1964–1966 national data-sets, the questions have also been repeated, along with others, in some more recent surveys of the Alcohol Research Group, including the 1984 national survey.

Those using this approach were critical of the "usual quantity" approach, pointing out that someone who drinks small amounts frequently and larger amounts infrequently would quite truthfully respond that the usual quantity consumed was one beer: "a person who drinks seven days a week and is drunk on only two of those days could not be regarded as one who 'usually' gets drunk when he drinks. Yet by using his usual drinking behavior this person becomes classified with others who drink daily and never have more than two drinks" (Fink, 1962; see also Knupfer, 1966). The method of asking proportions of drinking occasions on which particular quantities were used lent itself naturally to defining two dimensions of quantity of drinking for each beverage type: the "modal quantity", i.e., the amount consumed "more than half the time," and the "range", i.e., the amount consumed at least "once in a while." The summary measures derived from these measures (discussed below) were based on combinations of these two dimensions and the dimensions of frequency of drinking.

By the mid-1960s, however, as attention shifted from partitioning the general population by drinking patterns to measuring drinking-related problems and their correlates, Knupfer and her associates were growing increasingly uncomfortable with an upper-range category that started as low as five drinks. The 1964 reinterview of the San Francisco sample extended the range substantially by asking about "the times when you had the most to drink" in the last year, with an upper coding category of "12 or more" drinks, and found that substantial proportions of current drinkers—23% of men and 3% of women—reported having drunk this much (Room, 1968). The researchers in the Berkeley group also moved away from the "proportion of occasions" questions in favor of straightforwardly asking respondents how often they drank at different levels of consumption. The result, first used in a 1967 survey of San Francisco males, was a series of questions about how often the respondent drank at least 12, 8–11, and 4–7 drinks, as well as an overall frequency-of-drinking question (see Fig. 5). The different beverage types were combined in asking these questions, with respondents being given equivalents in terms of different bottle sizes for the number of drinks in question. The 1967 national reinterview study, in addition to using the beverage-specific "proportion of occasions" question series, also asked about the timing and amounts of drinking on the last two drinking occasions (Room, 1970*a*).

The 1968 national survey of males combined two methods by using the beverage-specific "proportion of occasions" questions for 5+, 3–4, and 1–2 drinks and then adding cross-beverage questions for 8–11 and for 12+ drinks. Whereas earlier surveys had simply asked the questions in the present tense, and the 1967 San Francisco and most later surveys in this tradition used a time period of 1 year, the 1969 survey used a 3-year reporting period. To maintain comparability with earlier surveys, the 1984 national adult survey also adopted this combination of two methods, but with a 1-year reporting period.

The first national survey financed under contract by the National Institute of Alcohol Abuse and Alcoholism (NIAAA)—carried out by Louis Harris and associates in

1949/1951 National college student drinking survey ($N$ = 15,747 from 27 colleges of all types and regions) (Straus and Bacon, 1953).

1951 Washington State adult general-population survey ($N$ = 478) (Maxwell, 1952, 1958).

1956 Cochrane, Ontario, adult survey (nonprobability) ($N$ = 281) (Gibbins and Duda, 1960; de Lint, 1960; Marcus, 1962).

1958 Iowa adult general-population survey (quota sample) $N$ = 1185) (Mulford and Miller, 1960).

1961 Iowa adult general-population survey (quota sample) ($N$ = 1213) (Mulford and Miller, 1963) (includes comparisons with 1958 survey above).

1963 National adult general-population survey ($N$ = 1515) (probability to the block level, then quota) (Mulford, 1964).

1964 Cedar Rapids, Iowa, adult general-population survey ($N$ = 524) (Mulford and Wilson, 1966).

1967/1968 Swedish national adult general-population survey ($N$ = 2110, aged 21–70) (McMillin, 1973) (reanalyzes data collected by the 1965 Swedish Parliamentary Committee for the Investigation of Alcohol and Temperance Policy — APU).

Fall 1972, spring 1973, autumn 1973, winter 1974, fall 1975 national surveys commissioned by NIAAA (respective $N$ = 1544, 1583, 1603, 1578, 1071) (the first four surveys were done by Louis Harris and Associates — studies 2224, 2318, 2342, and 2355 — and the fifth was the first of two Opinion Research Corp. surveys; each of them has a primary research report; the cited reports are reanalyses. The Harris surveys are probability to the block level, then quota samples) (Johnson et al., 1977; Noble, 1979, pp. 7–13; Rappeport et al., 1975).

1974/1975, 1975/1976, 1977, 1979 National household surveys of drug use commissioned by NIDA (respective $N$ = 3071, 2590, 3322, 5059 adults; 952, 986, 1272, 2165 youth aged 12–17) (Abelson and Atkinson, 1975; Abelson and Fishburne, 1976; Abelson et al., 1977, 1980).

1974 Metropolitan Boston adult general-population sample ($N$ = 795) (methodological study) (Gerstel et al., 1975; Harford and Gerstel, 1979; Harford, 1979).

1975 National adult general-population survey, NORC methodology study ($N$ = 1172) (probability frame, then quota sample) (Blair et al., 1977).

1975 Three small Wyoming communities — adult survey ($N$ = 127) (this study attempts a census of adults but seems to have low response rates) (Carman, 1977).

1976 Villages in three districts in Punjab State, India — age 15+ survey ($N$ = 3590) (Mohan et al., 1980).

1977/1978 Eastman region, Manitoba adult survey ($N$ = 1353) (a personal interview and a mail sample) (Murray, 1978).

1978 Wayne, Oakland, and Macomb Counties, Michigan (Detroit area) employed adult survey ($N$ = 1367) (telephone interview) (Parker et al., 1983).

1978 Four-city sample of Jewish, Irish Catholic, Italian Catholic, and Swedish Protestant families with adolescent children ($N$ = 980) (telephone screening with mail follow-up questionnaire in Boston, New York, Chicago, Minneapolis) (McCready et al., 1983; Greeley et al., 1980).

1979 National 6 adult general-population survey ($N$ = 1772) (Clark et al., 1981; Clark and Midanik, 1982).

1979/1980 Iowa adult general-population survey and two reinterviews (respective $N$ = 1535, 751, 685) (Fitzgerald and Mulford, 1981, 1984*a, b*).

Figure 2. General population studies using the Straus and Bacon series. This listing is focused on adult general-population samples in North America. For studies with multiple publications, citations are focused on those reporting amount of drinking.

1980 Baltimore telephone survey of adult women (*N* = 1084) (Celentano and McQueen, 1984).

1981 National survey of adult women (with a comparison sample of men) (*N* = 917 women, 396 men) (Wilsnack et al., 1984, 1984/1985).

c. 1982 Denver area adult twin pairs study (*N* = 346) (Gabrielli and Plomin, 1985).

1982 Baltimore, Chicago, and Greensboro, NC adult general-population study (*N* = 2109) (probability sampling in the three SMSAs with quotas at the block level) (2- and 4-week periods: how many drinking days, usual Q, total Q in 2 and in 4 weeks for each beverage type and altogether, also a diary method) (CSR, Inc., 1983; Wiliams et al., 1985).

1982/1984 Hispanic Health and Nutrition Examination Survey (Hispanic HANES) (*N* = about 16,000) (Hispanic-ancestry adults in regions with many Hispanics) (4-week period: how many drinking days, usual Q, total Q in 4 weeks for each beverage type and altogether) (for description and questionnaire, see Alcohol Epidemiology Data System, 1984).

1983 Health Interview Survey — nationwide survey (*N* = about 25,000) (conducted by National Center for Health Statistics for NIAAA) (2-week period: how many drinking days, usual Q, total Q in 2 weeks for each beverage type and altogether) (for description and questionnaire, see Alcohol Epidemiology Data System, 1984).

The next few questions ask you about your own use of various types of drinks. Will you please take this booklet (HAND RESPONDENT BOOKLET) and on the first page put a checkmark next to the answer that tells how often you *usually* have *wine.* Please be sure your checkmark is on the WHITE page.

Now please turn to the GREEN page and do the same for *beer.* . . . Now please turn to the PINK page and do the same for drinks containing *whiskey* or *liquor,* including scotch, bourbon, gin, vodka, rum, etc. . . . And now turn to the YELLOW page and please check how often you have *any* kind of drink containing *alcohol* — whether it is wine, beer, whiskey, or any other drink.

Booklet response categories: Three or more times a day; two times a day; once a day; nearly every day; three or four times a week; once or twice a week; two or three times a month; about once a month; less than once a month but at least once a year; less than once a year; I have never had wine/beer/whiskey or liquor/any kind of beverage containing alcohol

(INSTRUCTIONS TO INTERVIEWERS: Make sure the frequency of drinking reported on the last [yellow] page is not less than the frequency reported on any of the other pages. Resolve any inconsistencies before going on. Using the last [yellow] page of the booklet, . . . check the appropriate drinking category below: . . .

Never drank any alcoholic beverages/drinks less than once a year/all other categories.)

Think of all the times you have had *wine* recently. When you drink wine, how often do you have as many as five or six glasses: nearly every time/more than half the time/less than half the time/once in a while, or/never? When you drink *wine,* how often do you have three or four glasses: [same response categories]. When you drink *wine,* how often do you have one or two glasses: [same response categories].

(5–6, 3–4, and 1–2 drinks questions are repeated for beer, and then for "drinks containing whiskey or liquor.")

Figure 3. The Knupfer et al. "proportion of occasions" questions (1984), National 7 version.

1960 Berkeley, California, adult general-population sample (*N* = 569) (Knupfer et al., 1963).
1961 Southwestern Colorado "triethnic study" town adult general-population sample (*N* = 221) (Jessor et al., 1968).
1962 San Francisco adult general-population sample (*N* = 1268) (three drinks and four drinks are separated in this sample) (Knupfer and Room, 1964; Room, 1972—which also draws on the sample following and on National I and II).
1963/1964 San Francisco follow-up study: a subselection of the 1962 sample and their spouses (*N* = 970) (Williams, 1967).
1964 Hartford and West Hartford, Connecticut, adult general-population sample (*N* = 433) (Cahalan et al., 1965; Cahalan, 1968, 1969) (also a follow-up reported in the last two publications).
1964/1965 National 1 adult general-population sample (*N* = 2746) (Cahalan et al., 1969).
1967 National 2 follow-up study: a subselection of National 1 sample (*N* = 1359) (Cahalan, 1970) (901 of this sample were reinterviewed again as National 5 in 1974).
1969 National 3 survey of males aged 21–59 (*N* = 978) (Cahalan and Room, 1974; Room and Beck, 1974) (725 of this sample were reinterviewed again as National 4 in 1974).
1970/1971 Nelson, Kamloops, and Prince George, British Columbia, adult general-population samples (*N* = 849) (Cutler and Storm, 1973).
1971 National adult general-populaton survey (*N* = 1968) (probability to the block level, then quota) (Harris, et al., 1971; Room and Beck, 1974).
1972/1973 National survey of those aged 16+ employed half-time or more (*N* = about 1496) (Quinn and Shepard, 1974).
1973 East Baton Rouge parish adult general-population survey (*N* = 1963) (Rutledge et al., 1974).
1974/1975 Seattle pregnant women receiving prenatal care at two large hospitals (*N* = 1529) (Streissguth et al., 1977).
1975 Erie and Niagara Counties, New York, adult general-population sample (*N* = 1041) (Barnes and Russell, 1977, 1978).
1975 Boston metropolitan area adult general-population survey (*N* = 1043) (questions asked for three beverage types together) (Wechsler et al., 1978).
1976 Hillsborough County, Florida, north catchment area (*N* = 485) (Hogue, 1977).
1977 Boston SMSA adult general-population survey, telephone interview (*N* = 5314) (Hingson et al., 1981).
1978 Lake View district of Chicago adult general population survey (*N* = 328) (Rodin et al., 1979*a*, *b*).
1984 National 7 adult general-population survey (effective *N* = about 2300) (includes special samples of about 1500 Hispanics and 2000 blacks) (Hilton 1987*a*, 1987*b*; Caetano, 1986; Herd, 1985; Knupfer, 1987*a*).

Figure 4. General-population studies using the Knupfer et al. series. This listing is focused on adult general-population samples in North America. For studies with multiple publications, citations are focused on those reporting amount of drinking.

1970—used the beverage-specific "proportions of occasions" questions derived from the studies by Knupfer, Cahalan, and their associates (see Room and Beck, 1974). However, the five succeeding federally contracted surveys, carried out in 1972–1975 by Harris and by Opinion Research Corporation as evaluations of NIAAA's public service advertisement campaigns, shifted back to a version of the Straus and Bacon series on usual quantity of each beverage type (reanalyzed in Johnson et al., 1977; see Noble,

1979, pp. 7–13; Rappeport et al., 1975). By 1972 NIAAA was deeply committed to an alcoholism treatment monitoring and evaluation system (see references in Room, 1980), which had adopted a usual-quantity formulation in asking clients at intake about their drinking in the previous month (Armor et al., 1978, p. 303), and the reversion to usual-quantity questions in the general-population surveys probably reflected the influence of this monitoring and evaluation effort and the desire to collect general-population data in comparable form (see Chapter 3 in Armor et al., 1978).

Meanwhile, the four national surveys of drug use carried out under contract between 1974 and 1979 for the National Institute on Drug Abuse combined some elements of two traditions in their summary questions on amount of drinking, using both Straus and Bacon-type questions and questions about frequency of drinking 5+ drinks (Abelson and Atkinson, 1975; Abelson and Fishburne, 1976; Abelson et al., 1977, 1980).

In the last few years, there has been some convergence between the Berkeley Alcohol Research Group (ARG) tradition and that represented by RAND Corporation researchers and NIAAA contractors. Starting with the 1975 San Francisco and Marin studies, some ARG surveys have included questions about days of drinking at particular levels in the last 30 days, with higher quantities measured over the past year (Fig. 5). Polich and Orvis (1979) adopted a similar method, asking, for each beverage type, the amount drunk in a typical day during the last 30 days, while also asking the frequency of drinking 8+ drinks in the last year. The Sobells and associates (1980) have proposed and used on clinical samples a "Time-Line" method of eliciting data on drinking behavior, using a detailed reconstruction of the respondent's drinking in the context of life events over the last 30 days. Such a method amounts to being a variant "recent occasions" method. Most recently, Armor and Polich (1982) have recommended an approach in terms of frequency and usual quantity in the last 30 days, plus a series of questions asking how often the respondent had drunk 5–10 and 11+ drinks in the preceding 12 months.

The picture has been further muddied by two recent studies performed under NIAAA contract, which each used a hitherto unused time period and a new formulation for the alcohol consumption questions. The 1983 Health Interview Survey special questionnaire on drinking used a 2-week base period, asking for the usual number of drinks in a day on a drinking day in the period and for the total number of drinks in the period for each beverage, while the special Hispanic Health and Nutrition Examination Survey (Hispanic HANES) of 1982 used the same questions for a 4-week base period (Alcohol Epidemiology Data System, 1984).

So far, this discussion has focused on three traditions of asking about quantity of drinking, each of which asks the respondent to summarize his or her drinking patterns: the "usual quantity" approach, the approach in terms of the "proportion of occasions" at a given level, and the "frequency of specific levels of drinking" approach. As will be seen from Figures 2, 4, and 6, each of these methods has been used in a number of adult general-population surveys in North America. A few North American studies have also used the alternative method of the "listing of drinking occasions" in the last week (Figs. 7 and 8). The list of studies in Figure 8 is much shorter and is primarily composed of methodological studies and community surveys designed to maintain comparability in cross-national comparisons.

a. *1975 San Francisco and Marin version.* This version was designed to be self-administered. Note that it uses both a 1-month and a 1-year frame, picking up heavy drinking that did not occur in the last month.

Now, think of all the times and places when you might have something to drink. In the last 12 months, how often have you had some kind of drink containing alcohol (include beer, wine, liquor, or any other drink)?

Usually twice a day, or more often/only once a day/nearly every day/three or four times a week/once or twice a week/one to three times a month/less than once a month but at least once a year/have not drunk during the last year —SKIP to . . .

Think of your drinking last month. On how many days (out of the 30 or 31 days of the month) did you have at least one drink?

I had at least one drink on ___ days last month.

On how many of those days did you have *4 or more drinks** in the course of the day?

I had at least four drinks on ___ days last month.

On how many of those days did you have *8 or more drinks*** in the course of the day?

I had at least eight drinks on ___ days last month.

On how many of those days did you have *12 or more drinks**** in the course of the day?

I had at least 12 drinks on ___ days last month.

Now think of the *past 12 months.* How often did you have *eight or more drinks* in the course of a single day during the past 12 months?

Never in the past 12 months/1–6 times in the past 12 months/7–11 times in the past 12 months/1–3 times a month/once or twice a week/3 or 4 times a week/nearly every day/every day.

(IN SIDE BOXES:)
**4 drinks* is about 6 oz of liquor, or about a 6-pack or 2 qt of beer or a little less than a fifth of table wine or about 12 oz of sherry or port.
***8 drinks* is about ¾ pt of liquor, or about 4 qt of beer or about 1½ fifths of table wine, or about 1 fifth of sherry or port.
****12 drinks* is about 1 pt of liquor or about 5 qt of beer or about 2 fifths of table wine or more than 1 fifth of port or sherry.

b. *1979 National 6 version.* This version probably carried the subdivision of drinking quantities too far. Few other general-population studies have gone beyond a 12+ drinks level.

The next few questions are about the use of wine, beer, and liquor — all kinds of alcoholic beverages. Have you had *any* alcoholic beverages during the past 12 months?

Yes (CURRENT DRINKER)/Used to drink, stopped within past 12 months (CURRENT DRINKER)/No, have had no alcoholic beverages in the past year.

First of all, let me ask about your use of wine. How often did you drink wine (or mixed drinks containing wine) in the past 12 months?

Every day/five or six times a week/three or four times a week/once or twice a week/two or three times a month/about once a month/about 8–11 times a year/about four to seven times a year/two or three times a year/only once/never/don't know

Figure 5. The "how often *N*+ drinks" approach: 1975 San Francisco and Marin and 1979 National 6 versions.

Now think of all the times you've had wine in the past 12 months. During those 12 months, think of the *occasion* when you drank the most wine. What was that occasion?________

How many glasses of wine did you drink on that occasion? (PROBE, IF NECESSARY: If you're not sure, just your best guess will do.) NUMBER OF GLASSES:____ . . .

Now we'd like to ask you for your best estimates for your use of wine during the past 12 months. (ASK THE QUANTITY SERIES FOR WINE BEGINNING WITH THE QUANTITY RESPONDENT GIVES/ABOVE/AND CONTINUE TO ASK FREQUENCY OF ALL *LESSER* QUANTITIES.. . .)

Every day/five or six times a week . . .[categories as for overall frequency above]; these frequency categories are arranged in a matrix with the following quantity categories:

18 or more glasses/between 15 and 17 glasses/between 12 and 14 glasses/between 8 and 11 glasses/between 5 and 7 glasses/3 or 4 glasses/1 or 2 glasses

(The same series of questions is repeated for beer, and then for liquor.)

1967 San Francisco males aged 21–59 sample (*N* = 786) (4–7, 8–11, 12+ drinks) (Cahalan and Room, 1974, Chapter 8).

1969 National 3 males aged 21–59 sample (*N* = 978) (8–11, 12+ drinks) (Cahalan and Room, 1974).

1974 and 1980 California state adult general-population survey (*N* = 1020, 1037) (5+ drinks) (Cahalan et al., 1976; Cameron, 1981).

1975 San Francisco and Marin Counties, California, adult general-population survey (*N* = 1513, 979) (also 278 youths 12–17 in San Francisco) (4+, 8+, 12+ drinks) (Cahalan and Treiman, 1976*a, b*).

1974/1975, 1975/1976, 1977, 1979 National household surveys of drug use commissioned by NIDA (respective *N* = 3071, 2590, 3322, 5059 adults; 952, 986, 1272, 2165 youths aged 12–17) (5+ drinks) (Abelson and Atkinson, 1975; Abelson and Fishburne, 1976; Abelson et al., 1977, 1980).

1977/1978 Eastman region, Manitoba, adult survey (*N* = 1353) (a personal interview and a mail sample) (8+ drinks) (Murray, 1978).

1977, 1978, and 1980 Alameda, Contra Costa, and San Joaquin Counties, California, adult and youth surveys (adult *N* = 1534, 1542, 1436; youth *N* = 316, 308, 274) (1–2, 3–4, 5–6, 5+, 8+ drinks) (Wallack and Barrows, 1981, 1982/1983; Caetano, 1984).

1977 and 1982 Ontario omnibus surveys (*N* = 1454, 803) (5+ drinks) (Smart and Adlaf, 1982).

1979 National 6 adult general-population survey (*N* = 1772) (1–2, 3–4, 5–7, 8–11, 12–14, 15–17, 18+ drinks) (Clark et al., 1981; Clark and Midanik, 1982).

1979/1980 Iowa adult general-population survey and two reinterviews (*N* = 1535, 751, 685) (5+ drinks) (Fitzgerald and Mulford, 1981, 1984*a, b*).

1984 National 7 adult general-population sample (effective *N* = about 2300) (includes special samples of about 1500 Hispanics and 2000 blacks) (8–11, 12+) (Hilton, 1987*a*, 1987*b*; Caetano, 1986; Herd, 1985; Knupfer, 1987*a*).

Figure 6. Studies using a "how often *N*+ drinks" approach. This listing is focused on adult general-population samples in North America. For studies with multiple publications, citations are focused on those reporting amount of drinking.

a. *1984 National 7 version*

When was the very last time before today that you had *anything* at all containing alcohol to drink?____ days/weeks/months/years

What did you have to drink then:

wine only/beer only/liquor only/wine and beer/wine and liquor/beer and liquor, or/wine, beer, and liquor?

How many drinks did you have at that time? ____

Did you drink at your home, at someone else's home, at a restaurant or bar, or where?

Were you alone? yes/no

Were you with (your husband/your wife/the person you are living with)? yes/no

Take the very last time *before that* when you had *anything at all* to drink. How long ago was it from today? ____ days/weeks/months/years

How many drinks did you have at that time? ____

During the last year, what is the largest number of drinks you had at any one time?____

b. *1979 Contra Costa County version.* This listing-of-occasions questionnaire is elaborated from the generic WHO Community Response Study questionnaire used in Zambia, Mexico, and Scotland (Roizen, 1981), which in turn derives from the Dight (1976) survey in Scotland. The WHO generic instrument did not handle the occurrence of more than one occasion in a day clearly. The Contra Costa County questionnaire provided columns for three occasions on a day, arranged on a double page for each of the last 7 days. Those who had not had two occasions in the last week, but had had a drink in the last month, were asked about their last 2 drinking days. Before the series below, respondents had been asked, "How often you have a drink containing alcohol (a glass of beer, wine, a mixed drink, any kind of alcoholic beverage?" and "When was the last time you had a drink?"

We're also trying to get a clearer picture of people's drinking practices from day to day and from country to country. So now I need a little more detail about what, where, and when you had anything to drink during the last seven days. Let's start with yesterday — that is . . . (CIRCLE ONE CODE TO SHOW WHICH DAY OF WEEK YESTERDAY WAS)

Please think about what sort of day it was — where you were, what you were doing, any anything special that happened. (If you think it might help, please feel free to check your calendar or anything else that might help refresh your memory.)

Let's start with what you had to drink when you had your first drink that day. (And then what else did you have to drink that time?)

____Nothing that day/beer:____/wine:____/liquor:____/____can't recall. Can't even approximate.

And what time was it when you started your (first) drink (that time)? ____:____ a.m./p.m.

And about what time did you finish (your last drink/it) that time? ____:____ a.m./p.m.

Where were you when you had (those drinks/that drink) — at home, at a friend's home, in a bar, or what?

R's home/friend's home/bar or tavern/restaurant/other (specify:__________)

Who were you with (or were you alone)? (CODE ALL THAT APPLY)

Alone/spouse/other relative:__________/friend/other:__________

Figure 7. Recent drinking occasions methods: 1984 National 7 and 1979 Contra Costa County versions.

1974 Metropolitan Boston adult general-population sample ($N$ = 795) (daily drinking diary vs. weekly interview for 4 weeks) (Gerstel et al., 1975; Harford and Gerstel, 1979; Harford, 1979).

1978/1979 Canada Health Survey — nationwide adult samples (Hughes and Layne, 1982).

1978 Durham region, Ontario, adult general-population sample ($N$ = 1007) (Gillies, 1978 *a*, *b*).

1979 Contra Costa County, Calif. adult survey ($N$ = 484) (conducted in association with the WHO Study of Community Response to Alcohol-Related Problems) (Roizen, 1981).

1979 Adult general-population survey in two Middle Atlantic region communities ($N$ = 1002) (Solomon and Harford, 1984; Lubalin and Hornik, 1980).

1982 Baltimore, Chicago, and Greensboro, NC, adult general-population study ($N$ = 2109) (probability sampling in the three SMSAs with quotas at the block level) (diary and recall of drinking on each day for 2 weeks and for 4 weeks) (CSR, Inc., 1983; Williams et al., 1985).

Figure 8. Studies listing drinking occasions or days in last week. This listing is focused on adult general-population samples in North America with 1 week or multiple occasions listed. The 1967 National 2 and 1984 National 7 studies collected some information on the last two occasions (see Fig. 7). For studies with multiple publications, citations are focused on those reporting amount of drinking.

## 3. AGGREGATE MEASURES OF ALCOHOL CONSUMPTION

Whatever method of asking about amount of drinking is used, most studies move to aggregate the data from the different questions into summary measures or scores. It has been at this level of aggregate measures that most of the published North American discussions of measuring amount and patterns of drinking have been pitched. It has also been the level at which there has been the maximum of confusion—both because of failure to distinguish between methods of questioning and methods of aggregation and because of confused terminology and designations.

From the beginning there have been two main types of aggregate measures of amounts of drinking: single-dimensional orderings and multidimensional (mostly bidimensional) typologies. The choice of type and form of measure reflected a combination of influences on the investigator: substantive interests, presumptions about relations with correlates, and available or preferred analytical methods. Investigators whose main object was describing drinking patterns in the population tended to report amount of drinking in discrete categories (particularly in the days of analysis by countersorter), often using a typology. Frequently, such investigators have offered a "profile analysis" of the correlates of the different "types" of drinking pattern. On the other hand, investigators interested in using amount of drinking as a predictor in multiple regression or similar analyses tended to prefer at least an ordered and, if possible, a unidimensional measure of consumption.

Straus and Bacon's "Q-F" (Quantity-Frequency) Index, later adapted by Mulford and others, set the style of multidimensional typologies of amount of drinking, cross-classifying the dimensions of frequency and usual quantity of drinking. Other measures in this style, each with its own categories and construction rules, included the "F.Q." (Frequency–Quantity) measures of Knupfer and associates (1963) and the "QF"

(Quantity–Frequency) categorization of Edwards and associates (1972). Knupfer et al.'s "F.Q." was composed from three dimensions: frequency of drinking, modal quantity of drinking, and range of drinking, in terms of drinks per occasion.

Cahalan et al. (1969) used the same three component dimensions to compose the measure in the main text of *American Drinking Practices,* "Q–F–V" Quantity–Frequency–Variability), but this measure is actually an essentially unidimensional measure of the "heaviness" of drinking. As Bowman et al. (1975) point out, Cahalan et al.'s Q–F–V tends to give greater weight to quantity than to frequency, pushing infrequent heavy drinkers in the "heavy" category, particularly as compared with Straus and Bacon's Q-F.

Perhaps the most straightforward way of treating amount of drinking unidimensionally is to compute the total volume of drinking, i.e., how many liters of absolute alcohol (or some other measure) are consumed per given time period. The computation is simple for Straus and Bacon–style questions: for each beverage type, the number of occasions per time period is multiplied by the average quantity per occasion, and the results for the three beverage types are summed. For the Knupfer et al. style of questions, numerical proportions must be assigned also to the responses "once in a while," "less than half the time," "more than half the time," and "nearly every time." In the late 1960s, Jessor and associates (1968, pp. 483–486) and Cahalan and associates (Cahalan and Cisin, 1968; Cahalan et al., 1969, pp. 213–215) devised independent and different ways of computing a volume measure from the Knupfer et al. questions. (As a matter of record, since it has not been fully published, Fig. 9 gives the method of computation used by Cahalan and associates.)

Confusingly, Jessor et al. named their volume measure a "Q–F" (Quantity–Frequency) Index, and this name was adopted by NIAAA contract researchers from the RAND Corporation and elsewhere as a generic term for volume-of-drinking measures, although their "Q–F" volume measure (sometimes called "A–A") was usually based on Straus and Bacon–style questions, and the designation "Q–F" had previously been used for typologies rather than a unidimensional score (see, for example, Armor et al., 1978, p. 86; Polich and Orvis, 1979, p. 144.)

The primary initial use made by Cahalan and associates of their volume measure was as one dimension of a two-dimensional typology, "V–V" (Volume–Variability), of which the other dimension was the range of drinking (specifically, whether the respondent at any time drinks as many as five drinks at a sitting) (see Cahalan et al., 1969, pp. 211–224). Recently, Greenfield (1986) has proposed a new two-dimensional "Volume–Maximum Index," where the maximum quantity criterion slides up with increasing volume of drinking.

In other work, the Berkeley group has made use of yet another dimension originally derived from the Knupfer et al. question series: how often the respondent drinks five or more drinks, usually trichotomized between not at all, less than once a week, and at least once a week, with the last category denominated "Frequent Heavy Drinker" (Room, 1972; computation method from Knupfer et al. questions is in Fig. 10). The measure was a major component of the "Index of Frequent Intoxication" used in Cahalan's *Problem Drinkers* (1970, p. 28.) A "Quantity/Frequency typology" crossing the "frequency of heavy drinking" dimension with frequency of drinking has been used in a number of reports (see, for example, Cahalan et al., 1976; Cahalan and Treiman, 1976*a* (using 4+ drinks); Wallack, 1978; Caetano and Herd, 1984; Herd, 1985; Hilton, 1987*b*).

# 4. DIFFERENCES IN RESULTS WITH DIFFERENT QUESTION APPROACHES

There are surprisingly few empirical studies comparing results in general populations with different methods of questioning. Most such studies are based on asking a respondent to report drinking patterns by alternative methods in the same interview. Given that the study has other purposes as well, this approach has the advantage of being inexpensive. But it is an approach which tries the respondent's patience and which probably underestimates discrepancies between different methods, since respondents may attempt to maintain consistency in their responses.

## Comparing Summary and Recent-Occasions Methods

A number of studies have compared results between "recent occasions" questions and summary-pattern questions. The comparisons have usually focused on frequency of drinking or on volume of drinking. Such comparisons raise the complication of how to treat the relationship between the time since recent occasions—particularly since the last drinking occasion—and the average time between occasions (this issue is, of course, also intrinsic to the computation of a volume measure from recent-occasions measures). Let us consider two examples to pose the issue, assuming in both cases that interviews are randomly distributed in time—e.g., by day of the week. (1) For respondents who drink at regular intervals, say every fourth day, the average time since the last drinking occasion would be one-half the average time between occasions. (2) But for respondents who drink only on Friday and Saturday nights every week, the average time since the last occasion would be almost the same interval as the average time between occasions. In cultures where patterns like the latter example are frequent, assuming the time since the last occasion is equal to the average time between occasions may be a better choice in estimating frequency. Notice also that the problem is not solved by taking the time between the last two occasions as equivalent to the average time between occasions: With the "only on Friday and Saturday" pattern, using this interval would result in a substantial overestimate of frequency of drinking. Of course, the problem of the relationship between average frequency and the time since drinking occasions is considerably muted when many occasions are measured.

There have been several statistical discussions of this problem as it applies to measuring frequency and volume of alcohol consumption or purchases.* From statistical reasoning, Skog (1981) shows that an estimation based on the time between the last two occasions "will generally lead to overestimation of the individual consumption level," even for drinkers with a fairly regular pattern.

In a study of Australian university students, most of whom drank twice a week or less often, Margaret Sargent (1970) found 31% reporting a higher habitual frequency

*Two of these are relatively inaccessible: "Date of Last Purchase Technique," a 9-page note with no note of author or date from the Division of Prices and Cost of Living, Bureau of Labor Statistics, U.S. Department of Labor, referenced in Lamale, 1959, p. 137; Anders Ekholm, "Skevheten hos ett speciellt estimat av antalet dryckesganger per ar" (Bias in a certain estimate of the number of drinking occasions per year), Appendix II in Erland Jonsson and Tom Nilsson, *Samnordisk undersökning av vuxna mäns alkoholvanor* (A joint Nordic study of the drinking habits of adult males), mimeographed, 1969, referenced in Mäkelä, 1971, pp. 7, 31.

*Sittings per month:*

Chart for converting frequency of drinking to sittings per month:

| | |
|---|---|
| Three or more times per day | 90 |
| Two times a day | 60 |
| Once a day | 30 |
| Nearly every day | 22 |
| Three or four times a week | 15 |
| Once or twice a week | 7 |
| Two or three times a month | 2.5 |
| About once a month | 1 |
| Less than once a month, but at least once a year | 0* |
| Less than once a year or never | 0 |

*In the 1964 survey, these respondents were not asked the quantity questions, and so are assigned 0 volume. In other studies, when comparability with the 1964 data is not at stake, they are assigned a value of 0.5 sitting per month.

*Average number of drinks per sitting:*

For each beverage type, respondents were asked the proportion of times they drank 5–6 (in other studies "5 or more"), 3–4, and 1–2 drinks. The different drinking levels were assigned the following values:

5+ drinks = 6 drinks
3–4 drinks = 3.5 drinks
1–2 drinks = 1.5 drinks

In 1964 and in some other studies, respondents were not asked the proportion of times they drank at lower levels if they drank at a higher level "nearly every time" or "more than half the time." Numeric proportions are assigned to the three drinking levels according to the relative patterning of the responses to the levels, with the condition that the proportions for the three levels must add up to 1.0. According to the pattern of other responses, "nearly every time" is set at 1.0 for "5+ drinks" and at 0.8 for the lower quantities, "more than half the time" is set at 0.66, "less than half the time" ranges between 0.125 and 0.66, and "once in a while" ranges between 0.075 and 0.5. (Quite a few infrequent drinkers, for instance, reply "once in a while" to all three levels; they are assigned a ratio of 0.33 for each level.)

The chart below shows the average number of drinks per sitting that results from all possible combinations of codes, after the number of drinks has been multiplied by the assigned ratio for each drinking level and the results summed.

Response codes: EV: nearly every time; MH: more than half the time; LH: less than half the time; OW: once in a while; NE: never; IN: inapplicable.

| *5+ drinks* | *3–4 drinks* | *1–2 drinks* | *Average drinks per occasion* |
|---|---|---|---|
| EV | IN | IN | 6.00 |
| MH | IN | IN | 4.90 |
| LH | EV | IN | 4.00 |
| LH | MH | IN | 4.29 |
| LH | LH | EV | 2.15 |

Figure 9. Computation of volume—"Cahalan method," Knupfer et al. questions. (This method is used, but not fully spelled out, in Appendix 1 to Cahalan et al., 1969.) The overall volume measure, in drinks per month, is derived by summing the volumes for beer, for wine, and for spirits. The volume for each beverage type is derived by multiplying the number of *"sittings per month"* by the computed *average number of drinks consumed at a sitting.*

| *5+ drinks* | *3–4 drinks* | *1–2 drinks* | *Average drinks per occasion* |
|---|---|---|---|
| LH | LH | MH | 2.61 |
| LH | LH | LH | 3.63 |
| LH | LH | OW | 4.10 |
| LH | LH | NE | 4.75 |
| LH | OW | EV | 2.21 |
| LH | OW | MH | 2.70 |
| LH | OW | LH | 3.70 |
| LH | OW | OW | 3.90 |
| LH | OW | NE | 5.12 |
| LH | NE | EV | 2.40 |
| LH | NE | MH | 2.97 |
| LH | NE | LH | 3.75 |
| LH | NE | OW | 4.46 |
| LH | NE | NE | 6.00 |
| OW | EV | IN | 4.00 |
| OW | MH | IN | 4.29 |
| OW | LH | EV | 2.09 |
| OW | LH | MH | 2.42 |
| OW | LH | LH | 3.20 |
| OW | LH | OW | 3.65 |
| OW | LH | NE | 4.29 |
| OW | OW | EV | 2.15 |
| OW | OW | MH | 2.61 |
| OW | OW | LH | 3.45 |
| OW | OW | OW | 3.63 |
| OW | OW | NE | 4.75 |
| OW | NE | EV | 2.40 |
| OW | NE | MH | 2.97 |
| OW | NE | LH | 2.97 |
| OW | NE | OW | 3.75 |
| OW | NE | NE | 6.00 |
| NE | EV | IN | 3.50 |
| NE | MH | IN | 2.81 |
| NE | LH | EV | 1.90 |
| NE | LH | MH | 2.15 |
| NE | LH | LH | 2.50 |
| NE | LH | OW | 2.81 |
| NE | LH | NE | 3.50 |
| NE | OW | EV | 1.90 |
| NE | OW | MH | 2.15 |
| NE | OW | LH | 2.15 |
| NE | OW | OW | 2.50 |
| NE | OW | NE | 3.50 |
| NE | NE | EV | 1.50 |
| NE | NE | MH | 1.50 |
| NE | NE | LH | 1.50 |
| NE | NE | OW | 1.50 |
| NE | NE | NE | 0 |

Figure 9. *(continued)*

Codes:

| | | | |
|---|---|---|---|
| 2D | two or three times a day | EV | nearly every time |
| DL | once a day | MH | more than ½ the time |
| ND | nearly every day | LH | less than ½ the time |
| 3W | three or four times a week | # | any response |
| WK | once or twice a week | / | or |
| 2M | two or three times a month | | |
| / | or | | |

| FHD | BEVERAGE A | | | BEVERAGE B | | | BEVERAGE C | |
|---|---|---|---|---|---|---|---|---|
| code | frequency | prop. 5+ | prop. 3-4 | frequency | prop. 5+ | prop. 3-4 | frequency | prop. 3-4 |
| 3. Respondent drinks 5+ drinks approximately 4 or more days in a week: those who fit any of the following lines: | | | | | | | | |
| | 2D/DL | EV/MH | # | # | # | # | # | # |
| | ND | EV | # | # | # | # | # | # |
| | ND/3W | EV/MH | # | ND/3W | EV/MH | # | # | # |
| | WK | EV | # | ND/3W | EV | # | # | # |
| | 2D | # | EV | # | # | # | # | # |
| | DL | # | EV | DL | # | EV | # | # |
| | ND | # | EV | ND | # | EV | ND | EV |
| 2. Respondent drinks 5+ drinks approximately 2–3 days in a week: those who did not fit any line above, but fit any of the following lines: | | | | | | | | |
| | 3W | EV/MH | # | # | # | # | # | # |
| | ND | MH | # | # | # | # | # | # |
| | WK | EV/MH | # | WK | EV/MH | # | # | # |
| | 2D | # | MH | # | # | # | # | # |
| | DL | # | EV/MH | DL | # | EV/MH | # | # |
| | ND | # | EV/MH | ND | # | EV/MH | ND | EV/MH |
| 1. Respondent drinks 5+ drinks approximately one day per week: those who did not fit any line above, but fit any of the following lines: | | | | | | | | |
| | WK | EV/MH | # | # | # | # | # | # |
| | 2D/DL | LH | # | # | # | # | # | # |
| | ND | LH | # | # | # | # | # | # |
| | 3W/WK | LH | # | 3W | LH | # | # | # |
| | 2M | EV/MH | # | 2M | EV/MH | # | # | # |

Figure 10. Computation of "frequent heavy drinking" (Knupfer et al. questions). This measure, which is a relatively conservative estimate from the pattern of responses to frequency and quantity questions of how often the respondent drinks five or more drinks on an occasion, was first built on the 1967 National Survey.

The measure looks across the pattern for all three beverage types, using the frequency of drinking the beverage type and the proportions of drinking occasions on which 5+ and on which 3–4 drinks are consumed. Respondents are classed into the first category which applies to them. Note that "Beverage A" can be *any of* wine, beer, or spirits, and "Beverage B" can be *either* of the types not already defined as A. There are thus six permutations of each line, according to which of the three beverage types are being defined as "A" and "B." Respondents must fit *all* the conditions on a line to fall into that category. The specifications for codes 3 and 2 are quite tightly within the description for the category, those for code 1 a little looser.

and 21% a lower habitual frequency than implied by the time between the last two occasions. On the other hand, respondents were far more likely to report a larger quantity than a smaller quantity on their most recent drinking occasion in comparison to their modal quantity (56% vs. 6%; the 56% includes about 18% former drinkers giving a quantity for their last drinking occasion). Using college student and adult samples in North Carolina, Beatrice Rouse (1970) found different results; she reported respondents "were more likely to report more frequent drinks but smaller usual amounts in the past week" than when they gave an overall estimate of their drinking. The total volume "was usually larger when the overall estimate approach was used." (Rouse appears to have based the last-week estimates on the actual number of drinking occasions but a report of "usual quantity consumed" on drinking occasions in the week.) Using data from the 1967 U.S. National sample reinterview, Room (1970*a*) reported that a volume computation based on Knupfer et al.–type overall questions was more often higher rather than lower than a volume computed from the last two occasions (31% vs. 9%). [The computation assumed that time since the last occasion was half the average time between occasions. But the overall-estimate method also resulted in a higher volume more often than a computation based on only the time between the last two occasions (18% vs. 13%).] The volume estimate from the last two occasions was particularly likely to be lower for very frequent drinkers (in part because the minimum coding interval between occasions was 1 day). On the other hand, for infrequent heavier drinkers, the last two occasions were likely to result in a higher volume.

Mäkelä's results (1971) from national Finnish surveys supported the implication of Room's analysis that, compared to their overall estimate, frequent drinkers space out occasions whereas infrequent drinkers may telescope them (Table 1). Respondents in the surveys were asked about drinking occasions in a time period set by their reported overall frequency of drinking. Respondents who drink more often than once a month tended to report a higher frequency of drinking by the overall estimate than by listing occasions, while infrequent drinkers reported more occasions in a list than was implied by their overall frequency estimate. Time periods of about the length covered by the infrequent drinkers have commonly been involved in the findings in the survey research literature of a general "telescoping" tendency in respondents' dating of events (Neter and Waksberg, 1965). [Skog's argument (1981) concerning the likely statistical properties of the estimation of frequency from time intervals of occasions would predict a greater "overestimation" from recent occasions for infrequent drinkers.] Of course, in terms of an overall volume estimate, a stretching out by frequent drinkers would far outweigh a telescoping by infrequent drinkers.

Comparing interim periods and quantities reported for the most recent three occasions, Mäkelä (1971) also analyzed patterns of "forgetting," finding some tendency, except among very frequent drinkers, for higher quantities of consumption to be reported for more distant occasions, and for the time between occasions to rise (pp. 33, 49). This suggests that respondents may be differentially forgetting low-consumption occasions, which would offset at least to some extent infrequent drinkers' tendencies to telescope time.

Mention should be made of the findings of a 1950 methodological study of U.S. consumer expenditures, which compared several methods of reporting consumer expenditures on alcohol for home consumption. The respondents' estimate of annual expendi-

Table 1. Number of Drinking Occasions in Survey Period, by Drinking Frequency Groups[a]

| Drinking frequency, overall estimate | Time period asked about | Expected no. occas. | Reported occas., 1st wave, 1968 | Reported occas., 2nd wave 1969 |
|---|---|---|---|---|
| Daily | 1 week | 7 | 5.30 | 5.49 |
| A few times a week | 2 weeks | 5 | 3.60 | 3.58 |
| Once a week | 4 weeks | 4 | 3.33 | 3.74 |
| A few times a month | 2 months | 5 | 3.46 | 3.74 |
| Once a month or so | 4 months | 4 | 4.11 | 4.30 |
| Every two months or so | 8 months | 4 | 3.96 | 4.27 |
| 3 or 4 times a year | 12 months | 3½ | 3.84 | 3.30 |
| Once or twice a year | 12 months | 1½ | 2.05 | 2.32 |
| Less than once a year | 12 months | ½ | 1.24 | 1.44 |

[a]Source: Mäkelä (1971, pp. 9, 13).

tures was 108% of an estimate based on their memory of expenditures in the last week, and 114% of an estimate based on a week's diary (Lamale, 1959, p. 141.)

With data from a small treatment-population sample, Sobell et al. (1982) compared a "Time-Line (TL)" method of eliciting all drinking occasions in the last 30 days with a "usual quantities" method, finding that "when discrepancies occurred, the TL method as compared to the QF method always resulted in a greater number of reported (a) drinking days, (b) mean g of absolute ethanol consumed per drinking day, (c) low ethanol consumption days, (d) heavy ethanol consumption days, and (e) excessive ethanol consumption days."

Two methodologically oriented surveys commissioned by NIAAA have explored the relation between diary, recent occasions, and summary report methods. Using data from 1974 Boston general population sample, Harford (1979) compared responses on overall frequency of drinking with respondents' reports of specific drinking occasions over a 4-week period, provided either by once-a-week interviews or by filling out a daily drinking record (Table 2). On balance, Harford found that the summary judgment method provided a lower estimate of drinking frequencies, although the results were more equivocal when comparisons were limited to categories where there were no "ceiling" or "floor" effects—i.e., those drinking between three times a month and four times a week.

A more recent survey (CSR, Inc., 1983; Williams et al., 1985), carried out in three metropolitan areas (Baltimore, Chicago, and Greensboro, North Carolina), compared four different modes of data collection, each carried out for two periods, 14 days and 28 days: (1) a volume measure (daily absolute alcohol consumption) was estimated by asking respondents to report the total number of drinks of each beverage type consumed in the course of the reporting period; (2) a similar volume measure was estimated from the frequency of drinking and usual quantity per occasion of each beverage type; (3) respondents were asked to fill out a detailed 30-day drinking diary, with a payment of $20 for completion of the diary; (4) respondents were asked in an interview to recall

Table 2. Overreports, Matches, and Underreports of Overall Frequency by Sex and Type of Beverage (%)[a]

| | Summary overreports | | | Summary underreports | | |
|---|---|---|---|---|---|---|
| | 4+ days less | 1–3 days less | Matches | 1–3 days more | 4+ days more | Base $N$ |
| All respondents | | | | | | |
| Men | | | | | | |
| Beer | 12% | 16 | 34 | 21 | 18 | (270) |
| Wine | 6% | 18 | 53 | 21 | 2 | (278) |
| Spirits | 6% | 21 | 36 | 28 | 9 | (278) |
| Women | | | | | | |
| Beer | 4% | 12 | 60 | 17 | 7 | (317) |
| Wine | 7% | 23 | 45 | 20 | 5 | (354) |
| Spirits | 5% | 13 | 38 | 31 | 13 | (353) |
| Respondents drinking 3–16 days a month | | | | | | |
| Men | | | | | | |
| Beer | 4% | 20 | 31 | 21 | 24 | (149) |
| Wine | 13% | 43 | 26 | 13 | 6 | (70) |
| Spirits | 4% | 31 | 31 | 21 | 12 | (121) |
| Women | | | | | | |
| Beer | 9% | 38 | 29 | 13 | 11 | (85) |
| Wine | 14% | 39 | 32 | 5 | 9 | (148) |
| Spirits | 6% | 21 | 40 | 18 | 14 | (179) |

[a]Source: Harford (1979, pp. 6, 8).

drinking on each day of the period covered. Table 3 shows the results for total alcohol consumption by these four methods. In each comparison, the estimate is higher for the 14-day period than for the 28-day period. The two summary-patterns methods give slightly higher volumes than the diary method, with the volumes by the "usual quantity" method being a little higher than those from asking the total number of drinks in the period. Asking respondents to recall each day's drinking (a variant of the recent occasions method) seems to yield a somewhat higher volume than the "usual quantity" method.

On the other hand, Simpura's analysis (1987) of the 1984 Finnish national survey shows that a volume of drinking computed on Straus and Bacon-like "usual quantity" questions yielded a somewhat higher coverage of national sales (34%) than volumes based on the last week's drinking occasions (29%) or on a variable period including at least the last four drinking occasions (26%). However, the "usual quantity" computation, unlike the other two, did not exclude homemade beverage consumption.

## Comparing Different Summary Methods

Surprisingly few studies have compared results with the different methods of summary estimation of drinking patterns. Using a U.S. nationwide sample of males

Table 3. Daily Absolute Alcohol Consumption by Various Questions and Computation Methods, Baltimore, Chicago, and Greensboro Sample, CSR Inc. Study ($N$ = 2109)[a,b]

| | 14-day period ($N$ = 105) | 28-day period ($N$ = 98) |
|---|---|---|
| Computation on drinks in period | 1.16 | 0.71 |
| Computation on usual quantity × frequency | 1.22 | 0.77 |
| Diary | 1.06 | 0.69[c] |
| | ($N$ = 152) | ($N$ = 149) |
| Computation (on usual quantity × frequency?) | 0.63 | 0.55 |
| Daily recall (occasions in period) method | 0.69 | 0.68 |

[a]Source: CSR, Inc. (1983).
[b]All comparisons are for the same time period (either 14 days or 28 days); all respondents had apparently previously been interviewed with the same questionnaire prior to the diary or daily recall period. The study also involved manipulating several other conditions (administering forms one after the other, self-administered vs. interview form, follow-up readministration 5–7 days later, etc.), which may have interacted with the results shown.
[c]From Table 3 of CSR report; value in Table 2 is 0.87.

aged 21–59, Room (1971*b*) showed that adding questions on the frequency of drinking 8–11 and 12+ drinks to the Knupfer et al. series, which stopped at five and more drinks, raised the overall average volume of drinking by 16%. In the study of drinking among U.S. Air Force personnel conducted by Polich and Orvis (1979), adding questions on the frequency of drinking 8+ drinks for each beverage type in the last year to the Straus and Bacon-type "usual quantity" questions concerning the last 30 days raised the overall average volume of drinking by 36% (Armor and Polich, 1982). On the other hand, a computation based only on "frequency of particular quantities" questions was reported to result in an average overall volume of only 91% of the Straus and Bacon series (computed from Armor and Polich, 1982; the sample and questions used in these comparisons are not specified). Using a student sample at the University of Oregon ($N$ = 484), Gwartney-Gibbs (1982) compared an average daily volume computed by asking respondents the total number of beers, glasses of wine, and shots of liquor they had drunk in the "past week" with a volume computed from asking on how many days the respondent had drunk 1+, 4+, 8+, and 12+ drinks in the last 4 weeks. While the aggregate mean volume reports by the two methods were almost exactly the same—0.87 and 0.88 drinks per day, respectively—the distribution of responses by volume showed some differences: 31% had not had a drink in the last week (vs. 16% in the last 4 weeks), and 22% reported a daily volume of 1-1/2 or more drinks in the last week (vs. 19% in the last 4 weeks).

Drawing on data from annual nationwide surveys of the number of occasions of drug use among high-school seniors, Bachman and O'Malley (1981) found that for alcohol consumption, across the whole range of answers they could test (between 1 and 39 occasions in a year), respondents reported on the average 3.2 times as many drinking occasions in the last week as would be expected from their report of drinking occasions in the last year. The ratio seemed consistent from one class to the next and held also for marijuana use; for illicit drugs, the ratio was consistently lower, in the range 2.4–2.9. The authors relate these findings to the general finding from studies of the reporting of health events that underreporting increases relatively rapidly with the time since the event (Cannell et al., 1977).

The 1979 U.S. national survey of drinking ("National 6") used two alternative methods of asking about amount of drinking. For each beverage type, respondents were asked their frequency in the last year of drinking 18 or more drinks on an occasion, and then of 15–17, 12–14, 8–11, 5–7, 3–4, and 1–2 drinks. Respondents were also asked about their drinking of each beverage type in the last month, in terms of frequency and how much they usually had "at one time, on the average." From these two separate sets of questions, an overall volume in drinks per month was computed. Table 4 compares the results on these two measures. For each beverage type and overall, the "frequency of specific levels" approach yields a higher volume estimate more often than the "usual quantity" approach—38% higher in the case of the overall volume of drinking. In Table 5, distributions on the two measures of overall volume are cross-tabulated. The higher estimates by the "frequency of specific levels" approach arise in two ways: (1) a substantial proportion of the sample has had a few drinks in the last year, but reports no drinking in the last month; and (2) a high proportion of relatively heavy-drinking respondents—presumably particularly those who often drink more than their "usual" quantities—give a higher volume estimate by the "frequency of specific levels" approach.

Table 6 shows the correlations of the two volume estimates with each other, with a measure of the difference between them, and with selected demographic variables. A multiple regression of the five demographic variables in Table 6 on the volume–difference measure (multiple $r = 0.21$) found that a higher volume with the "frequency of specific levels" questions is modestly predicted by being male (beta weight 0.14), having less education (0.12), and being younger (0.12)—factors generally associated with relatively heavy, though not necessarily frequent, drinking.

Simpura (1987) also investigated the intercorrelations and correlates of volume scores computed from his three different questioning methods. The "usual quantity" estimate correlated 0.81 with the "period" estimate from four or so occasions; both

Table 4. Comparison of Volumes Computed from "Usual Quantity" and from "Frequency of Specific Levels" Questions, 1979 U.S. National Drinking Survey, $N = 1772$ (%) (Based on Weighted Data)

| | Wine | Beer | Liquor | Overall |
|---|---|---|---|---|
| 0 drinks on both measures | 54% | 51% | 50% | 33% |
| Higher by "usual quantity" questions | | | | |
| 3+ drinks/month higher | 7 | 10 | 10 | 17 |
| 0.1–2.9 drinks/month higher | 9 | 10 | 10 | 10 |
| Lower by "usual quantity" questions | | | | |
| 0.1–2.9 drinks/month lower | 21 | 12 | 17 | 14 |
| 3+ drinks/month lower | 9 | 17 | 13 | 26 |

Table 5. Overall Volume in Drinks per Month by the Two Methods, 1979 U.S. National Study, Corner Percentaging ($N$ = 1772, Weighted Data)

| Volume by "frequency of specific levels" questions | Volume by usual quantity questions | | | | | |
|---|---|---|---|---|---|---|
| | 0 | 0.1–17.4 | 17.5–44.9 | 45.0–119.9 | 120.0+ | Total |
| 0 | 33% | [a] | [a] | [a] | 0 | 33% |
| 0.1–17.4 | 10 | 25 | 2 | 1 | 0 | 38 |
| 17.5–44.9 | [a] | 4 | 6 | 1 | [a] | 12 |
| 45.0–119.9 | [a] | 1 | 3 | 5 | 1 | 10 |
| 120.0+ | [a] | [a] | 1 | 3 | 3 | 7 |
| Total | 44% | 31 | 12 | 10 | 3 | 100 |

[a]= less than 0.5%.

measures had a lower correlation with an estimate from the last week's drinking occasions, owing to the substantial number of respondents who had no drinking in the last week (0.67 with "period" estimate, 0.61 with "usual quantity" estimate; all correlations on logarithmically transformed measures).

## 5. DIFFERENCES IN RESULTS WITH DIFFERENT SCORES AND MEASURES

There is a somewhat more developed literature in this area, although it has been curiously noncumulative. Survey reports in the 1960s often presented different aggregations based on the same data; Cahalan et al.'s discussion on Volume-Variability in an

Table 6. Correlations of Overall Volume Measures and Overall Volume Difference with Demographic Variables, 1979 U.S. National Study ($N$ = 1772, Weighted Data)[a]

| | OVOLFSL | OVOLDIF | Gender | Education | Age | Income | Dry region |
|---|---|---|---|---|---|---|---|
| OVOLUSU | 0.58 | 0.13 | −0.20 | 0.00 | −0.06 | 0.04 | −0.03 |
| OVOLFSL | | 0.88 | −0.20 | −0.08 | −0.09 | −0.03 | −0.01 |
| OVOLDIF | | | −0.13 | −0.10 | −0.07 | −0.06 | 0.00 |
| Gender | | | | −0.01 | −0.00 | −0.09 | −0.04 |
| Education | | | | | −0.27 | 0.41 | −0.07 |
| Age | | | | | | −0.16 | −0.06 |
| Income | | | | | | | −0.11 |

[a]OVOLUSU = overall volume, based on "usual quantity in last month" questions; OVOLFSL = overall volume, based on frequency of specific levels in last year questions; OVOLDIF = OVOLFSL − OVOLUSU; dry region = dichotomy, dry regions (East South Central, West South Central, South Atlantic, West North Central, Mountain) = 1, all others = 0; Gender: 2 = female, 1 = male; Age in actual years, Income, and Education: higher score indicates higher level.

appendix to *American Drinking Practices* (1969), for instance, includes a comparison with the Quantity-Frequency-Variability variable used in the main text.*

*See also the comparison of Knupfer et al.'s F–Q with what became the Q–F–V index (pp. 10–14 of Cahalan et al., 1965). The report noted that the new measure was adopted because "it was shown to differentiate more sharply between the various groupings for age and family income than was true for the California drinker classifications" (p. 11).

There was also a great deal of unpublished experimentation, comparisons, and correspondence in this period. The few excerpts which follow give the flavor of these discussions between the Washington and Berkeley staffs.

Genevieve Knupfer to Ira Cisin and Don Cahalan, June 2, 1965, responding to the adoption of the Q–F–V index: "I am chagrined at the changes in the definition of the F.Q. index that you have made, as I have been carrying the torch for the importance of 'quantity,' and I thought we were all agreed. . . . The essence of the point might be put this way: we want an index that is more related to the blood alcohol level of the drinker than to the profit level of the alcoholic beverages industry. A light drinker as we defined it is one who never gets a high blood alcohol level. One cannot get to be a light drinker in our system by going on a binge once a month, whereas he can in your system. That is what I object to. Being slightly drunk three times a week is *more* drinking, not *less* drinking, than having a glass of wine at each meal, yet the latter type you have called a heavy, for no other reason that that they drink several times a day. . . ."

Don Cahalan to Genevieve Knupfer, June 21, 1965: "I am sure we will agree that no single index will be entirely satisfactory for all purposes. We intend to wring the maximum out of the national data from many standpoints, taking into account frequency, quantity per sitting, and type of beverage. We do intend to use the [Q–F–V] as one major index on which to report most of the principal group differences. We find it useful primarily because (1) it yields the most linear results for more groupings than any other single index, and (2) because while using the concept of intra-personal variation, it fits in well with other national and regional studies which use Q–F indices which are familar to the alcohol research fraternity and which permit certain comparisons from one study to another. At the same time, we recognize that it probably is not adequate to differentiate the (probably rare) very occasional binge drinker from the person who has a small amount of alcohol every day. . . ."

Robin Room to Vito Signorile, June 26, 1967, responding to a letter from Signorile concerning a "Rationalized F/Q Typology" Room had proposed in 1965 (Signorile had sent a proposed "Index of Frequent Intoxication" built because "Don Cahalan and I were interested in detecting any tendency toward binge drinking in the Hartford follow-up study"): ". . . when we built the Rationalized F/Q, we did not really intend it as a measure of the frequency of drinking amounts which hold the potential of intoxication. . . . Quite simply our reason for building it was that we had grown dissatisfied with our old F/Q scale. . . . Our basic indicator of drinking patterns provided inadequate means of differentiating the effects of frequency and quantity. . . . [In the new measure] the particular distinctions between levels of quantity were chosen partly with an eye to the possibility of intoxication, and partly to yield a partitioning of a general population with a respectably large N at each level of drinking. The distinction on frequency was made with some idea in mind of distinguishing between 'regular' and 'irregular' patterns, on the assumption that anything that happens less than one a week become more a 'special occasion' than a regular part of the respondent's routine. . . . Still, basically, both [indexes] are laboring very hard to overcome difficulties caused by questions on amount of drinking formulated long ago for different purposes. Both of our purposes would be much more simply served by questions of the form, 'how often would you say you drink X amount'."

Don Cahalan to Robin Room, July 27, 1967: "Our own opinion (Ira's, Vito's, and mine) is that the Q–F–V index used in [*American Drinking Practices*] is already outmoded. (Note the strictures expressed on [p. 17 of the book].) We believe that the best single measure thus far is the Volume-Variability Index which we (primarily Ira) developed *after* we had gone too far with the more traditional Q–F–V Index to scrap the whole analysis and start from scratch."

A few reports in the course of the 1970s focused on the differences between the "heavy" drinking category of the various aggregate measures. A 1971 report (Room, 1971*a*) showed that the prevalence of heavy drinking varied between 7% and 20% according to five different measures of heavy drinking built on the same questions in the same sample; altogether, 34% of the sample was defined as a "heavy" drinker by one or another of the measures. The paper also showed that the relationship between "heavy drinking" and social class could be completely reversed, depending on the heavy drinking measure that was chosen. Streissguth et al. (1977) studied the interrelations of Q–F–V, Volume–Variability (V–V), and "Jessor's AA" (a volume measure) in a sample of pregnant women—a sample mostly composed of relatively light drinkers—and found that, although the three measures identified much the same proportions as "heavy drinkers," there was considerable divergence in which members of the sample were thus identified—only 70% of those with over 1 oz absolute alcohol on the AA measure were "High Volume–High Maximum" (HVHM) drinkers, while only 70% HVHM drinkers met the 1-oz criterion on the AA, for instance. Noting that the "poor interrelationship" of the scores might be partly "due to the attempt to oversimplify relatively complex drinking activity by reducing it to a single scale or a small number of categories," the authors concluded that "it is probably advisable to use multiple alcohol assessments in a study of this type" (p. 418). Another report on a study of pregnant women (Little et al., 1977) proposed a new "A–A—Q–P" measure, composed of two dimensions: (1) overall volume (A–A), computed by Jessor et al.'s method, and (2) Quantity–Pattern (Q–P), a four-step measure of the frequency with which the respondent drinks five drinks on an occasion. [It will be noted that conceptually this dimension is related to the "Frequent Heavy Drinking" measure—see Fig. 10. However, Little et al. use considerably more liberal scoring criteria, assuming, for instance, that "once in a while" can be translated to 30% of the drinking occasions (p. 559).] Cross-tabulating the Q–P categorization with Q–F–V, V–V, and A–A categories, the authors concluded that Q–P "expresses the average frequency of massed drinking with greater precision than either" Q–F–V or V–V; for instance, "these indicators . . . fail to differentiate between weekly and monthly massed drinking, although weekly binging is a much more dangerous pattern than monthly intoxication on payday, for instance" (p. 560). A study based on an alcohol treatment sample (Bowman et al., 1975) proposed a two-dimensional "Volume–Pattern Index" where the "pattern" dimension was conceptualized in terms analogous to the standard deviation of the respondent's daily consumption. The relations between the "Volume–Pattern" grid and the categories of the Q–F, Q–F–V, and V–V measures were shown graphically. To the authors' surprise, the "Pattern" dimension was not related to five measures of social adjustment, although the Volume measure was. It was concluded that "pattern of intake may have a very different meaning for severe problem drinkers requiring hospitalization and for the social drinkers who were most numerous" in general-population studies.

The 1984 national survey of drinking conducted for the Alcohol Research Group by Temple University's Institute for Survey Research included questions on drinking from which several measures of the volume of drinking could be created:

1. A volume measure ("Cahalan method") computed as in Cahalan et al.'s Volume–Variability (but including a volume for all drinking at least once a year), based on

the Knupfer et al. questions on the proportion of consumption occasions for each beverage type on which 5+, 3–4, and 1–2 drinks were consumed.

2. A volume measure computed from the same questions, but according to the method specified in Jessor et al. (1968). (The metric in this computation is ounces of absolute alcohol per day, and in the other volume measures is drinks per month. Assuming 0.5 oz absolute alcohol per drink, all measures are converted to "drinks per month" by multiplying the Jessor-method result by 60.)

3. A volume measure ("optimum method") adding the extra volume attributable to questions on the frequency of drinking 8–11 and 12+ drinks to the volume computed in (1) above. Assuming that the 8–11 and 12+ drinks occasions would also have been reported as "5+" occasions—and thus already counted with a value of 6—the frequency of drinking 8–11 drinks was multiplied by 3.5, and the frequency of drinking 12+ by 7.0, to reflect the "extra" drinks, and these products were added to the volume computed in (1) above.

4. A volume measure ("last two occasions method") computed on the basis of the time since the last two drinking occasions and amount consumed on these occasions. The computation of volume in drinks per month added together the amounts for the last two occasions, divided by the number of days since the second-to-last drinking occasion, and multiplied by 30. This computation assumes that the time since the last occasion is the same as the time between occasions, which gives a volume estimate that usually will err on the side of overestimation (Skog, 1981).

Table 7 shows the means and standard deviations of these four volume measures. The aggregate volume estimate for the "last two occasions method" is only 76% of the estimate by the method used by Cahalan et al. (despite the inflationary estimation procedure used). On the other hand, adding two questions on the frequency of drinkiing 8–11 and 12+ drinks adds 13% extra volume to the estimate ("optimum method").

It will be seen that the "Jessor method" also results in a higher estimate, by 19%, than the "Cahalan method" (Fig. 9), although they are based on exactly the same questions. The differences between the Cahalan method and the Jessor method derive from two sources. (1) The Cahalan method assumes that all drinks have equivalent alcohol content (set at 0.5 oz absolute alcohol in Table 7), whereas the Jessor method assigns 0.6 oz to a glass of wine, 0.48 oz to a bottle of beer, and 0.675 oz to a liquor

Table 7. Means, Standard Deviations, and Median for Four Volume Measures 1984 National Drinking Survey (Drinkers Only, $N = 3647$, Weighted Data)

| Volume measures (drinks per month) | Mean | Standard deviation | Median |
|---|---|---|---|
| Cahalan method | 39.93 | 78.93 | 12.80 |
| Jessor method[a] | 47.82 | 92.94 | 16.80 |
| Optimum method | 45.18 | 94.67 | 14.05 |
| Last two occasions method | 30.31 | 62.40 | 8.57 |

[a]Multiplied by 60 to convert to drinks per month.

drink. While the Jessor method overestimates the proof strength of wine and liquor drinks today, it has been argued that wine and liquor drinks consumed at home frequently contain a greater volume of alcoholic beverage than assumed in the Cahalan method (Gross, 1983, pp. 126–132). (2) The Cahalan method distinguishes between all available response categories in assigning proportions of occasions to the 5+, 3–4, and 1–2 levels, while the Jessor method lumps "once in a while" with "less than half the time," and "more than half the time" with "nearly every time." The methods also differ in how the pattern of responses to the three levels is taken into account. The net result of the Jessor method is to give more weight to low-proportion responses such as "once in a while." In the Jessor method, for instance, a quantity consumed "nearly every time" has only twice the weight of a quantity consumed "once in a while," whereas in the Cahalan method the ratio varies between 4 : 1 and 10.6 : 1, according to the pattern of other responses. The main result of elevating the estimates of "once in a while" occasions is to push a substantial number of low-volume drinkers into the middle volume range (Table 8). Although there is a good deal of assumption involved in either method, it seems to me that the relative weights assigned to the response categories in the Cahalan method are closer to their probable meanings to the respondents. This, then, is a case in which, in my view, a higher volume estimate is not necessarily a better estimate.

Table 9 shows the intercorrelations of the four methods of estimating volume and their correlations with overall frequency of drinking, with frequency of drinking 8+ drinks, and with selected demographic variables. It will be seen that there is a very high intercorrelation between the Jessor-method, Cahalan-method, and optimum-method indices. Much of this interrelation must be attributed, of course, to the fact that they are aggregated in large part or in whole from the same questions and responses. The correlation of each of these three measures with the volume estimate based on the last two occasions is considerably lower, as might be expected on substantive as well as procedural grounds. The correlations with this volume estimate are, in fact, lower than those with the overall frequency question, which is not a component of any of the volume measures.

It will be noted in Table 9 that there is very little relation of any of the volume measures with age, education, or family income, while the relation with gender is moderate. Both overall frequency of drinking and frequency of drinking 8+ drinks show a stronger relationship with being male, while the frequency of drinking 8+ drinks is fairly strongly related to youth. We shall return to the issue of the strength of correlates of different drinking measures in Section 6.

## 6. DISCUSSION

Questions about amount of drinking are asked of many populations and with many purposes in mind. In picking our way through the implications of the material laid out here, it is perhaps best to work backward through the aggregate measures to the questions.

Table 8. Comparison of Volume Computation Methods, 1984 National Drinking Survey ($N$ = 5221, Weighted Data) (Corner Percentages)

| | Cahalan et al. method (drinks per month) | | | | |
|---|---|---|---|---|---|
| | 0 | 0.01–17.4 | 17.5–44.9 | 45+ | Total |
| Jessor et al. method (oz absolute alcohol per day) | | | | | |
| 0 | 31.1% | 0 | 0 | 0 | 31.1% |
| 0.01–0.21 | [a] | 29.9 | 0 | 0 | 29.9 |
| 0.22–0.99 | [a] | 8.1 | 12.0 | 2.6 | 22.7 |
| 1.0+ | 0 | 0 | 1.0 | 15.3 | 16.3 |
| Total | 31.1% | 38.0 | 13.0 | 17.9 | 100 |

[a]Multiply by 60 to convert to drinks per month.

Table 9. Correlations of Volumes Computed by Different Methods, and with Demographic and Other Measures, 1984 National Sample, Drinkers Only ($N = 3272$, Weighted Data)

| | Volume Jessor method | Volume optimum method | Volume last 2 occasions | Overall frequency | Frequency 8+ drinks[a] | Age | Education | Family income | Gender |
|---|---|---|---|---|---|---|---|---|---|
| Volume Cahalan method | 0.98 | 0.97 | 0.52 | 0.68 | 0.52 | −0.02 | −0.03 | 0.02 | −0.21 |
| Volume Jessor method | | 0.95 | 0.50 | 0.68 | 0.50 | −0.02 | −0.01 | 0.04 | −0.19 |
| Volume optimum method | | | 0.55 | 0.64 | 0.60 | −0.03 | −0.04 | 0.01 | −0.21 |
| Volume last 2 occasions | | | | 0.45 | 0.51 | −0.07 | −0.02 | 0.03 | −0.19 |
| Overall frequency | | | | | 0.42 | 0.01 | 0.04 | 0.10 | −0.27 |
| Frequency 8+ drinks | | | | | | −0.24 | −0.10 | −0.03 | −0.27 |
| Age | | | | | | | −0.15 | −0.07 | 0.02 |
| Education | | | | | | | | 0.42 | 0.02 |
| Family income | | | | | | | | | −0.07 |

[a]This measure takes as the "frequency of drinking 8+ drinks" whichever response to the 8–11 and 12+ drinks level is more frequent, except that if the two levels are drunk with equal frequency, they are raised one category—e.g., if both are drunk "once or twice a week," the "8+ frequency" is set at "three or four times a week."

## Aggregate Measures

*Volume of drinking* continues to exercise a strong attraction as a single overall measure of amount of drinking. It is easy to conceptualize, it captures all the drinking, and it has strong technical attractions: It is unidimensional and is, in principle, a continuous variable. It is the appropriate measure for the main check on the aggregate validity of survey data—alcohol sales data for the population surveyed. Work in the tradition of Ledermann has helped focus attention on the volume dimension. It is a comfortable measure for epidemiologists concerned with a variety of behavioral risk factors in morbidity and mortality, and indeed, the dimension may well be the most closely related to risk of long-term health consequences of drinking, such as cirrhosis.

Yet for many purposes, volume is an inappropriate or awkward measure, and, for that matter, for many purposes the individual's drinking cannot adequately be summarized by any single dimension. The argument can be seen laid out in 1926 in Pearl's *Alcohol and Longevity*. In an earlier study he had grouped the cases studied essentially on a dimension of volume of drinking, remarking that "I realize fully that in placing the moderate and temperate but *steady* daily drinker in the 'Heavy' category that I am going contrary to common opinion and the common usage of descriptive language," but defending the choice as "sound from a purely biological point of view." An English committee remonstrated that Pearl's classification did not reveal "whether moderate drinking, using the word moderate in its colloquial sense, is prejudicial to longevity. Are a daily pint or two of beer, or a daily bottle of claret, or a few glasses of whiskey and soda *per diem* harmful?" In his new study, Pearl therefore adopted a distinction between those who were "moderate in amount, steady in frequency" and those who were "heavy in amount, occasional as to frequency," noting that "surely it is in accord with common usage to call a person who gets drunk a heavy drinker. Also it is common usage to call a person who drinks a little but never gets drunk a moderate drinker" (p. 73). Pearl further remarked that "the basis of the present classification is the same as that which we use regarding drinking in everyday life. It is that of the immediate *effect* of the drinking on the drinker. If a person drinks enough to get drunk it is *prima facie* evidence that he is a heavy drinker" (p. 75).

The problem with a volume measure, then, is that it is relatively insensitive to differences in the patterning of drinking that are of social importance in terms both of correlates and of consequences. As can be seen in Table 9, volume of drinking is relatively insensitive to variations in the U.S. population by such significant social differentiations as age or social class: The less frequent and heavier drinking of the younger and the poorer is balanced by the relatively more frequent and lighter drinking of the middle-aged and middle class. More crucially, many of the adverse consequences of drinking—notably casualties and social problems—are fairly specific to heavy-drinking occasions. Knupfer (1984) has recently reemphasized this point: "The average amount a person drinks seems to us of little importance, from the point of view of social norm violation or driving accidents: what matters, we contend, is frequency of intoxication. Indeed, it is difficult to see what interest there is, unless one is doing some sort of market research, in average amounts or total amounts." It is for this reason that, as attention turned in U.S. studies in the mid-1960s to measuring drinking-related problems as well as drinking patterns, researchers began to seek typologies or measures with a dimension reflecting the drinking of significant amounts on an occasion.

It might be noted that the adequacy of a volume measure (number of cigarettes consumed in a given interval) is now questioned even in the current literature on tobacco smoking—where, given the nature of smoking habits and the emphasis on long-term health consequences, one might have expected it to have been seen as an adequate measure. "In times past," one of the participants (Fredericksen, 1983) at a recent conference on measurement in the field noted, "smoking rate (number of cigarettes per unit time) was considered to be an adequate descriptor of smoking behavior. . . . In recent years, it has been increasingly clear that this is a far too simplistic picture. . . . Overall it becomes apparent that while our concern is 'risk,' an adequate description of smoking must involve the assessment of what is smoked, the rate or temporal pattern of that consumption, and smoking topography (puff rate, puff size, interpuff interval, puff volume, etc." Similarly, contributors discussing the measurement of smoking among youth proposed that "less weight should be given to the quantity (i.e., absolute number) of cigarettes young people smoke. Instead, more attention ought to be put on the timing and situational patterns of youth's tobacco consumption" (Schinke and Gilchrist, 1983).

However patterns of drinking are measured and aggregated, U.S. survey reports on drinking have commonly cut the drinking population up into discrete *categories of drinking*. Such categorizations, often with relatively few cells, have been criticized by European researchers as often hiding the character of the overall distribution of consumption. It is clear, also, that comparisons of such categorized variables can be quite misleading when the focus is on changes in drinking (Caetano et al., 1982). Such categorizations were a necessity in the era, through the late 1960s, when most analysis was done on the countersorter, but categorizations are still commonly used for presentation in tabular and other analyses comparing statistics across parts of the sample. Behind the categorizations adopted are at least two implicit criteria: that the categories be describable and appear meaningful, and that each category include a decent-sized "chunk" of the sample. The latter criterion means that shifting patterns of drinking may render a particular categorization less useful because of shrinking "chunks": In the 1984 U.S. national sample, most high- and medium-volume drinkers at least occasionally drink 5+ drinks, so that the Volume–Variability measure defined on the 1964 U.S. national sample (Cahalan et al., 1969, Appendix I) no longer yields usable "chunks." Sometimes a third, more controversial criterion, of maximizing differences on or the linearity of relations with important correlates, also enters into consideration. One difficulty with categorizations is that different choices by researchers on where to set the boundaries of categories can make comparisons difficult or impossible, even when the underlying items or scores are comparable.

Despite their problems, categorizations remain useful in describing patterns of drinking in a population. The alternative—to work only with summary statistics—gives a far less detailed picture of patterns, and frequently leaves interesting patternings hidden.

Along with categorizations of volume and other single-dimensional variables, U.S. researchers have often used *drinking typologies* composed of two or more dimensions. Many of the early typologies, such as Q–F–V, while composed from several dimensions, added them together into a partly or wholly unidimensional measure, so that they amounted to weighted and categorized volume measures, in which some patterns of drinking (often those drinking relatively large amounts on an occasion) were given a

Table 10. Typology of Frequency of Drinking by Frequency of Drinking 5+ Drinks, 1984 U.S. National Drinking Survey ($N$ = 5221, Weighted Data) (Percentaged on Total Sample)

| | Frequency of drinking 5+ drinks | | |
|---|---|---|---|
| Overall frequency | Drinks 5+ once a week | Drinks 5+ less often | Does not drink 5+ |
| At least once a week | 11.2% | 12.5% | 12.0% |
| 1–3 times a month | | 6.3% | 12.3% |
| 1–11 times a year | | 1.7% | 13.6% |
| Abstainer | | | 30.2% |
| | | | 100% |

special weight. The advantage of such a weighted measure over a simple volume of drinking measure has not been systematically argued in the survey literature; it presumably parallels the tendency of some clinically based measures to assess a special "penalty" for binge drinking (Milton and Lee, 1967; Ewing, 1970). It might be added that, since the computation of volume itself frequently rests on a substratum of plausible, but arbitrary assumptions, the analyst's choices of assumptions often, in fact, amount to differential weights within what is conceptually a volume measure.

More recently, typologies have usually been constructed from the intersections of two distinct dimensions. The Volume–Variability index, for instance, is composed of a volume dimension and a dichotomous dimension of whether the respondent reports drinking 5+ drinks on an occasion at least once in a while. Many typologies include overall frequency of drinking as one dimension, often cut into categories according to the periods of everyday life—daily, weekly, and monthly. A typology that has often been used at the Alcohol Research Group (e.g., Cahalan et al., 1976; Wallack, 1978; Caetano and Herd, 1984; Hilton, 1987*a*) cross-cuts this with a trichotomous division on drinking 5+ drinks on an occasion—that the respondent does this at least once a week, that the respondent does it once in a while, or that the respondent does not do it at all. Such a typology makes a serviceable classification of current U.S. drinking patterns and complements, without duplicating, a drinking volume measure (Table 10; the "infrequent–high maximum" category—1–11 times a year, sometimes 5+—would often be combined with another category).

Whether or not typologies are used, the general tendency of the literature has been toward a *dimensional approach* to summarizing drinking patterns. There is an almost endless choice of dimensions for summarizing a behavior as complex as drinking. *Frequency* of drinking is perhaps the most commonly reported dimension. The logical complement to this would be *average drinks per occasion,* i.e., volume/frequency. This dimension has been little used, although it has an interestingly small relation with frequency of drinking in current U.S. data (Table 11). Various measures of *variability* have been proposed, but the most frequently used have been some form of *maximum quantity on an occasion,* which is easily interpretable but taps only one element of variability. There has been some convergence of different approaches on the *frequency*

Table 11. Average Number of Drinks per Occasion (Cahalan Method) by Overall Frequency of Drinking, 1984 National Drinking Survey, Current Drinkers Only (Total $N = 5221$, Weighted Data)

| | Overall frequency of drinking | | |
|---|---|---|---|
| Average drinks per occasion[a] | Nearly daily or more often | 1–4 times a week | Less than once a week |
| 4.4+ | 29.0% | 30.7% | 22.5% |
| 2.4–4.39 | 32.6 | 35.6 | 37.1 |
| 0–2.39 | 38.4 | 33.6 | 40.4 |
| ($N$) | (477) | (1084) | (1631) |
| Pearson's $r = 0.07$ | | | |

[a]Average number of drinks is computed from the volume–Cahalan method divided by the overall frequency (in occasions per month). Percentages are based on weighted data, $N$'s are unweighted.

*of drinking specified amounts* as a useful operational representation of "heavy drinking"; Finnish researchers, for instance, taking body weight into account, have used the frequency of drinking enough to reach a given blood alcohol level (Bruun, 1969), while U.S. researchers have tended to use the frequency of drinking five or more or eight or more drinks.

At least since the mid-1960s, U.S. survey research on drinking patterns in the general population has been primarily conducted in the context of studies of drinking-related problems. This tradition, which differs, for instance, from the Scandinavian tradition of studies of drinking patterns without much attention to drinking problems, has meant that primary attention has been paid to drinking dimensions and levels that might be regarded as "problematic." Although studies of clinical populations have sometimes been interested in the occurrence and proportion of small-quantity occasions, for instance, since this bears on discussions of addiction models, this dimension has not been prominent in general-population studies. Rather little attention has been paid in U.S. analyses, since the 1969 study by Cahalan and associates, to differential patterning by type of beverage, although even from a drinking-problems perspective there are some interesting differences in patterning between beer, wine, and spirits consumption (Room, 1976).

## Asking Questions about Drinking

It will be clear from the preceding discussion and data that much of what we think we know about asking questions about drinking is based on presumption and lore rather than on detailed quantitative studies. Given the substantial underestimation of aggregate alcohol consumption in survey data, the criterion usually offered for choosing between methods is whether the method yields a higher average volume of drinking (Midanik, 1982). Yet a higher volume estimate for a population as a whole is not necessarily the best criterion. A set of questions and method of aggregation that yield a high estimate may nevertheless be indefensible on logical or statistical grounds (see Skog, 1981). Also, a volume criterion assigns a primary role to frequent and heavier drinkers, giving little weight to the handling of the lighter and more infrequent drinkers who form the bulk of the population.

The choice of method should, in fact, depend on the main analytical purposes for which the data are being collected. As outlined earlier, there are only a few main choices of approach in asking questions about amount of drinking. But besides these main choices, there are many detailed decisions to be made by the researcher, some of which are discussed in the following sections.

Recent Occasions Questions. Quite a number of studies have asked about the last two drinking occasions (or about drinking occasions on the last two drinking days, which is not the same thing). As is apparent from the discussion and references above, there are severe statistical problems in using the last two occasions to estimate volume of drinking, mostly because of the difficulty of estimating the frequency of drinking. More generally, summarizing respondents' drinking on the basis of one or two occasions will be unreliable to the extent the respondents are not absolutely regular in their rhythm and amounts of drinking. Nevertheless, asking about recent occasions has several potential uses: It is a way of securing information on contexts of drinking; it can give a good sampling (though weighted toward infrequent drinkers) of drinking person–occasions; and it may yield reliable population estimates despite the unreliability at the individual level.

Several studies—notably the WHO Community Response Study in Mexico, Zambia, and Scotland (Roizen, 1981)—have asked about the occasion on which the respondent drank the most in the last month and the occasion on which the respondent drank the most in the last year. Such questions are potentially useful descriptively and, along with a frequency question, can form the minimum data needed for a frequency–maximum quantity typology.

Substantial studies using the recent-occasions approach usually enquire about the drinking days and/or occasions for at least the last week. This is the basic approach used for governmental surveys in Britain (Dight, 1976) and in the WHO Community Response Study. Such an approach excludes many drinkers in cultural situations, such as Zambia and Mexico, where many drinkers drink quite infrequently. Accordingly, respondents in the WHO study were asked about their last two drinking days, at a minimum (see Fig. 7b for the elaborated U.S. version of these questions). The Finnish approach to this problem has been to vary the time period asked about according to the reported overall frequency of drinking (see Table 1). As Mäkelä showed (1971), the drawback of asking about longer periods is the greater forgetting of occasions in earlier weeks.

At a minimum, such approaches ask about the amount and type of beverages consumed, and usually also the length of the drinking occasion, the setting, and the number and type of companions. The questioning involved in this method is often quite lengthy—on the average perhaps 20 min of interview time in the 1979 Contra Costa County survey. A less obvious cost of this method is the substantial programming job involved in collating and aggregating the "occasions" data into summary scores.

In my view, the extended recent-occasions or "survey period" approach yields a rich data-set for contextual analyses of drinking, but is not clearly superior to other approaches in characterizing the respondent's overall drinking patterns. This view is not shared by many European researchers, however: In Alanko's view, "the survey period approach gives unbiased estimates for most existing drinking styles and is thus the one to be preferred in actual survey work'' (Alanko, 1984, p. 220.)

Recent Period Summary Methods. A number of U.S. studies in recent years, particularly NIAAA contract studies, have asked about drinking in a fixed period of time—usually 30 days. Unlike the ''recent occasions'' methods, these studies ask the respondent to summarize his or her drinking in the period. A questionnaire used in 1975 Alcohol Research Group studies (Fig. 5a)—and since used in college drinking studies (Greenfield and Haymond, 1980; Greenfield et al., 1980; Greenfield, 1986)—asks respondents to report on how many days in the last month they had any drinks, 4 or more drinks, 8 or more drinks, and 12 or more drinks. A method originally used in clinical follow-up studies has been adopted by Armor and Polich and others (e.g., Polich and Orvis, 1979) for use in the general population. The method asks about drinking of each beverage type in the 30 days before the last drinking occasion: On how many days did the respondent drink that beverage, and what was the usual quantity? Adaptations for NIAAA contract studies use a 2-week period (1983 Health Interview Survey Supplement) and a 4-week period (Hispanic HANES study) and add a question about the total number of drinks of the beverage consumed during the period (Alcohol Epidemiology Data System, 1984).

These methods represent something of a hybrid between the ''recent occasions'' and other summary methods. Specifying responses to a particular time period perhaps puts the respondent in mind of specific drinking occasions and does put all responses on an equal time footing; many overall summary methods specify no time period beyond the use of the present tense. But the method runs the risk that the time period is not typical of the respondent's consumption over a longer period. The 1975 ARG questions (Fig. 5a) and the Armor and Polich (1982) recommendations partly remedy this by asking also about frequency of consumption of larger amounts over a 1-year period.

Recent questionnaires also often ask for the amount of beverage in the respondent's usual ''drink''; the differing sizes of drinks, particularly for wine and spirits, is increasingly seen as a major contributor to survey underestimation of drinking in the United States (see Gross, 1983, pp. 126–132). The questions about the total number of drinks in the time period in the new NIAAA formulations are presumably intended to recapture infrequent large amounts for the volume accounting, but it is difficult to believe that frequent drinkers really find it possible to add drinks across all occasions in a 30-day period.

Overall Summary (Customary Drinking) Methods. For the many nondrinking studies which want a summarization of the respondent's drinking, but which do not have the questionnaire time to spare for exhaustive questioning, a few overall summary questions are probably the best compromise. The Alcohol Research Group has had good results with just two questions added to ''caravan surveys'' in monitoring drinking practices in California:

> Now, please think of all the times during *the last* 12 months when you had something to drink. How often have you had some kind of beverage containing alcohol, whether it was wine, beer, whiskey, or any other drink? Just give me the letter A, B, C, or whatever fits your answer. . . .

About how often during the last twelve months would you say you had five or more drinks?*

Beyond this bare minimum, the refinements lie in many directions, as can be seen in the figures in this chapter. A majority of U.S. drinking surveys ask about beverage types separately, although there is no published study of how much difference this makes. Some studies provide tables of equivalence between "drinks" and common beverage container sizes; as noted earlier, some also ask about the average size of drinks. A fundamental difference remains between approaches soliciting the respondent's estimate of "usual quantity" and those requesting information about the drinking of specific amounts, although, as mentioned, some current studies compromise between the approaches. In my view, "usual quantity" is a flawed approach to asking about amount of drinking in the general adult population (in teenage populations and in treatment samples, where drinking may be more of an all-or-nothing proportion, "usual quantity" questions may work adequately—although see Harford, 1979). The Knupfer et al. "proportion of occasions" series represent an improvement, but except where comparability is needed, it seems preferable to ask about actual frequencies of different drinking levels. Respondents may be daunted by an overelaboration of levels of drinking: The 1979 national survey (Fig. 5b) asked, for each beverage type, about the frequency of drinking at the levels of 18+, 15–17, 12–14, 8–11, 5–7, 3–4, and 1–2 drinks; anecdotally, it seemed that such elaboration became self-defeating.

It is also an improvement to specify a time period to be covered—whether a year or a week. But in the choice of a time period, researchers seem to be faced with a paradox. As long as the respondent's frame of reference is remembering specific drinking occasions, the shorter the time period the better the recall. Yet the shorter the time period, the more potential for misclassification of respondents because the period is "unusual." On the other hand, there is little evidence that the time period specified makes much difference in the aggregate when the respondent is being asked about his or her customary behavior.

Future consideration of and work on improving questions on amount of drinking must also take into account the results of Blair et al.'s experimental study manipulating the form of questions about amount of drinking of beer, wine, and liquor in the last year. The study (Blair et al., 1977), carried out on a nationwide "probability sample with quotas" ($N$ = 1172), systematically varied the form of questions on three dimensions: open-ended vs. closed-ended questions; long questions (with at least 30 words) vs. short questions; and questions using words of the respondent's choice rather than standard wordings (the last variation was applied only to liquor). Higher annual volumes were reported in answer to open-ended, to long, and to familiarly worded questions. The cumulative effect was striking: Drinkers reported 208 drinks of liquor in the last year with a long, open, familiar question, as against 80 drinks with a short, closed, standard question.

*Response categories were: usually twice a day, or more often; usually once a day, sometimes twice; only once a day; nearly every day; three or four times a week; once or twice a week; two or three times a month; about once a month; 6–11 times a year; one to five times a year; *never* in the last year (the top response for 5+ drinks was "every day") (see Cameron, 1981).

In presenting in some detail the diversity of U.S. approaches to measuring and aggregating responses on amount of drinking, this chapter aims to bring some coherence to a field where too often researchers have paid little attention to others' methods, and in particular to contribute to a dialogue between North American and European researchers. There is by now an enormous investment in the different national traditions; for comparability over time it is inevitable that at least part of previous methods will be maintained. But perhaps in the future we may be able to move toward a cross-fertilization of methods that would allow more detailed cross-national analyses.

ACKNOWLEDGMENTS

Revised from a paper presented at the Alcohol Epidemiology Section meeting, 31st International Institute on the Prevention and Treatment of Alcohol Problems, Rome, Italy, June 2–7, 1985. Preparation of this chapter was supported by a National Alcohol Research Center grant (AA-05595) from the U.S. National Institute on Alcohol Abuse and Alcoholism to the Alcohol Research Group, Institute of Epidemiology and Behavioral Medicine, Medical Research Institute of San Francisco. Thanks are due to Gary Collins and DeeDee Davis for programming, to Carol Seiden and Reuben Kuszel for typing the tables, and to Tom Greenfield and Mike Hilton for their comments.

## REFERENCES

Abelson, H. I., and Atkinson, R. B., 1975, *Public Experience with Psychoactive Substances: A Nationwide Study among Adults and Youth,* Response Analysis Corp, Princeton, NJ.

Abelson, H. I., and Fishburne, P., 1976, *Nonmedical Use of Psychoactive Substances: 1975/6 Nationwide Survey among Youth and Adults,* Response Analysis Corp, Princeton, NJ.

Abelson, H., Fishburne, P., and Cisin, I., 1977, *National Survey on Drug Abuse: 1977,* DHEW Publ. No. (ADM) 78-618, USGPO, Washington, DC.

Abelson, H., Fishburne, P., and Cisin, I., 1980, *National Survey on Drug Abuse: Main Findings 1979,* DHHS Publ. No. (ADM) 80-976, USGPO, Washington, DC.

Alanko, T., 1984, An overview of techniques and problems in the measurement of alcohol consumption, *Res. Adv. Alcohol Drug Problems* **8**:209–226, 1984.

Alcohol Epidemiology Data System (AEDS), 1984, *Data Catalog, December 1984,* CSR, Inc., Washington, DC.

Armor, D. J., and Polich, M. J., 1982, Measurement of alcohol consumption, in: *Encyclopedic Handbook of Alcoholism* (E. M. Pattison and E. Kaufman, eds.), pp. 72–80, Gardner Press, New York.

Armor, D. J., Polich, J. M., and Stambul, H. B., 1978, *Alcoholism and Treatment,* Wiley, New York.

Auth, J. B., and Warheit, G. J., 1982/1983, Estimating the prevalence of problem drinking and alcoholism in the general population: An overview of epidemiological studies, *Alcohol Health Res. World* **7**:11–12.

Bachman, J. G., and O'Malley, P. M., 1981, When four months equal a year: Inconsistencies in student reports of drug use, *Public Opinion Q.* **45**:536–548.

Barnes, G. M., and Russell, M., 1977, *Drinking Patterns among Adults in Western New York State: A Descriptive Analysis of the Sociodemographic Correlates of Drinking,* Research Institute on Alcoholism, Buffalo, NY.

Barnes, G. M., and Russell, M., 1978, Drinking patterns in western New York State: Comparison with national data, *J. Stud. Alcohol* **39**:1148–1157.

Billings, J. S., 1903, Data relating to the use of alcoholic drinks among brain workers in the United

States, in: *Physiological Aspects of the Liquor Problem, Vol. 1* (J. S. Billings, ed.), pp. 307–338, Houghton Mifflin, Boston.

Blair, E., Sudman, S., Bradburn, N. M., and Stocking, C., 1977, How to ask questions about drinking and sex: Response effects in measuring consumer behavior, *J. Marketing Res.* **14**:316–321.

Bowman, R. S., Stein, L. I., and Newton, J. R., 1975, Measurement and interpretation of drinking behavior, *J. Stud. Alcohol* **36**:1154–1172.

Bruun, K., 1969, The actual and the registered frequency of drunkenness in Helsinki, *Br. J. Addiction* **64**:3–8.

Caetano, R., 1984, Ethnicity and drinking in Northern California: A comparison among whites, blacks and Hispanics, *Alcohol Alcoholism* **19**:31–44.

Caetano, R., 1986, Patterns and problems of drinking among U.S. Hispanics, in: *Report of the Secretary's Task Force on Black and Minority Health, Vol. 7: Chemical Dependency and Diabetes*, pp. 143–186, U.S. Department of Health and Human Services, Washington, DC.

Caetano, R., and Herd, D., 1984, Black drinking practices in northern California, *Am. J. Drug Alcohol Abuse* **10**:571–587.

Caetano, R., Suzman, R., Rosen, D., and Vorhees-Rosen, D., 1982, A methodological note on Quantity–Frequency categorizations in a longitudinal study of drinking practices, *Drinking Drug Practices Surveyor* **18**:7–12.

Cahalan, D., 1968, Correlates of change in drinking behavior in an urban community sample over a three-year period, Ph.D. dissertation, George Washington University, Washington, DC.

Cahalan, D., 1969, A multivariate analysis of the correlates of drinking-related problems in a community study, *Social Problems* **17**:234–247.

Cahalan, D., 1970, *Problem Drinkers*, Jossey-Bass, San Francisco.

Cahalan, D., and Cisin, I. H., 1968, American drinking practices: Summary of findings from a national probability sample: II. Measurement of massed versus spaced drinking, *Q. J. Stud. Alcohol* **29**: 642–656.

Cahalan, D., and Room, R., 1974, *Problem Drinking among American Men*, Monograph No. 7, Rutgers Center for Alcohol Studies, New Brunswick, NJ.

Cahalan, D., and Treiman, B., 1976*a*, *Drinking Behavior, Attitudes and Problems in Marin County*, Report C11, Alcohol Research Group, Berkeley, CA.

Cahalan, D., and Treiman, B., 1976*b*, *Drinking Behavior, Attitudes and Problems in San Francisco*, Report C10, Alcohol Research Group, Berkeley, CA.

Cahalan, D., Cisin, I. H., Kirsch, A. D., and Newcomb, C., 1965, *Behavior and Attitudes Related to Drinking in a Medium-Sized Urban Community in New England*, Social Research Group, Report No. 2, George Washington University, Washington, DC.

Cahalan, D., Cisin, I. H., and Crossley, H. M., 1969, *American Drinking Practices: A National Study of Drinking Behavior and Attitudes*, Monograph No. 6, Rutgers Center of Alcohol Studies, New Brunswick, NJ.

Cahalan, D., Roizen, R., and Room, R., 1976, Alcohol problems and their prevention: Public attitudes in California, in: *The Prevention of Alcohol Problems* (R. Room and S. Sheffield, eds.), pp. 354–404, State Office of Alcoholism, Sacramento, CA.

Cameron, T., 1981, *Alcohol and Alcohol Problems: Public Opinion in California, 1974–1980*, Report No. C31, Alcohol Research Group, Berkeley, CA.

Cannell, C. F., Marquis, K. H., and Laurent, A., 1977, *A Summary of Studies of Interviewing Methodology*, Vital and Health Statistics, Public Health Service, Series 2, No. 69, USGPO, Washington, DC.

Carman, R. S., 1977, Patterns of alcohol use in rural communities, Final Report on NIAAA Grant AA00622-01.

Celentano, D. D., and McQueen, D. V., 1984, Alcohol consumption patterns among women in Baltimore, *J. Stud. Alcohol* **45**:355–358.

Clark, W. B., and Midanik, L., 1982, Alcohol use and alcohol problems among U.S. adults: Results of the 1979 national survey, in: *Alcohol and Health Monograph No. 1: Alcohol Consumption and Related Problems*, pp. 3–52, DHHS Publ. No. (ADM) 82-1190, USGPO, Washington, DC.

Clark, W. B., Midanik, L., and Knupfer, G., 1981, *Report on the 1979 National Survey,* Alcohol Research Group, Berkeley, CA.

CSR, Inc., 1983, *Final Report: Validity/Reliability Study of Self-Reported Drinking,* NIAAA Contract No. ADM 281-81-0005, CSR, Inc., Washington, DC.

Cutler, R., and Storm, T., 1973, *Drinking Practices in Three British Columbia Cities: I. General Population Survey,* Alcoholism Foundation of British Columbia, Vancouver.

de Lint, J., 1960, *Four Comments on "An Exploratory Survey of Drinking in a Northern Ontario Community,"* Alcoholism (now Addiction) Research Foundation, Substudy 3-10-60, Toronto.

Dight, S. E., 1976, *Scottish Drinking Habits: A Survey Carried out for the Scottish Home and Health Department,* HMSO, London.

Duffy, J. C., 1982, The measurement of alcohol consumption in sample surveys, Presented at the Alcohol Epidemiology Section of the International Council on Alcohol and Addictions, Helsinki, July.

Duffy, J. C., 1984, Survey measurement of drinking behavior, Presented to the Workshop on Sample Surveys, Epidemiology Section, ICAA, Edinburgh, June.

Edwards, G., Chandler, J., and Hensman, C., 1972, Drinking in a London suburb: I. Correlates of normal drinking, *Q. J. Stud. Alcohol* Suppl. 6:69–93.

Ewing, J. A., 1970, Notes on quantity frequency studies on alcohol intake, with a comment and response, *Drinking Drug Practices Surveyor* **1**:8–15.

Fink, R., 1962, Survey method in the study of drinking behavior, Presented at the annual meetings of the Society for the Study of Social Problems, Washington, DC, August.

Fitzgerald, J. L., and Mulford, H. A., 1981, The prevalence and extent of drinking in Iowa, 1979, *J. Stud. Alcohol* **42**:38–47.

Fitzgerald, J. L., and Mulford, H. A., 1982, Alcohol consumption in Iowa 1961 and 1979, *J. Stud. Alcohol* **43**:1171–1189.

Fitzgerald, J. L., and Mulford, H. A., 1984*a*, Factors related to problem-drinking rates, *J. Stud. Alcohol* **45**:424–432.

Fitzgerald, J. L., and Mulford, H. A., 1984*b*, Seasonal changes in alcohol consumption and related problems in Iowa, 1979–1980, *J. Stud. Alcohol* **45**:363–368.

Fredericksen, L. W., 1983, Evaluation of smoking risk: Some proposed minimum standards, in: *Measurement in the Analysis and Treatment of Smoking Behavior* (J. Grabowski and C. S. Bell, eds.), pp. 90–95, NIDA Research Monograph 48, DHHS Publication No. (ADM) 83-1285, USGPO, Washington, DC.

Gabrielli, W. F., and Plomin, R., 1985, Drinking behavior in the Colorado adoptee and twin sample, *J. Stud. Alcohol* **46**:24–31.

Gallup, G. H., 1972, *The Gallup Poll: Public Opinion 1935–1971,* Random House, New York.

Gerstel, E. K., Mason, R. E., Piserchia, P. V., and Kristiansen, P. L., 1975, Final report: A pilot study of the social contexts of drinking and correlates, Project No. 23U-892, Research Triangle Institute, Research Triangle Park, NC.

Gibbins, R. J., and Duda, G. M., 1960, *An Exploratory Study of Drinking in a Northern Ontario Community,* Substudy 1-3 and D-60, Alcoholism (now Addiction) Research Foundation, Toronto.

Gillies, M., 1978*a*, *The Durham Region Survey: Alcohol Use Characteristics of the Survey Sample,* Substudy No. 997, Addiction Research Foundation, Toronto.

Gillies, M., 1978*b*, *The Durham Region Survey: A Preliminary Report,* Substudy No. 996, Addiction Research Foundation, Toronto.

Greeley, A. M., McCready, W. C., and Theisen, G., 1980, *Ethnic Drinking Subcultures,* Praeger Special Studies, Praeger, New York.

Greenfield, T. K., 1986, Quantity per occasion and consequences of drinking: A reconsideration and recommendation, *Int. J. Addictions* **21**:1059–1079.

Greenfield, T. K., and Haymond, C. J., 1980, *Typologies of College Student Alcohol Consumption: Instrument Development, Selected Results and Application,* Student Services Research, Report No. 1, Washington State University, Pullman, WA.

Greenfield, T. K., Korzmark, P. B., Haymond, C. J., Wyatt, C. J., and Gunns, D. A., 1980, *Patterns of Student Drinking: Characteristics, Experiences, Motivations and Problems in College,* Student Services Research, Report No. 2, Washington State University, Pullman, WA.

Gross, L., 1983, *How Much Is Too Much?: The Effects of Social Drinking,* Random House, New York.

Gwartney-Gibbs, P. A., 1982, Alcohol use at the University of Oregon, 1982: Implications for an alcohol education program, Working paper, August.

Harford, T. C., 1979, An examination of the consistency of self-reports of the frequency of drinking and social activity, Presented at the 25th International Institute on the Prevention and Treatment of Alcoholism, Tours, France, June 18–22.

Harford, T. C., and Gerstel, E. K., 1979, The consistency of weekly drinking cycles, *Drinking Drug Practices Surveyor* **14:**7–8.

Harris, L., and associates, 1971, *American Attitudes toward Alcohol and Alcoholics,* Study 2138, Louis Harris and Associates, New York.

Herd, D., 1985, The socio-cultural correlates of drinking patterns in black and white Americans: Results from a national survey, Ph.D. dissertation, Medical Anthropology, University of California, San Francisco.

Hilton, M., 1987*a*, Demographic characteristics and the frequency of heavy drinking as predictors of self-reported drinking problems, *Br. J. Addiction* **82:**913–925.

Hilton, M., 1987*b*, Drinking patterns and problems in 1984: Results from a general population survey, *Alcoholism: Clin. Exp. Res.* **11:**167–175.

Hingson, R., Scotch, N., Barrett, J., Goldman, E., and Mangione, T., 1981, Life satisfaction and drinking practices in the Boston metropolitan area, *J. Stud. Alcohol* **42:**24–37.

Hogue, R. C., 1977, *Drinking Behavior and Attitudes: An Alcoholism Needs Assessment for the North Catchment Area of Hillsborough County,* Northside Community Mental Health Center, Tampa, FL.

Hughes, F. K., and Layne, N., 1982, Drinking patterns in Canada: Variations in drinking frequencies and demographic characteristics of current drinkers, Presented at the annual meeting of the ICAA Alcohol Epidemiology Section, Helsinki, June.

Jessor, R., Graves, T. D., Hanson, R. C., and Jessor, S. L., 1968, *Society, Personality and Deviant Behavior: A Study of a Tri-Ethnic Community,* Holt, Rinehart and Winston, New York.

Johnson, P., Armor, D., Polich, M., and Stambul, H., 1977, *U.S. Adult Drinking Practices: Time Trends, Social Correlates and Sex Roles,* Report to NIAAA, RAND Corp., Santa Monica, CA.

Knupfer, G., 1966, Some methodological problems in the epidemiology of alcoholic beverage usage: Definition of amount of intake, *Am. J. Public Health* **56:**237–242.

Knupfer, G., 1984, The risks of drunkenness (or, ebrietas resurrecta): A comparison of frequent intoxication indices and of population sub-groups as to problem risks, *Br. J. Addiction* **79:**185–196.

Knupfer, G., 1987*a*, Drinking for health: The daily light drinker fiction, *Br. J. Addiction* **82:**547–555.

Knupfer, G., 1987*b*, New directions for survey research in the study of alcoholic beverage consumption, *Br. J. Addiction* **82:**583–585.

Knupfer, G., and Room, R., 1964, Age, sex and social class as factors in amount of drinking in an urban community, *Social Problems* **12:**224–240.

Knupfer, G., Fink, R., Clark, W. B., and Goffman, A. S., 1963, *Factors Related to Amount of Drinking in an Urban Community,* Drinking Practices Study Report No. 6, California State Department of Public Health, Berkeley, CA.

Lamale, H. H., 1959, *Study of Consumer Expensitures, Incomes and Savings Methodology of the Survey of Consumer Expenditures in 1950,* University of Pennsylvania Press, Philadelphia.

Little, R. E., Schultz, F. A., and Mandell, W., 1977, Describing alcohol consumption: A comparison of three methods and a new approach, *J. Stud. Alcohol* **38:**554–562.

Lubalin, J., and Hornik, J., 1980, *Survey of the Normative Structure of Drinking in a Community: Final Report,* SysteMetrics, Inc., Bethesda, MD.

Mäkelä, K., 1971, *Measuring the Consumption of Alcohol in the 1968–1969 Alcohol Consumption Study,* Report No. 2, Social Research Institute of Alcohol Studies, Helsinki.

Marcus, A. M., 1962, *Some Remarks on "An Exploratory Study of Drinking in a Northern Ontario Community,"* Studies in Alcohol Education, Research Memo 7, Alcoholism and Drug Addiction Research Foundation, Toronto.

Maxwell, M. A., 1952, Drinking behavior in the state of Washington, *Q. J. Stud. Alcohol* **13**:219–239.

Maxwell, M. A., 1958, A quantity–frequency analysis of drinking behavior in the state of Washington, *Northwest Sci.* **32**:57–67.

McCready, W. C., Greeley, A. M., and Theisen, G., 1983, Ethnicity and nationality in alcoholism, in: *The Biology of Alcoholism. 6. The Pathogenenesis of Alcoholism: Psychosocial Factors* (B. Kissin and H. Begleiter, eds.), pp. 309–340, Plenum Press, New York and London.

McMillin, J. D., 1973, Drinking patterns in Sweden, Ph.D. dissertation, Sociology, University of Southern Illinois, Carbondale (University Microfilms No. 74-6229).

Midanik, L., 1982, The validity of self-reported alcohol consumption and alcohol problems: A literature review, *Br. J. Addiction* **77**:357–382.

Milton, R. B., and Lee, R., 1967, A severity-of-drinking scale in chronic alcoholics, *Med. J. Aust.* **2** (16):727–729.

Mohan, D., Sharma, H. K., Sundaram, K. R., and Neki, J. S., 1980, Pattern of alcohol consumption of rural Punjab males, *Indian J. Med. Res.* **72**:702–711, Nov.

Mulford, H. A., 1964, Drinking and deviant drinking, U.S.A., 1963, *Q. J. Stud. Alcohol* **25**:634–650.

Mulford, H. A., and Miller, D. E., 1960, Drinking in Iowa: II. The extent of drinking and selected sociocultural categories, *Q. J. Stud. Alcohol* **21**:26–39.

Mulford, H. A., and Miller, D. E., 1963, The prevalence and extent of drinking in Iowa, 1961: A replication and evaluation of methods, *Q. J. Stud. Alcohol* **24**:39–53.

Mulford, H. A., and Wilson, R. W., 1966, *Identifying Problem Drinkers in a Household Health Survey*, Public Health Service Publication No. 1000, series 2, no. 16, USGPO, Washington, DC.

Murray, R. P., 1978, *Manitoba Health and Drinking Survey: The Social Epidemiology of Alcohol Abuse in Eastman Region*, Manitoba Health and Drinking Survey, Winnipeg.

Neter, J., and Waksberg, J., 1965, *Response Errors in Collection of Expenditures Data by Household Interviews: An Experimental Study*, Technical Paper No. 11, U.S. Department of Commerce, Bureau of the Census, Washington, DC.

Noble, E., ed., 1979, *Third Special Report to the U.S. Congress on Alcohol and Health: Technical Support Document*, DHEW Publ. No. (ADM) 79-832, USGPO, Washington, DC.

Parker, D. A., Kaelber, C., Harford, T. C., and Brody, J. A., 1983, Alcohol problems among employed men and women in metropolitan Detroit, *J. Stud. Alcohol* **44**:1026–1039.

Pearl, R., 1926, *Alcohol and Longevity*, Knopf, New York.

Pernanen, K., 1974, Validity of survey data on alcohol use, in: *Research Advances in Alcohol and Drug Problems, Vol. 1* (R. J. Gibbins et al., eds.), pp. 355–374, Wiley, New York.

Polich, J. M., and Orvis, B. R., 1979, *Alcohol Problems: Patterns and Prevalence in the U.S. Air Force*, Rand Corp., Santa Monica, CA.

Quinn, R. P., and Shepard, L., 1974, *The 1972–73 Quality of Employment Survey: Descriptive Statistics, with Comparison Data from the 1969–70 Survey of Working Conditions*, Survey Research Center, University of Michigan, Ann Arbor.

Rappeport, M., Labaw, P., and Williams, J., 1975, *The Public Evaluates the NIAAA Public Education Campaign*, Opinion Research Corp., Princeton, NJ.

Riley, J. W., Jr., and Marden, C. F., 1947, The social pattern of alcoholic drinking, *Q. J. Stud. Alcohol* **8**:265–273.

Rodin, M. B., Morton, D. R., and Becker, B. A., 1979*a*, *Lake View (Chicago) Survey on Community Dynamics and Drinking Behavior: Goals, Rationale, Procedures, and Statistics*, Project on Community Dynamics, Social Competence and Alcoholism in Illinois (Project No. 839), Technical Report No. 4, University of Illinois School of Public Health, Chicago.

Rodin, M. B., Morton, D. R., and Shimkin, D. B., 1979*b*, *Social and Psychological Correlates of Drinking in the Lake View Community (Chicago)*, Project on Community Dynamics, Social Competence and Alcoholism in Illinois (Project No. 839), Working Paper No. 6, University of Illinois School of Public Health, Chicago.

Roizen, R., 1981, *The World Health Organization Study of Community Responses to Alcohol-Related Problems: A Review of Cross-Cultural Findings*, Report C36 (Annex 41 of the WHO report), Alcohol Research Group, Berkeley, CA.

Room, R., 1968, Amount of drinking and alcoholism, Presented at the 28th International Congress on Alcohol and Alcoholism, Washington, September [abstract in *Proceedings of the 28th International Congress on Alcohol and Alcoholism, Vol. 1: Abstracts* (M. Keller and M. Majchrowicz, eds.), pp. 97–98, Secretariat, 28th International Congress, Washington, DC].

Room, R., 1970*a*, Amount of drinking measured by two methods in a national U.S. sample, *Drinking Drug Practices Surveyor* **2:**8–10.

Room, R., 1970*b*, Asking about amount of drinking, *Drinking Drug Practices Surveyor* **1:**16.

Room, R., 1971*a*, Measures of heavy drinking: The difference it makes, *Drinking Drug Practices Surveyor* **3:**3–6.

Room, R., 1971*b*, Survey vs. sales data for the U.S., *Drinking Drug Practices Surveyor* **3:** 15–16.

Room, R., 1972, Drinking patterns in large U.S. cities: A comparison of San Francisco and national samples, *Q. J. Stud. Alcohol* Suppl. 6:28–57.

Room, R., 1976, Beverage type and drinking problems in a national sample of men, *Drinking Drug Practices Surveyor* **12:**29–30.

Room, R., 1977, Measurement and distribution of drinking patterns and problems in general populations, in: *Alcohol-Related Disabilities* (G. Edwards, M. Gross, M. Keller, J. Moser, and R. Room, eds.), pp. 61–87, Offset Publ. No. 32, World Health Organization, Geneva.

Room, R., 1980, New curves in the course: A comment on Polich, Armor and Braiker, "The Course of Alcoholism," *Br. J. Addiction* **75:**351–360.

Room, R., and Beck, K., 1974, Survey data on trends in U.S. consumption, *Drinking Drug Practices Surveyor* **9:**3–7.

Rouse, B. A., 1970, Comparison of two bases of estimating indices of alcohol consumption: Drinking reported in the past week and overall estimate of drinking in the past year, *Drinking Drug Practices Surveyor* **2:**6–7.

Rutledge, C. M., Carroll, G. B., and Perkins, R. A., 1974, *A Socio-epidemiological Study of Alcoholism in East Baton Rouge Parish,* School of Social Welfare, Louisiana State University, Baton Rouge, LA.

Sargent, M., 1970, Methods of measuring drinking: Are reported habitual drinking and recent occasion drinking comparable? with an exchange, *Drinking Drug Practices Surveyor* **2:**3–6.

Schinke, S. P., and Gilchrist, L. D., 1983, Survey and evaluation methods: Smoking prevention among children and adolescents, in: *Measurement in the Analysis and Treatment of Smoking Behavior* (J. Grabowski and C. S. Bell, eds.), pp. 96–104, NIDA Research Monograph No. 48, DHHS Publication No. (ADM) 83-1285, USGPO, Washington, DC.

Simpura, J., 1987, Comparison of indices of alcohol consumption in the Finnish 1984 drinking habits survey data, Presented at the annual meeting of the Alcohol Epidemiology Section, International Council on Alcohol and Addictions, Aix-en-Provence, June.

Skog, O-J., 1981, Distribution of self-reported alcohol consumption: Comments on Gregson and Stacey, *Psychol. Rep.* **49:**771–777.

Smart, R. G., and Adlaf, E. M., 1982, *Trends in Alcohol and Drug Use among Ontario Adults: Report of a Household Survey, 1982,* Substudy No. 1234, Addiction Research Foundation, Toronto.

Sobell, L. C., Cellucci, T., Nivenberg, T. D., and Sobell, M. B., 1982, Do Quantity–Frequency data underestimate drinking-related health risks? *Amer. J. Pub. Health* **72:**823–828.

Sobell, M. B., Maisto, S. A., Sobell, L. C., Cooper, A. M., Cooper, T. C., and Sanders, B., 1980, Developing a prototype for evaluating alcohol treatment effectiveness, in: *Evaluating Alcohol and Drug Abuse Treatment Effectiveness: Recent Advances* (L. C. Sobell, M. B. Sobell, and E. Ward, eds.), pp. 129–150, Pergamon Press, New York.

Solomon, S. D., and Harford, T. C., 1984, Drinking norms versus drinking behavior, *Alcoholism: Clin. Exp. Res.* **8:**460–466.

Straus, R., and Bacon, S. D., 1953, *Drinking in College,* Yale University Press, New Haven, CT.

Streissguth, A. P., Martin, D. C., and Buffington, V. E., 1977, Identifying heavy drinkers: A comparison of eight alcohol scores obtained on the same sample, in: *Currents in Alcoholism, Vol. 2* (F. A. Seixas, ed.), pp. 395–420, Grune & Stratton, New York.

Wallack, L., 1978, *An Assessment of Drinking Patterns, Problems, Knowledge and Attitudes in Three Northern California Communities,* Report C21, Alcohol Research Group, Berkeley, CA.

Wallack, L., and Barrows, D. C., 1981, *Preventing Alcohol Problems in California: Evaluation of the Three Year "Winners" Program,* Report C29, Alcohol Research Group, Berkeley, CA.

Wallack, L. M. and Barrows, D. C., 1982/1983, Evaluating primary prevention: The California "Winners" alcohol program, *Int. Q. Community Health Education* **3**:307–335.

Wechsler, H., Demone, H. W., and Gottleib, N., 1978, Drinking patterns of Greater Boston adults: Subgroup differences on the QFV Index, *J. Stud. Alcohol* **39**:1158–1165.

Williams, G. D., Aitken, S. S., and Malin, H., 1985, Reliability of self-reported alcohol consumption in a general population survey, *J. Stud. Alcohol* **46**:223–227.

Williams, J., 1967, Waxing and waning drinkers, Presented at the annual meeting of the Society for the Study of Social Problems, San Francisco, August.

Wilsnack, R. W., Wilsnack, S. C., and Klassen, A. D., 1984, Women's drinking and drinking problems: Patterns from a 1981 national survey, *Am. J. Public Health* **74**:1231–1238.

Wilsnack, S. C., Wilsnack, R. W., and Klassen, A. D., 1984/1985, Drinking and drinking problems among women in a U.S. national survey, *Alcohol Health Res. World* **9**(2):3–13.

4

# Alcohol and the Family

## An International Review of the Literature with Implications for Research and Practice

JIM ORFORD

## 1. INTRODUCTION

In 1982 the present author wrote for WHO a paper entitled, "The Prevention and Management of Alcohol Problems in the Family Setting: A Review of Work Carried out in English-Speaking Countries." This was subsequently published in *Alcohol and Alcoholism* in 1983 (Orford, 1983). The present chapter represents an update of that earlier paper with an extension to cover literature from other countries and literature written in languages other than English.

Work from Britain, the United States, Canada, and Australia has been excluded from this review unless (1) the work was published since the earlier review was being prepared *and* it added substantially to the earlier literature, *or* (2) it referred to the indigenous, or nonwhite, population in one of those countries, *or* (3) its inclusion in the review was necessary in order to make a point that could not be made easily in any other way.

Otherwise an attempt has been made to review comprehensively the literature on alcohol and the family from around the world. Although the review is based on a computer literature search of Psychological Abstracts, Sociological Abstracts, Social Science Research, Medline, Excerpta Medica, and Commonwealth Agricultural Bureaux, plus a personal search of a wide range of recent journals available at the University of Exeter, there is no doubt that some relevant literature has been missed. More serious is the possibility that a whole perspective on the subject is missing. The author is conscious of the fact that a variety of widely divergent perspectives on this subject can be adopted—the social and cultural view of Section 4 is very different from the family

JIM ORFORD • Department of Psychology, University of Exeter, Washington Singer Laboratories, Exeter EX4 4QG, and Department of Clinical and Community Psychology, Exeter Health Authority, Larkby, Exeter EX2 4NU, United Kingdom.

psychology and psychiatry perspective of most of Section 2, for example. An economist, historian, or political scientist might have written a review with a very different balance. No doubt a psychogeneticist would have tackled this task in yet a different way.

A number of non–English language papers were translated into English for the reviewer. These are indicated in the reference list. This review also draws on a helpful summary of Eastern European work prepared for WHO by Boyadjieva (undated). In the case of all other non–English language work, this review has had to rely on abstracts.

The organization of the review into four main subsections was dictated by the material available. The largest amount fell into the following two subsections: marriage in disorder and distress, and intergenerational effects. This reflects the predominance of Western models of research on the nuclear family, the recent expansion of interest in the intergenerational transmission of drinking problems, particularly in the United States, and the concern in Eastern European countries over the socialization of youth and the increasing rate of family breakdown. Section 4, on social and cultural studies, has a much more even worldwide coverage, with work from Africa particularly well represented. Nevertheless, the amount of material with an alcohol focus is relatively small. Once again, Section 5, on prevention and treatment in the family setting, is dominated by work from the West. In particular, this reviewer discovered next to no work on the prevention and treatment of alcohol problems in the family outside Europe or North America. The final section considers the implications for future intervention and research.

## 2. MARRIAGES IN DISORDER AND DISTRESS

This section examines the findings of research that has focused on marriages that are disordered or distressed as a result of, or in association with, excessive drinking. Most of this work is about the marriages of alcoholics or problem drinkers and is carried out within the Western tradition of family psychology, psychiatry, or social work. The section begins with those studies that most clearly view marriage partners as victims of the stress associated with excessive drinking in a family member. It considers the nature of this stress and focuses in particular on marital violence and on separation and divorce (child abuse and neglect, and stress on children, are considered separately, in Section 3). This section then considers what is known about how partners cope with excessive drinking. This leads to a consideration of those studies that have taken an interactional or systems, rather than stress victim, perspective on alcohol and the family.

### Marital Hardship

For many years, studies from the United States (e.g., Bailey et al., 1962; Jackson and Kogan, 1963; Lemert, 1962; Moos and Moos, undated) and Britain (e.g., Orford et al., 1976) have been reporting that women married to men with identified drinking problems often describe a great deal of severe and long-lasting hardship (including economic insecurity, social embarrassment, reduction of social contact, failure of the husband to meet role obligations, rows and quarrels, a poor sex life and infidelity, possessiveness and jealousy directed toward the wife, damage to household objects or furniture, and physical violence in the family).

Although there are many hints that such hardship for wives married to excessively drinking husbands is a regularly recurring feature of family life elsewhere in the world, very few studies have focused on it. One such study, carried out by an American researcher, has focused on the experiences of wives in Finland (Wiseman, 1976*a,b*). She describes the many problems such women experience, including their husbands' recurring mood swings, physical aggression, and problems with money, sex life, and health. She comments that few wives in this situation in Finland obtained divorces, and while some succeeded in building separate lives focused on career and new friends, others experienced increasing isolation and despair.

From a group far removed from Europe or white North America, both culturally and geographically, namely an aboriginal community in rural New South Wales in Australia, comes a report which suggests that many of the problems described in European and North American literature are universal (Kamien, 1976). Kamien reports that the husband's drinking was regarded as the major family problem for the female head of 19% of the aboriginal households and was a moderate problem for another 28%. Alcohol-related family problems included loss of work, depletion of the family income, violence that resulted in a woman fearing for her own and her children's safety, and difficulties with the law. Kamien provides short statements from six wives, with whom wives in New York, London, or Helsinki would have little difficulty in identifying.

Although the proportion of those seeking help for drinking problems who are women has been reported to be as high as one in three in some reports from Britain and the United States, there has been a regrettable lack of research on husbands married to women excessive drinkers. Two studies from other countries, however, suggest that they could experience as much hardship as women married to men with drinking problems.

The first, a Bulgarian study, involved following up women with the ''alcohol dependence syndrome'' who had been admitted for treatment during the period 1980–1984 (Guerdjikova, 1984). Boyadjieva (undated) summarizes the findings as follows: In two-thirds of families the relations between the couples were either conflictual or formal, in some cases this being due to drinking behavior, in other cases leading to it; 31% of the women had divorced, 8% were abandoned by their husbands, and 13% were living legally with another man; the effects on the children were extremely unfavorable. The second report, from West Germany, compared the recent impact on their husbands of the problems of 20 alcoholic and 20 depressive women being treated in four psychiatric clinics in Baden–Wurttemberg (Lutz et al., 1980). When asked in detail about the 3 or 4 weeks before their wives' hospitalization, no differences between the two groups were found in the husbands' reports of their wives' efficiency and behavior toward other members of the family, nor in their reports of the effects on the husbands, the children, or others (the authors note, however, the near-zero correlations between husbands' and wives' accounts of these supposedly ''objective'' facts). Differences did emerge, however, in terms of the husbands' feelings of resignation (husbands of depressed women were more resigned, although this difference tended to disappear when this group's greater age and length of marriage were taken into account) and of subjective distress and blame. Husbands of alcoholic women were more distressed, particularly over effects on the marriage relationship (*Partnerschaftsverhalten*) and were more blaming of their wives for causing symptoms of disturbance in the husbands.

The only research known to the present author which has directly compared families containing husbands with drinking problems with those containing wives was a Swedish study which involved following up, for 6–12 years, patients treated in the 1960s (Dahlgren, 1979). As in the mainly North American studies reviewed by Jacob and Seilhamer (1982), this study also found that a high percentage (50%) of husbands of women problem drinkers had drinking problems themselves. Sixty percent of the marriages of women problem drinkers were described as "serious conflicts, divorce discussed," in comparison with 35% of the marriages of male problem drinkers. Thirty-nine percent of partners in the former group were described as "understanding" vs. 65% in the latter, and the percentages of partners who were "strongly disapproving" were 55% and 28%, respectively. Although the marriages of the women problem drinkers emerged as less satisfactory, with husbands less sympathetic than wives of male problem drinkers, percentages of marriages surviving intact at follow-up (32% and 35%, respectively) were similar.

Before considering the issue of marital violence in greater detail, it is worth reiterating two points made by the present author elsewhere (Orford et al., 1976; Orford, 1975). The first is that detailed research reported in the English language literature showed clearly that hardship of the kind considered here is of variable quantity. It is probably important not to make sweeping generalizations about alcohol-troubled marriages. Levels of marital disorder and distress vary greatly, even within samples of marriages recruited via treatment agencies (Orford et al., 1976). The impact of excessive drinking on the rest of the family is likely to depend on a number of variables, including the amount of drinking, its regularity, and the extent to which excessive drinking takes place at home rather than outside it (Jacob, 1988). The second point is that the kinds of hardship described by those who have studied families containing a member who is drinking excessively are unlikely to be unique to such families, but almost certainly occur also in families that are disordered and distressed for other reasons. There are dangers in viewing the subject of alcohol problems in the family as a specialism divorced from the study of marital problems generally.

## Alcohol and Marital Violence

The possible connection between excessive drinking and marital violence has attracted special research attention in Britain and North America over a number of years (e.g., Gayford, 1975; Byles, 1978; van Hasselt et al., 1985). Research supporting the existence of such a relationship is reported by van Hasselt et al. (1985), who found significantly higher Michigan Alcoholism Screening Test (MAST) scores for physically abusive husbands than for husbands from either maritally discordant but nonabusive or maritally concordant couples (this was confirmed by asking wives to complete the MAST independently but referring to the husbands' drinking).

Preliminary data from a recent interview study of young British adults in their late teens, twenties, or early thirties, who had had a parent with a drinking problem, show much higher rates of recalled family violence than was the case for a comparison group (Velleman, 1987). This was particularly the case for recalled parent-to-parent violence.

Again, however, the results of this study show that it is dangerous to generalize about families complicated by alcohol problems: By no means all subjects from such families reported violence between their parents (67% vs. 21% of the comparison group), and only a minority recalled violence that was serious (using an implement or object or leaving bruising or injury—29% vs. 7%), regular (at least once a month—27% vs. 5%), or maintained over a prolonged period during childhood (at least 3 years—48.5% vs. 6%).

Although, once again, there appear to be very few reports from elsewhere in the world that focus on alcohol and marital violence, there is every reason to think, from the few reports that do exist, that the existence of a connection between excessive alcohol use and marital violence would be widely endorsed. From Czechoslovakia, for example, Student and Matova (1969) reported that 30 of 40 wives of hospitalized alcoholics were maltreated by their husbands, and in 13 cases the husband's behavior was described as "rough." Kamien's (1975) account of excessive drinking among Australian aborigines and its impact on family life mentions violence repeatedly, and it is clear that both the author and most of the women who described their husbands' drinking were of the view that there was a causal link between drinking and marital violence. For example:

> A woman aged 22 years, said . . . "Usually he is okay when he's drunk. . . . Sometimes he picks and picks. Once he hit me and my four-year old son still hasn't got over it." A woman aged 57 years, said . . . "Whenever he gets drunk he picks up a lump of wood and starts to hit me. . . . The other day he kept hitting me so I picked up the carving knife and warned him I'd put it through him. . . ."

By no means everyone is agreed, however, that the connection between the two is so straightforward. For example, although Dobash and Dobash, in their detailed study of wife beating in Scotland, found that nearly 26% of the men who had assulted their wives were considered by the police to be drunk at the time of the attack, their general view is that drinking is largely used as an excuse:

> Although it may be comforting for all concerned to blame the problem on drinking and be done with it, this is simply not the case. Alcohol does provide the husband with a convenient excuse for his behaviour, or denial of it, and it may be comforting for the woman to see the problem as caused by some extraneous factor beyond the relationship or outside of the husband's usual self. In all of these ways it plays a complex role in wife beating, but it would be erroneous to accept the simplistic argument that the behaviour of men who beat their wives is dictated by drink. (Dobash and Dobash, undated, p. 27)

It is possible, however, that they underestimated the role of excessive drinking by asking women, not whether their husbands drank excessively, but rather whether the husband's drinking *per se* was a source of conflict leading to a particular assault (this was the case in 6% for typical assaults, and in 2% for the most recent assaults). There are also hints from their case descriptions that some husbands may have had serious drinking problems of which the interviewers were unaware (Dobash et al., 1977–1978).

The complexities of this matter are shown by another study, from the United States, in which battered women were asked to describe four violent incidents. Sixteen percent reported excessive drinking by their husbands during each of the four incidents. On the other hand, only 19% thought their husbands had not been drinking during any of the four, the majority showing an inconsistent pattern of alcohol use or excess across the four occasions (Eberle, 1982).

Like the Dobashes, Room (undated) has argued that alcohol is used by husbands as a "tactic of domination," within the family. Particularly where the traditional legitimacy of male domination has been undermined, Room suggests, alcohol serves to legitimize dominance and violence. Indeed, ". . . the mere threat to go drinking acquires the power that a raised stick would have: a drunken beating can be used to terrorize the subordinate party long afterwards, without any threat of violence needing to be uttered" (Room, undated, p. 5).

In closing this section on marital violence, it should be noted that the literature on the connection between alcohol and violence in general has been divided on the question of whether alcohol acts directly to disinhibit violent behavior, or whether it acts indirectly via expectations and other mechanisms of the kind to which the Dobashes and Room are referring.

Anthropological work reviewed by MacAndrew and Edgerton (1970) and experimental work using a "balanced placebo" design which separates the direct effects of alcohol and expectation (Kreutzer et al., 1984) have both suggested that expectation plays a large part. Recent evidence suggests that alcohol may play a genuinely disinhibiting role but only under conditions of personal threat (Taylor et al., 1976), a finding which is consistent with Room's hypothesis.

## Partners as a High-Risk Group

For many years research from the United States and Britain has been confirming that wives living with men with drinking problems are at risk of experiencing distress and disturbance themselves. In addition to the kinds of hardship already described, there is the uncertainty that many family members describe about knowing whether there really is a problem in the family or not, deciding whether it is a problem of their own making or of someone else's, deciding exactly what the problem is, and then deciding what is the best way to respond. These uncertainties were described in the classic research report by Joan Jackson (1954) more than 30 years ago.

Although, again, there has been less work of this kind on husbands of women with drinking problems, in the case of wives of men with drinking problems there is evidence that they experience relatively high levels of anxiety and of psychological and psychosomatic symptoms (Bailey, 1967; Orford, 1976). In support of the stress victim view of excessive drinking and marriage, there is the finding that such symptoms occur more frequently when a woman is living with an actively drinking problem drinker and that they decrease when the drinker stops drinking excessively or when the woman leaves her husband (Bailey, 1967). On the other hand, a more recent study found that the partners' symptomatology correlated significantly with the degree of harm *ever* caused by drinking, not with recent level of consumption or with whether the problem drinker was currently "wet" or "dry" (Steinglass, 1981).

The only study from the non–English-speaking world addressing this issue that is known to the present author is the study from Czechoslovakia already referred to (Student and Matova, 1969). Of the 40 wives in that study, 35 complained of mental disturbance developed during marriage. The main symptoms were: anxiety (26 wives), insomnia (24), tearfulness (21), increased tension (20), irritability (18), grief (18), headaches (17), disinterest in sex (16), tiredness (14), thoughts of suicide (13), weight loss (12), and loss of appetite (eight). Psychosomatic diseases were also present: eight wives suffered from chronic gynaecological conditions, seven from hypertension, and there were many cases of allergy. Again, consistent with the stress victim view is the finding that the intensity of the wives' disturbance was proportional to the degree of the husbands' "behavior defects" in family and sexual life. However, there are also hints of greater complexity: 65% of the Czechoslovakian wives are described by the authors as immature, dependent, and suffering inferiority complexes originating in their own family conditions, and 12 were divorced and seven pregnant before marriage, factors said to have contributed to their choice of husband and their ambivalent attitudes.

## Marital Separation and Divorce

In the North American literature, a link between excessive drinking and separation or divorce has long been accepted (e.g., Straus and Bacon, 1951; Kephart, 1954). Two more recent studies from the United States confirm the high frequency with which marital dissolution is attributed to excessive drinking. In one of these studies (Burns, 1984) the partner's drinking was mentioned as a cause of marital dissolution by 36% of divorced or separated women and 17% of men. This factor ranked sixth of 16 factors examined. It was one of the most strongly related to estimated time of breakdown in the marriage (more commonly mentioned by those nominating the first year of marriage as the time of onset of breakdown), and along with partner's cruelty, it was one of only two factors correlated with socioeconomic status (drinking much more frequently being a complaint in lower socioeconomic status groups). In the second of these studies, alcohol was cited as a major factor precipitating marital abuse by 67.5% of wives who decided to leave an abusive relationship (Strube and Barbour, 1984).

Many observers of families with alcohol problems have expressed surprise that so many marriage survive at all. Survival is less surprising, however, if one considers the heterogeneity of marriages complicated by excessive drinking, to which reference has already been made, as well as the many obvious barriers against marital dissolution. For example, in the study of abusive relationships just cited, drinking was almost as likely to be cited as a major factor precipitating abuse by those wives who decided to stay with their husbands (60%), but they were less likely to be employed, had on average been married longer, experienced greater economic hardship, and expressed greater affection for their husbands than did those wives who decided to leave (Strube and Barbour, 1984). Over 20 years ago, Levinger (1965) considered the factors that were likely to tip the balance in the direction of a decision to remain and included obligations to children, moral restraints, external pressure from relatives or the local community, legal difficulties, a wife's lack of independent income, and absence of anyone to take the partner's place.

Research linking excessive drinking and marital breakdown has also appeared in Eastern Europe, Switzerland, and Japan. From Switzerland, there is an investigation of 1350 married couples who were seeking divorce in the early 1960s (Hedri, 1971). Mentioned as a source of marital conflict by 20%, alcoholism ranked third of the first five factors to which conflict was attributed (the others being character clashes 49%; infidelity 35%; financial difficulties 18%; and sexual problems 16.5%). From Japan, there is the report that excessive drinking was involved in 37 of 47 cases of divorce conciliation at a Japanese family court: 34 husbands were diagnosed as alcoholic (Hayashi, 1978).

A number of recent reports display the concern that is felt about family breakdown in Eastern Europe and about the role that excessive drinking may play. In 1982, Sysenko explained the concern about the growing divorce rate in terms of its effect on family, cultural, and national life in the U.S.S.R.

> The negative social consequences of divorce are multifarious. Such a split creates disharmony amongst the population, a decline in the standard of upbringing of children, an increase in the incidence of nervous, psychological illnesses and alcoholism. The process of divorce destroys an extremely important type of social interaction—it severs bloodties which are vitally important in the life of each individual insofar as they greatly promote the continuity of cultural and spiritual traditions, the development of altruism, humanism and strengthening of basic collective principles. (Sysenko, 1982, p. 99, translated from Russian)

Sysenko analyzed the motives for divorce among 500 petitioners in Moscow in 1978. At 63% the husband's heavy drinking and alcoholism were mentioned by the highest percentage of women petitioners ($N = 345$), whereas the wife's heavy drinking was reported by only 4.5% of men petitioners ($N = 155$), far behind such factors as "personality clash" (24.5%). Sysenko found a major difference depending on the couple's social position: Heavy drinking and alcoholism was given as the basic cause of divorce by 59.5% of working class couples, but only 17.5% of professional class couples. Sysenko was conscious of the fact that there might be deeper, and unexpressed, reasons for divorce that required further study. Social changes, including the greater involvement of women in the workforce, might give rise to important changes in the function of the family and hence to a whole range of conflicts within marriage, he argued.

Sysenko noted that the divorce rate was considerably higher in the western part of the U.S.S.R., including the Baltic republic, than in other regions, and another paper, by Tiit (1982), is concerned with marital dissolution in the Estonian S.S.R. In this study, the interesting technique was used of comparing the aspects of marriage valued by 575 newly married couples recruited from seven registry offices in 1972, with the reasons for divorce given by 950 individuals (62% women, 38% men, including 150 couples) divorcing in the same districts in 1975. The rank order correlations between the frequencies of mentioning values (the newlyweds) and reasons for divorce (the divorcees) were positive and highly significant both for men (0.82) and for women (0.62); such values and reasons as "love," "mutual respect," and "faithfulness" ranked high both as marital values by those getting married and as reasons for divorce among those separating, while "common ideological and political views," "relations with the parents-in-law," and "financial security" ranked low on both occasions. Of particular interest for present purposes was the fact that "sobriety" showed one of the greatest shifts toward a high-rank position for divorcees compared with newlyweds. This was particularly the case for women: Newlyweds ranked "sobriety" only thirteenth out of 18 marital values, but divorcing women ranked its absence first as a reason for divorce. Indeed, in about half the applications completed by women, the husband's "addiction to drink" was either the primary or secondary motive for seeking a divorce. However, the complexity of the matter is recognized by Tiit, who comments:

> It should be stressed that according to our data women are very sensitive to their husband's habit of drinking: 68% of the women divorcees claimed that they were disturbed by their husband's drinking (although, as the same women admitted, part [sic] of the husbands were rather moderate drinkers). (Tiit, 1982, pp. 69–70)

Sysenko (1982) cited four other studies of reasons for divorce in Latvia, Lithuania, Kiev, and Grodnen, each of which suggests that three factors—husband's heavy drinking, unfaithfulness, and personality clash—led wives to petition for divorce in 60% or more of cases. In his review, Boyadjieva (undated) cites five further studies on this topic from the U.S.S.R., including one from the Ryazan region where divorce was attributed to the partner's drinking by 10% of divorcing men and 19% of divorcing women. Guerdjikova's study (1984), mentioned by Boyadjieva, also shows a high rate of divorce associated with alcoholism in wives in Bulgaria. Even within this literature, which mostly assumes that excessive drinking is the cause of marital breakdown, there is the occasional recognition that causal relationships may not be so straightforward. For example, Boyadjieva cites the opinions of Brennenstuhl and Wielguszewski (1980) from Poland, who wrote, on the basis of their therapeutic practice, that they considered interpersonal conflicts lead to excessive drinking, rather than the other way around. As part of the evidence, they cited a Polish study suggesting that a large number of divorces could be attributed to the compulsory treatment for alcoholism imposed on a husband, usually by his wife.

## Coping with Excessive Drinking in Marriage

One research direction that has developed in Britain and the United States concerns the tactics and strategies that family members use to try to cope with excessive drinking in their families. Using a Coping Questionnaire developed for the purpose by Guthrie and the present author (Orford and Guthrie, 1976; Orford et al., 1975), we found that wives of husbands in contact with a psychiatric treatment agency had used a number of coping strategies, including the following: pleading, threatening, and arguing; avoiding, keeping out of the way; withdrawing sexually; being indulgent (giving a drink to help with the hangover, going without to give the drinker money, etc.); controlling access to drink (pouring it away, making a rule not to allow it in the house, etc.); attacking or competing; taking greater control or responsibility (e.g., over money matters or child care); seeking outside help; and taking steps toward separation.

In her study of "home treatment," Wiseman (1980) focused on wives' earlier attempts to get their husbands (who by the time of the study had all undergone professional treatment) to stop or cut down their drinking. She suggested that attempts at coping escalate from logical reasoning, to nagging, to emotional pleading with threats to leave. When early, direct approaches of this kind fail, various indirect tactics are used, she claimed, including acting "normal" or "natural" in order to reduce stress and the likelihood of drinking, taking over the drinker's responsibilities, selecting "safe," nondrinking companions or visitors, manipulating the availability of money, controlling the alcohol supply, keeping the drinker busy, drinking with him, and, finally, beginning to feel that there is nothing she can do about the drinking. It is important to realize that Wiseman's sample was confined to women whose early attempts at "home treatment" had failed.

The Coping Questionnaire, referred to earlier, has also been used in research in the United States (James and Goldman, 1971; Schaffer and Tyler, 1979), India, and Japan. A study of the reported coping behavior of 46 wives of men receiving treatment for alcohol problems in Madras found that discord, fearful withdrawal, and avoidance were commonly used coping styles, as in Britain and the United States (Ranganathan and Chakravarthy, undated). On the other hand, competition (the wife drinking herself, pretending to be drunk, etc.), withdrawal within the marriage, and marital breakdown were less common than in previous research from the West. Ranganathan and Chakravarthy suggest that these differences are cultural and reflect such factors as censure on women's drinking and different women's roles in India than in the West.

In Japan, Hayashi (1978) used the Coping Questionnaire in the study of divorce conciliation, to which reference has already been made. Attack (discord) was the most frequently used coping style reported by wives in this study, with withdrawal, acting-out, protection, and safeguarding family interests being categories successively less used (in that order). Research is also being conducted in West Germany using the Coping Questionnaire (E. Stumm, personal communication, 1985).

In an edited volume about the drinking experiences of different cultural groups in the United States (Bennett and Ames, 1985), a number of contrasting examples are provided of how families cope with excessive drinking. For example, it is suggested that in rural Appalachia, intense family loyalty combined with a characteristic avoidance of direct confrontation leads to excessive drinking often being ignored or accepted except at times of crisis (Edwards, 1985). By contrast, Mexican–American wives in Southern California often maintain control over their husbands' drinking by not allowing their husbands to bring alcohol or their drinking friends into the home (Gilbert, 1985).

Before moving on, it must be pointed out that the coping approach to excessive drinking in the family illustrates, once again, the folly of treating alcohol and the family as a specialism (Orford, 1975). Coping with excessive drinking in the family may have much in common with coping with other problems or troubles, such as schizophrenia, depression, agoraphobia, dementia, and chronic illnesses and handicaps in partners or children (Orford, 1987). Of interest here, because of the association between excessive drinking and marital violence discussed earlier, is work on the coping responses of abused wives (Pfouts, 1978). Of particular relevance, also, are general typologies of coping behavior, including appraisal-focused vs. problem-focused vs. emotion-focused (Billings and Moos, undated; Folkman and Lazarus, 1980); or negotiation vs. optimistic comparisons vs. selective ignoring vs. resignation (Menaghan, 1982).

## Interactional and Systems Perspectives

The stress victim perspective on alcohol and the family assigns clear roles to different family members: one is the excessive drinker or "alcoholic" and the rest of the family are the victims of the stress this causes and they are themselves at risk of suffering ill effects as a result. There are a number of research findings in the English-language literature which are troublesome to such a view, however: As already mentioned, drinking is often heavy or excessive in a second member of the family, particularly when the wife is the identified "problem drinker"; role performance is sometimes reported to be nonideal even in the early months of marriage, and many partners appear to have married in the knowledge that their spouses were already heavy or excessive drinkers (Lemert, 1962; Orford et al., 1976); positive changes in drinking with treatment may positively affect the quality of marriage in certain ways, but may not have such an effect on marital roles (Orford et al., 1977); and wives' levels of stress and their current symptoms, although affected by their husbands' drinking, are not independent of their reports of abnormalities in their own families of upbringing (Kogan and Jackson, 1965).

Quite apart from the complex origin of family distress and disorder is the recognition by writers adopting the coping approach (Orford et al., 1975; Wiseman, 1980), as well as in the writings of Al-Anon (Harwin, 1982), that the reactions of family members may further compound problems which may initially have been attributable to excessive drinking. From outside the alcohol literature, Menaghan's conclusions about coping with marital problems strongly support a transactional model:

> . . . the strong link between level of problems and choice of coping efforts apparent in this analysis suggests a worsening spiral of marital role problems over time: as problems mount, typical coping choices may actually exacerbate distress. . . . Over time, initially higher problems, less effective coping strategies, and higher distress all increased later levels of marital problems. (Menaghan, 1982, p. 231)

A systems view of families with alcohol problems is described in a number of English-language reviews (Steinglass, 1976, 1982; Paolino and McCrady, 1977; Stanton, 1979; Kaufman, 1980). From this perspective, the use of alcohol in the family is purposive, adaptive, and meaningful. According to Steinglass (1982), writing from the United States, drinking behavior in the family system may serve two possible functions: (1) It may appear as a sign or signal of stress within the system and may be functional as a tension releaser or a way of recruiting help for the family, or (2) drinking behavior may function as an integral part of the system, maintaining, in homeostatic fashion, rigidly established repetitive patterns of behavior involving closeness or distance, dominance or submission.

The systems view of alcohol problems in the family has also been espoused by writers in Europe, for example, in West Germany (Hemmer, 1979) and Yugoslavia. Gacic (1978) and others, such as Lazic (1977) in Yugoslavia, have been particularly concerned to draw on general systems theory to understand conflicts and communication patterns within families where excessive drinking is a problem. Hemmer (1979), from West Germany, writes that the communication approach may be more suitable as a framework for the treatment of the earlier phases of alcoholism, but inadequate for the advanced stages. This is an interesting conclusion, particularly as it appears to be opposite to that reached by Kaufman and Pattison (1981), from the United States, who concluded from their review that the focus on family dynamics was necessary in the treatment of more disturbed families, whereas a more educational, relatively drink-focused, approach might be in order with "functional family systems" where affection remains relatively high.

An explicit interactional, transactional, or systems view of alcohol and the family appears to be confined to the United States, Canada, Yugoslavia, and a few other European countries, such as West Germany and Britain (Bennun, 1985). The perspective that has been termed here the "stress victim" view is dominant elsewhere, including most of Eastern Europe. Hints of the greater complexity of the matter than is implied by the stress victim view emerge in the research and writing of a number of Eastern

Europeans, however. Brennenstuhl and Wielguszewski (1980), from Poland, considered that excessive drinking was generally *consequent upon* interpersonal conflict rather than the other way round. Tiit's (1982) suggestion that wives in Estonia might be oversensitive to the issue of their husbands' drinking and Student and Matova's (1969) conclusion that some of their Czechoslovakian wives were ambivalent about their husbands' drinking partly as a result of their own personal histories are other examples. A further hint that different ways of understanding the role of excessive drinking in the family may be more or less acceptable to different members of families themselves comes from the Swedish follow-up study referred to earlier (Dahlgren, 1979). While only 20% of married male problem drinkers thought their problems were partly due to their partners (none thought they were wholly so), no less than 80% of married women problem drinkers felt this way (16% thought their alcohol problem wholly due to their partners).

Certainly controlled research of a psychological kind, which bears on interactional or systems views of alcohol in the family, has been confined almost exclusively to the United States. Steinglass has employed the unique research strategy of simultaneously admitting family members to an experimental residential treatment facility in which periods of drinking and abstinence are alternated and the effects on family interactions observed. Observations revealed dramatic, and often surprising, changes in patterns of interactional behavior during intoxication in comparison with those seen during sobriety. For example, ". . . a father and son who had been distant and highly critical of each other while sober expressed warmth, tenderness and closeness while drinking," and "a couple who described their alcohol symptoms as increasing their ability to relate to strangers were noted to become more distant and appear to wall themselves off from other couples once drinking began" (Steinglass, 1982, pp. 135, 139). These observations support the view that excessive drinking may serve some positive functions within the family, despite the seemingly harmful effects.

Other studies, confined to the United States so far, have observed couples interacting, but in a less naturalistic setting than the simulated home environment of the experimental ward used by Steinglass. In a pilot study carried out by Jacob and his colleagues, for example, eight families with a drinking problem (the husband–fathers being the identified problem drinkers in each case) and eight comparison families were recruited through newspaper advertisements (Jacob et al., 1981). Each family consisted of both parents and at least two children between 10 and 17 years old. The parents were observed interacting alone, and each parent was observed interacting with the two children together. The results are complicated but suggest that problem drinking fathers showed less leadership/assertiveness/problem-solving behavior than did control fathers, but that their wives exhibited relatively more of such directive influence than did control mothers.

Another study of this kind included a group with family problems other than excessive drinking, as well as a "nondistressed couples" control group. A number of differences were found in interactional behavior (only husbands and wives were involved in this study, again the husbands being the identified problem drinkers), but there were no differences between the couples with drinking problems and the nonalcoholic distressed couples, thus supporting the nonspecific hypothesis. The authors of this report summarize their findings by saying:

> Both alcoholic and distressed couples communicated significantly fewer rational problem-solving statements and engaged in more negative and hostile acts than did non-alcoholic, maritally satisfied couples. . . . These results suggest that at least some of the problematic marital communications noted in the literature on alcoholics are observed among distressed couples in general and may not reflect problems unique to alcoholics. (Billings et al., 1979, p. 193)

Later work by Jacob and his colleagues (1988) has included couples in which the husband has a psychological problem other than excessive drinking (depression), and in addition, it has recognized the heterogeneity of families complicated by excessive drinking. In particular, it has focused on two variables: whether drinking is steady or in binges, and whether it is predominantly at home or out of home. Very different findings have emerged in this research for two groups: binge-out-of-home (BO) and steady-in-home drinkers (SI). Within couples containing BO drinkers interaction was more negative than for other couples containing an excessively drinking husband and more negative than interaction within control couples. Interaction was also more negative and less task-focused and instrumental in drinking than in nondrinking conditions in the BO group. In the SI group, on the other hand, interaction was no more negative than for control couples, and it became significantly more *positive* in the drinking sessions.

Furthermore, the SI group showed a strong, *positive* correlation between amount of alcohol consumed in daily life over a 90-day period and marital satisfaction ratings of wives, and detailed sequential analysis for a small number of such couples showed that drinking by the husband was followed, if anything, by an *increase* in the wives' reported marital satisfaction. For binge drinkers, and for the BO group in particular, results were reversed: The correlations between alcohol consumption and marital satisfaction were not significant, but detailed sequential analysis suggested that husbands' drinking days were usually followed, a few days later, by decreases in wives' marital satisfaction. These results are quite preliminary, and further analysis is proceeding, but they support the view that families of alcoholics should not be treated as a homogeneous group, and that for some couples (particularly those with SI drinking husbands in Jacob's research) drinking may serve adaptive, functional purposes for the family in line with a systems view.

## Integrating the Stress Victim and Interactional Viewpoints

It is apparent, then, that work on families with drinking problems, often receiving treatment for those problems, has largely been carried out in the West. The stress victim view continues to be the dominant model, particularly, as in Eastern Europe, where there is concern over the causes of family breakdown. A family systems model is a serious contender, but there is scarcely any literature written from this perspective outside the United States and Yugoslavia. Controlled research on the interactional dynamics within families complicated by excessive drinking is almost entirely confined to the United States.

Certainly research does not enable us to choose between these two major viewpoints, which have led to different types of research and which appear to have different strengths and possible weaknesses. Systems thinking alone carries the danger of losing sight of the fact that families often experience stress and feel themselves to be victims of the excessive drinking with which they must learn to cope in the best possible way (although some schools of systems-oriented family therapy are more oriented than others toward the resolution of presenting problems). Stress victim thinking alone runs the risk of ignoring the interactional nature of family life and the possible family functions that continued excessive drinking may be serving.

The two models may be reconciled by giving relatively greater weight to one view or the other in different cases (e.g., Steinglass, 1976; Hemmer, 1979; Kaufman and Pattison, 1981). An alternative is to attempt a reconciliation in the form of a single theory. Wilson, in Britain, for example, has proposed a form of transactional model in which all family members (including the identified problem drinker) are seen as attempting to cope with the stress to which they are exposed, with all such reactions having repercussions for the rest of the family (Wilson, 1983). Such a view acknowledges both the importance of the drinking problem and the interdependence of parts within the whole family system.

Finney and Moos and their colleagues, in the United States, have also outlined a conceptual framework that reconciles the "widely discrepant" viewpoints on alcohol and the family (Finney et al., 1983). Their model takes into account not only drinking, but also other characteristics of both partners (such as anxiety, depression, and occupational functioning), incorporates other sources of environmental stress, and acknowledges that the partner's coping style mediates the effects of stressors and itself influences the family's functioning. Although these combined models of alcohol problems and the family originate in Western concerns and research styles, they may have greater application to an understanding of such problems elsewhere in the world than do either systems or stress victim models alone.

## Summary

The hardship of wives married to excessive drinkers has been recognized around the world, and the link between alcohol abuse and marital violence is well established, as is the status of wives as a group at high risk for psychological disturbance. However, none of these aspects of alcohol and the family has been much studied in detail outside North America and the United Kingdom. Even in those countries, hardship experienced by wives has been found to be variable in severity and is mostly not of a kind that is unique to marriages with drinking problems. Furthermore, there is controversy about the mechanism linking alcohol abuse and marital violence, and husbands of women who drink excessively have rarely been studied.

The link between excessive drinking and marital separation and divorce is also well established and in this case has been studied in a number of countries, including Switzerland and Japan and especially countries within Eastern Europe. One focus of study in India, Japan, and the United Kingdom, and across cultural groups within the United States, has been the ways in which partners cope with having a problem drinking spouse.

Work on problem drinking and marriage has generally taken a stress victim approach toward wives and other relatives of problem drinkers and has assumed a causal link from excessive drinking to such outcomes as marital violence and marital separation and divorce. Interactional and systems models of excessive alcohol use and the family have largely been confined to the industrialised English-speaking world and to Yugoslavia.

## 3. INTERGENERATIONAL EFFECTS

### Child Abuse and Neglect

Whereas in Britain and the United States there has been a far greater amount of research on excessive drinking and *marriage* than on children as the victims of the stress caused by parental drinking, this imbalance is less apparent elsewhere. The focus of some research and comment has been on the *physical* abuse of children. In 1978, for example, Straus noted that three French studies had estimated the rates of alcoholism in families responsible for child abuse at 30%, 50%, and 90% respectively. The same author also noted that excessive drinking appeared to play a smaller role in child abuse in Anglo–Saxon countries. A more recent French study (Bornstein et al., 1980) examined the psychiatric court evaluations of 31 child abusers: In only 20% was abuse thought to be a symptom of psychosis or neurosis, but 35% of abusers were judged to be "socially malajusted (alcoholism)."

A review of child abuse in West Germany (Gostomzyk, 1977) concluded that only a small percentage of abusers were psychopaths, and that in the majority of cases the child was abused when the offender was under a great deal of stress. Family crisis, alcoholism, social problems, unemployment, professional overwork, and social isolation were cited as examples of the kinds of stress that could give rise to abuse.

A South African study (Stricklin and Austad, 1982) investigated the reasons for removal of 52 2- to 16-year-old white children from their parental homes to a temporary reception center. Of the professionals involved in these cases, 59% attributed removal of the children to alcoholism, at least in part. The focus of this report was on the differences between the attributions of the professionals and of the parents. The latter tended to deny responsibility, and only 36% of fathers and 7% of mothers attributed removal to alcoholism. The same was true of 15% of the children interviewed. Forty-one percent of cases of alcoholism reported by professionals were among mothers, but no mothers attributed removal of their children to their own excessive drinking. In Edinburgh, Scotland, too, a survey of open social work cases has shown that families where a parent was thought to have a drinking problem were more likely to contain a child thought to be at risk of physical abuse (Lothian Regional Social Work Department, 1981).

Preliminary results from the writer's own study of young adult (16–35 years) offspring of problem drinking parents (Velleman and Orford, 1984) showed higher rates of reported parent-to-child violence during upbringing than for a comparison sample. However, the difference was less extreme than was the case for reported parent-to-parent violence (serious parent-to-child violence, 20% for offspring vs. 10% for comparisons; regular violence, 21% vs. 6%; violence over a prolonged period, 30% vs. 15%). An investigation of delinquents in the United States (Tarter et al., 1984*b*) found that those who had been physically abused as children (bodily assault on at least one occasion, unrelated to disciplinary action) were significantly more likely to have had an alcoholic father (55% vs. 16% of nonabused delinquents) and also to have had an alcoholic mother (18.5% vs. 3%).

Three articles from Czechoslovakia in the late 1960s and 1970s reported a link between parental excessive drinking and incest. In the first of these (Nedoma et al., 1969), chronic alcoholics were reported to form one of two major groups among 20 incest offenders, the victims of whose sexual abuse were mostly daughters. In the second report (Topiar and Satkova, 1974), alcohol intoxication, conflict between marital partners, aging and rejecting or threatening wives, and general disintegration of the family were given as the most frequent conditions responsible for 21 cases of incest between 14 fathers and their 4 to 16-year-old daughters. In the third report (Mokran and Kramer, 1976), most of the male perpetrators among 14 cases of confirmed incest, typically involving fathers and daughters, were described as ''aggressive, dominant and alcoholic.''

In the United States, although there is the occasional report linking excessive parental drinking and child abuse, such as that by Behling (1979) in which a history of alcoholism or alcohol misuse was found in at least one parent in 35 of 51 cases of child abuse at a mental hospital in California, direct evidence is sparse. In fact, Orme and Rimmer (1981) concluded that there was no satisfactory empirical data to support the existence of such a link. There is, however, much stronger evidence to support an association between parental excessive drinking and child *neglect*. One review from the United States defined child neglect as

> a condition in which someone responsible for the child either deliberately or by extraordinary inattentiveness permits the child to experience avoidable present suffering and/or fails to provide one or more of the ingredients generally deemed essential for developing a person's physical, intellectual and emotional capacities. (Polansky et al., 1975)

The same review estimated that child neglect was three times as prevalent as physical child abuse, and that ''the drug addict mother'' and ''alcoholism in one or both parents'' were foremost among high-risk situations giving rise to child neglect.

Studies of children as victims of parental excessive drinking in the United States, Britain, and Canada (e.g., Cork, 1969; Wilson and Orford, 1978; Wolin et al., 1979), including Cork's Canadian classic *The Forgotten Children* (Cork, 1969), have also highlighted the general neglect, rather than specific physical violence, that can occur. Chronic exposure to a poor family atmosphere, with much parental marital tension and discord, and disruption of joint family activities and rituals are among the kinds of stresses to which such children are particularly prone. Indeed, 98 of Cork's 115 children reported ''parental fighting and quarrelling'' as their main concern, in comparison with only seven who gave ''drinking'' or ''drunkenness'' as their main worry. In our own study young adults who had had parents with drinking problems frequently recalled such things as, ''arrangements going wrong,'' ''lack of social life for the family,'' ''being forced to participate in rows between parents,'' and ''having to take care of a parent'' (Velleman and Orford, 1985). Once again, it is important to be reminded, first of the heterogeneity to be found within a sample of children of alcoholics and their families, and second that most stresses in families with alcohol problems are unlikely to be specific to families complicated by excessive drinking.

In 1981, from Czechoslovakia, Matejcek reported in two parts, the results of a

Table 1. Matejcek's 1981 Czechoslovakian Study of Children's Family Circumstances

**Significant findings for 200 children of fathers registered at Prague alcoholic counseling centers compared with controls:**

1. Fathers relatively uninvolved with the child, both in the first year of life and currently (mothers' reports)
2. Mothers had more authority in the family (mothers' reports)
3. Mothers were the more consistent parents (mothers' reports)
4. Parents relatively disunited in bringing up their children (mothers' and fathers' reports)
5. More factors in the family that adversely affected the children's upbringing (mothers' and fathers' reports)
6. Fathers' relationships had worsened with their children as the latter had grown up (fathers' reports)
7. Fewer significant correlations between father and mother ratings of the children's personalities (suggesting a lack of consensus between parents)
8. Family circumstances below average (teachers' reports, 4–6 year-olds only)
9. Care of the children below average (teachers' ratings, significant at all age groups, but most significant for ages 4–6)
10. Family life relatively discordant (teachers' reports, significant at all ages, but most significant at ages 9–11 and 13–15)

major investigation which bears on this question of child neglect. Two hundred children from intact families in which the father had been registered at one of Prague's anti-alcoholic counseling centers in the years 1975 and 1976 were individually matched, on the basis of age, number of children in the family, position in the family, age of parents, and education of parents, with children without alcoholic parents. Teachers and parents were interviewed and the children were tested, the interviewers and examiners being blind to group membership. The children fell into three age groups: 4–6 years, 9–11 years, and 13–15 years.

The first part of Matejcek's report (1981*a*) concerned the home situation. A number of significant differences between the groups were found; these are summarized in Table 1. Matejcek concluded that the atmosphere for bringing up children was worse in families in which the father was an alcoholic. The father played a lesser role in bringing up the children, and this deficiency was not compensated for by an increased positive role on the mother's part. Despite statements to the contrary in some of the reports from Bulgaria and the U.S.S.R. (see below), the author's hypothesis that there would be a stronger bond between mother and child when the father was alcoholic was not upheld by the findings. The second of Matejcek's reports (1981*b*) concerned the children themselves and will be discussed later.

## Effects on Children and Adolescents with Problem Drinking Parents

This section will now consider research on the possible *effects* on children of having a parent with a drinking problem, first of all on offspring during their childhood and adolescence, and then (in a later subsection) in later adulthood. There has been an upsurge of interest in this topic in recent years, although most research comes from

Eastern Europe and the United States. Apart from a Swedish study of the short- and long-term effects of parental drinking problems (Nylander, 1960; Rydelius, 1981), there are only scattered studies from Western Europe, and apart from a small amount of work from Japan and some interest in the fetal alcohol syndrome in Australia, this author has found virtually no work on the subject outside Europe and North America.

Research from Eastern Europe. Bulgaria is one country where there has been a considerable interest in the effects on children. Research there has been summarized by Boyadjieva (undated). One study, reported in the early 1970s (Stankoushev et al., 1974), found a higher rate of neurotic behavior and memory and attention disturbances among children with an alcoholic parent than among controls. Four years later, another Bulgarian study (Christozov et al., 1978) investigated 50 children, aged between 4 and 15 years, with an alcoholic father, and attributed the high rate of neuroticism they found among these children to three pathogenic mechanisms: immediate stress, frustration, and deprivation. In the early 1980s, in a dissertation and a series of papers (Toteva, 1982*a,b*, 1984), the findings of a study of 220 children aged between 5 and 25 years were reported. This group of children, each of whom had a parent (usually the father) who had been treated for alcoholism, was compared with a control group of 110 children of healthy parents. Neurotic disturbances were found in 56% of the former vs. 22.5% of the latter; antisocial behaviour was registered in 23% vs. only 3% of the control group; suicidal tendencies were found in a substantial minority of the former and four children had attempted suicide [also from Bulgaria is a single case report (Christozov and Mumdzieva, 1978) of attempted suicide in a 6-year-old boy whose alcoholic father had attempted to kill his wife, and later committed suicide himself]. Testing for intelligence, memory, and attention showed, according to Boyadjieva's review (undated), that 60% of children with an alcoholic parent had IQs below 75 and 53% had disturbances in short-term memory. In a thesis (Boyadjieva, 1979) and in his review (Boyadjieva, undated), Boyadjieva has developed the theory that the presence in the family of a father with a drinking problem is a major stress factor for children, slowing down normal development, leading to lowered self-esteem and inferiority complexes, and hence in many cases to identify crises. The connection between parental alcoholism and childhood neurotic disorders continues to be investigated by Toteva (1985).

In the U.S.S.R., a major study was reported by Shurygin (1978) in which 74 children (aged from less than 1 year to 16 years) from 52 families where the father was suffering from chronic alcoholism and had received treatment were compared with an equal-sized comparison group. Shurygin reported that psychogenic disorders were almost six times as frequent among the former group. Twenty-eight were diagnosed as suffering from one or other variant of "patho-characteristological development." Shurygin describes in detail how the disorders, in particular the two commonest variants, grew out of the microsocial environment of the family. In 10 cases an "inhibited" variant was noted. In the early stages, behavior peculiarities were apparent only in the presence of the father: Children avoided their fathers totally, refused to go home, or hid from them. Later, this behavior generalized to the school, where teachers noticed increased pensiveness and silence in the children, who avoided the company of peers. As Shurygin (1978) puts it, such behavior is justified in the following way:

> I see what sort of father my friend has, how everything is peaceful with them. Then I go home and cry. Why are my mother and I so unhappy? So now I do not go to see my friend, and yes, I am ashamed of my father. (p. 1567, translated from Russian)

The second pattern of disorders described by Shurygin was the "temporary-excitable" variant. Eight children displayed this variant, which began with sullen, unwilling, and threatening behaviors, again specifically in the presence of the father. Once again, this behavior developed and generalized, and unless the problem was resolved by death or departure of the father, or by his cure, developed into symptoms of "social–pedagogic neglect" with a tendency to antisocial forms of behavior. A proportion of the children in Shurygin's study were followed over a period of 2 years or more, and if such a resolution of the family problem did occur, a reversal in the child's behavior was observed, with the inhibited children becoming more active, lively, tender, and accessible, and the "temporary-excitable" children becoming more balanced in mood, with the frequency of their outbursts lessening and their behavior becoming more easily corrected.

Shurygin's investigation was confined to what he termed the microsocial factor in the generation of childhood disorders. However, he pointed out that most Russian work has considered biological causes as fundamental in the transmission of problems or has at least considered biological and microsocial factors jointly. He cited work suggesting that parental drinking problems may be linked with the development of childhood epilepsy, as well as mental retardation. Several researchers, he pointed out, are examining the morphological and functional changes in the generative cells of parents as one of the probable reasons for the "inferiority" of the offspring. In his review, Boyadjieva (undated) also cited work from the U.S.S.R. suggesting a higher frequency of abortions and the possibility of damage prior to birth (the fetal alcohol syndrome). Other Russian workers have also suggested that parental alcoholism may be one of the factors related to childhood convulsions (Antonov and Shan'ko, undated).

In Poland, according to Boyadjieva (undated), there has been a small number of studies of children in alcoholic families. One such study (Strzembosz, 1979), found maladjustment in 64% of children in families where the mothers had drinking problems, and in another (Gerkowicz, 1976) a correlation was found between the duration of alcohol abuse and the degree of psychological disturbance in the children. In another Polish study, broken homes and criminal behavior resulting from alcoholism were discovered in the backgrounds of 80% of a sample of 50 8- to 16-year-old boys residing in a child custody center in Warsaw (Drecka et al., 1976). A study from the 1960s by Borzova (1967–1968) reported the results of administering tests, questionnaires, and interviews to 50 6- to 14-year-olds from alcoholic families who were attending a month's reeducational camp. A higher-than-expected incidence of neurotic symptoms and lower-than-expected intelligence levels were reported, and 82% of the children showed strong attachment toward the mother and minimal or no positive relation to the alcoholic father.

In Yugoslavia, there has been a greater interest in marriage and marital therapy than in the effects of drinking problems on children. However, in the early 1970s Dordevic and Dukanovic (1974) pointed to the frequent behavior and learning problems experienced by the children of 100 alcoholics at the Treatment Institute in Belgrade. Alcoholism as one of a number of negative factors in the backgrounds of epileptic schoolchildren, in comparison with nonepileptic controls, has also been reported from Yugoslavia (Plavec and Vukadinovic, 1976), and Boyadjieva (undated) has cited a Yugoslavian study (Veseb, 1973) of suicidal tendencies among the children of women alcoholics who had attempted suicide themselves.

In Czechoslovakia, there has been a long-standing interest in the effects of parental drinking problems on children. In the late 1960s, Freiovai (1966) studied over 500 families with a "morally impaired" child between 9 and 16 years of age, who was placed in a reeducation facility. In 27% alcoholism was found in one or both parents, and of 47 families with more than one child in the center, 53% had one or both parents alcoholic. Similarly, in 1979, Koznar et al. found alcoholism, along with incomplete and disharmonious families, mental illness, and criminal behavior, more common in the family backgrounds of adolescents with antisocial behavior problems than in the backgrounds of adolescents with neurotic problems or learning difficulties.

The second of Matejcek's reports from Czechoslovakia (1981*b*) examined intelligence, school performance and adjustment, and general adjustment in the 200 children whose fathers had been registered at the antialcoholic counseling center in Prague. On intelligence testing, Matejcek found a difference of seven IQ points in favor of the comparison group (almost wholly accounted for by a difference of eight points on verbal intelligence) in the oldest of the three age groups only (the 13- to 15-year-olds). There was no difference in parents' assessments, which in many cases were felt to be unrealistic. Teachers' assessments were much closer to the formal IQ test results, and pediatricians' ratings of intelligence (above average, average, below average) and schoolmates' nominations of most intelligent, most gifted, and quickest children both showed significant differences in favor of the comparison group. Children from alcoholic families were less likely to be chosen as best friends on a sociometric test. On a test of maladjustment, the difference between group means was significant overall; was particularly significant for the 9- to 11-year-olds ($p < 0.001$); was less significant for the 4- to 6-year-olds ($p < 0.02$); and the difference was not significant for the oldest age group. In a regression analysis, the most important variable predictive of maladjustment was gender, with boys showing higher scores than girls.

Other studies from Eastern Europe include a Czechoslovakian study of gypsy and nongypsy special schoolchildren in Western Bohemia (Machova and Gutvirth, 1981), which noted a high rate of unfavorable family circumstances, including alcoholism, especially among the gypsy children. From Slovenia there is a report (Sterle, 1970) of several differences in the family lives of 4- to 8-year-olds who dropped out of school, in comparison with control children, one factor being a higher rate of parental alcoholism. Finally, Boyadjieva (undated) found a small number of studies from Eastern Germany, of which the most conclusive appears to have been one reported in the mid-1960s by Parnitzke and Prussig (1966). They investigated 120 children with alcoholic fathers and found three times the rate of neuroticism than that found in control children. A second study from the 1970s (Farkasinszky et al., 1973) found that children with alcoholic parents had an increased level of anxiety as well as psychopathic character and social maladaption.

Research from Western Europe. From Western Europe, which on the whole has contributed rather less to this line of research on the effects of parental drinking problems on young children and adolescents, there is the occasional report in keeping with one of the major themes of the Eastern European research, namely that antisocial behaviour is something for which sons of parents with drinking problems are particularly at risk. For example, the records of a child psychiatric clinic in West Berlin showed boys with alcoholic fathers to be particularly likely to be attending with conduct disorders, while both boys and girls with alcoholic parents were likely to have emotional problems, especially if the problem drinking parent was the mother (Steinhausen et al., 1984).

An Austrian study (Mader, 1972) reported a high rate of family alcoholism among "adolescent dipsomaniac criminals," and from Switzerland (Fanai, 1969) there appeared a report that adolescents with personality disorders had a higher-than-average number of psychiatrically abnormal persons in their families, particularly alcoholics, who made harmonious family life impossible.

Of greater interest is a study from Zurich reported by Schmid et al. (1983), in which parental alcoholism is listed as one of nine psychosocial risk factors that differentiated 300 11-year-olds with learning difficulties from a contrast group of 200 children of the same age who were in the top third of their classes academically. Children in the former group had had the start of schooling postponed, and/or had had to repeat a class, and/or had been admitted to special classes or educated in special schools or homes for the handicapped.

In France, the main point of interest appears to have been suicide and attempted suicide. From that country there has been a report that a family history of alcoholism was one of five risk factors for adolescent suicide attempts among over 500 14- to 19-year-olds, who had been hospitalized after a suicide attempt in Lyon, Strasbourg, or Paris (Angel et al., 1978). Another study found parental alcoholism to be one possible factor in the etiology of suicide attempts among children under 12 years old, who constituted 10–15% of all child and adolescent suicide attempts in France (Marcelli, 1978). Yet another study reported that 10 of 130 adolescent suicide attempters had an alcoholic parent: No control data were reported to enable this figure to be interpreted, however (Duche et al., 1974). In all the families of 35 drug addicts who had made at least one suicide attempt, one or both parents were found to be alcoholics or users of psychotropic drugs in another study (Braconnier and Olievenstein, 1974). Finally, alcoholism and conflict were found to be more frequent among the parents of 28 6- to 16-year-old suicide attempters, in comparison with a group with psychosomatic problems (Moullembe et al., 1973).

In Portugal, de Mendonca carried out a study that was published in French in 1976. As it was "obvious" to him that maternal alcoholism had a very disturbing effect on the child, in view of the poisonous effect on the embryo, the fetus, and the nursing child, de Mendonca was interested in the effects on children when only the father had a drinking problem. He compared two groups of children, of 100 each, from the district of Coimbra, one group with alcoholic fathers and one without. In all cases the mothers were free of drinking problems and mental illness. The fathers in the former group had all been treated at an alcoholism treatment center, and the results were based on interviews with the mothers. There were some considerable differences between the two groups of families which make interpretation difficult. At the time of the study, children in the paternal alcoholism group were older (median age 8–9 vs. 6–7), their families were often of lower social status (96% vs. 32% in classes IV and V on a five-point scale, although de Mendonca argues that this was due to "social drift" and that the original levels of the two groups were similar), and they were from larger families (median number of children four vs. two).

Sizeable differences existed between the groups in terms of the mothers' reports of their children's early development and adjustment. In the paternal alcoholism group, breast feeding was more likely to have been prolonged to 1 year or more after birth (57% vs. 35%); developmental delays (first teeth, first steps, first words, and first sentences) were much more common; sphincter control was more often delayed; more infantile illnesses were reported (infectious, allergic, and neuropsychiatric); progress at school was much more likely to be poor (76% vs. 14% had had to repeat at least 1 year); and later neuropsychiatric symptoms of one kind or another were universal (vs. 24% of controls). Anxiety, fears, fear at night, anxiety crises, and insomnia were some of the commonest symptoms.

Although most children in both groups were under 10 years old, and the oldest only 12–13, mothers reported that 74% and 55% in the two groups, respectively, drank alcohol regularly. In the control group, a frequently cited reason given was that wine was a form of nourishment and was good for the child. In the paternal alcoholism group, 25% of mothers stated that the child was imitating the father, and 16% indicated that the father forced the child to drink.

de Mendonca (1976) attributed the differences he found partly to the child's anxiety which was reactive to the family atmosphere of conflict created by the father's drinking. However, he also took into account the toxic effect of the child's own alcohol consumption and in general was conscious of the etiological complexity of the matter:

> In our opinion the neuropsychological problems that we came across in the children of alcoholic fathers resulted from hereditary, social and psychological factors, which combined together cause certain basic deficiencies, be they organic or functional, in the child's nervous structures, onto which there grow, very exaggerated psychological manifestations of emotional imbalance. All these disturbing factors abound in the households where there is an alcoholic father. (p. 425, translated from French)

de Mendonca also formed the opinion that in some cases the birth of the children had revealed conflicts in the parents' relationship which had hitherto been lying dormant, and that in many instances the mothers had a profound need for affective compensation which they found in their children, toward whom they established a very restrictive and protective relationship. These observations are to be seen against the prevailing conservative traditions of the region which dictated that wives rarely worked outside the home, and families rarely split up.

Considerable interest in the transmission of disadvantages as a result of parental drinking problems has been shown in Sweden. Nylander's monograph (1960) compared 229 children from 141 families where the fathers were alcoholics with 163 control children. The groups were carefully matched and children were aged between 4 and 12 years old. Children in the former group, as in de Mendonca's (1976) and so many other studies, showed more frequent signs of mental ill health and a wider variety of symptoms than control children: 27% of boys and 30% of girls showed "mental insufficiency." Anxiety neuroses and depression were the commonest diagnoses, and rates were equally high among the three age groups, 4–6, 7–9, and 10–12 years. Apart from clear psychiatric diagnoses, stress symptoms such as headaches, stomachaches, and tiredness were very common, and children had often been investigated for physical conditions without any underlying organic reasons being confirmed. Of those children who were of school age, 48% (vs. 10% of control children) were considered by their teachers to be problem children at school. Among the youngest school-age boys (7–9 years) as many as 74% with alcoholic parents showed difficulty in adjusting. A long-term follow-up of this sample by Rydelius (1981) will be considered in more detail later.

Although there appear to have been no special studies of this subject in Japan, occasional mention has been made of a possible link between parental drinking problems and outcomes for children in that country. For example, one study of depressive symptoms among 14- to 22-year-olds claimed to establish a link between depression of behavior disorder type (as opposed to depression of inhibited, anxious, or withdrawn type) and families with dominant fathers or disorganized families with mentally ill or alcoholic parents (Nishimura et al., 1983). Another study describes a single case of childhood psychosis where the father had a serious drinking problem (Murata et al., 1976). Another cites alcoholism in one or both parents as one of several family background factors leading to juvenile delinquency (Takei et al., 1974), and again, the father's pronounced tendency toward alcoholism is mentioned as the first of a number of factors differentiating a sample of families where a majority of siblings were delinquent in comparison with families of similar socioeconomic status, but without delinquency (Ishihara and Ikegawa, 1974).

From the rest of the world, the only study relevant to this topic discovered by the present author is one from Brazil concerning suicide attempts (Cassorla, 1984). Broken homes, poor relationships between parents, and physical and mental diseases and alcoholism in the family were all found to be higher among 50 12- to 27-year-olds who had recently attempted suicide, in comparison with both normal and psychiatric controls.

In comparison, a great deal of research has been carried out on this subject in North America and Britain. This work has been reviewed on a number of occasions (e.g., el-Guebaly and Offord, 1977, 1979; Wilson, 1982; Velleman and Orford, 1984) and will be summarized only briefly here. In general, the results of this work have been in line with those from studies elsewhere, such as Nylander's (1960), de Mendonca's (1976), and Matejcek's (1981*b*). A higher risk of some ill effects, including negative attitudes to the problem drinking parent and to the parents' marriage, reading retardation and loss of concentration at school, and temper tantrums and fighting, seems to be a universal finding for young children. In studies of adolescents the findings are less consistent, with the occasional finding of no difference between offspring and controls (e.g., Kammeier, 1971), but most studies have reported an increased risk of ill effects, including delinquency or antisocial behavior, anorexia nervosa, and drinking and drug problems (Velleman and Orford, 1984). One study, from Ireland, found that family violence was important in distinguishing those families in which paternal alcohol problems were associated with childhood developmental problems from those without such problems (Keane and Roche, 1974).

## Adult Outcome for Children of Problem Drinking Parents: Retrospective Family Histories of Adults with Problems

A multitude of reports from clinical settings in Britain and North America have shown that excessive drinkers are particularly likely to report having had a parent who had a problem with drinking (Velleman and Orford, 1984; Cotton, 1979). Similar reports have come from many countries elsewhere, including Chile (Kattan et al., 1973), Iceland (Helgason and Asmundsson, 1975), Hungary (Laszlo, 1970), Yugoslavia (Djukanovic et al., 1978), and the U.S.S.R. (Paschenkov, 1976). For example, in the Icelandic study (Helgason and Asmundsson, 1975), 70 men under 30 years of age who had been convicted for public drunkenness at least twice within 1 month, and who lived in Reykjavik or vicinity, were matched for age, school attended, examination successes, and intelligence with 70 controls. Each young man was asked about family background, and a number of mothers were contacted to check on the answers. Significantly more fathers of the "alcohol abusers" than of the controls were reported to have been "excessive drinkers" (37% vs. 13%) and significantly fewer abstainers (17% vs. 34%). The authors also commented that their data suggested more psychiatric symptoms among mothers, although the latter had not been recognized as ill (the rate of excessive drinking among mothers was negligible). Significantly more abusers had experienced changes in family structure during childhood, mostly as a consequence of divorce, which was often related to the father's excessive drinking (53% vs. 23% at least one such change; 21% vs. 9% two or more changes; 12% vs. 3% three or more changes).

Djukanovic et al. (1978) reported on the retrospective accounts of 100 married male alcoholics attending a treatment unit in Belgrade, Yugoslavia. Although the absence of a control group makes it difficult to interpret the results, the authors were impressed that 27% of the men reported having lost one or both of their parents, through death, before the age of 18; that over half had lost one or both by death, separation, or divorce; that one-third had experienced frequent changes of guardian during childhood and early adolescence and that substitute parents were often inadequate; that 75% of the men reported relationships with parents being characterized by destructive conflict; that in 75% of cases one or more members of the parental family were excessive drinkers and in 42% alcoholic; and that 38% of the parental families exhibited other sociopathological phenomena (mainly criminality, suicide, and suicide attempts).

Although it has been suggested that total abstinence in the parental home, or a combination of abstinence in one parent and excessive drinking in another, predisposes to later excessive drinking in children [e.g., a paper from Belgium (Pelc, 1980)], the present author is not aware of any convincing evidence to support this view. However, there is some evidence from studies from Britain (Velleman and Orford, 1984; Hughes et al., 1985) and the United States (Vaillant, 1983) that the reverse may hold true, namely, that excessive drinking in a parent is followed by a raised incidence of total abstention or very light drinking in the offspring. One of these studies (Hughes et al., 1985) also found that abstaining, like excessive drinking, ran in families.

From the McCords' (1960) and Robins' (1966) work onward, including Vaillant's (1983) *The Natural History of Alcoholism,* there has accumulated evidence from studies in the United States that alcohol problems and criminality, both in the offspring's generation and in the previous generation, are linked in complex ways. A recent review from Finland (Pulkkinen, 1983) on the predictability of criminal behavior concluded that the pathogeneses of alcoholism and criminality are complex and interlinked developmental processes. A study from Yugoslavia (Cmelic and Brankovic, 1982) claims to distinguish primary and secondary "psychopathy" (a term that has ceased to have much currency in the English language literature) among chronic alcoholics and relates this categorization to a family history of alcoholism. In the same country it has been found that soldiers who resigned from the army were more likely to have had parents with alcoholic, psychopathic, and marital problems, in comparison with controls (Kapor et al., 1974). In another study from Yugoslavia (Kandic et al., 1969) an unfavorable family atmosphere with one parent alcoholic was reported in 50% of a sample of soldiers who committed delinquent acts in a state of acute drunkenness.

There is a suggestion from the findings of several studies from the United States (Lewis et al., 1983; Loranger and Tulis, 1985; Collins et al., 1985) that the process of intergenerational transmission may be different for women than for men. One line of research in the United States has suggested a link between family histories of excessive drinking (particularly in male members) and family histories of depression (particularly in female members) (e.g., Winokur, 1972). A French study has also found significantly more alcoholic men and depressed women in the family histories of alcoholic men than of controls, and the same in the family histories of depressed women than of controls (Bourgeois and Penaud, 1976).

The possibility that women with alcohol problems may have more negative factors in their family histories than do men with drinking problems is also raised by Bevia's study (which will be described in more detail in Section 4) of the families of woman alcoholics in Spain (Bevia, 1976). Over three-quarters of the women in his sample described childhoods "full of negative experiences" (p. 231), and 30% had lived in "intensely alcoholic families" (p. 231). He implied that these negative family experiences were greater than those found in comparable samples of men with drinking problems, although the data presented are not sufficient to establish this. A British study (Latcham, 1985) found a positive family history of alcoholism in 73 of 190 male alcoholics (32 fathers, six mothers, 23 brothers, one sister, two grandparents, eight uncles, one aunt), but in as many as 26 of 27 women (seven fathers, three mothers, 11 brothers, four uncles, one son). In the United States, Midanik (1983) has reported the prevalence of alcoholism and problem drinking among first-degree relatives of respondents in a national population survey. Women with alcohol problems, whether alone or in conjunction with depressive symptoms, reported higher rates of alcoholism or problem drinking in their immediate families (fathers, mothers, brothers, or sisters) than did men. Explanations suggested by the author are that women are more influenced by the home environment, or alternatively that a more severe family history of alcoholism is the necessary condition for women to eventually manifest alcohol problems. However, women overall more often reported positive family histories than men, which suggested to the author that women might be utilizing a less restricted definition and might therefore be more likely to classify their relatives (particularly male relatives) as alcoholics or problem drinkers.

Other work in the retrospective tradition that suggests a familial link between drinking and other kinds of psychiatric and psychological problems has been reported in studies from the United States, Yugoslavia, Czechoslovakia, and Switzerland. One report from the United States (Merikangas et al., 1985) is of interest because it is the first, to this author's knowledge, that mentions an increased risk of anxiety disorders in the blood relatives of individuals with alcoholism. This increased risk was linked to the presence of both an alcohol problem and an anxiety disorder in the identified alcoholics, suggesting to the authors that the latter's alcoholism might have resulted from the self-medication of anxiety symptoms. Another U.S. study from the same year (Kosten et al., 1985) found a link between reported parental drinking problems and reports of drinking problems, depression, and personality disorder among a sample of over 600 opioid addicts. Those with parental drinking problems also reported more disrupted childhoods.

From Yugoslavia is a report of the childhood recollections of over 200 schizophrenic patients, compared with those of members of a large general-population sample (Pozarnik, 1977). Family discord and an accumulation of two or three unfavorable family factors, of which alcoholism plus poor financial and housing conditions was the commonest combination, were found at a higher rate (62% vs. 38%) among the schizophrenic sample. In a study from Czechoslovakia (Sipova and Nedoma, 1972), 100 "depraved" women, who were investigated for suspected prostitution and venereal disease, were compared with 100 married women attending a prenatal clinic. The former more often reported the absence of a father during their upbringing, and more often described dissension in their families. Thirty percent reported at least one alcoholic parent. A report from the United States (Price et al., 1984) picks out parental fighting and excessive drinking as dominant themes in the memories of childhood recalled by a sample of 28 teenage male prostitutes. Finally, from Switzerland (Lobos, 1971) there is a report that parental alcoholism was one of a number of background factors among patients seeking help with marital troubles.

Among those who have themselves developed drinking problems in adult life, an association between an early onset and/or degree of severity of these problems and a positive family history of excessive drinking has frequently been reported (Schuckit, 1984*b*; Volicer et al,, 1984; Cook and Winokur, 1985). For example, from South Africa there is a report that among white, male patients hospitalized for the treatment of "secondary alcoholism" in Cape Town, age of onset was significantly negatively correlated with the severity of parents' drinking habits (Abelsohn and van der Spuy, 1978).

The possibility that birth order might in some way be predictive of later drinking problems has excited interest from time to time. However, findings are highly inconsistent [a positive finding linking penultimate birth order with alcohol problems among women in West Germany (Source unknown, 1984*b*), but a negative finding from Iceland, for example (Helgason and Asmundsson, 1975)]. Work in the alcohol field (Blane and Barry, 1973), and beyond it (Koch, 1956), has shown how very complex the apparently simple question of birth order turns out to be. For a start, research is rarely able to control for size of family, spacing of children, or gender of siblings.

Finally, in this section mention should be made of the much smaller amount of work that has been carried out on the family histories of spouses of drinkers. For example, Nici (1979) has produced some confirmatory evidence for the long-held view that daughters of problem drinkers are subsequently more likely to marry problem drinkers than are other women, and Djukanovic et al. (1978), in the study already referred to, have reported that wives of male alcoholics under treatment in Belgrade are as likely to have disturbed childhood backgrounds as are their husbands. Of the wives in their sample, 39% had lost one or both of their parents through death before the age of 18; many were exposed to emotional frustration during childhood and adolescence, in particular having been discriminated against by their mothers; and excessive drinking existed in 55% of their parental families and alcoholism in 24%. As noted earlier, the absence of a control group in this study makes interpretation difficult.

## Adult Outcome for Children of Problem Drinking Parents: Prospective and Community Studies

In comparison with the large number of retrospective studies of samples of people who have developed problems in adulthood, very few have adopted alternative strategies, such as prospective follow-up from childhood or the recruitment of community samples of adults who had parents with drinking problems. One of the most important is the 20-year follow-up, via public records, of the children who were the subjects of Nylander's (1960) Swedish study of the late 1950s. Significant findings from this study, reported by Rydelius (1981), are numerous; the more noteworthy are listed in Table 2. Compared with the carefully matched control group, children of fathers with drinking problems as a group appeared to have had a poor adulthood outcome.

However, Rydelius pointed out that the group of children originally recruited by Nylander were mostly of lower social status and the results cannot be generalized to other groups. He also pointed out that the results were much less clear for daughters of alcoholic fathers. For sons, the factors recorded in the original investigation which best predicted a poor adult outcome (registration in all three social registers—Social Service, Temperance, and Criminal Offences) were symptoms of aggression in the child and signs of neglect displayed as poor dental status.

Two family studies of hospital admissions are also relevant here. Through the National Archives, Karlsson (1985) traced a large number of the close relatives of men treated for alcoholism at the Icelandic mental hospital between 1881 and 1940. For fathers and sons of index cases, the risk of also having been admitted for the treatment of alcohol addiction was found to be five to six times that for the general population, for brothers 4.5 times, and for uncles and nephews 2.5 times. An Italian study (de Vanna and Fracasso, 1979) also found, among the children of patients diagnosed as having an "alcoholic psychosis" sometime between 1896 and 1976, a risk of alcoholic psychosis

Table 2. Rydelius' 1981 Swedish Follow-up Study

Significant findings for offspring of fathers with alcohol problems in comparison with controls:

1. Daughters had more children themselves
2. Sons were more likely to have had five or more changes of domicile
3. Daughters and sons were more likely to have had records with the Social Service Assistance Register
4. Sons were more likely to have had notifications on the Temperance Register
5. Sons were more likely to have had notifications on the Criminal Offences Register
6. Daughters and sons registered more days of sickness with the National Health Office
7. Daughters and sons made more visits to somatic clinics and hospitals (particularly poisonings, injuries and accidents for sons, and gynecological-obstetric problems for daughters)
8. Sons made more visits to psychiatric clinics and hospitals
9. Daughters and sons made more psychiatric visits for abuse of alcohol or drugs
10. Daughters and sons made more visits to somatic hospitals and clinics during which alcohol abuse or addiction was noted
11. Sons made more visits to somatic hospitals and clinics during which drunkenness was noted

about two times greater than in the general population and a risk for other forms of psychosis seven times greater.

Other studies from a number of countries are producing more optimistic findings. From Denmark, data are now available about the 19- to 20-year-old sons of alcoholic fathers included in a large cohort born in Copenhagen in 1959–1961 (Knop et al., 1985). A high-risk (HR) sample of 233 such young men was matched with a control group of 107, and the two groups were compared on school records, teacher ratings (obtained retrospectively from the last school attended; 44% response rate), and alcohol consumption in the preceding week (62% response rate). Although the HR young men had significantly more often repeated a school grade, been referred to a school psychologist, and attended a larger number of schools, and although they were rated by teachers as more "impulsive–restless" (especially fidgeting, restless, confused) and less "verbally proficient" (vocabulary, reading ability, and oral expression), last week's drinking showed no difference between the groups. Average consumption was 17 and 18 units in the HR and control groups, respectively (similar to Danish norms for that age group), and 36% and 34% had consumed more than 20 units in the week.

Another study of adulthood outcome is the recent investigation of 16- to 35-year-olds conducted by Velleman and the present author in Southwest England. The design of this study has been described elsewhere (Velleman and Orford, 1984), and preliminary results are becoming available (Velleman and Orford, 1985; Velleman, 1987). In brief, the results so far can be summarized as follows. Although our volunteer sample of 160 young adults who had had parents with drinking problems recalled substantially less childhood family happiness, cohesiveness, and stability, and considerably more family violence and disruption, than a comparison study of 80 young adults without parental drinking problems, relatively few differences in adulthood variables have emerged. This lends support to Rutter and Madge's (1976) important point that intergenerational discontinuities in psychological and psychiatric problems are numerous. Of the former group, more had left home at an early age and more had commenced using alcohol, cannabis, and in some cases other drugs, at an early age. As in the Danish study referred to earlier, levels of current drinking were similar, although more of the former admitted to having had drinking and drug problems and more were current abstainers from alcohol.

A Ph.D. thesis from Indiana University in the United States is also based on a volunteer sample of young adults who had parents with drinking problems, but is of special interest because it focuses on daughters (Benson, 1980). Women with fathers who had had drinking problems were compared with a group with paternal psychiatric problems and a third group reporting no paternal alcoholism or psychiatric problems. As in the Danish and English studies, no differences in alcohol consumption were found, and although the daughters of problem drinking fathers were found to be higher on nervousness and acting out, this was no greater than in the psychiatric group, and in general, the existence of a paternal drinking problem accounted for very little of the variance in outcome.

The complex nature of intergenerational effects is underlined by Karlsson's (1985) further finding that close relatives of hospitalized alcoholics were also more likely to be cited in *Who's Who in Iceland* and to have found employment in occupations requiring communication or socialization skills (such as professors, lawyers, clergymen, and parliamentarians). He speculates that the common factor in such successes might be "... a drive to get things done, to make one's influence felt, or to convert others to one's opinion" (pp. 187–188).

This question of intergenerational discontinuities—the routes whereby many offspring escape long-term harmful effects, and the sources of these people's resiliency—is now receiving the attention it deserves. Miller and Jang (1977) reported the results of a 20-year follow-up (by interview and record search) of 147 children of alcoholic parents and 112 matched controls derived from an original sample of over 300 poor, multi-problem urban families. At follow-up heavy drinking was more frequent in the former group (36% vs. 16%), but those whose alcoholic parent was of the opposite sex only were less likely to be in the heavy drinking group. In general, adulthood adjustment was less likely to be adversely affected if subjects had not experienced "socialisation failure" as children (11 items covering school performance, home adjustments, and disadvantaged home life).

In a more recent study from the United States (Werner, 1986), 49 members (22 male, 27 female) of a normal cohort of 700 Asian and Polynesian children born on the Island of Kauai, Hawaii, in 1955 were followed up (by interview and record search) to age 18. Forty-one percent of these offspring of parents with drinking problems had developed serious coping problems by that age. Girls were less likely to have developed such problems, and children of fathers were alcohol misuse were more resilient. Some success was obtained in predicting problems by age 18 on the basis of early characteristics of the child, qualities of the early care-giving environment, and low educational attainment at age 10. However, the sample is small, and like those of Rydelius (1981) and Miller and Jang (1977), most of these children grew up in chronic poverty and their families were of low socioeconomic status.

## Nonenvironmental Intergenerational Transmission

Most of the work reviewed in earlier sections has been based on the assumption that the mechanism that links parental drinking problems and ill effects in the offspring is an environmental one, involving the quality of parenting or quality of family life. However, mention has already been made, when reviewing the Russian work of Shurygin (1978) and the Portuguese work of de Mendonca (1976), that a number of authors recognize the likely complexity of the mechanisms involved and consider that biological or nonfamily environmental factors probably play a part.

One such biological mechanism is that involved in the fetal alcohol syndrome (FAS), which, it is now recognized, can occur in newborn infants as a result of heavy maternal alcohol intake during pregnancy. A great deal of research has been conducted on this subject in the United States (Streissguth, 1976) and Britain (Plant, 1984), and no attempt will be made to review this here. Suffice it to say that although the existence of the FAS and the contribution of alcohol to its etiology appear to be undisputed now, questions such as the risks associated with moderate drinking during pregnancy, and the precise ways in which alcohol, smoking, and dietary factors combine in producing these effects, are not so clearly answered (Poskitt, 1984; Barrison and Wright, 1984).

Relevant work has been reported from a number of other European countries also. In 1970, 13 cases of children aged between 3 and 12 years, displaying various behavioral, intellectual, psychosomatic, endocrine, and neurological disorders, were described in one French report (Laudinet and Kohler, 1970). Two theories were proposed to account for these disorders: direct or indirect action on the nutrition of the sex cells or the embryo, and disturbance of the child's social and affective development during the first few months of life. Other investigations employing the term "fetal alcohol syndrome" have been reported from France (Combes et al., 1980) and West Germany (Steinhausen et al., 1984; Majewski et al., 1978). In one of these (Majewski et al., 1978) the incidence of alcoholic embryopathy was found to increase progressively with prodromal, critical, and chronic phases of maternal alcoholism, and last-born children were found to be usually the worst affected. Similarly, from Holland, there is a report of a single family in which the degree of manifestation of the FAS in four siblings was found to be correlated with the intensity of maternal alcohol abuse during pregnancy (Spaans and Verspreet, 1981). Again, in a report from Switzerland (Fitze et al., 1978), there is an investigation of a single family in which the first child was normal and subsequent children, after the mother had developed alcoholism, were found to be increasingly abnormal. From West Berlin there is a report (Steinhausen et al., 1984) of a 3-year follow-up study of a group of children with FAS originally examined and tested for intellectual abilities when aged between 1 and 10 years. Significant improvements in psychiatric status and cognitive functioning were found. Other relevant work comes from Hungary (Bujdoso et al., 1980) and Tenerife (Falcon et al., 1980). Outside Europe, relevant work has been produced in Australia, where, for example, six cases have been reported from New South Wales (Collins and Turner, 1978) and seven from Western Australia (Walpole and Hockey, 1980).

More recently, a number of groups of researchers in the United States have compared neuropsychological functioning in offspring with and without problem drinking parents. Tarter and his colleagues, for example, have compared two groups of delinquent adolescent boys, with and without a biological father with a drinking problem (Tarter et al., 1984*a*; Hegedus et al., 1984). They found a significant difference in educational achievement. Although achievement was negatively correlated with family disorganization, the highest and most numerous correlations were found between educational achievement and neurological performance. The researchers suggested that some neuropsychological deficits might, therefore, *precede* rather than be a consequence of alcohol abuse in high-risk groups such as sons of alcoholic fathers. Schaeffer et al. (1984) examined neuropsychological functioning in a middle-aged sample including both alcoholics and nonalcoholics. Some members of both groups had a positive family history (parent, sister, or brother) of alcoholism. Both current alcoholism and positive family history were independently correlated with poorer neuropsychological performance. Finally, Ervin et al. (1984) studied intellectual and academic achievement among 100 children, aged from less than 3 years to 15 plus, 50 of whom had alcoholic fathers. The paternal alcoholism group achieved significantly lower IQ and educational achievement test scores. However, in this study only 19 of the 50 caretaking alcoholic fathers were also the children's biological fathers, and the authors of this report suggested that the results were probably attributable to a disruptive family life secondary to a parent's drinking problem.

Other studies have explicitly adopted a high-risk research strategy, studying the responses of adolescent or young adult offspring (usually sons) of biological parents (usually fathers) with alcoholism and comparing them with controls. Most of this work has been carried out in the United States and some in Denmark (e.g., Utne et al., 1977). Differences have been found in event-related brain potentials (Elmasian et al., 1982). stimulus augmenting (Hennecke, 1984), resting muscle tension levels after drinking (Schuckit et al., 1981), acetaldehyde levels after drinking (Schuckit and Rayses, 1979), task performance after drinking (Schuckit, 1980), heart rate reduction after alcohol placebo (Newlin, 1985), reports of childhood symptoms of hyperactivity (Lund and Landesman-Dwyer, 1979), and expectations of and subjective responses to doses of alcohol (O'Malley and Maisto, 1985; Schuckit, 1984*a*).

Some results have been negative and inconsistent, however. For example, higher acetaldehyde levels after drinking have not alway been confirmed (Goodwin, 1984), reports on symptoms of hyperactivity did not show differences between groups in one study (Tarter et al., 1985*b*), and another study found no difference in the rate of disappearance of blood alcohol (Utne et al., 1977).

Along with these high-risk studies, Scandinavian twin studies (Kaij, 1960; Partanen et al., 1966), and adoption studies carried out by Goodwin and colleagues in Denmark (e.g., Goodwin et al., 1973, 1977), by Bohman and colleagues and others in Sweden (Bohman and Sigvardsson, 1980), and elsewhere, have all aroused interest in the possibility that there may be a genetic component in the transmission of some forms of alcohol problem from one generation to the next. One line of research that is of particular relevance to the present review concerns ethnic differences and family resemblances in the degree of flushing in response to small doses of alcohol, a response that might partly explain the comparatively low rate of alcohol problems among the Chinese and other groups from the Far East (Goodwin, 1979). Some of this research has been carried out in Hawaii, where it has been possible to compare the responses of people whose ancestry is Chinese, Taiwanese, Japanese, Korean, or Causasian (Schwitters et al., 1982; Johnson et al., 1984; Park et al., 1984).

Research bearing on the genetic transmission hypothesis has been reviewed on a number of occasions (e.g., Davies, 1982; Murray and Stabenau, 1982; Tarter et al., 1985*a*; Goodwin et al., 1974). Conclusions include the following:

> The general conclusion from the evidence must be that a genetic component is clearly implicated in alcoholism. In other words *to some degree*, alcoholism can probably be transmitted from one generation to the next by a genetic mechanism. Its effect is to *increase the probability* that offspring will encounter problems with alcohol in later life. . . . it seems likely that what we are talking about is not a constitution which *determines* alcoholism, but continuous distribution of "predisposition," ranging from "high" to "low" which does not make an alcoholic outcome inevitable. (Davies, 1982, pp. 77–78).

> The family, twin, and adoptive studies concur in finding more evidence for male drinking being under genetic influence than female drinking. One of the reasons why researchers have been slow to elucidate the exact nature of the genetic predisposition is that they have been looking for simple answers. Any successful etiologic model must obviously take into account environmental factors such as price and availability of alcohol, plus the effects of occupation and family attitudes to alcohol. It is, furthermore, unwise to assume that the same genetic factors contribute to an individual's likelihood of becoming dependent on alcohol as influence, for example, the same individual's chances of committing a crime while drunk. For these reasons polygenic models have been suggested in which multiple

> genetic factors interact with powerful environmental influences at several different levels. (Murray and Stabenau, 1982, pp. 142–143).

In another review, Goodwin et al. (1974) have concluded that there are two separable forms of alcoholism: one familial, characterized by a positive family history, early age onset, and a severe course, and the other nonfamilial, which may more often be associated with other adult psychiatric disorders.

In the introduction to their recent report of a study of the drinking habits of 1742 individuals from 572 families containing twins, Clifford et al. (1984) wrote, ". . . the fact remains that the best predictor of drinking problems in any individual is a family history of alcohol-related problems, though the extent to which this is due to imitation or inheritance remains uncertain" (p. 64). In their own study they showed that the estimate of heritability for alcohol consumption (excluding nondrinkers) varied between 28% and 49%, depending on the model employed and whether or not the cohabitation history of twin pairs was taken into account. They conclude by saying: "The statistical analyses presented in this paper show clearly that environmental influences play a large role . . . , and should alert the behavioural scientists to the complexity of such influences" (p. 78).

## Summary

Although there have been many reports from Europe and North America, in particular, suggesting a link between parental excessive drinking and physical and sexual abuse of children, this link has yet to be conclusively established. A link with child neglect is better established as a result of research which includes a major study from Czechoslovakia.

There has been a considerable amount of work on the effects of parental problem drinking on children and adolescents who are still living at home. From non–English-speaking countries this work has mainly come from Eastern European countries and from Sweden. Suicide among children and adolescents has been a particular focus in France. The conclusion of this work is in agreement with research from English-speaking countries: there is widespread and convincing evidence of a raised incidence of childhood problems—emotional, conduct, learning, and physical—among children of problem drinking parents.

The likely consequences for offspring as adults have been studied in many parts of the world, but mainly through the retrospective study of offspring who have already developed alcohol problems themselves. It is apparent that the process of intergenerational transmission is complex; that the transmission of alcohol problems is intertwined with the development of criminality, depression, and other forms of deviance or disorder; and that the processes may be different for women than for men. There have been few prospective studies or studies that employ community samples, and those that have been carried out have taken place in Scandinavian countries as well as in the United States and the United Kingdom. The results are contradictory. Several such studies have found little difference between offspring and controls in terms of certain outcomes, such as current adulthood level of drinking. Others, notably a major study from Sweden, have found a higher frequency of negative adulthood outcomes among offspring. Several of these studies have been confined to offspring from lower socioeconomic status families living in poverty.

Nonenvironmental mechanisms of intergenerational transmission include investigations of the FAS (reports from several European countries, Australia, and North America), studies of high-risk adolescent or young adult offspring (largely sons) of known problem drinkers (largely in the United States), twin and adoption studies of possible genetic transmission mechanisms (Scandinavia, United States, and United Kingdom), and studies of abnormal, probably inherited, flushing responses to alcohol in Asia and among Asian immigrants in the United States.

## 4. SOCIAL AND CULTURAL STUDIES

### Alcohol and the Family in Social and Cultural Context

The work of Ablon (1979) provides a bridge between the two, otherwise totally separate, worlds of the clinician and the anthropologist. She has concerned herself with families, living on the West Coast of the United States, that contain a member with a drinking problem. At the same time, she has been at pains to point out the social and cultural meanings of excessive alcohol use within families. Her research is therefore in the tradition of those such as Bales (1962), Snyder (1962), and Pittman (1967), who have considered the drinking behavior of specific groups, such as Irish and Jews, in the context of the norms governing the family lives of members of those groups. She points out that models of alcohol and the family, such as the systems model of Steinglass and his colleagues, although they may be highly sophisticated, have no particular place for cultural considerations. She writes:

> A holistic perspective allowing the delineation of cultural prescriptions and expectations regarding behaviours and attitudes directly and indirectly related to drinking patterns can offer a significant new dimension to the systems model. For example, in a study I recently have completed dealing with a middle-class Catholic population, alcohol abuse appears to be integrally related to a total family cultural system which enforces massive social controls over most aspects of individual and family life. Excessive drinking, which creates ongoing family turmoil, allows men one of the few avenues through which to register their frustrations resulting from these controls. . . . Rather than viewing spouses as persons driven by individual pathological needs, one might see them as actors caught up in a cultural paradigm which in this case constitutes the homeostatic theme which perpetuates heavy drinking and related untoward social consequences through the generations. (Ablon, 1979, p. 198).

Ablon and Cunningham (1981) provide case histories from a 4-year anthropological study carried out by interview and participant observation with Irish–, German–, and Italian–Americans in Southern California. These illustrate, they suggest, the way in which the constricted emotional and sexual life and the dutiful commitment to a marriage on the part of the wives despite their husbands' heavy drinking, which was described by Bales (1962) for the Irish in Ireland, has continued among Irish–Americans in West Coast America. The two cases described are interesting because the husbands had experienced quite serious alcohol problems, although their marriages had remained intact and neither was receiving treatment for an alcohol problem. In discussion, the authors stress the cultural aspects: male models of often-absent-at-work or silent fathers and female models of competent, dominant wives and mothers who keep the family going, little premarital sexual experience, acceptable heavy drinking among young men before marriage, and poor communication and intimacy during marriage.

Although Ablon and Cunningham stress the cultural factors in these cases, they could well be used as illustrations of interactional or system factors. In the first case ("The Ryans") excessive drinking appeared to be serving the function of keeping the partners at a distance (they neither went to parties or on holidays together, nor slept together), while in the second case ("The Flanagans") the wife was reported as saying that her husband was in fact *more* pleasant when drinking.

In the anthropological tradition, but from a totally different cultural setting, are studies of the consumption of beer in African family and social life (Wolcott, 1974; Hagaman, 1980; Hedlund and Lundahl, 1984; Acuda, 1985). Wolcott's (1974) study was of the African beer gardens of Bulawayo in Zimbabwe (then Rhodesia). He described several ceremonial uses to which the Ndebele put beer drinking, including a number connected with family life, such as the ritual washing of burial implements in beer, brewing for occasions such as the birth of a first child, the "beginning of womanhood" of a daughter, drinking at the time when a suitor paid the Lobolo payment to the bride's father, and at the special ceremony held 1 year after the death of a male head of household. Opinions differed, and were often strongly held, on the question of whether municipally brewed beer, sold to urban Africans in the beer gardens, was suitable for use for such ceremonial purposes. It was particularly those who maintained substantial rural contacts who tended to deny this possibility. For those who held to these opinions, nothing could replace beer brewed in the traditional fashion, at home, in the rural areas.

Hagaman (1980) drew attention to the general neglect by anthropologists of beer production and drinking as a serious focus for research and reported on her observations of beer and its use among a small group of people in Northern Ghana whom she referred to as the LoBir. Not only was beer, among these people, a necessary and sacred accompaniment to almost all rituals and ceremonial occasions, but it also served as a vital source of cohesion in an otherwise rather dispersed and loosely organized group of people. The main drinking setting was the home, and the main drinking time the afternoon. Families would take turns hosting such parties, and it would be their responsibility to provide beer, which was an essential ingredient. It was Hagaman's observation that receiving a visitor but being unable to locate or buy the beer necessary for the expression of hospitality was a source of much embarrassment for a household. Being unable to receive guests in the proper manner could lead to being ostracized, which might be taken as a sign of witchcraft or deviance. Beer was essential to social exchange of all kinds. In an otherwise impoverished diet, beer also had an important nutritional function, and in an area inhabited by all kinds of parasites it was relatively safe to drink as a liquid.

Hedlund and Lundahl (1984) have also considered the way in which beer drinking and beer brewing reflect economic and social patterns in rural Zambia, in particular among the Ngoni groups of Chipata district. Hedlund and Lundahl say that most authors who have written about central African beer drinking have regarded the functions of drinking

> . . . as a mode of integrating the community, of confirming authority and social relations, of maintaining individual reciprocal relations, and of redistributing surpluses from wealthy households, which thus obtain a reputation for generosity and concomitant social prestige. (p. 62)

One of the most important aspects was the cooperation between different families in agricultural work, which was then rewarded by free beer from the organizing family. Most households brewed at least once during the season to obtain labor for the heaviest agricultural tasks. Hence, beer parties tied kin and friends together, gave security and continuity for the future for both families and village, and were a symbol of cooperation and unity. In the process the family arranging such a party also contracted a debt in terms of labor which had to be reciprocated when others arranged similar parties.

Acuda (1985), reviewing alcohol and alcohol problems research from East Africa, also mentions anthropological studies, mostly reported between the 1950s and the 1970s, dealing with the importance of home-brewed beer drinking in social life.

Numerous other social scientists touch on the subject of alcohol and the family while writing generally about the subject of alcohol use or in the course of a general account of a particular social group, community, or culture. Indeed, it is probably true to say that the specific topic of alcohol and the family is far more often touched on than explicitly studied and written about, particularly by those who take a social or cultural perspective. Nevertheless, despite the absence of a direct focus on the issue of alcohol and the family, the close enmeshment of alcohol use and family life around the world is described again and again. To give only a few examples, mention may be made of Waddell's (1975) description of the use of alcohol among the Papagos Indians of Arizona; Price's (1975) review of drinking patterns among a variety of North American Indian groups (both Waddell and Price describe the social context of Indian drinking, with the family serving as both an important means of social control and an area of life that gives rise to tension which may be expressed during drinking occasions); Figueroa-Rosales' (1971) description of family, work, and social pressures toward excessive drinking in Mexico; Komorowska's (1980) review of the nature of Polish family gatherings on feast days historically and in the present, in which the use of alcohol features prominently; de Silva's (1983) account of the Buddhist attitude to alcohol which extends, he tells us, to a stated preference for teetotalism in a prospective bridgegroom in marital advertisements in Sri Lanka; Fiallo et al.'s (1979) study of 100 alcoholic patients in Cuba for whom the home was the preferred place of drinking; and Andorka et al.'s (1970) account of alcoholism and culture in Hungary in which the microculture of the parental family is stated to be one of the main settings offering unrestrained drinking as a solution for life problems.

## Sex Roles, Alcohol, and the Family

A theme that recurs throughout the social and cultural literature on alcohol and the family is that of male vs. female sex roles and sex differences. Hagaman (1980), for example, in her study of beer and its use among the LoBir, concluded that beer production formed an important basis of power among women who controlled both its brewing and its distribution. Brewing was strictly a woman's occupation and it brought her both status and money. Even mensturating and parturient women, who were not supposed to touch grain or beer themselves, initiated the brewing of beer, supervised others, and retained control and "ownership" of the beer itself and its distribution. Women gained reputations as good brewers. While some beer was distributed free to children, to lovers, and sometimes to female coresidents or relatives, all the rest was sold, mostly to the men of the house or nearby residencies, or at market. Men who were related to the brewers either by blood or by marriage did not take precedence in buying beer, and those who were short of money borrowed from those who had it. As the latter were mostly sisters, mothers, and wives, they thus incurred long-standing and perpetual debts to women.

Hedland and Lundahl (1984) also described the traditional role of women in producing beer among the Ngoni in Zambia, as well as the changes that came about as a result of increased outmigration, mainly of men, to work in urban areas. The new social order, they say, made it possible for women to utilize their old roles as beer brewers in an increasingly entrepreneurial fashion. Wolcott (1974), writing specifically about urban, largely male, beer drinking among the Ndebele in then Rhodesia, suggests that traditional male and female roles were very separate and the urban beer gardens served the function of enabling men to get together away from home, which they could not otherwise easily do. Wolcott also reported that in his survey, over 80% of women claimed to do no drinking at all, and this was nearly always the case if the husband did not drink. However, like survey researchers in Europe and North America, he suspected that answers given by women to survey questions about drinking might represent a greater underestimate than was the case for men.

The distinct roles of male and female members of families in the production or purchasing, the consumption, and the reaction to others' consumption of alcohol are a regularly recurring theme in literature from nonindustrialized countries or about nonindustrialized peoples. For example, 20 years ago, Maccoby (1966) described the relationship between the sexes in a Mexican village. As he described it, the underlying tension between a basically patriarchal society and increasingly strong matriarchal tendencies was particularly acute in families where the husband was alcoholic. In their well-known review, *Drunken Comportment,* MacAndrew and Edgerton (1970) provide us with several other historical and present-day examples.

The role of Australian aboriginal women in coping with their husbands' drunkenness in the rural New South Wales community studied by Kamien (1975) has already been mentioned. A survey of the drinking habits of men and women in this community found an extreme discrepancy between drinking reported by the sexes. In the 20- to 40-year age group, where the differences were most extreme, over 75% of women claimed to drink nothing (vs. 3% of men), while over 60% of men reported drinking more than 80 g of alcohol a day (vs. only one woman in a sample of 81). Kamien describes how boys as young as 7 years old would learn to imitate the drunken behavior of older men in preparation for achieving adult male status.

Dorschner (1983) also has much to say about sex roles and drinking in his report of the drinking of Daru and other alcoholic beverages by the Rajputs of Northern India, whose drinking and drug-taking habits had previously been described by Carstairs (1954) and others. In this cultural group with its distinct sex roles, facing violence, fighting, and fearfulness were part of the masculine identity, while the woman's life was cloistered, centering on the performance of routine daily tasks. Within this context, alcohol was part of the man's world only, and men would drink in all-male groups out of sight of the female members of their families. The purity and innocence attributed to women and children precluded them from drinking, and part of the woman's role was to lecture her husband about the evils of drink and the frivolity of wasting scarce money on it. It was reported to Dorschner that many Rajputs beat their wives on returning home after drinking.

Similarly Suwaki (1985) has remarked on marked and continuing sex differences in rates of alcohol problems in Japan. These he attributes to traditional, cultural restraints on drinking among women, but points out that, with rising rates of women in employment and rising divorce rates, there is a growing concern in that country about the possibility of increasing female alcoholism.

Not that it is necessary, of course, to look outside Europe or North America to find traditional sex role structures described in the context of alcohol and the family. An "ethno-socio-psychiatric" study of alcoholism among sailors from Brittany in France is a case in point (Bourg et al., 1981). On the basis of interviews with 16 wives of such sailors, the authors considered some of the social and historical factors affecting sex roles and excessive drinking. These included a definite matriarchal family structure traceable to Celtic origins; the idealization and dominant role of the wife's mother in the former's life compared with the distant and relatively unimportant role of her father and husband; as well as the importance of the sea in the economic life of the region and in its religion, legends, and myths. Husbands were often absent, both physically and psychologically, and deaths of menfolk at sea were common in the wives' family histories. There was clearly a large subjective element in the interpretation of the interviews involved in this study, and the comments of a discussant in a following paper make it clear that opinions differ about the importance of a matriarchal family structure in Brittany. The discussant is more inclined to attribute the greater significance to the sea than to the mother (la *mer* rather than la *mère*).

That regional differences exist within developed countries in these respects is also illustrated by a study of drinking habits in the Acadian Peninsula, a rural area of Canada. Rates of excessive drinking showed a male-to-female ratio of 23-to-1 in comparison with a ratio for the whole province and for Canada as a whole of 5-to-1. Rates of alcoholism and "hazardous drinking" were similar for male and female teenagers, but the sex differences increased with increasing age (Frigault, 1979).

A study comparing the nature and origins of female alcoholism, in comparison with male, among a predominantly lower-socioeconomic group in a rural area in southern Spain (Bevia, 1976) is also relevant here. Among this group, characterized by frequent illiteracy and economic hardship, a woman's status is, according to the author of this report, highly dependent on the male head of the household to which she is attached. In this climate of female dependence, alcoholism, which is relatively rare amongst women, generally arises as a result of some special circumstances, such as excessive drinking or other negative experiences in childhood, alcoholism among husbands, or promiscuity or prostitution. Contrary to the findings of Moos and Moos (undated) in the United States, this report suggests that alcoholism in women in this area has a more severe effect on marriage and carries a great risk of marital breakdown.

A study of farm women in Poland, the German Federal Republic, Austria, France, and Sweden found that, like Breton seamen's wives (Bourg et al., 1981) and Irish-Americans in California (Ablon and Cunningham, 1981), most European farm women did not believe in divorce. However, they did believe that the strongest grounds for divorce was alcoholism in the husband. Although in the majority of cases the dominant partner in the marriage was the husband, with the responsibility for house and children falling on the woman, there were trends away from traditional peasant roles and toward more urban lifestyles in all countries studied, even though *rates* of change varied markedly (Kozakiewicz, 1982).

Although in developed countries and areas attention has turned in recent years to the particular stresses and sex-role conflicts that may give rise to alcohol problems among women [see Wagner (1979) for a West German example and Leland (1982) for a review of sex-role conflict and alcohol problems in the United States], it should not be thought that traditional divisions in the drinking habits of the sexes are a thing of the past, confined to peasant, rural, and underdeveloped parts of the world. A recent participant observation study of public houses in one English village (Hunt and Satterlee, 1985) suggests that stigma still attaches to the unaccompanied woman drinker. The approved role for a woman in a public drinking setting is still, according to these observations at least, that of someone who accompanies a male member of her family or a male to whom she is attached, who is not expected to take part in buying rounds of drinks for others, and who will probably drink less than her male companions.

Reference has already been made to Bennett and Ames's (1985) edited volume *The American Experience with Alcohol: Contrasting Cultural Perspectives*. This book provides a number of illustrations of marked gender differences in drinking behavior in the family. These include heavy drinking as exclusive male behavior, taken as a sign of virility and manhood, among Polish Americans (Freund, 1985); tension between heavy drinking as a sign of maleness and as a sign of cultural identity, on the one hand, and puritan attitudes, usually conveyed by the female members of the family, in Irish–Americans (Stivers, 1985); and the sex-segregated family lives of Mexican–Americans in California, with men drinking in all-male company away from home (Gilbert, 1985). In each case the sexual divisions were most strongly marked in first-generation immigrants to the United States, were less marked in the second generation, and were less easy to detect thereafter.

## Social Change

A theme of many of these contributions on the social and cultural context of alcohol use within the family, and on sex roles, is social change and the way it has affected the relationship between the family and drinking. A constant theme of Wolcott's (1974) description of the African beer gardens of Bulawayo was the increasing sophistication of the rural Africans and their drinking. Hedlund and Lundahl (1984) described the transition, in rural Zambia, from the provision of beer in a system of reciprocal exchange between families, to one in which women could utilize their old roles as beer brewers in a wider entrepreneurial fashion, and thence to one in which drinking was increasingly taking place outside the family setting. Similarly, Acuda (1985) cites work from Uganda which described rapid social change and a shift away from traditional drinking served by women in the home and paid for later, to drinking in bars or other drinking houses in trading centers, a shift accompanied by a change from predominantly mixed sex drinking to largely single sex drinking, with an increase in displays of public drunkenness. Acuda (1983) has also described the effects of rapid social change in Kenya. These changes included large-scale migration from rural areas to towns and cities, the consequent separation of family members when husbands were forced to leave families in order to work, and a move from extended family life to nuclear families. Like many other authors, Acuda believes that these changes have reduced family and other controls on drinking and have hence contributed to an increased risk of excessive drinking. He also comments that, with increased education and financial independence, women are now freer to drink alone outside the home, and there is concern, for example, about secret and excessive drinking among female students at the University of Nairobi. Tunisia is another country in which increases in rates of psychiatric problems, including alcoholism, have been attributed to rapid sociocultural changes (Ammar, 1972).

The breakdown of complicated kinship and family networks extending throughout tribal groups is one of the components of social change held responsible for excessive drinking among Australia aboriginals, according to Santamaria (1983). Mohan et al. (1978) also attribute alcohol abuse (although it is not clear from their report whether any distinction is being made between use and abuse) among university students in Delhi, India, to rapid social and economic change. This change appeared to have had the greatest effect on the "urban elite," a small segment of the student population who had been reared in nuclear rather than "joint" families and whose parents were generally more affluent and better educated. Students who were abusing alcohol were also more likely to be residing in a hostel or in private lodgings rather than at home and, in the case of male students, were more likely to have dated girls—a departure from the traditional Indian norm. Over 20 years ago, Yang (1967) studied university students in Taipei, Taiwan, and described the conflict between the traditional values which were instilled into children—filial piety, hard work, frugal living, and the avoidance of social vices, including drinking, gambling, sexual indulgence, and the use of drugs—and the demands on young people to fit into a role within a modern society for which traditional child training did not prepare them. O'Connor's (1978) study is another that documents the conflict experienced between traditional family norms governing drinking and the more permissive ways of the peer group in a country (England in this case) to which an immigrant group (from Ireland) was becoming acculturated.

In the 1960s, however, Graves (1967) made the point that although anthropologists had generally found acculturation to be associated with a weakening of family and other social controls, the opposite might sometimes be the case. In his own research he compared the alcohol consumption and rates of drunkenness of Indians, Spanish–Americans, and Anglo–Americans in one southwestern community in the United States. According to two measures of degree of acculturation, he was able to show that the more acculturated Spanish–Americans had more broken marriages and less frequent church attendance, and drank more and more frequently got drunk, than the less acculturated Spanish–Americans, but that relationships with acculturation were opposite for the

Indians, for whom greater acculturation was associated with more stable family life, greater church attendance, and *less* excessive drinking.

Drinking on the part of the husband was one of the main stated reasons for divorce in the U.S.S.R., according to Sysenko's (1982) study, but in his view there were more substantial and serious causes of marital conflict. One such factor to which he alluded was the increasing involvement of women in social production, marking an important change in the function of the family and giving rise to a whole range of conflicts in marital relationships. Italy is another country where changes in women's social and work roles have been seen as accounting in part for recent (the authors were writing in 1974) increases in female alcoholism (Rizzola and Rosadini, 1974). Guntern (1975) has also attempted to unravel the effects of social changes and individual and family factors in alcohol consumption in a mountain village in Switzerland. It is difficult to separate the effects of generation and of aging in this study, but once again the author makes the observation that the alcohol consumption of women has increased in direct relation to the increase in their status in the business world. Finally, Glatt (1973), writing about middle-class London Jews, offers the observation that within this group, with its traditionally low rate of alcohol problems, alcoholism appears to be more likely for those with few ties to their families and Jewish background.

## Family Diet and Malnutrition

We have already discussed studies that highlight the importance of home brewing in African societies, for example, in Ghana and Zambia, and at least one of these (Hagaman, 1980) makes specific mention of the importance of beer in an otherwise impoverished diet. A survey among the Kisii in rural west Kenya (Acuda, 1985) is another African study which comments on the percentage of homes in which alcohol is brewed. Indeed, one vantage point from which to view the subject of alcohol and the family is that of family diet, family expenditure, and—of obvious importance in the Third World—the role of alcohol use in malnutrition.

Two studies known to the present author have focused on the role of family drinking habits in child malnutrition in countries in Africa. The first involved an interview with the guardians of 92 malnourished children admitted to the pediatric department of a regional hospital in Tenga, Tanzania (Gupta and Mwambe, 1976). Most of the children were between 1 and 2 years of age. Although the authors of this report were also concerned with factors such as family size (the majority of families had more than three children at home) and the failure to identify these families when they attended the routine under-5 clinic, the report focused on social problems. Malnutrition could not be attributed to family poverty in this sample, but two-thirds had social problems, among which family instability associated with a parental drinking problem was given special mention. Drinking was considered to be a problem in 35% of these families, and this was largely confined to the Christian group, who constituted the minority in this largely Moslem sample.

In the second of these studies, parents of 200 malnourished children admitted to the Children's Hospital in Lusaka, Zambia, were interviewed (Khan and Gupta, 1979). Most of the children were between 1 and 3 years of age. An alcoholic family was considered to be a factor adversely affecting the child's health in 11.5% of cases, but in a total of 41% of cases, mothers complained that their husbands drank local beer and spent most of the family's money on alcohol. The authors comment, "In the African society, the father himself either brings the food ration for the family or else gives a small allowance to his wife. . . . The rest of the income is used by the father" (p. 44). However, in this report, unlike the one from Tanzania (although one author, Gupta, is common to the two reports), the overall conclusion is that malnutrition was due to sheer family poverty. The majority of families came from urban slums and periurban areas and just over half of the breadwinners were employed as casual laborers: Near-famine conditions in 1972–1973 had been followed by an escalation in the price index and an increase in the percentage of admissions to the Children's Hospital who were found to be malnourished (from 1–2% to over 9%).

A study from Chile is another which mentioned alcoholism in the family as a factor associated with severe malnutrition in babies (Alvarez and Wurgaft, 1982), and at least two other studies from South America mentioned a possible link between poor diet and the consumption of alcoholic drinks, although neither made specific reference to the family. One, from Brazil (Desai et al., 1980), referred to the poor diet of 100 families of the "new class of migrant workers" in periurban slums and their large consumption of empty-calorie food such as carbonated drinks and alcoholic beverages. The other, from Bolivia (Esquef, 1972), urged education to prevent the very poor dietary habits, including much use of coca and alcoholic drinks, among peasants of the highland areas.

Before leaving this all too brief section on the role of alcohol in malnutrition in the Third World, there is a final comment from one Chilean report that housewives, who are presumably the major guardians of family diet and health, can give valid and reliable information about the alcohol use of all members of the family (Tapia et al., 1966).

Of course, alcohol and diet is also of interest in Western industrialized countries. For example, concern has been expressed that alcohol-derived energy may be replacing other forms of calorific intake among secondary-school children in Marseilles in France, particularly those whose mothers work (Bresard and Chabert, 1974).

## Concern over Youthful Excessive Drinking

Another starting point for research on alcohol and the family has been excessive drinking among adolescents and even children. This is often thought to be increasing rapidly, and its origins are frequently attributed to unsatisfactory aspects of family life. In this area more than any other, however, many opinions have been stated but relatively little good research has been carried out.

Concern appears to have been particularly strongly felt in Eastern Europe. In the U.S.S.R., the Institute of Sociological Research called, some years ago, for an intensification of preventive work against alcoholism among children and adolescents and an increased emphasis on family-based recreation (Arkhipov, 1974). The role of unhappy families was highlighted in a study of the early signs of alcoholism in 100 boys who were pupils of a special boarding school (Butorina et al., 1978), and the Institute of Defectology reported that in about 86 families in which parents suffered from syphilis, the children lacked desire to attend school and lacked interest in "everything but alcoholic beverages" (Yavkin, 1976). From Bulgaria there was a report of a questionnaire study of over 1000 students aged 16–18 (Bozanov, 1980). Low parental control and disturbed emotional climate in the home were among the factors thought to be favorable to the spread of "negative phenomena in youth," such as alcohol, tobacco, and other drug use. A study of 300 under-age alcoholic migrants in Yugoslavia (Source unknown, 1981) was motivated by concern with alcoholics, the main category of "degraded, non-human disordered persons." A link between alcoholism in girls and prostitution was claimed, and special importance was attached to the deficient family and the role of the father in the etiology of youthful alcoholism. Another Yugoslavian report (Grcic et al., 1981) described adolescent alcoholism as a symptom of disturbed family relationships during a passing phase of adolescence. Compared to controls, the fathers of 23 boys treated at the Prague antialcohol clinic in Czechoslovakia (Meskova et al., 1978) were found to exercise control by methods involving the inducement of guilt and continuous anxiety in their sons; the fathers saw their sons as ungrateful; whatever the latter did was bad in the fathers' eyes, and they treated their sons with mistrust and frequently threatened punishment.

Equal concern has been expressed in Western Europe, particularly in West Germany and Austria. One author, for example, in the late 1970s (Jenner, 1978), attributed the dramatic increase in the "disease," especially among the young, and the total social disintegration and "social death" to which it could lead to the mechanization of human life, the lack of constancy in relationships, and the decline of intimate conversation among families (*das Gesprach zwischen Ich und Du*). In 1981, in a paper on alcohol abuse in adolescents, Kluge and Strassburg considered evidence for the origins of the "alarming alcohol abuse in children and adolescents." They concluded that families were the most important transmitters of drinking behavior; that parents acted as behavioral models; and that previous research (particularly that by Malhotra, 1976) suggested that "incomplete families" put children at risk of excessive alcohol abuse; but that the emotional climate in the home was of still more crucial significance. Maternal attitudes they concluded to be of greater importance than paternal, permissive maternal overconcern being singled out for special mention.

In a Swiss study of over 4000 20-year-old men, heavier consumers of alcohol and drugs not only described themselves more frequently as men with personal difficulties and psychosomatic disturbances, but they had also tended to separate earlier from their families (Hell et al., 1976). In Belgium, concern has also been expressed about problems connected with alcohol consumption, especially among young people, and the relevance of family circumstances has been discussed (Deraeck, 1982); a French paper from the early 1970s (Quidu et al., 1974) blamed juvenile public drunkenness or driving while intoxicated among juveniles on dominant mothers and passive fathers (on the basis of very small numbers).

There are sporadic reports from elsewhere in the world. For example, a report by Oshodin (1984) provides the results of a survey of 500 secondary-school students in Benin City, Nigeria. Motivated by awareness of "alarming increases" in commercial brewing and distilling of alcohol with no consideration for the repercussions for health, Oshodin was concerned to find out what role parents had in encouraging drinking among young people. As in developed countries, most students (60%) indicated that their first experience of alcohol had been at home, many during traditional festivities, but many others had received alcohol as medicine (usually with herbs) administered by their parents. Three-quarters were often offered alcohol by their parents, and in the case of the minority who were of the traditional African religious faith, this was often in the form of native gin. Oshodin cited a report to the effect that children under 10 years of age in Nigeria have suffered from alcohol poisoning as a result of the administration of combinations of alcohol and herbs. [A British report (Bradford, 1984) has also drawn attention to alcohol poisoning in young children, although this was thought to be largely due to lack of supervision of young children who were inadvertently poisoned with alcohol which had not been kept out of their reach.] Oshodin concluded that parents in Nigeria were major contributors to the early stages of alcohol abuse amongst teenagers, and that this could lead to more serious alcohol problems later.

Mohan et al.'s (1978) study of drug abuse (alcohol and tobacco being the most frequently abused drugs) among students in Delhi has already been referred to. Correlations with father's income, education, and place of residence (with students from *higher*-status families being more prone to drug abuse) were found for males only.

A study from Colombia (Morales and Atilano, 1977) investigated the use of drugs, alcohol, and tobacco in nearly 3000 secondary-school students in Barranquilla and found patterns of drug use to be correlated with a number of variables, including relationships with family. Chanfreau et al. (1979) studied 9-year-old children from state and private schools in Chile. Children were given questionnaires and mothers were interviewed. Of the children, 80% had already drunk alcohol and 63% of mothers acknowledged this. Most of the beverages were sweet and low in alcohol—for example, *Chicha,* a sweet beverage made from fermented grapes, or red wine diluted with water and sweetened with sugar. Fifty percent were used to drinking with their parents. More girls than boys abstained (31% vs. 11%). On average, each child had experienced one or two symptoms of intoxication, such as sleepiness or dizziness. Most had received either no particular parental opinions, or mainly negative opinions from mothers, and if they had received positive views about drinking, these had mainly been from their fathers. Of the mothers, 10% said they had taught their children positive aspects of drinking; 50% said they had not spoken about it to their children; and the rest had emphasized the dangers.

There have been numerous studies of youthful drinking and its correlates in Britain (e.g., Orford et al., 1974), the United States (e.g., Jessor and Jessor, 1977), Australia (Sargent, 1979), and elsewhere in the English-speaking world. In general, the results are consistent in showing positive correlations between parents' drinking and their children's drinking, although the size of these correlations is usually overshadowed by the degree of relationship between a young person's drinking and that of his or her peer group (Orford, 1985*a*). Only a few items from this large literature will be mentioned here. Two studies from the United States may be picked out: One took the novel approach of asking students to identify specific *situations* in which they believed they were expected to drink (a sample of 99 students identified 224 such situations) (Fontane and Layne, 1977); the second, of 200 13- to 15-year-olds, reached the interesting conclusion that a raised alcohol consumption in this group was related to *lack* of parental emotional tension and/or a *high* degree of parental control (Teusch, 1980). From Australia, a study of university students in Queensland is of interest because the authors concluded that their results were a reflection of changing roles for women: They found a greater discrepancy between the views of daughters and their parents than between those of sons and *their* parents, and greater discrepancies between the views of mothers and their children than between the views of fathers and *their* children, mothers having less favorable attitudes toward heavy drinking (Wilks and Callan, 1984).

Other studies from the United States and Britain have particular relevance for this review because they included a comparison of racial, ethnic, or national groups. Sue et al. (1979) questioned 23 Chinese, 24 Japanese, and 77 Caucasian–American students in Seattle about their own drinking and about their parents' attitudes. Asian–Americans drank less and had less positive attitudes toward drinking and reported less positive attitudes toward drinking and drunkenness on the part of their mothers, whose influence on their own drinking was considered to be the most important. Three measures of the degree of assimilation of the Asian students into the American culture were used, and two of these showed that students who were the most assimilated drank more.

A similar comparative investigation was O'Connor's (1978) study of Irish, Anglo–Irish (brought up in England by Irish immigrants), and English 18- to 21-year-olds and their parents. Anglo–Irish young people were exposed to some of the same abstinence norms to which the Irish youngsters were exposed, but were exposed to much the same permissiveness in their peer group as were the English youngsters. There were also more very heavy drinkers, both young men and women, among the Anglo–Irish group.

Finally, an important demonstration of the general principle that correlates of drinking can vary considerably from sample to sample was provided by the findings of Byron and Blight (Source unknown), who reported that black adolescents were more likely to be heavy users of alcohol when both their natural parents were present, but that the *opposite* was true for white adolescents.

## Summary

There appears to have been a general neglect of the topic of alcohol and the family within anthropology. Nevertheless, the fact that alcohol use and family life are closely interlinked is often remarked upon, and there has been a small number of anthropological studies of the ceremonial, family, and community roles of alcohol beverage production and consumption in African countries. Within a different research tradition, there has also been work in the United States examining the influence of cultural background on the development and maintenance of drinking problems in families of certain immigrant groups.

Sex roles and alcohol use in the family is a recurring theme. Distinct male and female roles is a feature of reports of work from nonindustrialized countries or areas. The pattern of adult males as drinkers and female partners as abstainers or light drinkers (and sometimes beer producers) and copers with their menfolk's excessive drinking recurs from Australian aborigines to Northern Indian villages and is preserved in reports from Japan, Brittany, and other rural parts of Europe and Canada, and to some degree in reports from other parts of the world.

Social change is a further recurring theme. Social change has been held responsible for the breakdown of family rituals and other social controls that hold drinking in check. Alternatively, social change may itself be stressful or may expose those who experience it to conflicting, traditional and modern, norms and pressures. Effects are likely to be complicated: Acculturation may lead to more or less family stability, depending on the circumstances, and the sexes may be affected differently.

Malnutrition among young children has been attributed to parental excessive drinking in reports from African countries and from South America.

Finally, concern over youthful heavy or problem drinking, and a possible link with deficiencies in parenting or in family life, has often been referred to in reports from Western Europe, Nigeria, and especially from countries within Eastern Europe. Causation is usually assumed to operate directly from a family deficiency to youthful problem drinking, but methods of research in this area have generally been poor, and results are likely to be complex, involving multiple interactions with a number of variables, including sex and race.

## 5. PREVENTION AND TREATMENT IN THE FAMILY SETTING

### Prevention Aimed at Parents and Children

In the earlier review of work carried out in English-speaking countries (Orford, 1983*a*), the present author drew attention to the almost total neglect of the subject of primary prevention of alcohol problems in the family setting. Of those alcohol prevention projects reviewed by Staulcup et al. (1979), only three involved the family at all, and none of these fell within that subgroup of projects which had been subject to satisfactory evaluation. Elsewhere (Orford, 1982), the present author has argued that since drinking usually begins in the family setting (Davies, 1982), and since the conditions for imitation, contagion, and acquiring relevant attitudes and values are all highly present in the family, and since there is evidence that parental and offspring drinking behaviors are correlated (see above), then alcohol-related health education for young people should be carried out in the family context and should involve parents.

The same call has been heard in other parts of the world. On the basis of their research with 9-year-olds in Chile, Chanfreau et al. (1979) concluded that the family should be the focus of alcohol education programs. They agreed with Jahoda and Crammond (1972), who concluded, on the basis of their research in Scotland, that parents should be educated in alcohol-related matters and should be encouraged to discuss alcohol use with their children as openly and as early as possible. Similarly, Oshodin (1984) concluded, from his research on parental influences on teenagers' alcohol use in Nigeria, that alcohol education programs for parents and young people should be set up.

From all the evidence reviewed earlier in Section 3, "Intergenerational Effects," it must be concluded that families containing problem drinking parents should be a particular target for preventive work designed to prevent the high rate of drinking and other problems expected to appear within the offspring from such families. One report from New Zealand (Wells, 1984) has estimated a maximum potential reduction in alcoholism of nearly 50% if all current alcoholic parents could be treated in such a way as to prevent the transmission of alcohol problems to their children. The evidence also suggests that there may be identifiable subgroups of offspring, such as those who are showing antisocial or delinquent behavior, or those who have been physically abused, who are particularly at risk and may be especially important as targets for preventive work. Nevertheless, as this author has pointed out previously (Orford, 1985*b*), children of problem drinking parents have been almost totally neglected in the design and delivery of treatment services both in English-speaking countries and elsewhere. With the exception of Gacic's form of family therapy in Belgrade (Gacic, 1980), there are, to this writer's knowledge, no evaluative reports of family treatments for alcohol problems which routinely attempt to involve children.

There have, however, been a number of suggestions about, and reports of early attempts at, involving high-risk children in treatment, either with or without their parents. For example, Ptacek (1983) has described his approach to the care of children from families affected by alcoholism in Czechoslovakia. This approach includes holidays with children, regular monthly club meetings, intensive work with whole families, and a 14-day rehabilitation camp. The first camp was held in 1976. Of 74 children between 7 and 14 years old, 49 attended one, 13 twice, eight three times, and four (one of whom became an instructor) four times or more. The program at the camp was based on the Robinson Crusoe story, with activities, psychopantomime, music therapy, psychotherapy, group relaxation, and reading from the book itself.

In her international review of alcohol problems prevention programs, Moser (1980) also mentioned a form of family treatment in Yugoslavia which included clubs for treating alcoholics where guidance was given to family members, including children. Similarly, Boyadjieva (undated) referred in his review to "leading–restructuring therapy," designed to respond to those youth crises that are particularly common among young people with parents with drinking problems, and which involved not only the young people, but also their parents. There is no indication that this approach has yet been evaluated, however. From Iceland, too, has come a call for social, psychiatric, and medical help for boys who are already in adolescence, showing signs of asocial alcohol abuse, and for their families (Helgason and Asmundsson, 1975), although there is no mention of such treatment having been provided.

As is the case with most other sections of this chapter, more work has been carried out on this topic in the United States than elsewhere. Much of this work is reviewed by Russell et al. (1985) in their comprehensive review of the literature on children of alcoholics, carried out for the Children of Alcoholics Foundation in the United States.

Over 10 years ago, in the United States, aggressive outreach was being recommended to locate and assist children of problem drinking parents before the children's problems became too severe (Hindman, 1975–1976). Identifying and working with children in the school setting or in other institutions or groups serving youth was considered by this author to be a promising approach. More recently, in the same country, a screening test for identifying children of alcoholics has been developed (Dicicco et al., 1984). This consists of the single question "Have you ever wished that either one or both of your parents would drink less?" In one survey in schools in one town in Massachusetts, 30% of both boys and girls in junior and senior high schools answered this question in the affirmative. Those who did were more likely to opt for an after-school (children from alcoholic family) group which focused on the effects of alcoholism on the family, on the child's relationship with others, and on means of surviving and coping with an alcoholic parent. They were also more likely to have had parents who had given up drinking, and they themselves were more external in their locus of control and lower in certain aspects of self-esteem (Dicicco et al., 1984).

Another intervention program, carried out in a Boston neighborhood, is described by Homonoff and Stephen (1979). This started with a request from an Al-Anon mother, and those involved were recruited largely by word of mouth and personal recommendation (advertising and agency referrals were not found to be very successful). By the time of their report, the authors had run nine time-limited groups serving a total of 55 children, either between 6 and 8 years old or between 9 and 11 years old. The aim of these groups was to educate about alcoholism and its effects on the individual and the family. Use was made of collage, plays, and puppets, and according to the authors, the children talked openly and with perception. The authors concluded that alcohol counselors ". . . tend to ignore how much the young children of alcoholics see, hear and understand about alcoholism and how deeply they are affected by it" (p. 926). The author's advice to children included: avoid confrontation, resist interfering in arguments, escape to your room or a friend's or relative's house, don't protect the alcoholic, assert your own needs for nurture and security, and take responsibility for tasks that are appropriate to your age. Much of this advice is similar to that contained in advice books directed specifically at children of alcoholics (e.g., Seixas, 1980). Thirty-three of the children had graduated to longer-term activity-therapy groups. The Homonoff and Stephen approach also included concurrent parent groups.

Seixas and Levitan (1984), in the United States, have described the setting up of a counseling group for *adult* children of alcoholic parents. Group members, who were recruited via newspaper advertisements, met weekly for eight sessions per cycle. They were asked to visit at least one Al-Anon meeting, and where basic information was felt to be lacking, the disease model of alcoholism was described, with an overview of AA, Al-Anon, and Alateen. The authors described how group members (almost all women in the first group) felt relieved to be able to talk about their experiences with others who shared them, and to be able to face common issues such as trusting others, knowing whether their parent really was an alcoholic, guilt, bad experiences at holiday times, feelings of grief about a parent whose competence had declined as a result of having a drinking problem, their own drinking and drug-taking habits, and their own abilities as parents. Although it is too early for the approach to have been evaluated systematically, the authors believe they are just beginning to meet an enormous need for resources designed to serve adult children of alcoholics.

A special case of prevention in the family setting is the prevention of alcohol-related damage to the unborn fetus. Access to expectant mothers, unlike some other risk groups, is relatively straightforward, although this depends on the state of antenatal care services in different countries. In Britain, research has been published on the screening for alcohol consumption of a large number of expectant mothers (Plant, 1984), and in the United States, there has been a number of attempts to intervene, with the aim of reducing the consumption of mothers thought to be particularly at risk (e.g., Little et al., 1980; Rosette et al., 1978). Probably the most ambitious project was that undertaken in Seattle by Little et al. (1980).

All these programs, especially those that attempt to identify and work with children or adolescents with problem-drinking parents, must face certain ethical issues, considered by Russell et al. (1985) in their review, including the dangers of victimizing young people who have had parents with drinking problems by focusing on them and, in many cases, wrongly assuming that they are at special risk.

Finally, the setting up of self-help groups for parents of young people who have already become drug and alcohol abusers has been reported from the United States (Galanter et al., 1984). Galanter et al. describe this as a national movement of recent origin, and they have presented the results of a survey of 135 members attending a national conference. Almost all were white, married, and had attended college. Almost three-quarters were women, and the family members about whom they were most concerned were mostly boys in their early teens. Forty-one percent were most concerned about alcohol use, and 40% about marijuana use, but discipline problems were reported as commonly as drug use problems.

## Partners as a High-Risk Group

Evidence of the hardship to which partners of people with drinking problems are exposed was reviewed in Section 2, "Marriages in Disorder and Distress." Despite such evidence, this author knows of no systematic attempt to offer treatment services for this group independently of treatment received by the problem drinking members of their families. The self-help group Al-Anon is an exception, as its membership is open to those whose problem drinking relatives have not sought treatment. Harwin (1982) reported that in 1982 there were more than 16,500 Al-Anon groups in 70 countries. She described the complex philosophy of Al-Anon captured in the expression "detach with love": ". . . what the phrase . . . suggests is that the individual must try to unravel the tight knot of symbiosis, whereby the spouse's entire life revolves around futile attempts to change the alcoholic" (pp. 232–233).

Clearly, Al-Anon has a message for partners, and this appears to involve the recommendation to avoid controlling or explicitly coping behaviors (Orford, 1983*b*). One of the few studies of Al-Anon, in the United States, found that the longer wives had been members, the less likely they were to use negative coping strategies, which included coaxing, nagging, pleading, covering up, and pouring drink away (Gorman and Rooney, 1979).

Relatively little is known about the impact of Al-Anon, although one fact that does emerge from two studies from the United States (Gorman and Rooney, 1979; Ablon, 1974) is that the typical member is white, middle-class, and aged between 30 and 50. Thus the groups as presently constituted may miss many partners who are at risk. Although Al-Anon has taken root in many countries, it would be of value to identify the countries it had not spread to and why, and also the degree to which the format taken has varied depending on local circumstances.

In view of the very large numbers of family members who seek advice or assistance without, or prior to, or instead of the problem drinking members of their families seeking help, not to mention the large numbers who do not actively seek help for one reason or another, it is very disappointing that there have been so few studies of advice or treatment for partners alone. Others have pointed to the same gap in the family treatment research that has been reported (Harwin, 1982). In the United States, Kaufman and Pattison (1981), for example, in their analysis of the way family treatment methods can be applied to families with a drinking problem, allow for the possibility that it may be necessary to work with a wet family system for some time in order to motivate the nondrinking members to remain in treatment, even if the problem drinker drops out or has not yet been involved.

Thomas and Santa (1982) have also described their conception of unilateral family therapy for single members of families where alcohol abuse is a problem. They recommend working with the non-problem-drinking partner if the problem drinker is not available. According to Thomas and Santa, such treatment has three aims: strengthening the ability to cope with the distress of the partner's excessive drinking; strengthening family relationships using the non-problem-drinking spouse as mediator; and, where feasible, facilitating greater sobriety. The latter aim can sometimes be achieved by inducing the problem drinker to seek help and/or by providing the spouse with methods for encouraging alternatives to drinking and by reducing behaviors that inadvertently encourage drinking. Similarly, the present author and colleagues (Orford et al., 1975) have suggested that research on partners' coping methods (see Section 2, "Marriages in Disorder and Distress") could be applied in the formulation of advice to partners alone. Our work suggested that some forms of reacting, for example, those involving attacking the drink itself (finding out where it is hidden, pouring it away, making a no-drink rule in the home), might be better than others—a result that clearly conflicts with the advice generally given by Al-Anon according to Harwin's (1982) description.

## Partners' Involvement in Treatment

Writers from a number of countries have suggested that the treatment of problem drinking is more effective if family members can be involved. Consequently, they have argued that treatment agencies should do their utmost to involve family members. Such suggestions have come from Yugoslavia (Despotovic, 1974; Stankovic and Timotijevic, 1980), Portugal (de Mendonca, 1976), West Germany (Source unknown, 1984*c*), Brazil (Source unknown, 1984*a*), and Switzerland (Gutschmidt and Maag, 1978), as well as from numerous sources in North America and Britain. The involvement of family members in Danshukai, a Japanese form of self-help movement for problem drinkers, has been described (Omori and Imazu, 1979; Suwaki, 1983). Among the basic tenets of Danshukai, according to Suwaki (1983), is the necessity of family cooperation, particularly from wives, if the alcoholics are to continue abstaining (apart from this insistence on family involvement, Danshukai has similar beliefs to AA). Wives and children usually belong to the same Danshukai as their husbands and fathers (Suwaki, 1983).

Arguments for the inclusion of family members rest not only on the expected benefits for the problem drinking member of the family, whose motivation may be enhanced thereby (Stankovic and Timotijevic, 1980), but also on the direct benefits which may accrue to the participating family members and the positive indirect effects which the inclusion of nondrinking parents may have on children in the family (de Mendonca, 1976). In the United States, both Kaufman and Pattison (1981) and Singer (1985) have pointed out the importance of attempting to reestablish family contacts, even in the case of problem drinkers who appear to have few such contacts currently. It is rare to find reports, such as one from Belgium (Bradfer, 1974), that consider family intervention to have been ineffective.

Several studies tend to confirm this view that treatment of drinking problems proceeds more effectively if a partner can be involved. One, from the United States, found that men with drinking problems persisted longer in treatment if their wives were attending a concurrent group (Ewing et al., 1961), and both this study and another from Edinburgh (Smith, 1969) reported greater improvement for men whose wives were involved in concurrent treatment. In the former study, 50% of eligible wives volunteered for the group program that was offered, but none of the husbands of women with drinking problems did so. Fridman et al. (1976) have also reported from Yugoslavia that abstinence among a group of male patients treated for alcoholism was correlated with an active, as opposed to passive, attitude toward treatment on the part of their wives. Some wives were treated individually, others in a group, and it was in the latter subsample that significant improvements in family relationships were found.

It is, of course, possible that the results of these studies were due simply to the better prognosis for men whose wives were willing to be involved. Married status has itself been found to be predictive of a more favorable outcome for drinking problems, both in the United States (Costello, 1980) and in Japan (Yamane, 1978). In addition, there is evidence from other research in the United Kingdom and the United States that prognosis is better when marriages are more cohesive or engaged (Orford et al., 1976; Steinglass et al., 1985; Stanetti, 1976). McCrady et al.'s (1979) study is the only one to date that might have resolved the question of whether partner involvement is associated with better outcome because of the partner's preexisting attitudes or family cohesion or because involvement itself is beneficial. They assigned patients at random to one of two groups who received couples' and individual treatment for both partners (in one group partners were jointly hospitalized, in the other treatment was received as outpatients) or to a third group in which the non-problem-drinking partners were not involved in treatment. All three groups showed marked changes, on both drinking and marital criteria; unfortunately, the numbers were too small to allow any definite conclusions about partner involvement.

## Treatment of Couples and Families

Evaluative research on treatment methods that involve partners of problem drinkers (although rarely their children) has been reviewed on a number of occasions (Harwin, 1982; Steinglass, 1982; Orford, 1985*b*). Methodological problems in such research are formidable, and few definite conclusions are possible. What is immediately apparent from these reports, however, is that a range of family treatments has been employed, and that with a few exceptions from Britain, Canada, and Yugoslavia, all this work has been carried out in the United States.

Group treatment for wives, running concurrently with treatment for their problem drinking husbands (paralleling the AA and Al-Anon model), was the subject of research in the 1950s and 1960s (Ewing et al., 1961; Smith, 1969; Gliedman et al., 1956), but has since received little attention. The two better-evaluated projects, one from the United States (Ewing et al., 1961) and one from Scotland (Smith, 1969), reported positive results, but the investigators found that only a proportion of partners, sometimes quite a small proportion, agreed to participate.

Conjoint group treatment, involving several couples simultaneously, has received more research attention than any other method (Burton and Kaplan, 1968; Corder et al., 1972; Cadogan, 1973; Gallant et al., 1970; Steinglass, 1979; O'Farrell et al., 1985), and three of these projects were better evaluated than the others (Corder et al., 1972;

Cadogan, 1973; O'Farrell et al., 1985). The structure of conjoint treatment has varied from once-weekly, open, outpatient groups (Cadogan, 1973), to intensive, 4-day, conjoint treatment at the end of a month's treatment for the problem drinker (Corder et al., 1972), and an intensive research and treatment program involving conjoint hospital admission (Steinglass, 1979). On the whole, the authors of these reports on conjoint couples treatment were more successful in involving at least some husbands of women with drinking problems, and the evidence for the value of conjoint treatment must be considered quite positive. There have been reports of the use of couples groups in East Germany (Bach et al., 1972), and a second German report has also appeared (Henle, 1977), but neither included a systematic evaluation.

Interest has turned in recent years toward forms of marital or family therapy in which a single couple or single family is seen individually by one or more therapists. Family therapy for families troubled by excessive drinking in at least one member has been urged by many writers, not only in the United States (e.g., Kaufman and Pattison, 1981; Janzen, 1977) and Britain (Wilson, 1982; Ritson, 1982), but also in such countries as Yugoslavia (Gacic et al., 1980), West Germany (Matakas et al., 1978), and Mexico (Serrano, 1977), and in Scandinavia (Hansen, 1978). Unfortunately, there has only been a small number of evaluative studies (Hedberg and Campbell, 1974; Meeks and Kelly, 1970; Gacic, 1980; Bennun, 1985, 1988), each with some limitations, and many questions remain unanswered. For one thing, there are many forms of family therapy, based on different theoretical principles, with additional important variations in such factors as the length of therapy and the composition of the client group (for example, whether children are included) and the therapist team.

An important source of variation within the kinds of family treatments evaluated in these studies of conjoint group therapy, or marital or family therapy, has been the degree to which the treatment focus is on drinking and its effects or on more general aspects of marital or family functioning. The main focus in the conjoint group treatments has in all cases been marital conflict, problem-solving, interactional behavior and communication, rather than drinking *per se*. In at least two instances (Burton and Kaplan, 1968; Steinglass, 1979), the focus was explicitly taken off excessive drinking itself. In Britain, Bennun has described two alternative approaches to family therapy with alcoholics: Problem-solving therapy focuses directly on drinking and attempts to modify it through the active participation of family members, while the alternative systemic approach aims to alter the functioning of the whole family system and thereby effect change in the problem drinker (Bennun, 1985). Results from the same author are available which suggest that each approach can produce definite changes in drinking despite the very different treatment focus (Bennun, 1988). There also exist, in the literature from the United States, single case reports suggesting that "marital relationship enhancement therapy" can produce positive changes in drinking, despite its lack of direct focus on drinking (Waldo and Guerney, 1983), but also a single case report suggesting that marital therapy alone was ineffective and that treatment should include a major component that focuses directly on drinking (Dinaburg et al., 1977).

From Canada, Zweben and Pearlman (1983) have presented in detail the methodological issues involved in setting up a controlled evaluation of marital systems therapy for couples in which one partner is abusing alcohol. They refer to the establishment of an appropriate balance in treatment between attending to the presenting problem of drinking and the underlying family dynamics as "a current dilemma confronting practitioners in the family field . . ." (p. 63). They themselves believe that a marital systems approach should not imply a deemphasis on the presented problem, and in their own study they have made a concerted effort to ensure that ". . . problems related to alcohol abuse remain the primary source of concern throughout the treatment process" (p. 64).

In her review of treatment approaches, Harwin (1982) identified a group of evaluated family treatment programs that she termed "ecological" (Pattison, 1965; Davis and Hagood, 1979; Hunt and Azrin, 1973). These had been aimed at a rather different target group than had been the case for most family group and marital and family therapies, and they included multiple-problem families, single-parent families with young children, and, in the case of the best evaluated [by Hunt and Azrin (1973)], some single men for whom one aim was to build up "synthetic families." The focus of these treatments had also been rather different, being much more on problems of child care, household management, job seeking, and family and legal problems, rather than on family interaction. According to Harwin's review, these programs showed considerable promise, although in most cases they involved quite intensive treatment.

## Families and Nonspecialist Agencies

Almost all the work reviewed in the foregoing section on family treatment has been conducted in specialist agencies or by people with a specialist interest in alcohol problems. However, a widely held view, certainly in Britain, is that the large bulk of family alcohol-related problems masquerade as a range of health and social problems and present, if at all, at a variety of nonspecialist agencies (Department of Health and Social Security, 1978; Orford, 1987*b*).

In the United States, there have been a number of studies of family alcohol-related problems as they present to general medical agencies. One such study (Roberts and Brent, 1982) found a higher rate of visiting a physician on the part of 90 members of families containing someone with an alcohol problem (excluding the identified problem drinker) than was the case for a matched group of 90 patients from other families (9.7 visits vs. 6.5 visits per year) and a greater number of distinct diagnoses (an average of 6.3 vs. 4.5 diagnoses per person per year). Of 25 categories of diagnosis, 20 were more frequent in the alcohol group, and six of these differences were significant: trauma (30% vs. 14%), gastrointestinal (31% vs. 12%), neurosis (19% vs. 2%), other mental and psychological disorders (36% vs. 7%), endocrine, nutritional, and metabolic (15% vs. 3%), and genitourinary (19% vs. 4%).

Another study of this kind asked patients at a university-based family practice center to complete the Michigan Alcoholism Screening Test (MAST) about themselves and a modified form of the test about their families (Leckman et al., 1984). Whereas men were more likely than women to have scores indicating an alcohol problem themselves (34% vs. 10%), the reverse was the case for positive family MASTs (38% vs. 24%). The authors comment that nearly 40% of patients with a positive family MAST had complaints (e.g., anxiety, depression, fatigue) that could be attributed to the family disruption caused by drinking problems, and another 21% had medical problems (e.g., insomnia, gastritis, irregular menstrual periods, headaches, colitis) that might be exacerbated by stress. Nevertheless, in only 12.5% of the practice records of those patients with positive family MASTs was use of alcohol by a family member mentioned.

Another study produced negative results (Roghmann et al., 1981). This study found *less* use of a health maintenance organization by the families of 69 identified alcoholics and 98 high-risk patients (who gave positive answers to questions about daily drinking and gave some evidence of concern about either their own drinking or that of others in the family) in comparison with a matched control group.

In Britain, Wilkins examined those factors in a general medical practitioner's patient's history or presentation which distinguished patients found on a screening interview to have possible alcohol problems from other patients (Wilkins, 1974). These included a number of factors, such as family disharmony, children with mental or psychosomatic disease or suffering from neglect, or one family member suspecting another of having a drinking problem, which would only be apparent from the presentation of a non-problem-drinking member. Ritson (1982) has listed a number of other front-line or contact agencies in Britain that might meet families at a time of crisis related to the excessive drinking of a family member. In addition to general medical practitioners, his list included members of the primary health care team, such as district nurses and health visitors, and also social workers, teachers, child guidance workers, marriage counselors, the police, women's refuge workers, lawyers, Samaritans, and clergy. The survey of the current case loads of social workers in a local authority social services department in Edinburgh, Scotland (Lothian Regional Social Work Department, 1981), has already been mentioned. Although the survey was on a small scale, 17 of 40 cases were thought by their social workers to be at least partly alcohol-related, and these were more likely to be those where a child was thought to be at risk. Alcohol-related cases were more likely to be long-term cases that had been open for at least a year at the time of the survey and were thought likely to remain open for some time to come. From the United States, Ehline and Tighe (1977) have made the same point about the high frequency of alcohol-related problems in a social service agency, drawing on a survey of their own case loads to support this observation.

An interview study of 275 general medical practitioners in 12 different countries (from Africa, Asia, Australasia and the Pacific, Europe, and South and Central America) shows that awareness of alcohol-related family problems among general practitioners is by no means confined to countries such as the United States and the United Kingdom (World Health Organization, 1984). Practitioners were asked about 12 alcohol-related problems, including intoxication, dependence syndrome, work problems, family problems, financial problems, and road accidents. Sixty-three percent considered that there were many family problems in their countries. Only intoxication achieved a higher percentage (68%). When asked whether they often provided help for people with such problems, family problems achieved the highest percentage (41%).

## Summary

From several parts of the world there have been calls that alcohol education be delivered in a family context and should involve parents. More specifically, a few programs have been reported which involve the identification of high-risk children of problem drinking parents. These have largely been confined to reports from Eastern

European countries, where programs are more activity based, and from the United States, where programs are more often based on a group psychotherapeutic format. Means of identifying high-risk children have sometimes been crude, and all such programs must face ethical issues, including the possibility of victimization and overprediction. At least one special program for adult children of alcoholics has been reported from the United States.

There has been little research on treatment for partners without or instead of their problem drinking spouses. The self-help organization Al-Anon, which has spread to many countries, is an exception, and in addition, there have now been a number of reports from the United States of unilateral therapy or working with part of the family which may not include the identified problem drinker.

Partners' involvement in the treatment of problem drinkers has been called for and described in reports from a number of countries, including Japan. However, research on the question of whether such involvement leads to better outcome is currently inconclusive and confined to the United Kingdom and the United States.

Research on the treatment of couples and families has largely been confined to the United States, with some reports from Canada, the United Kingdom, and Yugoslavia. Concurrent groups for problem drinkers and for their partners has received some research attention in the past. There has also been research on conjoint groups for several couples together, and research on this form of treatment has largely obtained positive results. There have been few evaluative studies of the more recent developments in family therapy. One issue is whether the focus in treatment should be on drinking and its effects or on family interaction and problem solving, and research to date suggests that these are alternative, equally effective approaches. An ecological approach to family treatment has been identified as an alternative model which has a more practical focus on a family's day-to-day concerns. It remains a completely open question which type of approach to the treatment of families with alcohol-related problems will be most effective outside the United States and similar industrialized countries.

## 6. IMPLICATIONS FOR FUTURE INTERVENTION AND RESEARCH

### The Need for Good Cross-Cultural Research on Alcohol and the Family

As is the case in psychology generally (Connolly, 1985; Moghaddam and Taylor, 1986), there is a danger of imposing on the rest of the world Western models of alcohol and the family. As this review has shown, nearly all the specialized research that has focused on alcohol and the family has been concerned with *excessive* drinking or alcoholism and has been reported from North America or Western or Eastern Europe. Research on treatment involving partners of problem drinkers has been even more restricted geographically, being confined largely to the United States, with a little work from Yugoslavia, Britain, and Canada. Of the different perspectives on the subject of alcohol and the family which were identified in the author's earlier review (Orford, 1983*a*), *the stress victim* and *systems* perspectives are the two that have been dominant in the North American and European research. The first of these has the longer history and has generally been predominant, particularly in Eastern Europe, where there has been special concern with intergenerational effects and the socialization of youth.

Neither of these perspectives takes much note of the cultural context. A small amount of research from North America and Europe has, however, taken a *cultural* perspective. Some of this has explicitly adopted a cultural patterning view, stressing the need to appreciate the historical and cultural roots of family life and of drinking (Ablon, 1979; Ablon and Cunningham, 1981). This and other work (e.g., O'Connor, 1978; Graves, 1967; Sue et al., 1979) has studied minority or immigrant groups and has considered the degree of their acculturation or assimilation and the extent of their drinking and family controls on drinking. Other work has hinted at, and sometimes focused on, sex roles in the family and the ways these are changing, particularly in hitherto more traditional parts of North America (e.g., Frigault, 1979), Western Europe (e.g., de Mendonca, 1976; Bourg et al., 1981), and Eastern Europe (e.g., Kozakiewicz, 1982).

Research on the subject from Africa (Wolcott, 1974; Hagaman, 1980; Hedlund and Lundahl, 1984; Acuda, 1985) has often been anthropological, and the cultural perspective has therefore been dominant. The role of the family in the home production of alcoholic beverages, and the role of drinking in family and community life, have been clearly delineated. Although their origins are very different—the African research rooted in anthropological concern with norms, customs, and social change, and the North American and European research in an interest in the treatment or prevention of alcoholism—there is clearly much common ground among Ablon's study of Irish–Americans in California (Ablon and Cunningham, 1981), Graves's study of American Indians and Spanish–Americans (1967), O'Connor's research on Irish immigrants to England and their children (1978), Hagaman's study of the LoBir in Ghana (1980), and Hedlund and Lundahl's study of the Ngoni in Zambia (1984).

What is now required is good cross-cultural research which has alcohol use in the family as one major focus, but which at the same time places alcohol use and family life within the wider social and cultural context. This research should combine the strengths and insights of previous research from the different traditions mentioned earlier: family psychology and psychiatry in the West; comparisons of groups with different ethnic and geographical origins now living in Western countries; and African studies of the role of alcohol production and consumption in families. Specific suggestions about such research include the following:

1. It should include samples that differ in the degree of their industrialization, the degree of their urbanization, and the degree to which their societies are rapidly changing. It should also include immigrant groups differing in rates of assimilation to the host culture [recent research from outside the alcohol field in Britain (Cochrane, 1983) has shown that different immigrant groups, those from the Caribbean, Ireland, India, and Pakistan, differ greatly in rates of mental ill health and in the ways they deal with such problems]. Such research should pay particular attention to the ways in which family controls on drinking are eroded or enhanced as a result of industrialization, urbanization, social change, and assimilation.

2. This research should consider carefully the various functions of alcohol beverage production and consumption in family life, bearing in mind some of the economic, social, and ritual functions stressed in the African research (Wolcott, 1974; Hagaman,

1980; Hedlund and Lundahl, 1984; Acuda, 1985), the historical–cultural norms of family life and alcohol consumption identified by Ablon (1979; Ablon and Cunningham, 1981), and the way in which some drinking patterns may be disruptive of family life while others may serve a homeostatic function for families (Jacob, 1988).

3. Sex roles in the family, and the ways in which these may be undergoing change, should constitute a major focus of such research. The role of drinking in families when the wife is thought to be an excessive drinker should be studied and compared with families where the husband is thought to be drinking excessively.

4. The ways in which family members cope with, or react to, excessive drinking in the family (e.g., Orford et al., 1975; Finney et al., 1983) should be studied, as well as the way this differs depending on the nature of the culture and the gender of the excessive drinker. Particular attention should be given to marital separation as a result of excessive drinking (e.g., Levinger, 1965; Sysenko, 1982) and the extent to which separation is more or less an option depending on culture and gender.

## The Need to Carry Out Well-Evaluated Projects to Help High-Risk Offspring of Problem Drinking Patients

Although this research has largely been confined to North America and Europe (both East and West), one of the most consistent findings of all the research on alcohol and the family is that the offspring of alcoholics or problem drinking parents are at risk in various possible ways. These include

1. The fetal alcohol syndrome as a risk to those infants whose mothers drink excessively during pregnancy (e.g., Bujdoso et al., 1980; Walpole and Hockey, 1980).
2. Malnutrition in infants as a risk, particularly in some parts of the world, when parents drink excessively (Gupta and Mwambe, 1976; Khan and Gupta, 1979; Alvarez and Wurgaft, 1982).
3. Possibly a raised risk of physical child abuse when parents drink excessively (e.g., Mokran and Kramer, 1976; Behling, 1979; Orme and Rimmer, 1981), although a specific link has not been completely confirmed and this requires more research. In addition, some work from Eastern Europe (e.g., Mokran and Kramer, 1976) has suggested a link between parental excessive drinking and child sexual abuse.
4. Child and adolescent offspring of problem drinking parents are at a high risk for a range of impairments and problems, including developmental delays, learning difficulties and cognitive impairment, emotional problems manifesting as nervousness and physical disorders for which no medical causes can be found, antisocial behavior, and deliberate self-harm. There is widespread evidence from a number of countries concerning these increased risks (e.g., Matejcek, 1981*a,b*; Nylander, 1960; Boyadjieva, 1979; de Mendonca, 1976), although there is considerably more research on offspring with problem drinking fathers than there is on offspring with problem drinking mothers.
5. Offspring who had parents with drinking problems are probably more at risk for

> drinking and other problems as adults. The evidence for this statement comes from the occasional prospective follow-up study of offspring identified in childhood (Rydelius, 1981), retrospective studies of adults who have already developed problems (e.g., Cotton, 1979; Djukanovic et al., 1978) recent research on the responses to alcohol of young adult offspring of biological parents with alcoholism (e.g., Newlin, 1985; O'Malley and Maisto, 1985; Schuckit, 1984*a*), and adoption and twin studies (e.g., Bohman and Sigvardsson, 1980; Clifford et al., 1984). However, there are clearly complex interactions between adult drinking problems and problems of other kinds, including antisocial behavior, depression, anxiety states, and even schizophrenia (e.g., Pulkkinen, 1983; Lewis et al., 1983); there is evidence that the intergenerational transmission process may be different for women and men (e.g., Bourgeois and Penaud, 1976; Bevia, 1976); and some recent studies that have recruited adult offspring by such means as advertising (Velleman and Orford, 1984; Benson, 1980), or which have examined the fate of such offspring by examining publicly available records (Karlsson, 1985), have suggested that adult outcomes may not be particularly negative, and in some cases may be more than usually positive.

Although in the process of intergenerational transmission, the relative contributions made by genetic mechanisms, specific environmental effects (the transmission of attitudes toward drinking, for example), and general environmental processes (parental discord, lack of family cohesion, or child neglect, for example) are not clear, there is sufficient evidence to conclude that the sons and daughters of parents with drinking problems are at special risk at different points in their development and should be the targets of special attempts at prevention. There is also enough evidence to suggest that certain subgroups of offspring are particularly at risk: infants whose mothers drank excessively during pregnancy; young children and adolescents in families where there is violence; adolescent or young adult offspring who are already displaying excessive drinking, drug-taking, or antisocial behavior; and adults who were themselves physically abused or neglected as children.

Thought should be given to designing prevention programs in this area. These will presumably vary in nature, depending on local circumstances and customs, including the extent of development of health and education services in different parts of the world. However, this review as well as the author's earlier review (Orford, 1983*a*) has drawn attention to a number of general issues that need to be addressed in designing any prevention project in this field. One is whether offspring need to be reached directly, or whether they can be influenced by the successful treatment or education of their parents (Wells, 1984). A second question is whether such a project can reach its intended target? There is some evidence that self-help and other family approaches in the alcohol field may be reaching only higher-status groups (Galanter et al., 1984; Gorman and Rooney, 1979; Ablon, 1974). The capacity of different forms of intervention to reach members of different social status, religious, racial, and cultural groups within a country is an important issue. It seems likely that a single form of preventive intervention will have difficulty in reaching certain sections of the target population in a particular country, and that different forms of response will need to be designed for different groups. Interventions for immigrant and indigenous minority groups may need particularly careful thought.

Another general, and important, issue is the extent to which prevention projects in this field should be specialized (seeking to influence children of problem drinking parents in particular), and to what extent they should be nonspecialized in design and delivery. On the one hand, there is considerable evidence that the problems experienced by members of families where excessive drinking is a problem are not specific to such families, but are shared with other families in distress and disorder (Orford et al., 1976; Orford, 1975; Billings et al., 1979; Cork, 1969), and that many family alcohol problems present and can be effectively dealt with by nonspecialist agencies (e.g., DHSS, 1978; Orford, 1987*b*; Wilkins, 1974). On the other hand, a number of specialist projects, for reaching and helping child, adolescent, and adult offspring of problem drinking parents, have been described in the United States and in Eastern Europe (Ptacek, 1983; Moser, 1980; Seixas and Levitan, 1984). Careful thought should be given to the appropriateness of developing such projects in other parts of the world. In the earlier review (Orford, 1983*a*) the present author raised similar questions about whether alcohol-related family health education should be specialized or integrated with wider considerations, and whether preventive programs aimed at high-risk adolescents, for example, should be alcohol-specific or should be part of more general preventive and compensatory programs for young people at risk.

## Research and Intervention with Partners at Risk

Whether partners are viewed primarily as victims of the stress caused by the problem drinking of their spouses, or whether they are seen as part of an interacting family system in which excessive drinking serves a homeostatic or distress-signaling function, that partners of identified problem drinkers themselves experience high levels of distress and are at high risk for the development of psychological symptoms, and that their marriages are at high risk of breakdown, are all conclusions that are well established from research in Eastern and Western Europe, from North America, and to a lesser extent from elsewhere (e.g., Wiseman, 1976*a,b*; Kamien, 1975; Dahlgren, 1979; Hayashi, 1978; Sysenko, 1982). The present review has, nonetheless, highlighted a number of research and intervention issues that require attention in future work. These include the following:

1. The supposed link between excessive drinking and marital violence requires further exploration. Although there is convincing evidence that problem drinking in married men is associated with particularly high levels of marital violence (Gayford, 1975; Byles, 1978; van Hasselt et al., 1985; Velleman, 1987; Student and Matova, 1969), whether this association is due to a directly disinhibiting effect of alcohol or whether it is due to expectation or to the function of excessive drinking as an excuse for violence against women is not clear (Dobash and Dobash, 1987; Eberle, 1982; Room, undated).

2. The importance of partners' involvement in treatment for alcohol problems requires further confirmation. Although there is evidence that strongly suggests the importance of partners' involvement in treatment (e.g., Despotovic, 1974; Smith, 1969; Fridman et al., 1976), the possibility that the positive results obtained when partners are

involved are due to selection factors cannot be ruled out (Bromet and Moos, 1977; McCrady et al., 1979). In view of the important implications of this finding for service delivery in different parts of the world, it is important that it be confirmed.

3. Evidence is required on the applicability of different forms of family treatment for different countries. This review has shown that, among the many types of family treatment that have been applied to families with alcohol problems, three different foci receive differing degrees of attention. While some family treatments focus most on excessive drinking and its effects and control, others focus much more on family communication, conflict, and cohesion (Bennun, 1988; Waldo and Guerney, 1983; Dinaburg et al., 1977; Zweben and Pearlman, 1983). Both here and in the earlier review (Orford, 1983*a*), the present reviewer drew attention to innovative family treatment approaches that placed greater emphasis in a third direction. These were the interventions that Harwin (1982) referred to as "ecological," since they tended to involve socially or economically deprived groups, were more likely to make use of paraprofessional staff, and were more practical in their approach. In addition to counseling on excessive drinking and family communication, they involved advice and assistance on health and home and child care and advice and referral to other appropriate agencies on financial, legal, and welfare matters. The orientation of these interventions, coupled with the nonspecialized approach, might make them better candidates for use in nonindustrialized parts of the world. However, this presently remains an assumption and clearly requires putting to the test.

4. Interventions need to be developed that are targeted at partners whose problem drinking spouses are not in treatment. The present review has identified this as a gap in the delivery of professional services in the West (Harwin, 1982; Orford, 1983*a*; Gorman and Rooney, 1979; Ablon, 1974; Thomas and Santa, 1982). In the earlier review (Orford, 1983*a*) the development of recommendations about the most adaptive ways of coping with excessive drinking in the family, based on work using the Coping Questionnaire (Hayashi, 1978; Orford and Guthrie, 1976; Orford et al., 1975; James and Goldman, 1971; Schaffer and Tyler, 1979), was suggested as one potential way forward. The spread of Al-Anon and its adaptability to different cultural environments is another (Orford, 1983*a*; Gorman and Rooney, 1979; Ablon, 1974), as is the development of written self-help materials. This general line of intervention is given great encouragement by the development of ideas on unilateral family therapy (Thomas and Santa, 1982), and by the development of cooperative counseling in Newcastle, England (Yates and Thorley, 1988).

Once again, there are important general issues to do with reaching the intended high-risk group, and the balance of specialist and nonspecialist interventions. The possibility that nonspecialist social and health agencies might be most likely to be consulted by high-risk partners of problem drinkers was raised in the earlier review (Orford, 1983*a*), and further evidence has been presented in the present review (Roberts and Brent, 1982; Leckman et al., 1984; Roghmann et al., 1981; Wilkins, 1974; Ehline and Tighe, 1977). On this important point, the earlier review had this to say:

> A notion of a holistic, ecological or systems approach to family health is spelt out in a number of WHO papers (1979, 1980), as is the need to train workers in a family approach to care, and the need to integrate the family more into the health education process . . . (WHO, 1973). . . . there are disadvantages of viewing alcohol and the family as a topic

> separate from other aspects of family health and well-being. This question may become more salient when applications to developing countries are considered. (p. 119)

The integration of alcohol and the family studies into the mainstream of social and medical science, and the integration of treatment and prevention approaches for families troubled by excessive drinking into the wider field of family health and social care, may be the best ways of advancing this topic in the long run. An international perspective gives added strength to this point of view.

## ACKNOWLEDGMENTS

The writing of this review was supported by the World Health Organization, Division of Mental Health, Geneva, for whom it was prepared in 1986. I am particularly grateful to Dr. N. Sartorius and Mr. Marcus Grant for their support of this project at WHO. I would also like to thank several people who translated articles into English for me: K. Cutts (Spanish), M. Fry (Czech and Serbo-Croat), J. Proud (French), Z. Wavell and C. Yates (Russian), and K. Wright (German). I would also like to acknowledge the help received from Mr. David Salter at the University of Exeter, who carried out computer literature searches. Finally, considerable thanks are due to Liz Mears and Joan Fitzhenry, who undertook the arduous tasks of typing draft and final versions of the review and compiling the reference list.

## REFERENCES

Abelsohn, D. S., and van der Spuy, 1978, The age variable in alcoholism, *J. Stud. Alcohol,* **39:**800–808.

Ablon, J., 1974, Al-Anon family groups: Impetus for learning and change through the presentation of alternatives, *Am. J. Psychotherapy* **28:**30–45.

Ablon, J., 1979, Research frontiers for anthropologists in family studies. A case in point: Alcoholism and the family, *Hum. Org.* **38:**196–200.

Ablon, J., and Cunningham, W., 1981, Implications of cultural patterning for the delivery of alcoholism services: case studies, *J. Stud. Alcohol* (**Suppl. 9**)**:**185–206.

Acuda, W., 1983, Alcohol and rapid socio-economic change, in: *Drug Use and Misuse* (A. Arif and J. Jaffe, eds.), pp. 77–83, Croom Helm, London.

Acuda, S. W., 1985, International review series: Alcohol and alcohol problems research. 1. East Africa, *Br. J. Addict.* **80:**121–126.

Alvarez, M., and Wurgaft, B., 1982, Labor factors of the father (or head of household) and infant malnutrition in Santiago, Chile (Sp), *Int. Sociol. Assoc.,* Assoc. paper. (Abst. no. 122982 Sociol. Absts.)

Ammar, S., 1972, Epidemiological overview of mental illness in Tunisia: Clinical, statistical, and sociocultural study of the last decade (Fr), *Information Psychiat.* **48:**677–718. (Abst. no. 11237 Psycinfo.)

Andorka, R., Buda, B., and G-Kiss, J., 1970, Alcoholism and culture in Hungary (Fr), *Toxicomanies* **3:** 371–381. (Abst. no. 05127 Psycinfo.)

Angel, P., Taleghani, M., Choquet, M., and Courtecuisse, N., 1978, An epidemiological approach to suicide attempts by adolescents: Some answers from the environment (Fr), *Evolution Psychiatr.* **43:** 351–367. (Abst. no. 140586 Sociol. Absts.)

Antonov, I. P., and Shan'ko, G. G., undated, Convulsive states in children (Ru). (Abst. no. 05455 Psycinfo.)

Arkhipov, B. S., 1974, Sociological research in the work of the Oblast Party committee (Ru), *Sotsiol. Issledovaniya* **1:**110–116. (Abst. no. J4335-0 Sociol. Absts.)

Bach, O., Feldes, D., Kriegel, A., and Smolinsky, B., 1972, Group therapy with married couples (Ge), *Psychiatrie Neurol. Med. Psychol.* **24:**90–97. (Abst. no. 09462 Psycinfo.)

Bailey, M. B., 1967, Psychophysiological impairment in wives of alcoholics as related to their husbands' drinking and sobriety, in: *Alcoholism: Behavioral Research, Therapeutic Approaches* (R. Fox, ed.), pp. 134–144, Springer, New York.

Bailey, M. B., Haberman, P., and Alksne, H., 1962, Outcome of alcoholic marriages: Endurance, termination or recovery, *J. Stud. Alcohol* **23:**610–623.

Bales, R. F., 1962, Attitudes toward drinking in the Irish culture, in: *Society, Culture, and Drinking Patterns* (D. J. Pittman and C. R. Snyder, eds.), pp. 157–187, Wiley, New York.

Barrison, I. G., and Wright, J. T., 1984, Moderate drinking during pregnancy and foetal outcome, *Alcohol Alcoholism* **19:** 167–172.

Behling, D. W., 1979, Alcohol abuse as encountered in 51 instances of reported child abuse, *Clin. Pediatr. Phila.* **18:**87–91. (Abst., *J. Stud. Alcohol,* 1979, 40, 629.)

Bennett, L. A., and Ames, G. M., 1985, *The American Experience with Alcohol: Contrasting Cultural Perspectives.* Plenum Press, New York.

Bennun, I., 1985, Two approaches to family therapy with alcoholics: Problem-solving and systemic therapy, *J. Subst. Abuse Treatment* **2:**19–26.

Bennun, I., 1988, Treating the system or symptom: Investigating family therapy for alcohol problems, *Behav. Psychother.* **16:**165–176.

Benson, C. S., 1980, Coping and support among daughters of alcoholics. Unpublished Ph.D. thesis, Indiana University, Bloomington, IN.

Bevia, F. J. O., 1976, La familia de la mujer alcoholica, *Actas Luso-Espanolas Neurol. Psiquiatria Cliencias Afines* **4:**227–238. (Trans. into English for this review.)

Billings, A. G., and Moos, R. H., undated, Psychosocial processes of recovery among alcoholics and their families: Implications for clinicians and program evaluators. Unpublished paper. (Dept. of Psychiat. and Behav. Sciences, VA and Stanford Univ. Med. Center, Palo Alto, CA).

Billings, A. G., Kessler, M., Gonberg, C. A., and Weiner, S., 1979, Marital conflict resolution of alcoholic and non-alcoholic couples during drinking and non-drinking sessions, *J. Stud. Alcohol* **40:** 183–195.

Blane, H. T., and Barry, H., 1973, Birth order and alcoholism: A review, *Q. J. Stud. Alcohol* **34:**837–852.

Bohman, M., and Sigvardsson, S., 1980, Negative social heritage, *Adoption Fostering* **101:**25–31.

Bornstein, S., Martel, J., Ruat, A., and Harlay, A., 1980, Les auteurs de sevices a enfants (The perpetrators of maltreatment of children). *Ann. Med. Psychol.* **138:**930–952. (Abst. no. 69-03653 Psycinfo.)

Borzova, E., 1967–1968, Problems of mental development of children in the alcoholic family, *Psychol. Patopsychol. Dietata* **3:**153–160. (Abst. no. 11112 Psycinfo.)

Bourg, M., Vanhoove, D., Barreau, A., and Faidherbe, D., 1981, The wife of the alcoholic sailor: An ethno-socio-psychiatric study of alcoholism amongst Breton sailors (Fr), *Ann. Med.-Psychol.* **139:** 1014–1023. (Trans. into English for this review.)

Bourgeois, M., and Penaud, F., 1976, Alcoholism and depression: Statistical inquiry into familial antecedents of depression and alcoholism in a group of alcoholic men and depressed women (Fr), *Ann. Med.-Psychol.* **2:**686–699. (Abst. no. 01051 Psycinfo.)

Boyadjieva, M., 1979, *Crisis Situations in Youth.* Narodna Mladej, Sofia. (Cited by Boyadjieva, undated.)

Boyadjieva, M., undated, Alcoholism and the family: Review of the literature in some socialist countries. Prepared for WHO. (Dept. of Alcoholism, Sofia.)

Bozanov, A., 1980, Studies on tobacco smoking, alcohol and drug use and abuse among students from the upper school courses (Bul). *Hig. Zdraveopaz. (Bulgaria)* **23:**343–348. (Abst. no. 81075127 Excerpt. Med.)

Braconnier, A., and Olievenstein, C., 1974, Attempted suicide in actual drug addicts (Fr), *Rev. Neuro-psychiatrie Infantile Hyg. Ment. Enfance* **22**:677–693. (Abst. no. 04225 Psyinfo.)

Bradfer, J., 1974, Comparative study of therapeutic results and of clinical and psychosocial data from a medico-social guidance center for alcoholics (Fr), *Acta Psychiatr. Belg.* **74**:617–629. (Abst. no. 08473 Psycinfo.)

Bradford, D. E., 1984, Alcohol and the young child, *Alcohol Alcoholism* **19**:173–175.

Brennenstuhl, W., and Wielguszewski, J., 1980, Psychotherapia rodzinna w poradiu alwykowej. *Problemy Alkoholizmy* **27**:10, 5–6 (cited by Boyadjieva, undated.)

Bresard, M., and Chabert, C., 1974, Diet and way of life of a group of secondary schoolchildren in Marseilles (Fr), *Cahiers Nutrit Dietet.* **9**:75–95. (Abst. no. 474701 CAB Absts.)

Bromet, E., and Moos, R. H., 1977, Environmental resources and the post-treatment functioning of alcoholic patients, *J. Health Soc. Behav.* **18**:326–338.

Bujdoso, G., Bergou, J., and Somogyi, E., 1980, Health damage in children of parents with chronic alcoholism: data from an anthropologic study (Hu), *Morphol. Igazsagugyi Orv.* **20**:30–35. (Abst. no. 80112287 Excerpt. Med.)

Burns, A., 1984, Perceived causes of marriage breakdown and conditions of life, *J. Marriage Fam.* **46**: 551–562.

Burton, G., and Kaplan, H. M., 1968, Group counselling in conflicted marriages where alcoholism is present: clients' evaluation of effectiveness, *J. Marriage Fam.* **30**:74–79.

Butorina, N. E., Movchan, N. G., Kazakov, V. S., and Rybakova, L. P., 1978, Traits of initial symptoms of alcoholism in adolescents: Sociopsychological and clinical aspects (Ru), *Nevropatol. Psikhiat. Im. S. S. Korsakova (USSR)* **78**:1569–1572. (Abst. no. 79051611 Excerpt. Med.)

Byles, J. A., 1978, Violence, alcohol problems and other problems in disintegrating families, *J. Stud. Alcohol* **39**:551–553.

Byron and Blight. Source unknown. Abstract available in Psyinfo, Dec. 1981.

Cadogan, D. A., 1973, Marital group therapy in the treatment of alcoholism, *Q. J. Stud. Alcohol* **34**: 1187–1194.

Carstairs, S., 1954, Daru and bhang: Cultural factors in the choice of intoxicant, *Q. J. Stud. Alcohol,* **15**: 220–237.

Cassorla, R. M., 1984, Family characteristics of youngsters attempting suicide in Campinas, Brazil: a comparative study with normal and psychiatric youngsters (Port), *Acta Psiquiatr. Psicol. Am. Lat.* **30**:125–134. (Abst. no. 1696578 Medline.)

Chanfreau, D., Furhmann, I., Lokare, V. G., and Montoya, C., 1979, Drinking behaviour of children in Santiago, Chile, *J. Stud. Alcohol* **40**:918–922.

Christozov, C., and Mumdzieva, D., 1978, Suicide: A problem in early childhood, *Pediatriya (Sofia)* **17**:526–532. (Abst. no. 79077301 Excerpt. Med.)

Christozov, C., Achkova, M., and Shoilekova, M., 1978, Psychological transformation of the father's alcoholism into the picture of child neuroses, in: *Alcoholism and Smoking,* (A. Maleev, ed.), Medizina & Fizkultura, pp. 93–97 (cited by Boyadjieva, undated.)

Clifford, C. A., Hopper, J. L., Fulker, D. W., and Murray, R. M., 1984, A genetic and environmental analysis of a twin family study of alcohol use, anxiety, and depression, *Genet. Epidemiol.* **1**:63–79.

Cmelic, S., and Brankovic, M., 1982, Da li je alkoholizam hereditarno oboljenje? (Se-Cr), *Soc. Psihijat.* **10**:57–60. (English Abst.)

Cochrane, R., 1983, *The Social Creation of Mental Illness,* Longman, London.

Collins, E., and Turner, G., 1978, Six children affected by maternal alcoholism, *Med. J. Aust.* **2**:14, 606–608.

Collins, G. B., Kotz, M., Janesz, J. W., et al., 1985, Alcoholism in the families of bulimic anorexics, *Cleveland Clin. Q.* **52**:65–67. (Abst. no. 85127493 Excerpt. Med.)

Combes, J. C., Bosvieux, G., Aumeras, C., et al., 1980, Fetal alcohol syndrome (Fr), *Ann. pediatr.* **27**: 527–530. (Abst. no. 81002572 Excerpt. Med.)

Connolly, K., 1985, Can there be a psychology for the Third World? *Bull. Br. Psychol. Soc.* **38**:249–257.

Cook, B. L., and Winokur, G., 1985, A family study of familial positive vs. familial negative alcoholics, *J. Nerv. Ment. Dis.* **173**:175. (Abst. no. 1608597 Medline.)

Corder, B. F., Corder, R. F., and Laidlaw, N. D., 1972, An intensive treatment program for alcoholics and their wives, *Q. J. Stud. Alcohol,* **33:**1144–1146.

Cork, R. M., 1969, *The Forgotten Children: A Study of Children with Alcoholic Parents,* Alcoholism and Drug Addiction Research Foundation of Ontario, Toronto.

Costello, R. M., 1980, Alcoholism treatment effectiveness: Slicing the outcome of variance pie, in: *Alcoholism Treatment in Transition.* (G. Edwards and M. Grant, eds.), pp. 113–127, Croom Helm, London.

Cotton, N. S., 1979, The familial incidence of alcoholism: A review, *J. Stud. Alcohol,* **40:**89–116.

Dahlgren, L., 1979, Female alcoholics. IV. Marital situations and husbands, *Acta Psychiatr. Scand.* **59:** 59–69.

Davies, J. B., 1982, The transmission of alcohol problems in the family, in: *Alcohol and the Family* (J. Orford and J. Harwin, eds.), Croom Helm, London.

Davis, T. S., and Hagood, L., 1979, In-home support for recovering alcoholic mothers and their families: The family rehabilitation co-ordination project, *J. Stud. Alcohol* **40:**313–317.

de Mendonca, M. M., 1976, Etude pedopsychiatrique sur des enfants de pere alcoolique, *Rev. Neuro-psychiatr. Infantile* **25:**411–428. (Trans. into English for this review.)

de Silva, P., 1983, The Buddhist attitude to alcoholism, in: *Drug Use and Misuse* (G. Edwards, A. Arif, and J. Jaffe, eds.), pp. 33–41, Croom Helm, London.

de Vanna, M., and Fracasso, G., 1979, Il rischio di morbilita specifico in figli di psicotici alcoolisti, *Minerva Psichiatr.* **20:**165–168. (English Sum.)

Department of Health and Social Security, 1978, Pattern and Range of Services for Problem Drinkers: Report of an Advisory Committee, Her Majesty's Stationery Office, London.

Deraeck, G., 1982, Alcohol consumption by adolescents in their free time (Du), *Sec. J. Source: Redoc* **15:**82. (Abst. no. 1702482 CAB Absts.)

Desai, I. D., Garcia Tavares, M. L., Dutra de Oliveira, B. S., Douglas, A., Duarte, F. A. M., and Dutra de Oliveira, J. E., 1980, Food habits and nutritional status of agricultural migrant workers in Southern Brazil, *Am. J. Clin. Nutr.* **33:**702–714. (Abst. no. 1215157 CAB Absts.)

Despotovic, A., 1974, Alcoholism, drug addiction and the family (Se-Cr), *Psihijatrija Danas* **6:**191–202. (Trans. into English for this review.)

Dicicco, L., Davis, R., and Orenstein, A., 1984, Identifying the children of alcoholic parents from survey responses, *J. Alcohol Drug. Educ.* **30:**1–17.

Dinaburg, D., Glick, I. D., and Feigenbaum, E., 1977, Marital therapy of women alcoholics, *J. Stud. Alcohol* **38:**1247–1258.

Djukanovic, B., Fridman, V., Milosavljevic, V., Vasev, C., and Ljububratic, D., 1978, Les familles parentales des alcooliques et de leurs epouses, *Rev. Alcoolisme* **24:**245–250. (Trans. into English for this review.)

Dobash, R. E., and Dobash, R. P., 1987, Violence towards wives, in: *Coping with Disorder in the Family* (J. Orford, eds.), Croom Helm, London.

Dobash, R. E., Dobash, R. P., Cavanagh, C., and Wilson, M., 1977–1978, Wife beating: The victims speak, *Victimology: Int. J.* **2:**608–622.

Dordevic, M., and Dukanovic, B., 1974, Effect of alcoholism on emotional relations in the family (Se-Cr), *Sociologija* **16:**473–488. (Trans. into English for this review.)

Dorschner, J., 1983, Rajput alcohol use in India, *J. Stud. Alcohol* **44:**538–544.

Drecka, M., Mazurczak, M., and Puzynska, E., 1976, Psychiatric and psychological characteristics of children remaining in the child custody center in Warsaw (Pol), *Psychiatria Polska* **10:**403–412. (Abst. no. 12476 Psycinfo.)

Duche, D., et al., 1974, Attempts at suicide by adolescents (Fr), *Rev. Neuropsychiatrie Infantile Hyg. Ment. Enfance* **22:**639–656. (Abst. no. 04232 Psycinfo.)

Eberle, P. A., 1982, Alcohol abusers and non-users: A discriminant function analysis of differences between two sub-groups of batterers, *J. Health Soc. Behav.* **23:**260–271.

Edwards, G. T., 1985, Appalachia: The effects of cultural values on the production and consumption of alcohol, in: Bennett and Ames (1985, Ref. 51*a*).

Ehline, D., and Tighe, P. O., 1977, Alcoholism: Early identification and intervention in the social service agency, *Child Welfare* **56:**584–592.

el-Guebaly, N., and Offord, D., 1977, The offspring of alcoholics: A critical review, *Am. J. Psychiatry* **134**:357–365.

el-Guebaly, N., and Offord, D., 1979, On being the offspring of an alcoholic: An update, *Alcoholism: Clin. Exp. Res.* **3**:148–157.

Elmasian, R., Neville, H., Woods, D., et al., 1982, Event-related brain potentials are different in individuals at high and low risk for developing alcoholism, *Proc. Natl. Acad. Sci. USA* **79**:241. (Abst. no. 83076337 Excerpt. Med.)

Ervin, C. S., Little, R. E., Streissguth, A. P., and Beck, D. E., 1984, Alcoholic fathering and its relation to child's intellectual development: A pilot investigation, *Alcoholism: Clin. Exp. Res.* **8**: 362–365.

Esquef, L. de, 1972, Dietary habits of the peasant of the Bolivian Highlands, *Nutr. Newsletter* **10**:16–20. (Abst. no. 070076 CAB Absts.)

Ewing, J. A., Long, V., and Wenzel, G. G., 1961, Concurrent group psychotherapy of alcoholic patients and their wives, *Int. J. Group Psychother.* **11**:329–338.

Falcon, J., Domenech, E., Bueno, A., and Moya, M., 1980, Foetal, alcoholic syndrome: Study of three sisters, two of whom are twins (Sp), *Rev. Esp. Pediat.* **36**(211):35–42. (Abst. no. 80165071, Excerpt. Med.)

Fanai, F., 1969, Progress and prognosis of degeneration: Catamnesis of adolescents with disturbed social behavior, *Psychiatria Clin.* **2**:1–13. (Abst. no. 10815 Psycinfo.)

Farkasinszky, T., et al., 1973, Entwicklungsstorungen den Personlichkeit bei Kindern Alkoholiker, *Alcoholism* **9**:3–8. (Cited by Boyadjieva, undated.)

Fiallo, S. A., Rolando, C. H., Olive, G. E., and Perez, M. J., 1979, Psychological and social aspects in alcoholism (Sp), *Rev. Hosp. Psiquiat. Habana* **20**:51–61. (Abst. no. 79215720 Excerpt. Med.)

Figueroa-Rosales, R., 1971, Alcoholism and its relation to aspects of social and community development, *Rev. Med. Psicol.* **6**:244–250. (Trans. into English for this review.)

Finney, J. W., Moos, R. H., Cronkite, R. C., and Gamble, W., 1983, A conceptual model of the functioning of married persons with impaired partners: Spouses of alcoholic patients, *J. Marriage Fam.* **45**:23–34.

Fitze, F., Spahr, A., and Pescia, G., 1978, Fetal alcohol syndrome: Follow-up of a family (Ge), *Praxis* **67**(37):1338–1354. (Abst. no. 78404721 Excerpt. Med.)

Folkman, S., and Lazarus, R. S., 1980, An analysis of coping in a middle-aged community sample, *J. Health Soc. Behav.* **21**:219–239.

Fontane, P. E., and Layne, N. R., 1977, The family as a context for developing youthful drinking patterns. Series: MISSA 0021. (Abst. no. 57301-0 Sociol. Absts.)

Freiovai, E., 1966, Alcoholism of parents and moral impairment of school-age youngsters, *Czeskoslovenskai Psychiatrie* **62**:188–192. (Abst. no. 12134 Psycinfo.)

Freund, P. J., 1985, Polish American drinking: Continuity and change, in: Bennett and Ames (1985, Ref. 51*a*).

Fridman, V., Fligic, M., and Petrovic, D., 1976, The role of wives in the development of positive treatment motivation (Yug), *Socijalna Psihijatrija* **4**:301–308. (Abst. no. 10089 Psycinfo.)

Frigault, J. A., 1979, Evaluation of the nature and extent of the alcoholism problem in the Acadian Peninsula (Fr), *Toxicomanies (Canada)* **12**:65–76. (Abst. no. 80036369 Excerpt. Med.)

Gacic, B., 1978, General system theory and alcoholism (Se-Cr), *Psihijatrija Danas (Yugoslavia)* **10**: 309–316. (Abst. no. 79156443 Excerpt. Med.)

Gacic, B., 1980, Experiences in evaluation of the family therapy of alcoholism: the Institute for Mental Health in Belgrade. Paper presented at 26th International Institute on the Prevention and Treatment of Alcoholism, Cardiff. (Center for Family Therapy and Alcoholism, Institute for Mental Health, Belgrade.)

Gacic, B., Sedmak, T., Ivanovic, M., Gardinovacki, I., and Gacic, R., 1980, Familial treatment of alcoholism as a modality of psychiatry in the community, *Toxicomanies* **13**:217–224. (Abst. no. 1169418 Social Scisearch.)

Galanter, M., Gleaton, T., Marcus, C. E., and McMillen, J., 1984, Self help groups for parents of young drug and alcohol abusers, *Am. J. Psychiatry* **141**:889–891.

Gallant, D. M., Rich, A., Bey, E., and Terranova, L., 1970, Group psychotherapy with married couples: A successful technique in New Orleans alcoholism clinic patients, *J. Louisiana State Med. Soc.*

Gayford, J. J., 1975, Wife battering: A preliminary study of 100 cases, *Br. Med. J.* **1:**194–197.

Gerkowicz, T., 1976, Wplyw alkoholizmu rozicow na zdrowie dziecka (Pol), *Problem Alcoholizmy* **23:** 7–8. (Cited by Boyadjieva, undated.)

Gilbert, M. J., 1985, Mexican–Americans in California: Intracultural variation in attitudes and behavior related to alcohol, in: Bennett and Ames (1985, Ref. 51*a*).

Glatt, M. M., 1973, Jewish alcoholics and addicts in the London area (Fr), *Toxicomanies* **6:**33–39. (Abst. no. 01207 Psycinfo.)

Gliedman, L. H., Rosenthal, D., Frank, J. D., and Nash, H. T., 1956, Group therapy of alcoholics with concurrent group meeting of their wives, *Q. J. Stud. Alcohol* **17:**655–670.

Goodwin, D. W., 1979, The cause of alcoholism and why it runs in families, *Br. J. Addict.* **74:**161–164.

Goodwin, D. W., 1984, Studies of familial alcoholism: A review, *J. Clin. Psychiatry* **45:**14–17.

Goodwin, D. W., Schulsinger, F., Hermansen, L., Guze, S. B., and Winokur, G., 1973, Alcohol problems in adoptees raised apart from alcoholic biological parents, *Arch. Gen. Psychiatry* **28:**238–243.

Goodwin, D. W., Schulsinger, F., Moller, N., Hermansen, L., Winokur, G., and Guze, S. B., 1974, Drinking problems in adopted and nonadopted sons of alcoholics, *Arch. Gen. Psychiatry* **31:**164–169.

Goodwin, D. W., Schulsinger, F., Knop, J., Mednick, S., and Guze, S. B., 1977, Alcoholism and depression in adopted-out daughters of alcoholics, *Arch. Gen. Psychiatry* **34:**1005–1009.

Gorman, J. M., and Rooney, J. F., 1979, The influence of Al-Anon on the coping behaviour of wives of alcoholics, *J. Stud. Alcohol* **40:**1030–1038.

Gostomzyk, J. G., 1977, Kindermisshandlung [child abuse], *Off. Gesundh. Es.* **39:**279–288. (Abst. no. 78092111 Excerpt. Med.)

Graves, T. D., 1967, Acculturation, access, and alcohol in a tri-ethnic community, *Am. Anthropol.* **69:** 306–321.

Grcic, R., Kastel, P., Bonevic, K., and Kacarevic, R., 1981, Therapy of dependent diseases: Adolescent alcoholism (Se-Cr), *Psihijatrija Danas* **13:**117–123. (Abst. no. 68-08365 Psycinfo.)

Guerdjikova, Z., 1984, Social consequences of problem drinking in women, Bulletin NINPN, Sofia, (in press). (Cited by Boyadjieva, undated.)

Guntern, G., 1975, Changement social et consommation d'alcool dans un village de montagne, *Schweiz. Arch. Neurol. Neurochir. Psychiatrie* **116:**353–411. (English sum.)

Gupta, B., and Mwambe, A., 1976, Study of malnourished children in Tanga, Tanzania. I. Socioeconomic and cultural aspects, *J. Trop. Pediatr. Environ. Child Health* **22:**268–273.

Gutschmidt, G., and Maag, F., 1978, Alcoholism in professional drivers (Ge), *Z. Unfallmed. Berufsk. (Switzerland)* **71:**92–96. (Abst. no. 79008586 Excerpt. Med.)

Hagaman, B. L., 1980, Food for thought: Beer in a social and ritual context in a West African society, *J. Drug Issues* **10:**203–214.

Hansen, D., 1978, Family therapy for alcoholic parents, Borjeson, B. book review (Sw), *Nordisk Psykologi* **30:**272–274. (Citation no. 882445 Social Scisearch.)

Harwin, J., 1982, Alcohol, the family and treatment, in: *Alcohol and the Family* (J. Orford and J. Harwin, eds.), Croom Helm, London.

Hayashi, S., 1978, Alcoholism and marriage: Family court divorce conciliation, *Jpn. J. Stud. Alcohol* **13:**177–190.

Hedberg, A. G., and Campbell, L., 1974, A comparison of four behavioural treatments of alcoholism, *J. Behav. Ther. Exp. Psychiatry* **5:**251–256.

Hedlund, H., and Lundahl, M., 1984, The economic role of beer in rural Zambia, *Hum. Org.* **32:**61–65.

Hedri, A., 1971, Marital crises in prosperous families (Ge), *Ztschr. Psychother. Med. Psychol.* **21:**35–38. (Abst. no. 08855 Psycinfo.)

Hegedus, A., Alterman, A., and Tarter, R., 1984, Learning achievement in sons of alcoholics, *Alcoholism: Clin. Exp. Res.* **8:**330–333.

Helgason, T., and Asmundsson, G., 1975, Behaviour and social characteristics of young asocial alcohol abusers, *Neuropsychobiology (Switzerland)* **1**(2):109–120. (Abst. no. 76136151 Excerpt. Med.)
Hell, D., Battegay, R., Muhlemann, R., and Dillinger, A., 1976, How alcohol and drug consumers see themselves: a personal and social self-assessment (Ge), *Arch. Psychiatr. Nervenk.* **221**:345–360. (English sum.)
Hemmer, C., 1979, The problem of alcoholism from the viewpoint of a communication theory approach (Ge), *Soziologenkorrespondenz* **6**:71–91. (Abst. no. 138961 Sociol. Absts.)
Henle, I., 1977, The tragedy of the Labdakides: unescapable fate of an alcohol diseased family? (Ge), *Praxis Kinderpsychol. Kinderpsychiatrie* **26**:46–52. (Abst. no. 03956 Psycinfo.)
Hennecke, L., 1984, Stimulus augmenting and field dependence in children of alcoholic fathers, *J. Stud. Alcohol* **45**:486–492.
Hindman, M., 1975–1976, Children of alcoholic parents, *Alcohol Health Res. World* Winter:2–6.
Homonoff, E., and Stephen, A., 1979, Alcohol education for children of alcoholics in a Boston neighborhood, *J. Stud. Alcohol* **40**:923–926.
Hughes, J., Stewart, M., and Barraclough, B., 1985, Why teetotallers abstain, *Br. J. Psychiatry* **146**: 204–205.
Hunt, G., and Satterlee, S., 1985, The pub, the village and the people, *New Directions Study Alcohol Group* **8**:18–54.
Hunt, G. M., and Azrin, N. H., 1973, A community reinforcement approach to alcoholism, *Behav. Res. Ther.* **11**:91–104.
Ishihara, T., and Ikegawa, S., 1974, Family structure associated with offense in brothers and sisters (Ja), *Jpn. J. Crim. Psychol.* **10**:41–52. (Abst. no. 01274 Psycinfo.)
Jackson, J. K., 1954, The adjustment of the family to the crisis of alcoholism, *J. Stud. Alcohol* **15**:562–586.
Jackson, J. K., and Kogan, K. L., 1963, The search for solutions: Help-seeking patterns of families of active and inactive alcoholics, *J. Stud. Alcohol* **24**:449–472.
Jacob, T., 1988, Alcoholism and family interaction: Clarifications resulting from subgroup analyses and multi-method assessments, in: *Understanding Major Mental Disorder* (M. K. Hahlweg and M. J. Goldstein, eds.), Family Process Press, New York.
Jacob, T., and Seilhamer, R. A., 1982, The impact on spouses and how they cope, in: *Alcohol and the family* (J. Orford and J. Harwin, eds.), Croom Helm, London.
Jacob, T., Ritchey, D., Cvitkovic, J. F., and Blane, H. T., 1981, Communication styles of alcoholic and non-alcoholic families when drinking and not drinking, *J. Stud. Alcohol* **42**:466–482.
Jahoda, G., and Crammond, J., 1972, *Children and Alcohol: A Developmental Study in Glasgow*, Her Majesty's Stationary Office, London.
James, J., and Goldman, M., 1971, Behaviour trends of wives of alcoholics, *Q. J. Stud. Alcohol* **32**: 378–381.
Janzen, C., 1977, Families in the treatment of alcoholism, *J. Stud. Alcohol* **38**:114–130.
Jenner, C., 1978, On the development of alcoholism among young people and women (Ge), *Osterr. Arzteztg.* **33**:693–696. (Trans. into English for this review.)
Jessor, R., and Jessor, S., 1977, *Problem Behavior and Psycho-social Development. A Longitudinal Study of Youth*, Academic Press, New York.
Johnson, R. C., Nagoshi, C. T., Schwitters, S. Y., Bowman, K. S., Ahern, F. M., and Wilson, J. R., 1984, Further investigation of racial/ethnic differences and of familial resemblances in flushing in response to alcohol, *Behav. Genet.* **14**:171–178. (Abst. no. 1497353 Medline.)
Kaij, L., 1960, Studies on the etiology and sequels of abuse of alcohol. Thesis, University of Lund, Sweden.
Kamien, M., 1975, Aborigines and alcohol, *Med. J. Aust.* **1**:291–298.
Kammeier, M., 1971, Adolescents from families with and without alcohol problems, *Q. J. Stud. Alcohol* **32**:364–372.
Kandic, B., Jovicevic, M., and Vujosevic, K., 1969, Forensic and psychiatric aspects of expertise of military personnel delinquency performed in the state of acute drunkenness (Se-Cr), *Vojnosanitetski Pregled* **26**:227–230. (Abst. no. 16924 Psycinfo.)

Kapor, G., Vujosevic, K., and Brankovic, M., 1974, Sociomedical factors influencing resignations from the army (Se-Cr), *Vojnosanitetski Pregled* **31:**79–83. (Abst. no. 04215 Psycinfo.)

Karlsson, J., 1985, Mental characteristics of families with alcoholism in Iceland, *Hereditas* **102:**185–188.

Kattan, L., et al., 1973, Characteristics of alcoholism in women and evaluation of its treatment in Chile (Sp), *Acta Psiquiatrica Psicol. Am. Lat.* **19:**194–204. (Abst. no. 11368 Psycinfo.)

Kaufman, E., 1980, Myth and reality in the family patterns and treatment of substance abusers, *Am. J. Drug. Alcohol Abuse* **7:**257–279.

Kaufman, E., and Pattison, E. M., 1981, Differential methods of family therapy in the treatment of alcoholism, *J. Stud. Alcohol* **42:**951–971.

Keane, A., and Roche, D., 1974, Developmental disorders in the children of male alcoholics, in: *Proceedings of 20th International Institute on the Prevention and Treatment of Alcoholism, Manchester,* ICAA, Lausanne.

Kephart, W. M., 1954, Drinking and marital disruption: A research note, *Q. J. Stud. Alcohol* **15:**63–73.

Khan, A., and Gupta, B., 1979, A study of children in Children's Hospital, Lusaka, *J. Trop. Pediatr. Environ. Child Health* **25:**42–45.

Kluge, K. J., and Strassburg, B., 1981, Alcohol abuse in adolescents: A means of discarding inhibitions (Ge), *Praxis Kinderpsychol. Kinderpsychiatrie* **30:**24–32. (Trans. into English for this review.)

Knop, J., Teasdale, T. W., Schulsinger, F., and Goodwin, D. W., 1985, A prospective study of young men at high risk for alcoholism: School behavior and achievement, *J. Stud. Alcohol* **46:**273–278.

Koch, H. L., 1956, Some emotional attitudes of the young child in relation to the characteristics of his siblings, *Child Dev.* **27:**393–426.

Kogan, K. L., and Jackson, J. K., 1965, Some concomitants of personal difficulties in wives of alcoholics and non-alcoholics, *J. Stud. Alcohol* **26:**595–604.

Komorowska, J., 1980, Feasting now and in the past, *Przeglad. Socjologiczny* **32:**181–195. (Abst. no. 135894 Sociol. Absts.)

Kosten, T. R., Rounaville, B. J., and Kleber, H. D., 1985, Parental alcoholism in opioid addicts, *J. Nerv. Ment. Dis.* **173:**461. (Abst. no. 1738621 Medline.)

Kozakiewicz, M., 1982, The rural woman and social change (Pol), *Wies Wspolczesna* **26:**73–82. (Abst. no. 1711105 CAB Absts.)

Koznar, J., Matijek, G., and Uhrova, A., 1979, Results of retrospective study of the family conditions of problem children in counselling (Cz), *Ceskoslovenska Psychol.* **23:**365–374. (Abst. no. 03350 Psycinfo.)

Kreutzer, J., et al., 1984, Alcohol, aggression and assertiveness in men: Dosage and expectancy effects, *J. Stud. Alcohol* **45:**275.

Laszlo, C., 1970, The internalization of deviant behaviour patterns during socialization in the family (Hu), *Demografia* **13:**386–393. (Abst. no. 10221-0 Sociol. Absts.)

Latcham, R. W., 1985, Familial alcoholism; evidence from 237 alcoholics, *Br. J. Psychiatry* **147:**54–57.

Laudinet, S., and Kohler, C., 1970, New reflections on the descent of alcoholic parents (Fr), *Psychiatrie Enfant* **13:**273–305.

Lazic, N., 1977, A systematic approach to solving the problem of an "unending struggle" between marital partners, *Psihijatrija Danas (Yugoslavia)* **9:**449–457. (Abst. no. 05577 Psycinfo.)

Leckman, A. L., Umland, B. E., and Blay, M., 1984, Alcoholism in the families of family practice outpatients, *J. Fam. Pract.* **19:**205–207.

Leland, J., 1982, Sex roles, family organisation and alcohol abuse, in: *Alcohol and the Family* (J. Orford and J. Harwin, eds.), Croom Holm, London.

Lemert, E. M., 1962, Dependency in married alcoholics, *J. Stud. Alcohol* **23:**590–609.

Levinger, G., 1965, Marital cohesiveness and dissolution: An integrative review, *J. Marriage Fam.* **27:**19–28.

Lewis, C. E., Rice, J., and Helzer, J. E., 1983, Diagnostic interactions: Alcoholism and antisocial personality, *J. Nerv. Ment. Dis.* **171:**105–113.

Little, R. E., Streissguth, A. P., and Guzinski, G. M., 1980, Prevention of fetal alcohol syndrome: A model program, *Alcoholism* **4:**185–189.

Lobos, R., 1971, Sociopsychiatric aspects of marital troubles (Ge), *Schweiz. Arch. Neurol. Neurochir. Psychiatrie* **109:**367–397. (Abst. no. 04697 Psycinfo.)

Loranger, A. W., and Tulis, E. H., 1985, Family history of alcoholism in borderline personality disorder, *Arch. Gen. Psychiatry* **42:**153. (Abst. no. 85148359 Medline.)

Lothian Regional Social Work Department, 1981, Alcohol-related problems in current social work cases. Unpublished paper, Social Work Dept., Edinburgh.

Lund, C., and Landesman-Dwyer, S., 1979, Pre-delinquent and disturbed adolescents: The role of parental alcoholism, in: *Currents in Alcoholism* (M. Galanter, ed.) Grune & Stratton, New York. (Cited by Goodwin (216).)

Lutz, M., Appelt, H., and Cohen, R., 1980, Belastungsfaktoren in den Familien alkoholkranker und depressiver Frauen aus der Sicht der Ehemanner [Distress factors in the families of alcoholic and depressive women from the point of view of the husbands], *Social Psychiat.* **15:**137–144. (Trans. into English for this review.)

MacAndrew, C., and Edgerton, R., 1970, *Drunken Comportment: A Social Explanation,* Nelson, London.

Maccoby, M., 1966, War between the sexes in a Mexican rural community, *Rev. Psicoanal. Psiquiatriia Psicol.* **4:**54–76. (Abst. no. 02436 Psycinfo.)

Machova, J., and Gutvirth, J., 1981, Family environment of special school children (Cz), *Psychol. Patopsychol. Dietata* **16:**352–360. (Abst. no. 68-03769 Psycinfo.)

Mader, R., 1972, Alcoholism in adolescent criminals: A comparative study from 1965/66 to 1969/70, *Acta Paedopsychiatr.* **39:**2–11. (Abst. no. 01306 Psycinfo.)

Majewksi, F., Bierich, J. R., and Seidenberg, J., 1978, Incidence and pathogenesis of alcoholic embryopathy (Ge), *Monatsschr. Kinderheilkunde* **126:**284–285. (Abst. no. 989279 CAB Absts.)

Malhotra, M. K., 1976, Alkohol bei Schulern im Kreis Mettmann, in: *Offentliches Gesundheitswesen, 1976,* pp. 226–245. (Cited by Kluge and Strassburg (284).)

Marcelli, D., 1978, Suicidal attempts of the child: Statistical and general epidemiological aspects (Fr), *Acta Paedopsychiatr.* **43:**213–221. (Abst. no. 05661 Psycinfo.)

Matakas, F., Koester, H., and Leidner, B., 1978, Which treatment for which alcoholics? A review (Ge), *Psychiatr. Prax.* **5:**143–152. (Abst. no. 78395026 Excerpt. Med.)

Matejcek, Z., 1981*a*, Children in families of alcoholics. I. The rearing situation (Cz), *Psychol. Patopsychol. Dietata* **16:**303–318. (Trans. into English for this review.)

Matejcek, Z., 1981*b*, Children in families of alcoholics. II. Competency in school and peer group (Cz), *Psychol. Patopsychol. Dietata* **16:**537–560. (Trans. into English for this review.)

McCord, W., and McCord, J., 1960, *Origins of Alcoholism,* Stanford University Press, Stanford, CA.

McCrady, B. S., Paolino, T. J., Longabough, R., and Rossi, J., 1979, Effects of joint hospital admission and couples treatment for hospitalized alcoholics: A pilot study, *Addict. Behav.* **4:**155–165.

Meeks, D. E., and Kelly, C., 1970, Family therapy with the families of recovering alcoholics, *Q. J. Stud. Alcohol* **31:**339–413.

Menaghan, E., 1982, Measuring coping effectiveness: A panel analysis of marital problems and coping efforts, *J. Health Soc. Behav.* **23:**220–234.

Merikangas, K. R., Leckman, J. F., Prusoff, B. A., Pauls, E. L., and Weissman, M. M., 1985, Familial transmission of depression and alcoholism, *Arch. Gen. Psychiatry* **42:**367–372. (Abst. no. 1623383 Medline.)

Meskova, H., Mecir, J., and Pihrtova, S., 1978, Paternal element in boys treated at the antialcoholic clinic in Prague (Cz), *Cesk. Psychiatr.* **74:**402–405. (Part trans. into English for this review.)

Midanik, L., 1983, Familial alcoholism and problem drinking in a national drinking practices survey, *Addict. Behav.* **8:**133–141.

Miller, D., and Jang, M., 1977, Children of alcoholics: A 20 year longitudinal study, *Social Work Res. Abst.* **13:**23–29.

Moghaddam, F. M., and Taylor, D. M., 1986, The state of psychology in the Third World: A response to Connolly, *Bull. Br. Psychol. Soc.* **39**:4–7.

Mohan, D., Prabhakar, A. K., Mohun, M., and Chitkara, 1978, Factors associated with the prevalence of drug abuse among Delhi university students, *Indian J. Psychiatry* **20**:332–338.

Mokran, A., and Kramer, R., 1976, Incest and incestuous behaviour in forensic practices (Cz), *Ceskoslovenska Psychiatrie* **72**:320–323. (Abst. no. 13885 Psycinfo.)

Moos, R. D., and Moos, B. S., undated, The process of recovery from alcoholism comparing family functioning in alcoholic and matched control families, Unpublished manuscript, Department of Psychiatry and Behavioral Sciences, VA, and Stanford University Medical Center, Palo Alto, California.

Morales Bedoya, A., and Atilano Vergara, J., 1977, A survey of drug dependence in the student population of Barranquilla (Sp), *Rev. Colombiana Psiquiatria* **6**:276–296. (Abst. no. 13601 Psycinfo.)

Moser, J., 1980, *Prevention of Alcohol-Related Problems: An International Review of Preventive Measures, Policies, and Programmes,* Alcoholism and Drug Addiction Research Foundation, Toronto.

Moullembe, A., et al., 1973, Essay on suicide: A theoretical and a clinical approach (Fr), *Bull. Psychol.* **27**:804–943. (Abst. no. 09861 Psycinfo.)

Murata, T., et al., 1976, A case report and conference discussion concerning a boy suffering from a psychogenic psychosis (Ja), *Jpn. J. Child Psychiatry* **17**:223–235. (Abst. no. 1381 Psycinfo.)

Murray, R. M., and Stabenau, J. R., 1982, Genetic factors in alcoholism predisposition, in: *Encyclopedic Handbook of Alcoholism* (E. M. Pattison and E. Kaufman, eds.), pp. 135–144. Gardner Press, New York.

Nedoma, K., Mellan, J., and Pondelickova, J., 1969, Incest pedophiliac delinquency, *Ceskoslovenska Psychiatrie* **65**:224–229. (Abst. no. 16958 Psycinfo.)

Newlin, D. B., 1985, Offspring of alcoholics have enhanced antagonistic placebo response, *J. Stud. Alcohol* **46**:490–494.

Nici, J., 1979, Wives of alcoholics as "repeaters," *J. Stud. Alcohol* **40**:677–682.

Nishimura, R., Masui, R., Tsuno, R., and Ushijima, S., 1983, Depressive states in adolescents (Ja), *Kyushu Neuropsychiatry* **29**:85–92. (Abst. no. 71-09701 Psycinfo.)

Nylander, I., 1960, Children of alcoholic fathers, *Acta Paediatr. Scand.* **49**(Suppl. 121).

O'Connor, J., 1978, *The Young Drinkers: A Cross-National Study of Social and Cultural Influences,* Tavistock, London.

O'Farrell, T. J., Cutter, H. S., and Floyd, F. J., 1985, Evaluating behavioral marital therapy for male alcoholics: Effects on marital adjustment and communication from before to after treatment, *Behav. Ther.* **16**:147–167.

O'Malley, S. S., and Maisto, S. A., 1985, Effects of family drinking history and expectancies on responses to alcohol in men, *J. Stud. Alcohol* **46**:289–297.

Omori, I., and Imazu, H., 1979, A survey of Danshukai (similar to Alcoholics Anonymous in USA) throughout Japan (Ja), *J. Transport. Med. (Tokyo)* **33**:264–271. (Abst. no. 8003351 Excerpt. Med.)

Orford, J., 1975, Alcoholism and marriage: The argument against specialism, *J. Stud. Alcohol* **36**:1537–1563.

Orford, J., 1976, The study of the personalities of excessive drinkers and their wives, using the approaches of Leary and Eysenck, *J. Consult. Clin. Psychol.* **44**:534–545.

Orford, J., 1982, The prevention of drinking problems in the family, in: *Alcohol and the Family* (J. Orford and J. Harwin, eds.), pp. 241–259, Croom Helm, London.

Orford, J., 1983*a*, The prevention and management of alcohol problems in the family setting: A review of work carried out in English-speaking countries, *Alcohol Alcoholism* **19**:109–122.

Orford, J., 1983*b*, Coping patterns in the alcoholic family. Paper presented at Symposium on alcoholism, Queen's University, Belfast, June 17, Northern Ireland Council for Postgraduate Medical Education. Dept. of Psychology, Univ. of Exeter.

Orford, J., 1985*a*, *Excessive Appetites: A Psychological View of Addictions,* Wiley, Chichester, England.

Orford, J., 1985*b*, Alcohol problems and the family, in: *Research Highlights in Social Work 10. Approaches to Addiction* (J. Lishman, ed.), Kogan Page, London.

Orford, J., ed., 1987*a*, *Coping with Disorder in the Family*, Croom Helm, London.

Orford, J., 1987*b*, The need for a community response to alcohol-related problems, in: *Helping the Problem Drinker: New Initiatives in Community Care* (T. Stockwell and S. Clement, eds.), Croom Helm, London.

Orford, J., and Guthrie, S., 1976, Coping behaviour used by wives of alcoholics: A preliminary investigation, in: *Alcohol Dependence and Smoking Behaviour* (G. Edwards, M. A. H. Russell, D. Hawks, and M. MacCafferty, eds.), pp. 136–143. Saxon House, Westmead, Hants.

Orford, J., Waller, S., and Peto, J., 1974, Drinking behaviour and attitudes and their correlates amongst English university students, *Q. J. Stud. Alcohol* **35:**1316–1374.

Orford, J., Guthrie, S., Nicholls, P., Oppenheimer, E., Egert, S., and Hensman, C., 1975, Self-reported coping behaviour of wives of alcoholics and its association with drinking outcome, *J. Stud. Alcohol* **36:**1254–1267.

Orford, J., Oppenheimer, E., Egert, S., Hensman, C., and Guthrie, S., 1976, The cohesiveness of alcoholism-complicated marriages and its influence on treatment outcome, *Br. J. Psychiatry,* **128:** 318–339.

Orford, J., Oppenheimer, E., Egert, S., and Hensman, C., 1977, The role of excessive drinking in alcoholism-complicated marriages: A study of stability and change over a one-year period, *Int. J. Addict.* **12:**471–495.

Orme, T. C., and Rimmer, J., 1981, Alcohol and child abuse: A review, *J. Stud. Alcohol* **42:**273–287.

Oshodin, O. G., 1984, Parental influences upon alcohol use by teenagers in Benin City, Nigeria, *J. Roy. Soc. Health* **104:**106–110.

Paolino, T. J., and McCrady, B. S., 1977, *The Alcoholic Marriage: Alternative Perspectives,* Grune & Stratton, New York.

Park, J. Y., Huang, Y., Nagoshi, C. T., et al., 1984, The flushing response to alcohol use among Koreans and Taiwanese, *J. Stud. Alcohol* **45:**481–485.

Parnitzke, K. H., and Prussig, O., 1966, Kinder alkoholsuchtiger Eltern, *Psychiatr. Neurol. Med. Psychol.* **18:**1–6. (Cited by Boyadjieva, undated.)

Partanen, J., Bruun, K., and Markkanen, T., 1966, *Inheritance of Drinking Behavior: A Study on Intelligence, Personality and Use of Alcohol of Adult Twins,* Finnish Foundation for Alcohol Studies, Helsinki.

Paschenkov, S. Z., 1976, Specificity of familial forms of alcoholism (Ru), *Sovetskaiya Med.* **11:**76–79. (Abst. no. 014079 Social Scisearch.)

Pattison, E. M., 1965, Treatment of alcoholic families with nurse home visits, *Fam. Proc.* **4:**75–94.

Pelc, I., 1980, Aetiopathogenic elements of alcoholism (Fr), *Acta Psychiatr. Belg.* **80:**138–148. (Abst. no. 81042315 Excerpt. Med.)

Pfouts, J. H., 1978, Violent families: Coping response to abused wives, *Child Welfare* **57:**101–111.

Pittman, D. J., 1967, *Alcoholism,* Harper & Row, New York. (Cited by Ablon (232).)

Plant, M., 1984, Drinking amongst pregnant women: Some initial results from a prospective study, *Alcohol Alcoholism* **19:**153–157.

Plavec, S., and Vukadinovic, M., 1976, Some problems of schooling and social status of epileptic children in the schools of the Crnomerec community (Se-Cr), *Neuropsihijatrija* **24:**49–53. (Abst. no. 03979 Psycinfo.)

Polansky, N. A., Hally, C., and Polansky, N. F., 1975, Profile of neglect: a survey of the state of knowledge of child neglect, DHEW (USA) Publ. 75-23037. (Abst. no. 76109914 Excerpt. Med.)

Poskitt, E. M., 1984, Foetal alcohol syndrome, *Alcohol Alcoholism* **19:**159–165.

Pozarnik, H., 1977, Family circumstances of preschizophrenic patients (Se-Cr), *Psihijat. Danas* **9:**495–499. (Abst. no. 79032238 Excerpt. Med.)

Price, J. A., 1975, An applied analysis of North American Indian drinking patterns, *Hum. Org.* **34:**17–26.

Price, V., Scanlon, B., and Janus, M., 1984, Social characteristics of adolescent male prostitution, *Victimology: Int. J.* **9:**211–221.

Ptacek, P., 1983, Experience of the care of children from families affected by alcoholism (Cz), *Psychol. Patopsychol. Dietata* **18**:245–249. (Part trans. into English for this review.)

Pulkkinen, L., 1983, Predictability of criminal behavior (Fin), *Psykologia* **18**:3–10. (Abst. no. 70-12940 Psycinfo.)

Quidu, M., et al., 1974, On several cases of public drunkenness in delinquent juveniles (Fr), *Rev. Neuropsychiatrie Infantile Hyg. Ment. Enfance* **22**:737–751. (Abst. no. 10550 Psycinfo.)

Ranganathan, S., and Chakravarthy, C., undated, Coping behaviour of wives of alcoholics. Unpublished paper, Ranganathan Clinical Research Foundation, Madras.

Ritson, E. B., 1982, Organisation of services to families of alcoholics, in: *Alcohol and the Family* (J. Orford and J. Harwin, eds.), Croom Helm, London.

Rizzola, N., and Rosadini, I., 1974, Family and social determinants of female alcoholism (It), *Neuropsichiatria* **30**:71–78. (Abst. no. 10036 Psycinfo.)

Roberts, K. S., and Brent, E. E., 1982, Physician utilisation and illness patterns in families of alcoholics, *J. Stud. Alcohol* **43**:119–128.

Robins, L., 1966, *Deviant Children Grown Up: A Sociological and Psychiatric Study of Sociopathic Personality,* Williams & Wilkins, Baltimore.

Roghmann, K. J., Roberts, J. S., Smith, T. S., Wells, S. M., and Wersinger, R. P., 1981, Alcoholics' vs. nonalcoholics' use of services of a health maintenance organisation, *J. Stud. Alcohol* **42**:321–322.

Room, R., undated, Alcohol as an instrument of intimate domination. Unpublished manuscript, Univ. of California at Berkeley, Berkeley.

Rosette, H. L., Ouellette, E. M., Weiner, L., and Owens, E., 1978, Therapy of heavy drinking during pregnancy, *Obstet. Gynecol.* **51**:41–46.

Russell, M., Henderson, C., and Blume, S., 1985, *Children of Alcoholics: A Review of the Literature.* Children of Alcoholics Foundation, Inc., New York.

Rutter, M., and Madge, N., 1976, *Cycles of Disadvantage: A Review of Research,* Heinemann, London.

Rydelius, P., 1981, Children of alcoholic fathers: Their social adjustment and their health status over 20 years, *Acta Paediatr. Scand.* (Suppl. 286):10–85.

Santamaria, J. N., 1983, Australia: Alcohol and the aboriginals, in: *Drug Use and Misuse* (G. Edwards, A. Arif, and J. Jaffe, eds.) pp. 93–100, Croom Helm, London.

Sargent, M., 1979, *Drinking and Alcoholism in Australia: A Power Relations Theory,* Longman Cheshire, Melbourne.

Schaeffer, K. W., Parsons, O. A., and Yohman, J. R., 1984, Neuropsychological differences between male familial and nonfamilial alcoholics and nonalocholics, *Alcoholism: Clin. Exp. Res.* **8**:347–351.

Schaffer, J. B., and Tyler, J. D., 1979, Degree of sobriety in male alcoholics and coping styles used by their wives, *Br. J. Psychiatry* **135**:431–437.

Schmid, W., et al., 1983, Genetical, medical and psychosocial factors as cause of learning difficulties in a cohort of 11-year-old pupils (Winterthur study) (Ge), *Acta Paedopsychiatr.* **49**:9–45. (Abst. no. 71-09856 Psycinfo.)

Schuckit, M. A., 1980, Biological markers: metabolism and acute reactions to alcohol in sons of alcoholics, *Pharm. Biochem. Behav.* **13**:9–16. (Cited by Goodwin (216).)

Schuckit, M. A., 1984*a*, Subjective responses to alcohol in sons of alcoholics and controls, *Arch. Gen. Psychiatry* **41**:879–887.

Schuckit, M. A., 1984*b*, Relationship between the course of primary alcoholism in men and family history, *J. Stud. Alcohol* **45**:334–338.

Schuckit, M. A., and Rayses, V., 1979, Ethanol ingestion: Differences in blood acetaldehyde concentrations in relatives of alcoholics and controls, *Science* **203**:54–55.

Schuckit, M. A., Engstrom, D., Alpert, R., et al., 1981, Differences in muscle-tension response to ethanol in young men with and without family histories of alcoholism, *J. Stud. Alcohol* **42**:918–924.

Schwitters, S. Y., Johnson, R. C., Johnson, S. B., and Ahern, F. M., 1982, Familial resemblances in flushing following alcohol use, *Behav. Genet.* **12**:349–352. (Abst. no. 69-02979 Psycinfo.)

Seixas, J., 1980, *How to Cope with An Alcoholic Parent,* Canongate, Edinburgh.

Seixas, J., and Levitan, M., 1984, A supportive counseling group for adult children of alcoholics, *Alcoholism Treat. Q.* **1:**123–132.

Serrano, F., 1977, Family psychotherapy in ISSSTE medical institutions (Sp), *Neurol. Neurocir. Psiquiatrica* **18:**173–177.

Shurygin, G. I., 1978, Concerning a psychogenic pathological personality formation in children and adolescents in families with fathers suffering from alcoholism (Ru), *Zhurnal Nevropatologii Psikhiatrii Imeni S S Korsakova* **10:**1566–1569. (Trans. into English for this review.)

Singer, M., 1985, Family comes first: An examination of the social networks of skid row men, *Hum. Org.* **44:**137–142.

Sipova, I., and Nedoma, K., 1972, Family setting and childhood in socially and sexually depraved women (Cz), *Ceskoslovenska Psychiatrie* **68:**150–153. (Abst. no. 05297 Psycinfo.)

Smith, C. G., 1969, Alcoholics: Their treatment and their wives, *Br. J. Psychiatry* **115:**1039–1042.

Snyder, D. R., 1962, Culture and Jewish sobriety: The in-group out-group factor, in: *Society, Culture, and Drinking Patterns* (D. J. Pittman and C. R. Snyder, eds.) pp. 188–225, Wiley, New York.

Source unknown, Dec. 1981, Yugoslavian article. (Abst. available in Sociol. Absts.)

Source unknown, Oct. 1984*a,* Brazilian article. (Abst. available in Psycinfo.)

Source unknown, Oct. 1984*b*, West German article. (Abst. available in Psycinfo.)

Source unknown, Oct. 1984*c*, West German article. (Abst. available in Sociol. Absts.)

Spaans, C., and Verspreet, F. A., 1981, The foetal alcohol syndrome: Four patients in one family (Du), *Nederl. Tijdschr. Geneesk.* **125:**452–454. (Abst. no. 1402307 CAB Absts.)

Stanetti, F., 1976, Alcoholism relapses: Relationship and prognostic significance of the patient's personality, social factors, and course of treatment (Yug), *Socijalna Psihijatrija* **4:**347–406. (Abst. no. 10105 Psycinfo.)

Stankoushev, T., Chinova, L., and Rasboinikova, E., 1974, On some peculiarities in the psychological development and in the behaviour of children with alcoholic parents, *Pediatria (Sofia)* **13:**25–29. (Cited by Boyadjieva, undated.)

Stankovic, Z., and Timotijevic, I., 1980, Family of the alcoholic during treatment of alcoholism (Se-Cr), *Psihijatrija Danas* **12:**287–291. (Abst. no. 67-12881 Psycinfo.)

Stanton, M. D., 1979, Family treatment approaches to drug abuse problems: A review, *Fam. Process* **18:**251–280.

Staulcup, H., Kenwood, K., and Frigo, D., 1979, A review of federal primary alcoholism prevention projects, *J. Stud. Alcohol* **40:**943–968.

Steinglass, P., 1976, Experimenting with family treatment approaches to alcoholism 1950–1975: A review, *Fam. Process* **15:**97–123.

Steinglass, P., 1979, An experimental treatment program for alcoholic couples, *J. Stud. Alcohol* **40:** 149–182.

Steinglass, P., 1981, The impact of alcoholism on the family and on relationships between degree of alcoholism and psychiatric symptomatology, *J. Stud. Alcohol* **42:**288–303.

Steinglass, P., 1982, The roles of alcohol in family systems, *Alcohol and the Family* (J. Orford and J. Harwin, eds.), Croom Helm, London.

Steinglass, P., Tislenko, L., and Reiss, D., 1985, Stability/instability in the alcoholic marriage: The interrelationships between course of alcoholism, family process, and marital outcome, *Fam. Process* **24:**365–383.

Steinhausen, H., Gobel, D., and Nestler, V., 1984, Psychopathology in the offspring of alcoholic parents, *J. Am. Acad. Child Psychiatry* **23:**465–471.

Sterle, V., 1970, School and home (S1), *Clovek-Sola-Delo* **3:**13–16. (Abst. no. 07544 Psycinfo.)

Stivers, R., 1985, Historical meanings of Irish-American drinking, in; Bennett and Ames (1985, op cit).

Straus, P., 1978, Les parents maltraitants: Abord psychologique, abord sociologique [Child abusing parents: Psychological and sociological approach], *Soins* **23:**13–17. (Abst., *J. Stud. Alcohol* 1979, **40:**630.)

Straus, R., and Bacon, S. D., 1951, Alcoholism and social stability: A study of occupational integration in 2023 male clinic patients, *Q. J. Stud. Alcohol* **12:**231–260.

Streissguth, A. P., 1976, Maternal alcoholism and the outcome of pregnancy: A review of the fetal alcohol syndrome, in: *Alcohol Problems in Women and Children* (M. Greenblatt and M. A. Schuckit, eds.), Grune & Stratton, New York.

Stricklin, A., and Austad, C. S., 1982, Perceptions of neglected children and negligent parents about causes for removal from parental homes, *Psychol. Rep.* **51**:1103–1108.

Strube, M. J., and Barbour, L. S., 1984, Factors related to the decision to leave an abusive relationship, *J. Marriage Fam.* **46**:837–844.

Strzembosz, A., 1979, Stopien przystosowania spolecznego dzieci alkoholicow z waszawy objetych przed 10 laty postepowaniem opiekunczym (Pol), *Problemy Alkoholizmu* **26**:11–14. (Cited by Boyadjeiva, undated.)

Student, V., and Matova, A., 1969, Development of mental disorders in the wives of alcoholics (Cz), *Ceskoslovanoka Psychiatrie* **65**:23–29. (Trans. into English for this review.)

Sue, S., Zane, N., and Ito, J., 1979, Alcohol drinking patterns among Asian and Caucasian Americans, *J. Cross-Cult. Psychol.* **10**:41–56.

Suwaki, H., 1983, Japan: Danshukai and Naikan, in: *Drug Use and Misuse* (G. Edwards, A. Arif, and J. Jaffe, eds.) pp. 115–120, Croom Helm, London.

Suwaki, H., 1985, International review series: Alcohol and alcohol problems research. 2. Japan. *Br. J. Addict.* **80**:127–132.

Sysenko, V. A., 1982, Divorce: Dynamics, motives and consequences, *Sotsiologicheskie Issledovaniya* **9**:99–104. (Trans. into English for this review.)

Takei, M., Sei, T., Kikuchi, T., and Hasoe, T., 1974, The relationship between "delinquent formation space" on juvenile delinquency and the family with special reference to the approach frame (Ja), *Jpn. J. Crim. Psychol.* **10**:52–62. (Abst. no. 01299 Psycinfo.)

Tapia, P. I., et al., 1966, Sociocultural patterns of alcohol ingestion on Chiloei Island. Preliminary report: Some methodological problems, *Acta Psiquiaitri. Psicol. Am. Lat.* **12**:232–240. (Abst. no. 01452 Psycinfo.)

Tarter, R. E., Hegedus, A., Goldstein, G., Shelly, C., and Alterman, A., 1984*a*, Adolescent sons of alcoholics: Neuropsychological and personality characteristics, *Alcoholism: Clin. Exp. Res.* **8**:216–222.

Tarter, R. E., Hegedus, M. P., Winstein, N. E., and Alterman, A. I., 1984*b*, Neuropsychological, personality, and familial characteristics of physically abused delinquents, *J. Am. Acad. Child Psychiatry* **23**:668–674.

Tarter, R. E., Alterman, A. I., and Edwards, K. L., 1985*a*, Vulnerability to alcoholism in men: A behavior-genetic perspective, *J. Stud. Alcohol* **46**:329–356.

Tarter, R. E., Hegedus, A. M., and Gavaler, J. S., 1985*b*, Hyperactivity in sons of alcoholics, *J. Stud. Alcohol* **46**:259–261. (Abst. no. 1713917 Medline.)

Taylor, S. P., Gammon, C. B., and Capasso, D. R., 1976, Aggression as a function of the interaction of alcohol and threat, *J. Pers. Soc. Psychol.* **34**:938–941.

Teusch, R., 1980, The drinking habits of teenagers in relation to parental behavior (Ge), *Psychol. Erziehung Unterricht* **27**:193–201. (Abst. no. 05708 Psycinfo.)

Thomas, E. J., and Santa, C. A., 1982, Unilateral family therapy for alcohol abuse, *Am. J. Fam. Ther.* **10**:49–58.

Tiit, E., 1982, Risk factors leading to marital dissolution in the Estonian SSR, *J. Divorce* **5**: 61–73.

Topiar, A., and Satkova, V., 1974, Behavior of delinquents, victims of incest, and their fathers (Cz), *Ceskoslovenska Psychiatrie* **70**:55–58. (Abst. no. 05555 Psycinfo.)

Toteva, S., 1982*a*, Neurotic symptoms in children with alcoholic parent. On the suicidal risk in children of Alcoholics, *Sofia, Bull. NINPN*, **10**:104–109. (Cited by Boyadjieva, undated.)

Toteva, S., 1982*b*, On the suicidal risk in children of alcoholics, *Sofia, Bull. NINPN* **10**:85–92. (Cited by Boyadjieva, undated.)

Toteva, S., 1984, Psychological disturbances and social desadaptation in children with alcoholic parent. Dissertation, Sofia. (Cited by Boyadjieva, undated.)

Toteva, S., 1985, A katamnestic follow-up study of children with neurotic disorders, brought up in a family with one parent suffering from alcoholism, *Nevrol. Psikhiatr. Nevrokhir. (Bulgaria)* **24:**10–14. (Abst. no. 852133194 Excerpt. Med.)

Utne, H. E., Hansen, F., Vallo, R., et al., 1977, Ethanol elimination rate in adoptees with and without parental disposition toward alcoholism, *J. Stud. Alcohol* **38:**1219–1223. (Cited by Goodwin, 1984, *op cit*).

Vaillant, G., 1983, *The Natural History of Alcoholism,* Harvard University Press, Cambridge, MA.

van Hasselt, V. B., Morrison, R. L., and Bellack, A. S., 1985, Alcohol use in wife abusers and their spouses, *Addict. Behav.* **10:**127–135.

Velleman, R., 1987, A study of the relationship between childhood, family and parental experiences, parental drinking problems and adult adjustment. Unpublished Ph.D. thesis, University of Exeter, U.K.

Velleman, R., and Orford, J., 1984, Intergenerational transmission of alcohol problems: hypotheses to be tested, in: *Alcohol Related Problems: Room for Manoeuvre,* (N. Krasner, J. S. Kadden, and R. J. Walker, eds.), pp. 97–113, Wiley, Chichester.

Velleman, R., and Orford, J., 1985, Making sense of what adults who had a problem drinking parent say about their childhood experience, *New Directions Stud. Alcohol (UK)* **10:**29–58.

Veseb, C., 1973, Suicidal attempts in women alcoholics, *Alkoholizam Godina (Belgrade)* **13:**79. (Cited by Boyadjieva, undated.)

Volicer, L., Volicer, B. J., and d'Angelo, N., 1984, Relationship of family history of alcoholism to patterns of drinking and physical dependence in male alcoholics, *Drug Alcohol Depend.* **13:**215–222. (Abst. no. 1395479 Medline.)

Waddell, J. O., 1975, For individual power and social credit: The use of alcohol among Tucson Papagos, *Hum. Org.* **34:**9–15.

Wagner, C., 1979, The origins of alcohol dependency among women, with particular reference to the situation of the woman in the family and society (Ge), *Soziologenkorrespondenz* **6:**121–146. (Abst. no. 139183 Sociol. Absts.)

Waldo, M., and Guerney, B. G., 1983, Marital relationship enhancement therapy in the treatment of alcoholism, *J. Marriage Fam. Ther.* **9:**321–323.

Walpole, I. R., and Hockey, A., 1980, Fetal alcohol syndrome: Implications to family and society in Australia, *Aust. Paediatr. J.* **16:**101–105. (Abst. no. 1349000 CAB Absts.)

Wells, J. E., 1984, Treatment as primary prevention: A model to explore the possible preventive effect of treating alcoholic parents, *Community Health Stud.* **8:**343.

Werner, E. E., 1986, Resilient offspring of alcoholics: A longitudinal study from birth to age 18, *J. Stud. Alcohol* **47:**34–40.

Wilkins, R. M., 1974, *The Hidden Alcoholic in General Practice,* Elek, London.

Wilks, J., and Callan, V. J., 1984, Similarity of university students' and their parents' attitudes toward alcohol, *J. Stud. Alcohol* **45:**326–333.

Wilson, C., 1982, The impact on children, in: *Alcohol and the Family* (J. Orford and J. Harwin, eds.), Croom Helm, London.

Wilson, C., 1983, Interactions in families with alcohol problems. Unpublished M. Phil. Diss., University of London.

Wilson, C., and Orford, J., 1978, Children of alcoholics: Report of a preliminary study and comments on the literature, *J. Stud. Alcohol* **39:**121–142.

Winokur, G., 1972, Depressive spectrum disease: Description and family study, *Compr. Psychiatry* **13:** 3–8.

Wiseman, J. P., 1976*a*, The other half: Wife of an alcoholic in Finland. I. Early diagnosis and therapeutic strategies on the home front, *Alkoholipolitiikka* **41:**62–72.

Wiseman, J. P., 1976*b*, Alkoholistien vaimot. II. Elaminen alkoholistin kaussa [The wives of alocholics. II. Living with an alcoholic], *Alkoholipolitiikka* **41:**109–117. (Abst. *J. Stud. Alcohol* 1979, **40:**50).

Wiseman, J. P., 1980, The "home treatment": The first steps in trying to cope with an alcoholic husband, *Fam. Relat.* **29:**541–549.

Wolcott, H. F., 1974, *The African Beer Gardens of Bulawayo: Integrated Drinking in a Segregated Society,* Rutgers Center of Alcohol Studies: New Brunswick, NJ.

Wolin, S. J., Bennett, L. A., and Noonan, D. L., 1979, Family rituals and the recurrence of alcoholism over generations, *Am. J. Psychiatry* **136:**589–593.

World Health Organization, 1973, Report of consultation on family health, November, WHO, Geneva.

World Health Organization, 1979, Studies of the determinants and consequence of family health. A draft discussion paper on the need for action-oriented research on the changing features of family health, WHO, Geneva.

World Health Organization, 1980, The work of WHO concerning family health, in: *Biennial Report of the Director–General for 1978–79,* WHO, Geneva.

World Health Organization, 1984, *Management of Alcohol-Related Problems in General Practice,* WHO, Geneva.

Yamane, Y., 1978, A long-term follow-up study of alcoholics (Ja), *Tokyo Jikeikai Med. J.* **93:**458–474. (Abst. no. 79102026 Excerpt. Med.)

Yang, M. M., 1967, Child training and child behavior in varying family patterns in a changing Chinese society (Ch), *Nat. Taiwan Univ. J. Sociol.* **3:**77–83. (Abst. no. G5887-0 Sociol. Absts.)

Yates, F., and Thorley, A., 1988, The evaluation of a 'cooperative counseling' alcohol service which uses family and affected others to reach and influence problem drinkers, *Br. J. Addict.* **83:** 1309–1319.

Yavkin, V. M., 1976, Psychopathoid conditions in syphilitic patients' children (Ru), *Defektologiya* **3:** 22–29. (Abst. no. 10631 Psycinfo.)

Zweben, A., and Pearlman, S., 1983, Evaluating the effectiveness of conjoint treatment of alcohol-complicated marriages: Clinical and methodological issues, *J. Marriage Fam. Ther.* **9:**61–72.

# 5

# The Origins of Modern Research and Responses Relevant to Problems of Alcohol

## A Brief History of the First Center of Alcohol Studies

MARK KELLER

Because alcohol had sometimes been used as an anesthetic, it came to be studied in the Laboratory of Applied Physiology at Yale University by the great physiologist Yandell Henderson and his associate Howard W. Haggard as one of the drugs of interest for the alleviation of pain.

## 1. THE 1930s

Beginning in the early 1930s, researchers in this laboratory published a series of important papers on the effects of alcohol. After the law in the United States that had prohibited commerce in alcoholic beverages was rescinded in 1933, a widespread renewed public concern about alcohol developed, especially over its effects on drinkers. The Laboratory at Yale then began to receive many requests for "scientific" knowledge about alcohol. Haggard, who had succeeded Henderson as Professor of Physiology and Director of the Laboratory, realized that he and the other physiologists and biochemists on his staff did not have the knowledge to answer many of the inquiries, which involved social, psychological, and even economic and political issues. Alcohol in drink was not just a physicochemical substance.

Although Haggard had graduated from the Yale Medical School with the M.D. degree, he had not chosen to practice as a physician. His interests were in research and education. Thus, he broadcast the first unsponsored public radio program on health and authored the popular *Devils, Drugs and Doctors*. When, in 1937, the Research Council on Problems of Alcohol was formed, he was invited to serve on its Scientific Advisory Committee. He supported the Council in obtaining a grant, from the Carnegie Corpora-

MARK KELLER • Rutgers University, Piscataway, New Jersey 08854.

tion, for a review of the biological literature on effects of alcohol. The grant was then assigned to the New York University College of Medicine, where the staff of Norman Jolliffe had already begun some preliminary documentation in the desired direction. Jolliffe was therefore named Medical Director of the review project.

Jolliffe's first step was destined to have enormous influence on everything connected with alcohol and alcoholism—in research and education, public attitudes, and treatment—that would happen in the next 50 years or more: He drove from New York City to Worcester, Massachusetts, and there persuaded E. M. Jellinek to become the executive director of the projected review.

With the documentalist from Jolliffe's staff at his right hand, and a newly hired staff of multilingual abstractors—mostly physicians and psychologists—and with the resources especially of the library of the New York Academy of Medicine, Jellinek completed the essential review task in some 16 months (September 1939–December 1940). A vast volume of facts had been abstracted and systematically entered in a newly designed, subject-indexed, mechanically retrievable archive. But the grant fund was exhausted, and many months of work remained to be done in writing and editing the review.

## 2. THE *QUARTERLY JOURNAL OF STUDIES ON ALCOHOL*

It was Howard W. Haggard who demonstrated the foresight and capacity to solve this problem. While the project was hardly midway, in early 1940, he founded, at Yale in the Laboratory of Applied Physiology, the *Quarterly Journal of Studies on Alcohol.* The *Journal* would provide, among other contents, a medium for publication of the emerging reports from the review then in progress (Jellinek and Jolliffe, 1940; Jellinek and McFarland, 1940). Now he invited Jellinek to come to Yale, with his staff, there to complete the review. Haggard, perhaps the most popular professor at Yale,* was able to raise the financial support for this costly undertaking among alumni families. He had in mind, however, that members of the review staff would participate in other work at the Laboratory.†

Work in formulating reviews, especially of the medical aspects of the effects of alcohol, progressed steadily. They were published in the first two volumes of the *Quarterly Journal of Studies on Alcohol* (1940–1942) and assembled in a volume published by Yale University Press (Jellinek, 1942*a*).

While the grand literature review and some research on drugs other than alcohol absorbed Jellinek at first, he did not neglect the wider interest in alcohol of Haggard, his boss, and of the Research Council, where he was now vice-chairman of the Scientific

*His course in physiology was known among the collegians as Sex I and Sex II.

†Indeed, Jellinek there designed an ingenious study of the effects of various drugs, used in combination in commercial "pain killers" (other than alcohol), which proved of great value to pharmaceutical manufacturers as well as to the Laboratory. Historically, it is possible that this was the first "double blind" experiment (Jellinek, 1946). In addition, both Martin Gross and Giorgio Lolli of the review staff became regular participants in the physiological researches at the Laboratory. Other staff who followed Jellinek to Yale and participated in the alcohol-related developments were Gertrude Gross, a psychiatrist, Anne Roe, a psychologist, and Vera Efron and Mark Keller, documentalists.

Advisory Committee. Based on the lacunae in knowledge that the review indicated, as well as on broader social considerations, he prepared a concise outline of desirable research directions for the Research Council (Jellinek, 1942*b*).

The Council was never very successful in raising money to support the desired researches. Haggard was. He assigned Laboratory staff to some of these researches—Leon Greenberg, a physiologist who at that time invented the first portable automatic breath-alcohol testing machine (Greenberg and Keator, 1941); David Lester, a chemist–biochemist–physiologist–psychologist; and Giorgio Lolli, a physician–physiologist with inclinations toward psychiatry. Jellinek assigned Anne Roe to analyze and report on the laws and content of education about alcohol in public schools (Roe, 1942, 1943). He added a scholarly former law-school dean to the staff with an assignment to study the origins of alcohol control law (Baird, 1944–1948) and an economist of the Council of Churches to analyze the economic costs of alcohol-related problems (Landis, 1945).

Early in 1943, a young Yale sociologist who had become interested in the people jailed for public drunkenness heard that somewhere on the campus was a laboratory where they knew something about alcohol. He went there to inquire and met E. M. Jellinek. Thus the Laboratory of Applied Physiology acquired a sociologist—his name was Selden D. Bacon—who was soon outlining the foundations for studies of drinking in all sorts of populations and settings, as well as drunkenness or alcoholism (Bacon, 1943, 1944).

Finished with the study of education in the schools, Anne Roe was assigned a new task: Jellinek thought it was time to analyze the possible role of heredity in alcoholism by means of a study of out-adopted children. More publications were soon forthcoming (Roe, 1944; Roe and Burks, 1945).

While Haggard and Jellinek were editors of the *Quarterly Journal of Studies on Alcohol*, its production, as well as the abstracting and subject indexing of the world scientific literature on alcohol, was in the hands of a multilingual staff of professional editors and documentalists. To their task Jellinek added the development and maintenance of another of his original ideas: *The Classified Abstract Archive of the Alcohol Literature*. From this *Archive* it now became possible with little effort to extract bibliography or abstracts or specific information on nearly limitless detailed topics relevant to alcohol. An announcement offering this service to the scientific–scholarly community was published in the *Journal*. Soon requests were coming from scientists, scholars, and activists from all over the world.

The editorial office of the *Journal* and *Archive* held a rich library useful to the entire staff of the Laboratory. It was Selden Bacon's idea that a formal library should be constituted—to ensure the safety of its contents and its systematic management and growth. A librarian was added to the staff of the developing Documentation and Publication Division.

Starting with the original bibliography of other 5000 items which formed the basis of the grand literature review (Jellinek, 1942*a*), the documentation staff proceeded to develop in the library a Master Catalog of the Alcohol Literature. This Catalog contains a full-reference card for every article and book published since 1472 that could be classified as scientific, scholarly, or historical. The current total is almost 250,000 cards. The Master Catalog became the basis of the several volumes of the *International Bibliography of Studies on Alcohol* published hitherto (Keller, 1966, 1968, 1980).

Education was very much on the mind of both Haggard and Jellinek. Haggard had only to mention the desirability of public education for Jellinek to produce effective ideas. One was a series of *Lay Supplements of the Quarterly Journal of Studies on Alcohol*. Jellinek himself wrote the first ones; others were composed by various members of the staff, to a total of 14. Hundreds of thousands were eventually sold, especially after the series title was changed to *Popular Pamphlets on Alcohol Problems*.

Professional as well as popular education was forwarded by an increasing volume of inhouse publication. Besides numerous separate books, a technical monograph series eventually numbered 14 volumes.

## 3. THE SUMMER SCHOOL OF ALCOHOL STUDIES

One of Jellinek's grandest and most fruitful ideas was the Summer School of Alcohol Studies. Already early in 1943 plans for program and space in the University were under discussion, and Jellinek was recruiting students as well as faculty. He was able to interest and influence Dr. Ernest Cherrington, a scholarly dean in the service of the Protestant churches. As a result, of the 80 students in the first class, which met for 6 weeks in July and August 1943, many were persons connected with the churches; many were former temperance workers.*

The lectures of the second session of the Summer School were recorded and published in a book, *Alcohol, Science and Society*, that became a classic of the alcohol-studies field and was reprinted five times, for a total sale of over 50,000 copies (Jellinek et al., 1945).† Gradually, the character of the student body changed to include personnel from all the disciplines, professions, and social and political interests relevant to alcohol use and problems. In the 1980s, among 500 students who attend the same Summer School at Rutgers University, the representation from the alcoholism treatment and rehabilitation field is most noticeable.

## 4. THE YALE PLAN CLINICS

Ideas were the constant product of the fertile Jellinek mind. We must learn how to treat alcoholism, he declared: how to treat different sorts of alcoholics by appropriate different methods. To do this, we need our own clinics—outpatient clinics—for most alcoholics do not need hospitalization. It was a very expensive idea, but Haggard liked it. So did all the staff. To attract all sorts of alcoholics, to bar none, even the Skid Row derelict, the alcoholism clinics should be free, Jellinek theorized. The chief documentalist argued for letting every patient pay what he could afford—some nothing, some

*Norman Jolliffe lectured on the diseases of chronic alcoholism (Jolliffe, 1945). When he had concluded, one of the students stood up in the aisle of the lecture hall and, parading his belly pompously, asked, "Doctor, you have described the ills that plague the chronic drunkard. Can you tell us what ills may affect the chronic abstainer?" Without a moment's hesitation, Jolliffe replied, "Sometimes they suffer from pressure of the halo!"

†A "revisited" volume under the same title has recently been published (White et al., 1982).

25¢ a visit, some even $5. Jellinek prevailed, and Haggard raised the money for free clinics.

Two Yale Plan Clinics were opened: in New Haven just off the campus and in Hartford (Jellinek, 1944). The Skid Row folk did not come. Bacon had enlisted a newly graduated student in sociology as assistant: Robert Straus. He was sent to Skid Row to drum up patients for the clinic in New Haven. He was nice and persuasive, and he did succeed in enticing a few Skid Rowers. But they did not return after initial interviews. The Yale clinicians had not yet learned how to make the Skid Row folk feel at home in the near-campus environment.*

To operate the clinics, Giorgio Lolli was appointed medical director, and Raymond G. McCarthy, originally an educationist, as executive director. McCarthy (1946) soon assumed the role of lay therapist (the term "alcoholism counselor" was not yet invented) and conducted the first group therapy sessions. Gertrude Gross assumed the duties of chief psychiatrist, and soon other physicians, nurses, and auxiliary staff had to be added as the popularity of the Yale Plan Clinics burgeoned.

The alcohol-related activities at the venerable Yale University excited much public interest and media attention. Such an event as a representative of the liquor industry and an officer of the Woman's Christian Temperance Union simultaneously attending the same School of Alcohol Studies at Yale was entertaining gossip for newspapers and fuel for articles in popular magazines. The Yale Plan Clinics were even more piquant. Everything about them seemed "news" to the media—as if treatment for alcoholics were a new invention. Writers and photographers came for days and weeks.

The Clinics were so successful and popular that the Center was persuaded to open clinics in three additional cities. Five Yale Plan Clinics, treating a growing intake of alcoholics without any fee, were obviously a severe drain on the Center's financial resources. It became difficult to support them. Fortunately, in 1949 the Connecticut State Legislature established the Connecticut Commission on Alcoholism, with a mission that included treatment of alcoholics. The Commission therefore gladly took over the five Yale Plan Clinics for its own.† The Yale Center was thus relieved of that financial albatross, but for the time being was without its own clinical program.

Already in the 1940s all these activities jointly had so enlarged the staff of the Yale Laboratory of Applied Physiology that the nonbiologists outnumbered the normal staff several times. Obviously, the alcohol-related program needed an independent identity. An understanding Yale administration, under President James Roland Angell, approved the creation of a Section of Studies on Alcohol as a division of the Laboratory of Applied Physiology. Thus, some of the early publications were designated *Memoirs of the Section of Studies on Alcohol*. Soon this somewhat awkward title, again with the blessings of the Yale administration, was changed to a name to which the fame came to be attached: the Yale Center of Alcohol Studies.

To give the concluding lecture at the first session of the Summer School, Jellinek had invited the founding father of Alcoholics Anonymous (AA), "Bill" Wilson. To the second session in 1944, on Wilson's advice, came a clever and charming young woman,

*But one of the Skid Row near-patients became sufficiently attached to Bob—if not to sobriety—to become the subject of a unique 27-year follow-up and of an equally unique book (Straus, 1974).

†The Center's chief sociologist, Selden D. Bacon, who had been active in persuading the legislature to create the Commission, was appointed by the Governor as its first chairman.

Marty Mann, the first woman alcoholic who had achieved sobriety in his New York AA group. She proposed to the Yale leadership that it was not enough to educate professionals, in the Summer School and by scholarly publication; the general public must be educated. In agreement with her proposal, the Yale Center sponsored the formation of the National Committee for Education on Alcoholism and supported it and housed it in the Laboratory of Applied Physiology for some 5 years. Under the direction of Marty Mann, whose background was in "public relations," aided by Yale sponsorship and a Yale address for respectability, and with some financial support from the Yale Center, the Committee flourished. After a few years it became independent as the National Council on Alcoholism and moved its headquarters to New York.

The social sciences too flourished in the Yale Center. Under the direction and inspiration of Selden Bacon, a ground-breaking series of studies was carried out, by a growing staff of scientists augmented by graduate students, of the drinking ways of numerous ethnic as well as other special populations, in the United States and in a few other countries.*

Long ago, still at the original literature review in New York, Jellinek had discovered that one vital and fascinating fact was not available anywhere in the scientific or other sources: How many alcoholics are there? Then and there, in 1940, after exhaustive study of the possibly relevant indicators in all the literature of many countries, he devised the to-be-famous Jellinek Estimation Formula: $A = (PD/K)R$ (Jellinek, 1951; Keller, 1965). In the alcohol studies field during the next decades, especially after Popham (1956) demonstrated its validity, this formula had the status of an Einsteinian $E = MC^2$. Eventually the stability of the constants in the formula failed and other methods of estimation had to be tried—thus far without notable success (Keller, 1975*b*).

## 5. THE YALE PLAN FOR BUSINESS AND INDUSTRY

It was Jellinek who stimulated interest in the occurrence and important effects of alcoholism in industry with an early estimate (Jellinek, 1947). His lead was followed by many studies (Bacon, 1951), and notably in one of the leading industries in the United States, eventually reported by "Observer" and Maxwell (1959). The pseudonymous coauthor of that fundamental study was the personnel director of that industry. His identity had to be masked lest the company be identified and the public learn how many alcoholics were serving them in that industry. This secrecy tells what a delicate and almost unapproachable subject alcoholism was in the 1940s and still in the 1950s. But sociologists of the Center of Alcohol Studies probed in their sphere as assiduously as the physiologists and biochemists in their laboratories. One consequence of the resulting revelations was that it became possible to persuade a few large industries to initiate alcoholism-related programs—advised and guided by the experts of the Yale Center. Thus, the Yale Plan for Business and Industry was devised and applied in several

*A few of the historically most influential, in that they whetted the interest of many followers, warrant mention: McCarthy and Douglass (1949); Straus and Winterbottom (1949); Williams and Straus (1950); Landman (1952); Straus and Bacon (1953); Skolnick (1954, 1957); Snyder (1954); Lolli et al. (1958); Sadoun et al. (1965).

industrial experiments by Ralph Henderson and Selden Bacon (1953) with the collaboration of other members of the growing Center staff.

By 1950—only a decade after the informal beginning of the Center of Alcohol Studies—a worldwide interest in study and activity around the problems of alcohol had been aroused. What was to be another great center was launched in Canada: The Ontario Addiction Research Foundation. Now the World Health Organization was ready to become involved, provided a suitable leading person could be found. No one could have been better suited than E. M. Jellinek, with his universal expertise in alcohol problems and his command of many languages. In 1951, then, Jellinek moved on to the international front and Haggard appointed Selden D. Bacon to the directorship of the Yale Center. Soon after this, Haggard retired as director of the Laboratory of Applied Physiology. It will become immediately apparent why a new director of that institute was never appointed.

A flukish fate now intervened in the history of the Center. Yale University acquired a new president who did not know science and whose image of Yale did not include certain nonclassical institutions. Among those that he sought to abolish, in some cases with success, was, of course, the Laboratory of Applied Physiology and especially its unseemly child the Center of Alcohol Studies.* In the next 10 years the Center had to expend much effort to survive at Yale. Only the leadership and skills and Yale background of Selden Bacon could have held off the president of the University so long. In spite of the fact that the Center's activities in the 1950s continued to glamorize the University in the nation and, indeed, in the world, by 1960 it was obvious that at Yale the Center was doomed.

## 6. THE MOVE TO RUTGERS

Faced with the question, not to be or to be, to disband or try to transfer as an institution to another university, the scientific–academic staff was unanimous for survival. Bacon then shrewdly released a public announcement that the Center would move from Yale. It excited front-page national newspaper headlines. Several universities immediately expressed interest. After complex negotiations with several of the inquirers, the entire Center—minus only one scientist—moved early in 1962 to Rutgers University. A logical transition was achieved: The physiology, biochemistry, and psychology laboratories became a division of the Center of Alcohol Studies, instead of the Center being a division of the Laboratory of Applied Physiology. At Rutgers, too, with adequate space in a new building, and with increased staff, the Documentation Division, including the library, could be developed as the primary source of alcohol-related knowledge in the world (Keller, 1964, 1972).

Two important new sources of support were instrumental in facilitating the transit of so large and complex an institute: the National Institute of Mental Health, under the direction of Robert Felix and his deputy Stanley Yolles, provided funds especially for the documentation activity as well as for a number of specific researches; and the

*For added pique, the distressing alcohol studies were located on gracious Hillhouse Avenue, practically across the street from the president's official residence.

Christopher D. Smithers Foundation, through its president, Brinkley R. Smithers, provided major funds for a new building for the Center on the Rutgers science campus.

This account has not attempted to detail the studies in the social sciences, in sociology and psychology, economics and epidemiology, education and treatment, that engaged the Center's staff during its developmental and maturational years, nor the variety of experimental studies in the Center's laboratories, from biochemistry to experimental psychology, and from physiology to enzymology. The record is in volumes of publications. This account has depicted, rather, the broad range of activities in which the staff of the Center engaged. From this it is possible to consider and evaluate the importance of its original and innovative approach and the impact and significance of that approach to alcohol problems in society and, indeed, in the world.

Probably the most important feature of the Center was the fact that it was a multidisciplinary organism from the beginning. That feature must be credited to the insights of Norman Jolliffe, Howard W. Haggard, and E. M. Jellinek, who in the 1930s recognized that alcohol problems were too complex to be understood or dealt with from the perspective of any one profession, whether medicine or law or education or any other, or of any one scientific discipline, whether physiology or sociology or psychology or any other. This understanding inspired the development of what they thought of as an interdisciplinary institute in which lawyers and educationers and economists and sociologists and psychologists worked and studied cooperatively side by side with physiologists and biochemists and enzymologists and experimental psychologists, as well as physicians and nurses and psychiatrists and historians and documentalists—in short, an interdisciplinary center. Many years later an editorialist in *Science* (Long, 1971) proposed a brand-new reform: "Interdisciplinary problem-oriented research in the university." The interdisciplinary problem-oriented Center of Alcohol Studies had been created by Haggard and Jellinek 30 years earlier.

Back of that ambitious and, in 1941, still untried idea was an assumption that these mixed characters would develop and carry out joint, that is, interdisciplinary, studies. Actually, for the most part, the physiologists did physiology, the psychologists did psychology, the sociologists did sociology, the psychiatrists did their thing, and so forth. Nevertheless the ideal was not entirely lost. Sometimes several disciplines did collaborate on important experiments—as in the study of effect of alcohol on higher-order problem solving by experimental psychologist Carpenter, educator Moore, sociologist Snyder, and clinical psychologist Lisansky (1961). More important, and what proved the value of the idea, was that the mix of disciplines in the same institute, with recognition of mutual concern about a common problem field, resulted in much interdisciplinary discussion, much mutual questioning and learning, and a consequent enrichment of the type of questions that even those working in their own exclusive discipline or profession tended to ask, enrichment, too, of the kind of inferences that tended to be drawn from the outcome of researches (Keller, 1975*a*).

## 7. IMPACT OF THE CENTER ON RESEARCH, EDUCATION, TREATMENT, AND PREVENTION

The existence and the manifest success and influence of the Center stimulated attempts to form other centers of alcohol studies and eventually led the National Institute on Alcohol Abuse and Alcoholism (which in 1970 replaced the National Institute of Mental Health as federal government financial supporter of alcohol-related activities) to sponsor and support the creation of several centers of alcohol studies in separate locations in the United States. In spite of the advice of a consultant from the Rutgers Center, the National Institute specified that the new Centers of Alcohol Studies should not be multidisciplinary but each should specialize.*

The influence of the Yale and Rutgers Center of Alcohol Studies on the alcohol-problems field is concretely evident in several developments. When the *Journal of Studies on Alcohol* was founded (*Quarterly* was deleted from its name when the frequency of its publication was increased), the only other scientific journal specialized to alcohol studies was the *British Journal of Inebriety* (now the *British Journal of Addiction*). More than a dozen journals devoted to studies of alcohol or alcohol and other addictive drugs are published now. Similarly, the fundamental bibliographic publications emanating from the Center (Keller and Efron, 1956; Keller, 1966) have been matched and supplemented by specialized bibliographies from other sources (Popham and Yawney, 1967; Polacsek et al., 1970, 1972; Barnes and Price, 1973; Heath and Cooper, 1981). Books about alcohol problems in the 1930s and early 1940s were few and mainly autobiographical or concerned with immediate policy issues of the postprohibition condition. The Memoirs and Monographs and Popular Pamphlets series of the Yale Center initiated a trend. Libraries were so poorly provided with objective books about alcohol issues that, on Jellinek's advice, many of the newly established state alcoholism agencies stocked academic as well as public libraries with publications of the Yale Center. In the 1980s books on any alcohol-related topic are published in abundance by commercial as well as academic presses, reflecting the vast increase of public interest in alcohol problems as well as the growth of the field.

A particularly important feature of the documentation program was the publishing of duplicate sets of the Classified Abstract Archive. At the initiative of the World Health Organization, as recommended by Jellinek, complete sets of the Archive were provided in 1953 to a number of depository libraries and government bureaus in 16 countries. Additional depositories, in research and teaching libraries in other countries and in the United States, eventually brought the total of Archive depositories to over 90. Each depository received initially over 6000 19.1 × 16.8 cm cards imprinted with bibliography and abstracts, each edge-notched according to the detailed Archive topical code, and was provided semiannually with duplicates of all new additions from the world current literature (Keller et al., 1953, 1965).

Here a regrettable reduction of function must be recorded: After the retirement of the original chief of the Center's Documentation Division, the National Institute on Alcohol Abuse and Alcoholism chose to withdraw its support of that activity at Rutgers and to take it over as its own—carried out on its behalf by commercial contractors, with a competence that must be judged by users. Though the Classified Abstract Archive was thus discontinued, the Center's library remains the most complete repository in the world of documentary knowledge about alcohol, with unique resources, historic and current, in collections of books, reprints, and journals, as well as card catalogs and topical bibliographies.

*The advantage of this single-minded sort of center is best understood in the councils of governmental bureaucracies.

When the Yale Center initiated its study of alcohol education in the schools, that education was entirely under the influence of the old Temperance Movement; in some states, by law, it was education on "the evils of alcohol." There followed a decided revision of focus in the direction of objectivity and educational standards, and with stimulus from the Center's chief educationist, Raymond G. McCarthy, a society of professional educators on alcohol and drugs was founded.

The Center was significantly influential in persuading the Connecticut State Legislature to establish a State Commission on Alcoholism. It was the first such commission, with a then generous budget. Before long, one state after another was establishing a commission on alcoholism.

The Summer School of Alcohol Studies was original and unique when founded at Yale in 1943. There are today more than a dozen summer schools of alcohol studies.

When the Yale Plan for Industry was projected, there were only two industry alcoholism programs in the country, so private, so unheralded, that the Yale faculty did not know of their existence and thought themselves utterly original in their idea. Dozens of alcoholism programs in industry flourish today, with an organization of several hundred "alcoholism counselors" specialized to industry programs.

The treatment of alcoholism, and hospitals specializing in that field of medicine, were well developed in the United States in the 19th century. When the Constitution was amended to prohibit commerce in alcoholic beverages, they closed up, went out of business; apparently they thought that there would be no more alcoholics! Yet most of the tens of thousands of alcoholics seen by physicians and admitted to hospitals in the early 1930s (Jolliffe, 1936) had become alcoholics during the prohibition years. They hardly received any treatment for their alcoholism, however. Though alcohol could not be suppressed, alcoholism was relegated to incognition. Undoubtedly the burgeoning of Alcoholics Anonymous in the early 1940s contributed to the growth of interest in alcoholism and alcoholics. The Center's Yale Plan Clinics, subject of unremitting publicity in the popular press, soon became the models for numerous similar and other treatment facilities that never lacked for patrons—and supporters.

As for research, the study of alcohol, and of alcoholism, had been substantially neglected during the first third of the 20th century. Indeed, it was almost as if there were something disreputable about the subject. People in academic institutions preferred to ignore it, perhaps in reaction to the offensive and growing influence of the antialcohol movement (Bacon, 1967). The courage of a few scientists and scholars in the 1930s brought the subject out of limbo, as it were. Following the favorable reception of the activities and published researches that emanated from the first Center of Alcohol Studies, along with the availability of new financial support—chiefly from governmental sources—research in the alcohol-problems field has subsequently engaged scientists in all relevant disciplines, and publication has flourished in proportion. Simultaneously, increased research and actions were stimulated in other countries, particularly in Canada, England, and the Scandinavian lands, including Finland.

This, then, is the chief social as well as scientific contribution and influence of the original Center of Alcohol Studies—that each of its activities and undertakings became a model, quickly popularized and adopted or adapted, in more or less likeness, throughout the land, and abroad as well.

It is interesting to note that in no case did the staff of the Yale Center initiate any of its pioneering activities with the intention or expectation of creating a model. That undesigned outcome reflects only the insight of the Center's staff in perceiving what was needful for coping with the problems of alcohol. Thus, the invention at Yale of the Alcometer (Greenberg and Keator, 1941)—the first portable breath-alcohol testing machine, first tentatively tried by the Connecticut State Police—has likewise been followed by the development of increasingly sophisticated instruments that police all over the world now use to identify drivers who are "under the influence."

The Center of Alcohol Studies initially set for itself four ideal aims to be cultivated: research, education, treatment, and prevention. The foregoing history has indicated how the first three ideals were realized. The fourth, which ultimately is the most important, was hardly advanced. Of course, it can be contemplated that the first three promote the last. That remains to be demonstrated. For while it is easy to render lip service to prevention, how to do it has hardly become apparent. Indeed, it is not even apparent that most people are agreed on what is to be prevented: Alcoholism? Drunkenness? Drinking? Alcohol? Of course, some perceive that by "preventing" alcohol all alcohol problems must disappear. It is not apparent, however, that alcohol can be eliminated from a population that desires to drink, whether moderately or immoderately. In the unavoidable presence of alcohol, it is not yet apparent how the related problems can be prevented. The learned, clever, wise, well-meaning folk in the Center of Alcohol Studies thought often and much about prevention. But they were unable to devise workable experiments in that direction. Their best thoughts contemplated education and consequent alterations in the social mores about drinking. Perhaps they were as wise as anyone can be. But during the time span of this history they could not demonstrate their rightness. Prevention is waiting to be researched. Research in prevention is waiting for the sort of long-term commitment of financial support that only rich private foundations can provide.

It remains to tell, to complete this brief history of the early Center of Alcohol Studies, that its second director, Selden Bacon, being required by University rule to retire as Director (in 1975), though not as Professor of Sociology, he was succeeded in this function for a brief interim by John A. Carpenter, and subsequently and to the present by Peter B. Nathan. Under this new regime, not only have traditional programs been continued at Rutgers, but at last it has been possible to revive the clinical program, with Barbara S. McCrady as Clinical Director, while under the direction of Gail G. Milgram, the education program has been broadened to include not only the greatly expanded Summer School, now offering over 30 separate courses each year, but also a series of year-round graduate courses that attract students from many departments and schools.

## 8. CONCLUSION

From the preceding history it seems possible to identify the critical events that in the mid-third of the 20th century moved the study of alcohol and its effects, including alcoholism and its treatment, from neglect to efflorescence.

The critical motivants were the two pertinent questions asked by two brilliant scientist–researchers in the mid-1930s: Norman Jolliffe's "Why are they drinking that way?'' and Howard W. Haggard's ''What is alcohol doing in the organism?'' To these questions were soon added E. M. Jellinek's and Selden D. Bacon's explorations of the possible avenues for achieving scientifically valid answers and possible means of applying existing scientific knowledge in the real world. The aims and efforts of these pioneers came to focus in the creation of the original Center of Alcohol Studies. It must be recognized that their aims were soon partly overwhelmed in the real world by the interactions of Alcoholics Anonymous and the National Council on Alcoholism, effecting an overwhelming attention to alcoholism and its treatment, with some consequent slighting of the fundamental scientific questions and answers. In the political world of a humane society this deviation is only natural. It remains, for those who understand that effective remedies and permanent solutions depend ultimately on study and resolution of the fundamental questions, to persist in their fundamental tasks, even while cooperating in the temporary ameliorations mandated by membership in the humane society, as well as by dependence on its support.

## REFERENCES


Bacon, S. D., 1943, Sociology and the problems of alcohol; foundations for a sociologic study of drinking behavior, *Q. J. Stud. Alcohol* **4**:402.

Bacon, S. D., 1944, The sociological approach to the problems of alcohol, *Fed. Probation* **8**(4):20.

Bacon, S. D., 1951, Alcoholism and industry, *Civitan Mag.* **31**(7):3.

Bacon, S. D., 1967, The classic temperance movement of the U.S.A.; impact today on attitudes, action and research, *Br. J. Addict.* **62**:5.

Baird, E. G., 1944, 1945, 1946, 1948, The alcohol problem and the law, *Q. J. Stud. Alcohol* **4**:525; **5**: 126; **6**:335; **7**:110, 271; **9**:80.

Barnes, T. H., and Price, S., 1973, *Interaction of Alcohol and Other Drugs,* Supplement 1, Addiction Research Foundation, Toronto.

Carpenter, J. A., Moore, O. K., Snyder, C. R., and Lisanky, E. S., 1961, Alcohol and higher-order problem solving, *Q. J. Stud. Alcohol* **22**:183.

Greenberg, L. A., and Keator, F. W., 1941, A portable automatic apparatus for the indirect determination of the concentration of alcohol in the blood, *Q. J. Stud. Alcohol* **2**:57.

Heath, D. B. and Cooper, A. M., 1981, *Alcohol Use and World Cultures: A Comprehensive Bibliography of Anthropological Sources,* Bibliographic Series, No. 15, Addiction Research Foundation, Toronto.

Henderson, R. M., and Bacon, S. D., 1953, Problem drinking; the Yale Plan for business and industry, *Q. J. Stud. Alcohol* **14**:247.

Jellinek, E. M., ed., 1942*a*, *Alcohol Addiction and Chronic Alcoholism,* Yale University Press, New Haven, CT.

Jellinek, E. M., 1942*b*, An outline of basic policies for a research program on problems of alcohol, *Q. J. Stud. Alcohol* **3**:103.

Jellinek, E. M., 1944, Notes on the 1st half year's experience at the Yale Plan Clinics, *Q. J. Studies Alcohol* **5**:279.

Jellinek, E. M., 1946, Clinical tests on comparative effectiveness of analgesic drugs, *Biometrics Bull.* **2**: 87.

Jellinek, E. M., 1947, What shall we do about alcoholism? *Vital Speeches* **13**:252.

Jellinek, E. M., 1951, Estimates of the number of alcoholics and rates of alcoholics per 100,000 adult population (20 years and older) for certain countries, in: *Report on the First Session of the Alcoholism Subcommittee, Annex I* (World Health Organization Committee on Mental Health), World Hlth Org. Tech. Rep. Ser., No. 42, Geneva.

Jellinek, E. M., and Jolliffe, N., 1940, Effects of alcohol on the individual; review of the literature of 1939, *Q. J. Stud. Alcohol* **1:**110.

Jellinek, E. M., and McFarland, R. A., 1940, Analysis of psychological experiments on the effects of alcohol, *Q. J. Stud. Alcohol* **1:**272.

Jellinek, E. M., Haggard, H. W., and Keller, M., eds., 1945, *Alcohol, Science and Society,* Quarterly Journal of Studies on Alcohol, New Haven, CT.

Jolliffe, N., 1936, Alcoholic admissions to Bellevue Hospital, *Science* **83:**306.

Jolliffe, N., 1945, Alcohol and nutrition; the diseases of chronic alcoholism, in: *Alcohol, Science and Society* (E. M. Jellinek, et al., eds.), pp. 73–82, Quarterly Journal of Studies on Alcohol, New Haven, CT.

Keller, M., 1964, Documentation of the alcohol literature; a scheme for an interdisciplinary field of study, *Q. J. Stud. Alcohol* **25:**725.

Keller, M., 1965, The Jellinek formula for the rate of alcoholism, *AA Grapevine,* February: 29–34.

Keller, M., ed., 1966, 1968, 1980, *International Bibliography of Studies on Alcohol,* Vol. I, II, III, Rutgers Center of Alcohol Studies, New Brunswick, NJ.

Keller, M., 1972, A special-library information-center model for a societal-problem field, in: *Proceedings of the ISLIC International Conference on Information Science* (L. Vilentchuk and G. Haimovic, eds.), Vol. 1, pp. 121–129, National Center of Scientific and Technological Information, Tel-Aviv.

Keller, M., 1975*a,* Multidisciplinary perspectives on alcoholism and the need for integration; an historical and prospective note, *J. Stud. Alcohol* **36:**133.

Keller, M., 1975*b,* Problems of epidemiology in alcohol problems, *J. Stud. Alcohol* **36:**1442.

Keller, M., and Efron, V., 1956, *A Bibliography on Alcohol Problems,* Pennsylvania Department of Public Health, Harrisburg.

Keller, M., Efron, V., and Jellinek, E. M., 1953, *Manual of the Classified Abstract Archive of the Alcohol Literature,* Quarterly Journal of Studies on Alcohol, New Haven, CT.

Keller, M., Efron, V., and Jellinek, E. M., 1965, *CAAAL Manual; a Guide to the Use of the Classified Abstract Archive of the Alcohol Literature,* Rutgers Center of Alcohol Studies, New Brunswick, NJ.

Landis, B. Y., 1945, Certain expenditures on account of inebriety, *Q. J. Stud. Alcohol* **6:**59.

Landman, R. H., 1952, Studies of drinking in Jewish culture; III, Drinking patterns of children and adolescents attending religious schools, *Q. J. Stud. Alcohol* **13:**87.

Lolli, G., Serianni, I., Banissoni, F., and Luzzatto-Fegiz, P., 1958, *Alcohol in Italian Culture; Food and Wine in Relation to Sobriety among Italians and Italian Americans,* Yale Center of Alcohol Studies, New Haven, CT.

Long, F. A., 1971, Interdisciplinary problem-oriented research in the university, *Science* **171:**961.

McCarthy, R. G., 1946, Group therapy in an outpatient clinic for the treatment of alcoholism, *Q. J. Stud. Alcohol* **7:**98.

McCarthy, R. G., and Douglass, E. M., 1949, *Alcohol and Social Responsibility; a New Educational Approach,* Crowell, New York.

Observer and Maxwell, M. A., 1959, A study of absenteeism, accidents and sickness payments in problem drinkers in one industry, *Q. J. Stud. Alcohol* **20:**302.

Polacsek, E., Barnes, T. [H.], Turner, N., Hall, R. [J.], and Tyminski, S., 1970, *Interaction of Alcohol and Other Drugs; an Annotated Bibliography,* Addiction Research Foundation, Toronto.

Polacsek, E., Barnes, T. [H.], Turner, N., Hall, R. [J.], and Weise, C., 1972, *Interaction of Alcohol and Other Drugs; an Annotated Bibliography,* 2nd ed., revised, Addiction Research Foundation, Toronto.

Popham, R. E., 1956, The Jellinek alcoholism estimation formula and its application to Canadian data. *Q. J. Stud. Alcohol* **17:**559.

Popham, R. E., and Yawney, C. D., 1967, *Culture and Alcohol Use; a Bibliography of Anthropological Studies,* Addiction Research Foundation, Toronto.

Roe, A., 1942, Legal regulation of alcohol education, *Q. J. Stud. Alcohol* **3:**433.

Roe, A., 1943, *A Survey of Alcohol Education in Elementary and High Schools in the United States*

(Memoirs of the Section on Alcohol Studies, Yale University), Quarterly Journal of Studies on Alcohol, New Haven, CT.

Roe, A., 1944, The adult adjustment of children of alcoholic parents raised in foster homes, *Q. J. Stud. Alcohol* **5**:378.

Roe, A., and Burks, B., 1945, *Adult Adjustment of Foster-Children of Alcoholic and Psychotic Parentage and the Influence of the Foster-Home* (Memoirs of the Section on Alcohol Studies, Yale University), Quarterly Journal of Studies on Alcohol, New Haven, CT.

Sadoun, R., Lolli, G., and Silverman, M., 1965, *Drinking in French Culture* (Monographs of the Rutgers Center of Alcohol Studies, No. 5), Rutgers Center of Alcohol Studies, New Brunswick, NJ.

Skolnick, J. H., 1954, A study of the relation of ethnic background to arrests for inebriety, *Q. J. Stud. Alcohol* **15**:622.

Skolnick, J. H., 1957, The stumbling block; a sociological study of the relationship between selected religious norms and drinking behavior, Yale University Doctoral Dissertation, New Haven, CT.

Snyder, C. R., 1954, Culture and sobriety; a study of drinking patterns and sociocultural factors related to sobriety among Jews, Yale University Doctoral Dissertation, New Haven, CT.

Straus, R., 1974, *Escape from Custody; a Study of Alcoholism and Institutional Dependency as Reflected in the Life Record of a Homeless Man,* Harper & Row, New York.

Straus, R., and Bacon, S. D., 1953, *Drinking in College,* Yale University Press, New Haven, CT.

Straus, R., and Winterbottom, M. T., 1949, Drinking patterns of an occupational group: Domestic servants, *Q. J. Stud. Alcohol* **10**:441.

White, H. B., Gomberg, E. S., and Carpenter, J. A., eds., 1982, *Alcohol, Science and Society Revisited,* University of Michigan Press, Ann Arbor.

Williams, P. H., and Straus, R., 1950, Drinking patterns of Italians in New Haven; utilization of the personal diary as a research technique, *Q. J. Stud. Alcohol* **11**:51, 250, 452, 586.

6

# Drugs, Alcohol, and Aging

EDITH S. LISANSKY GOMBERG

## 1. DEMOGRAPHICS OF THE ELDERLY

Although developmental psychology used to stop abruptly after infancy, childhood, and adolescence had been described, there has been, for some decades now, increasing awareness and increasing research activity in the biological, psychological, and social aspects of adult life: young adults, middle-aged adults, elderly adults. The last group, defined here as 65 and older, is one stage (obviously the last stage) in the lifespan, and demographic data have pointed up the fact that this group represents an increasing proportion of the population of developed nations. In the early 1980s, this age group constituted 9.3% of the Canadian population (*Fact Book on Aging in Canada*, 1983) and 11–12% of the U.S. population (*A Profile of Older Americans*, 1986). Demographers predict an increasing proportion of elderly in the population, projecting their speculations into the early decades of the 21st century.

We speak of "the elderly" or "the pensioners" or "retirees" as though these are homogeneous groupings. Most research attention has, in the past, concentrated on the differentiation between sick and well, on morbidity and mortality, although the relatively healthy segment of the older population represents a wide range of behaviors, habits, cognitions, personalities, attitudes, values, and even health status (Rowe and Kahn, 1987). Some hold the view that heterogeneity is even wider in this age group than in others. Whether this concept is valid or not, it is clear that everyone ages biologically, psychologically, and socially at different intraindividual and interindividual rates. Developmental unevenness exists for children, adolescents, and young adults, and it exists for older adults as well.

Part of the challenge of gerontology is to study and differentiate between "normal" aging and "abnormal" aging, and the assumption that *all* aging processes involve loss and impairment is being questioned. Rowe and Kahn (1987) distinguish between *usual*

---

EDITH S. LISANSKY GOMBERG • School of Social Work, and Alcohol Research Center, Department of Psychiatry, School of Medicine, University of Michigan, Ann Arbor, Michigan 48104.

aging and *successful* aging. *Usual* aging is normative in affluent societies and involves the heightening of the effects of aging by "extrinsic" factors. In *successful* aging, loss and impairment may be minimized by factors such as nutrition, exercise, continued activity, and social involvement. Successful aging, seen in the late work of major creative artists, was described recently as ". . . art born in the fullness of age" (Russell, 1987).

It hardly seems necessary to examine cross-cultural data and compare traditional agricultural societies with industrialized societies, as suggested by Rowe and Kahn (1987), to make this distinction. Within Canada and the United States, women are longer-lived than men, and the greater longevity of women may well be explained not only in terms of biological and physiological sex differences, but in terms of different role behaviors which encourage women to pay more attention to their health, to maintain activity in domestic roles, and to remain socially involved—thus increasing the likelihood of *successful* aging. It has been hypothesized that the greater longevity of women is linked to sex role and to greater adaptability to change (Gomberg, 1979).

The older population is indeed heterogeneous, and we may start with *age differences*. Persons defined as elderly may be of any age between 65 and 95, a 30-year, three-decade span. We speak now of "the frail elderly," meaning the oldest in that age group who have more or less difficulty in maintaining themselves. There has already been a classification into "young old" and "old old," and there is likely to be further subdivision.

There are *racial* and *cultural variations* in the aging process and the development of a research area called ethnogerontology (Jackson, 1985). Ethnic study includes not only those groups called "minorities," but variations in behaviors and customs among people whose families originate in different European, Asian, and African countries, and elderly people who practice different religions (Gelfand and Barresi, 1987). Membership and participation in different ethnic subgroups play a major role in social networking, community participation, and the use of health services (Gelfand, 1982). There are also regional differences in the percentage of elderly in the population, in life styles, and in services available in the different provinces and states of Canada and the United States.

Examining the *marital status* and the *economic status* of the elderly shows interesting *gender differences*. In 1985, older men were twice as likely to be married as older women. For the United States, the percentages were 77% of the men and 40% of the women. For Canada, the same is true: In Toronto, for example, the 1981 census showed 76% of men, 65 and older, to be married, and 36.1% of the same age women (*A Socio-Demographic Profile of the Elderly,* 1984). In the United States, 51% of all older women are widows and there are five times as many widows as widowers. The *Fact Book on Aging in Canada* (1983) sums it up: ". . . Most older men are married while most older women are widowed." Marital status is, of course, associated with living arrangements: 41% of older women and 15% of older men in the United States live alone. The same holds true for the Canadian elderly (Stone and Fletcher, 1981). The *economic status* of the elderly is a complex subject embracing earned income, social security, pensions, housing arrangements, and the definition of poverty level. But one aspect of economic status that stands out clearly is *gender difference*. Older women have higher rates of poverty than older men in the United States: 16% and 8%, respectively.

Since older people living alone or with nonrelatives are more likely to be poor than older people living with relatives, and since women are more likely to be in the former group, the results are predictable. One survey (Old, Alone and Poor, 1987) states flatly that poverty among elderly Americans living alone is primarily the poverty of widowed women; such poverty increases with age and is highest among U.S. minorities.

One aspect of the economic status of older people that has had much research and media attention is the economics of maintenance of the Social Security system. The increasing percentage of the population represented by the pensioners of the Social Security system, plus a diminishing workforce making payments into the system, has raised the specter of ultimate system collapse. Intergenerational tension and the burden of support of the elderly prompted the Gerontological Society of America to sponsor a work about "Ties that Bind, the Interdependence of Generations" (Kingston et al., 1986).

There is association by older people among age, economic status, health, marital status, living arrangements factors, and the utilization of health services (Shanas and Maddox, 1985). Equally clearly, there is an association between the same demographic factors and the use of medication and alcohol by older people.

## 2. PSYCHOSOCIAL ISSUES FOR THE ELDERLY

Some age-related psychosocial adaptations are related to use of medication and alcohol by older persons. In a sense, all such age-related adaptations, including the question of whether the older person lives alone or with others, is relevant to alcohol use and nonuse (Johnson and Goodrich, 1974; Branch, 1977; Monk et al., 1977; Barnes, 1979; Meyers et al., 1982; Alexander and Dutt, 1988). The age-related psychosocial adaptations to be discussed include (1) role and status change; (2) increase in chronic illness; (3) cognitive changes, such as sensory loss and memory problems; (4) retirement and work; (5) widowhood; (6) social networks and social supports; and (7) loss, affect, and life satisfaction.

### Role and Status Change

Status is the sum of all statuses a person occupies, a collection of rights and duties. When the rights and duties are exercised and performed, that is role. Rosow (1985) describes the diminution of status of the elderly and its accompanying consequences: Roles become increasingly tenuous and decrements in status are largely irreversible. Rosow (1985) summarizes the role/status of the elderly in these points: (1) Role loss excludes older people from significant social participation and devalues them; (2) old age is the first stage of life with systematic status loss for an entire cohort; (3) persons in American society are not socialized for aging; (4) since no age role is specified, the lives of older people are socially unstructured; (5) role loss deprives people of their social identity.

This seems a very negative, ethnocentric position. It is true that there are traditional, preliterate societies where older people have the greatest social power (Guttman,

1976). In such societies (granted that there is a smaller proportion of elderly survivors than is true in industrialized societies), the labor of the elderly is a necessity, and the experience of older people is often valued and commands respect.

But I would argue that in both American and Canadian society, the role and status of older persons is currently in flux. The abolition of mandatory retirement in many occupations and a growing literature on the older worker suggest that change may be in progress. Labor force participation of men aged 55–64 has declined in the last three decades, but labor force participation of women in the same age group has increased (Robinson et al., 1985). As a voting force in the United States, older persons in lobbying organizations and in percentages who vote exercise influence over legislation (Binstock et al., 1985). For those older women who are not in the workplace (and for those who are), domestic role responsibilities continue, and indeed, there is increasing recognition of the significant role of caretaker of the sick, elderly, and disabled, a role taken largely by older women (*Exploding the Myths: Caregiving in America,* 1987).

Two aspects of role should be considered: societal contribution and personal fulfillment. A sizable portion of the elderly population continues to make societal contribution in full-time and part-time jobs, in volunteer work, and in helping roles within the family. The bonds that seem to exist between young children and older people have been developed (and need further development) in jobs such as school helper and day care assistant. If ''caretaker'' role is defined as a societal contribution, there is a large portion of the elderly population working at that role. As for personal fulfillment, there is a relevant observation by Robinson et al. (1985) that work and leisure are becoming less distinct as retirees move in and out of the workplace, often seeking working arrangements that provide a satisfying combination of work and leisure. And while contemporary Western culture does not set a high value on the contemplative life, the fact remains that older people may now have more time and opportunity to pursue both quiet and active interests, including genealogy, golf, fishing, elderhostels, arts and crafts, and travel. Some opt for more passive leisure time and spend time watching television—but that is hardly confined to older people!

## Increase in Chronic Illness

In 1986, 31.2% of people 65 years and older in the United States reported their health to be ''fair'' or ''poor,'' and 50.4% of people in that age group reported that they had a chronic or serious illness (Special Report, 1987). The number of days in which activity is restricted because of illness or injury increases with age, and the number and length of hospital stays increase. In 1984, the 11–12% of the population 65 or over accounted for 31% of total personal health care expenditures (note that this includes the institutionalized elderly). Most people over 65 have at least one chronic medical condition. These are, in the order of occurrence: arthritis (53%), hypertension (42%), heart disease (34%), cataracts (23%), orthopedic impairment (19%), visual impairment (14%), arteriosclerosis (12%), cerebrovascular disease (10%) and diabetes (10%) (*A Profile of Older Americans,* 1986). The occurrence of chronic medical conditions among the Canadian elderly is similar, although the percentages vary slightly (Simmons-Tropea et al., 1986). Hearing disorders, listed among major health problems of the elderly, appear twice as frequently among older men as older women. The Canadian prevalence data also include mental disorders (12%) and dental problems (8%).

Among the young old, 65–74 years of age, 14% need assistance in self-care and home management, and this increases to 26% for the 75–84 group, and to 48% of those 85 and older. Note, however, that half of the most elderly are managing self-maintenance, and that of Americans 65 and older, 68% rate their health as "good" or "excellent." If more education on nutrition, exercise, and preventive health care is made available to the elderly, it is anticipated that the medical status of those over 65 will improve. The picture is mixed: The increase in chronic illness does increase with aging, and the capacity to prevent or ameliorate illness among older persons is improving.

## Cognitive Changes

This is an area in which stigma and prejudice directed toward older people appear most frequently; e.g., "he's senile," or "she's lost her marbles." It is commonly believed that dementia is a normal, everyday component of aging. Yet the encyclopedic *Handbook of the Psychology of Aging* (1985) includes no less than eight chapters dealing with different aspects of the mental processes of older adults. Three chapters deal with sensory phenomena, one with reaction time, one with memory, one with language skills, one with "intelligence and cognition," and one with problem solving and complex decision making.

Slowing of reaction time or reduced "speed of behavior" with increased age is apparently one of the areas of agreement, although little is known about its causes or consequences (Salthouse, 1985). In current studies of memory, there is more sophistication about the multivariate nature of memory; the fact is that no one hypothesis can adequately account for observed age differences (Poon, 1985). Deficit hypotheses alone do not account for the variability in the observed performances of older adults.

Psychologists who devised psychological tests (Terman and Merrill, 1937; Wechsler, 1958) were convinced of the decline of abilities with age, Wechsler stating that ". . . most human abilities . . . decline progressively . . . after ages 18 and 25." Such decline was studied with measures of sensory acuity and reaction time. The view of intelligence as unitary also contributed little to the subject, but more recent views of *intelligence,* seen as the summation of a number of factors, offer a more valid picture of change with aging. Indeed, Labouvie-Vief (1985) has noted that currently it is clear that decrement, stability, even growth, may occur ". . . over the adulthood period." There is no simple decline of intellectual functioning with age (Baltes and Nesselroade, 1973; Horn, 1976; Horn and Donaldson, 1976; Baltes and Schaie, 1976; Botwinick, 1977; Labouvie-Vief, 1985). There is current research on the question whether or not loss with aging may be reversible (Baltes and Willis, 1981; Schaie and Willis, 1986).

Part of the changing perception of cognitive loss is a methodological shift. Cross-sectional studies have suggested more loss than have longitudinal studies which indicate that decline occurs at a much later age than was originally thought. That there are cohort effects must go without saying, and progressive cohorts are more educated; educational achievement plays a significant role in maintenance of intellectual abilities in aging (Green, 1969).

The issue of cognitive change is particularly relevant to discussion of the effects of alcohol on older persons. The combined effect of age changes and heavy intake of alcohol is a major issue with old problem drinkers. Indeed, it has been hypothesized that alcohol effects and aging effects are similar ("premature aging"), although this hypothesis has mixed support.

## Retirement and Work

Public policy developments on employment and retirement are pushed from different directions, one favoring early retirement and the other favoring flexible retirement policies. Employer concerns about retirement vary according to industry and occupations involved, the labor supply and demand, and general economic conditions (Robinson et al., 1985). The individual decision to retire seems to be based on two sets of factors: individual factors, e.g., income and health, and institutional factors, e.g., labor market conditions.

Several trends in retirement should be noted. Blue-collar status vs. white-collar status is one influence; amount of schooling seems to be negatively correlated with retirement rates (Sheppard, 1976). The nature of the work performed, whether rigidly fixed or involving variety, autonomy, and responsibility, plays a role in retirement decisions (Jacobsohn, 1972). Data suggest that the lower the skill level, the greater the propensity to retire. In a survey of white men, 50 and older, respondents were asked if they would retire if provided with adequate income; 45% of the blue-collar workers and 24% of the white-collar workers said they would (Sheppard, 1976). The question of retirement has been further complicated by the rising proportion of women in the workforce and the retirement decision made in a husband/wife working family.

There is an interesting gender difference in the limited data available on gender comparisons of response to retirement. Atchley (1976) found women in the workplace to have as much difficulty as men—or even more—in adapting to retirement. This is supported by Fox's (1985) findings that retirement is associated for women with ". . . lower feelings of psychological well-being." For women who have held jobs for most of their adult lives, social contact outside the family is more linked to "positive affect balance" than it is for housewives.

## Widowhood

The loss of a spouse represents a major stress, social and psychological. Inevitably, it is more frequently experienced by older people. In addition to the emotional response of grief and mourning, there are decisions to be made. One question is whether to continue living in the same house; another is one's income status. When marital status shifts to widow/widower, there are inevitably new aspects of interpersonal dealings, of social role to be considered. The large proportion of all marriages that end in divorce and the large number of households headed by a single parent suggest that marital loss or marital shift is a situation not unique to the elderly. For younger persons, however, adjusting to a new nonmarried role, there is the possibility of new relationships as they reenter the dating/mating scene. The choices are obviously narrower for older persons, particularly older women.

Among the elderly, there is a different rate of remarriage for widowers and for widows. One obvious consequence of sex differences in longevity rates is that older men have a larger pool of women available to choose from, and men who participated in a marital interdependency seem more likely to look for another wife. The situation is more complicated than that: It has been traditional for men to marry women younger than themselves, whereas there is only now beginning to be more acceptance of marriages where the wife is older. Men come out both better and worse in spouse loss. Although it is true that they remarry more frequently, widowers also tend to respond negatively, particularly within the first 6 months to 2 years after the loss. They have higher rates of morbidity (Verbrugge, 1979), of mortality (Gove,. 1975), and of suicide (Berardo, 1970). It is only in recent years that social scientists have begun to explore the question of loneliness (Peplau and Perlman, 1982; Vinick, 1983).

## Social Networks and Social Supports

In a frequently cited study of Alameda County, California, Berkman and Syme (1979) reported that over a 9-year period, "... people who lack social and community ties are at a substantially increased risk of dying." There is, however, little support for the idea that the relationship between social networks, social supports, and health status is different for *older* people (Kasl and Berkman, 1981; House et al., 1982; Minkler, 1985).

Is it true, as frequently assumed, that increasing social isolation is a concomitant of old age? The majority of people over 65 live with other family members, including spouses, and although the percentage is higher for men, 79%, there are still 59% of elderly women living with family (Sussman, 1976). Nor does living alone necessarily mean social isolation. A large proportion of elderly people live alone but close to their children, and there is evidence that a large proportion of older people prefer that arrangement. Berkman (1985) described a Social Network Index which includes marriage, contacts with extended family and close friends, church membership, and other group affiliations. Berkman concludes that isolated, disconnected people who have recently lost an intimate relationship are at increasing mortality risk, but that there is no indication that the elderly are more vulnerable in this regard.

There are methodological problems. The definition and measurement of social support is the first problem, and most definitions exclude "instrumental or tangible support" (Minkler, 1985). The qualitative aspects of family life and other relationships have been neglected (Aizenberg and Treas, 1985). Most reported data ignore ethnic differences, although there is evidence that black widows and widowers are less likely to live alone than their white counterparts (Chevan and Korson, 1972). The phrase "role reversal" refers to parent–child relationships and surfaces in the literature, although little is understood about this complex phenomenon. And with increasing institutionalized support networks, e.g., retirement communities and government health care, how will these networks affect the relationships and supports of older people?

Of direct relevance is the relationship between social supports and high-risk-health practices. Among all age groups, there is evidence that more isolated people are more likely to smoke, drink heavily, engage in minimal physical activity, and be overweight. The relationship between lack of social and community ties and heavy drinking is clearer among men than women (Berkman, 1985). What is not clear is whether people drink heavily because they are isolated or whether their social networks become eroded by their heavy drinking—antecedent, concomitant, or consequence?

## Losses, Affect, and Life Satisfaction

There are many points of view about the affective responses and optimal adjustment of the elderly. One group's view is "gloom and doom": Aging is *loss,* loss of spouse, job, cognitive skills, and social networks. Hardly surprising that under these conditions, the most common affective disorder in late life is depression. A variant of this view is *disengagement* (Cumming and Henry, 1961), a theory that precipitated a debate among gerontologists. In this theory, aging is viewed as withdrawal both by the aging person and by society, so that distance and disengagement are the end result. The theory has received little support (Burrus-Bammel and Bammel, 1985).

A more neutral position about aging emphasizes *continuity* in activity and in behavioral patterns over time (Zborowski, 1962), and there is some evidence to support this view. Findings are that participation in activity during earlier years is related to current level of activity of older persons. There is also *activity theory,* which assumes a positive relationship between activity and life satisfaction. The greater the role loss, the less the life satisfaction; successful aging is therefore characterized by activity and by resistance to diminution of the social world (Burrus-Bammel and Bammel, 1985). Finally, there are gerontologists who hold a Pollyannish viewpoint, that aging releases creative talents and abilities that have lain dormant during adult life.

Obviously, there is heterogeneity among older persons. The simplest rule-of-thumb, on the basis of available evidence, is that people who were sensitive and alert to their environments, responsive to others, and interested in a variety of activities and subjects will deal with the adjustments of aging better than those who displayed minimum ability in interpersonal relations and problem solving.

Do affective responses change over time and are there characteristic personality changes associated with growing old? The evidence is inconclusive (Schulz, 1985), but one may assume that the repertoire of emotional response of older persons is not very different from the repertoire of emotional response in other age groups. More research is needed about the manifestations of affect in different age groups. Negative feelings, e.g., depression, guilt, anxiety, and loneliness, and positive feelings, e.g., self-confidence, serenity, and acceptance of other human beings, seem to change little over time. Anger, rage, and hostility change little. The lifetime patterns of habitual emotional response do not appear to change as the person ages, although they may vary. Available biological data, when older and younger people are compared, indicate that older people manifest ". . . higher levels of arousal when confronted with novel stress-inducing situations" and tend to take longer to return to baseline (Schulz, 1985). The intensity and duration of some emotional responses appear to increase with age.

Examples of some stable personality patterns that seem to hold up through the life cycle have recently been investigated and defined. These are anxiety level, friendliness, and eagerness for new experience (Costa and McCrae, 1980; Conley, 1983, personal communication). Conley confirms the stability of these patterns in the data from a longitudinal study of married couples interviewed in 1935, 1955, and 1980 and suggests that some traits make certain life crises more probable (Goleman, 1987). Costa has stated that there is no evidence of any universal age-related crises and that "more emotional" people experience more crises throughout their lives (Goleman, 1987).

As far as is known, ego defense mechanisms remain the same, although the degree to which they are utilized may change through the lifespan. It is commonly asserted, for example, that the elderly use the mechanism of denial more than do other groups.

Several national surveys have produced some information about the mood and morale of older people. In an extensive study of mood states over a wide range, the frequency of happy, sad, or neutral moods showed no differences when young and old are compared (Cameron, 1975). Age-related differences in feelings of life satisfaction or sense of well-being have been studied with the same result: No differences are found in "subjective well-being" in comparison of older and younger persons. Subjective feelings of well-being are most strongly related to health, followed by socioeconomic status, amount of social interaction, marital status, housing, and availability of transportation, for older adults. It is also of interest that older people are less likely than younger respondents to describe themselves as "very happy," although older persons are more likely to report higher levels of overall life satisfaction (Campbell et al., 1976).

Are older people more depressed than younger people? The most common affective disorder of late life is depression (Weinstein and Khanna, 1986). Estimates vary widely and depend on the criteria of depression. Some community surveys report depressive symptoms in 30–65% of persons over 60, but the full symptom complex of major depression, as defined in DSM-III, appears in up to 6%, and depressions severe enough to warrant intervention are estimated to occur in 10–15% of older persons (LaRue et al., 1985). Affective disorders are estimated to account for approximately half of psychiatric hospital admissions of older adults, most of these being first admissions. Unipolar depression is the usual clinical diagnosis. Are such disorders related to age-related losses? On this question, opinion is divided. Some view elderly depression as secondary to physical, social, and economic difficulties, losses that are inevitable in the aging process (Blazer and Williams, 1980). Klerman (1976) has argued that the diagnosis of "reactive depression" among older people is an oversimplification. He argues that there are biological factors, coping mechanisms developed in early life, and environmental demands for adaptation that need to be considered, and that depression is not a response simply to the "stresses" of aging.

## 3. MEDICATION

Drugs of medication include prescription drugs (for medical conditions), over-the-counter (OTC) drugs, and psychoactive drugs. *Pharmacokinetics* involves the study of the time course of absorption, tissue distribution, metabolism and excretion of drugs and their metabolites from the body, and the relationship of drug disposition to the intensity and duration of effects. Studying the effects of age on pharmacokinetics produces information about the mechanism of altered pharmacodynamics in the elderly. *Pharmacodynamics* is described as the physiological and psychological response to a drug (Vestal and Dawson, 1985). Pharmacodynamics concerns itself with the greater or lesser response in elderly persons to particular drugs, independent of pharmacokinetic effects. Different psychoactive drugs, for example, may show different pharmacodynamic effects; e.g., response of older people to some of the benzodiazepines seems to be enhanced (McCormack and O'Malley, 1986).

It is, by now, a cliché: Although the elderly comprise 11–12% of the American population, they receive 25–30% of the prescriptions. In the United States, the population 65 and older spends 20–25% of the total national expenditure for drugs, and in the United Kingdom, the elderly 12% of the population spends 30% of the national expenditure for medication (O'Malley et al., 1980).

What are the most commonly prescribed and nonprescribed medications? Chien et al. (1978), in a survey of people 60 and older living in the community, found this order: analgesics (67%), cardiovascular preparations (34%), laxatives (31%), vitamins (29%), antacids (26%), and antianxiety drugs (22%). OTC drugs accounted for 40% of medications used, and 83% of the respondents reported taking two or more medications. Guttman (1977*b*), in a similar community study, found the most frequently used medication to be cardiovascular agents (61%), with sedatives and tranquilizers next (17%), followed by antiarthritic agents (12%) and gastrointestinal agents (11%). Two-thirds of Guttman's respondents reported use of OTC drugs, of which analgesics were most commonly used (52%). In sum, nonnarcotic analgesics were the most commonly used OTC drug, and cardiovascular agents and psychoactive substances the most commonly prescribed medications. Data for older persons in other countries are similar (Vestal and Dawson, 1985).

There is some evidence that older persons are significantly more susceptible to adverse drug reactions than younger patients (Siegel, 1982; Goldberg and Roberts, 1983; Schmucker, 1984; Vestal and Dawson, 1985). There are more hospital admissions among older patients with adverse drug reactions, but the drug response will be related to the presence and severity of chronic disease (more among older people), to the use of medication (more among older people), to the interaction of drugs (more among older people), and to patterns of alcohol usage.

Whether the medication is prescribed or bought from pharmacy shelves by the customer, what are some of the problems associated with the self-administration of medication? These usually relate to the use of prescription drugs, since the directions-for-use involved in OTC drugs come from either the packaging or the pharmacist. Most discussions of medication and the elderly deal with *noncompliance;* i.e., the patient does not comply with instructions. Noncompliance may involve:

Nonuse, in some cases not obtaining the prescription
Partial use, in which the patient begins but does not continue the course
Self-directed medication in which the patient decides on the dosage
Self-directed medication in which the patient buys and uses an OTC drug with the prescribed drug
Incorrect dosage: less or more than prescribed
Improper timing or sequencing of medications
"Drug swapping," shared medication

There are probably other patterns of noncompliance (Gaeta and Gaetano, 1977; Solomon et al., 1978; Raffoul et al., 1981; Kendrick and Bayne, 1982). The question is whether this phenomenon is *drug misuse*. Most discussions of elderly medication attribute the noncompliance to impairment processes in older people: This may be described as impairment of vision, hearing, memory, or even "dementia" or "senility." A pharmaceutical company publication for physicians, directed toward "encouraging medical compliance'' (Sandoz, 1977), described the older patient as ''. . . often forgetful . . . needing more time to understand . . . loss of hearing.'' The advice to physicians, to give instructions as clearly, simply, and slowly as possible, might well be applied to medication practice with *all* age groups.

Is noncompliance a simple matter of the mental impairment of the elderly? A sizable proportion of all prescriptions written are not brought to a pharmacy at all, estimated as perhaps 30% of all those written (Woolley, 1983); one reason clearly is that the expense of the medication may be too much for the person's budget. But there are other questions about noncompliance and, up to now, psychosocial issues have been ignored. To what extent are matters of control, autonomy, and self-determination in decision making involved? To what extent are issues of denial of illness and aging involved? Might self-destruction wishes be implicated? These questions have been raised (Gomberg, 1987), but the psychodynamics of older persons in making decisions and in action are not much studied. There are interpersonal interactions involved, too; one author points out that compliance is not so much a function of patient satisfaction with the patient–physician encounter as it is a function of ''. . . the quality of communication'' between patient and physician (Lampe, 1985). And might the current cohort of elderly be more respectful of medical authority than future cohorts?

The economics of medication—the costs of prescription drugs—is another issue. A recent pilot study of medication drug use and misuse with a Veterans Administration outpatient clinic sample (Gomberg, Hsieh and Adams, forthcoming) reports *hoarding* as the misuse most frequently reported, and this is clearly linked to concerns about access to medication.

A recent national survey by the American Association of Retired Persons (1984) reported most frequent noncompliance to manifest itself ''. . . when consumers stop taking a prescription drug mid-process.'' Forty percent of the respondents experienced side effects, and half of those reported that neither physician nor pharmacist discussed potential side effects. In spite of this, most respondents look to physicians as the primary source of information but are quite passive in patient–physician interaction. Very few ask about nondrug alternatives.

This problem of *drug misuse* or *noncompliance* is usually a problem of *underuse*. While noncompliance might result in overdose or drug interactions, the main issue appears to be underusing medication. There is a question whether such underutilization of medication is not an adaptive, defensive maneuver of older persons. Of course, people die because of inadequate medication, but they also die from overmedication and drug interactions. One way of avoiding adverse drug reactions and adverse drug interactions is underutilization. How frequently is noncompliance a mistake of impaired vision or memory and how frequently is it a decision made by the older person? There is no information on this question.

A recent discussion of detection of medication misuse by older people (Lesage and Zwygart-Stauffacher, 1988) suggests that older people ''. . . have the right to make final decisions concerning their drug intake.'' The older patient is the one who must weigh potential benefits against adverse side effects; unfortunately, the passivity implied by the responses in the American Association of Retired Persons survey (1984) suggests that there is a good deal of education to be done.

This brings us to the question of *drug interactions*. It has been pointed out that the more drugs taken, the greater the likelihood of adverse reaction (Hall, 1986). Some warnings about drug interactions are printed on the container in which the medication is sold. Drug interaction is a complex subject, including drug–drug interaction, drug–nutrient interaction, drug–laboratory test interaction, and drug–alcohol interaction (Simonson, 1984). And there is a pharmacodynamic response, which may be called drug–patient interaction, in which an adverse drug reaction occurs, based on individual sensitivity to a specific type of drug. Drug interaction, as commonly used, refers to adverse effects of combining two substances. For older people, the combination of medication and alcohol may present problems (Hubbard et al., 1979).

There is an issue about *polypharmacy:* Do older persons receive prescriptions more than necessary? This is a question of medical practice, of education about gerontology, about advancing knowledge in chemotherapy and in the nature of chronic diseases of older persons. The question has been raised about the gender differential in the prescribing of psychoactive drugs for women and for men (Cooperstock, 1976), and the same question may be raised about age differentials. Do older persons receive prescriptions more readily than younger persons? It is indisputable that older persons have more chronic illnesses and that great advances have been made in the chemotherapy of disease. What defines "more than necessary"? The question needs examination: Are other alternatives set aside because it is simpler to write a prescription? Ouslander (1986), who is himself a physician, points out that while four out of five older persons have at least one chronic illness, many such illnesses ". . . can be managed without drug therapy." Has the significant role of self-maintaining health measures, such as nutrition, exercise, and social activity, been emphasized enough in health maintenance of older people?

### Over-the-Counter Drugs

OTC drugs frequently purchased and used by older persons include analgesics, laxatives, and antacids. All medications may have negative effects when used immoderately, and packages usually contain directions and warnings. A question has been raised about special labeling for the elderly, but the consensus seems to be that it would be preferable to label by *specific medical condition* rather than by age (Eckian, 1985). It is not clear whether older people purchase and use OTC drugs more than do other age groups. One view is that ". . . compared with other age groups, the elderly do not use OTCs excessively" (Jones-Witters and Witters, 1983). Others estimate that the percent of the elderly using such nonprescription medication may be as high as 75% or higher (Simonson, 1984). One may say that OTC medication, particularly analgesics, receives wide usage by older persons. This does not, incidentally, include home remedies such as herbal teas, soups, and other concoctions whose effectiveness may be dismissed as "old wives' tales" or as placebo effects. Such home remedies should be studied more extensively (Boyd et al., 1984).

## 4. PSYCHOACTIVE DRUGS

Older persons have a higher rate of prescription and usage of psychoactive drugs, e.g., tranquilizers, sedatives, and hypnotics, than other age groups (Warheit et al.,

1976; Levenson, 1981). Hospital admission is thought to be more related to adverse drug reactions among the elderly than among younger age groups. But if drug-related crises in emergency rooms (ER) are examined, older persons contribute a modest percentage because most ER drug crises are younger persons presenting with overdose and other medical crises of "street drug" use, drug mixtures, or suicide attempts. It is important to note that when an older person is seen in the ER, it is likely to be a *psychoactive* drug which is involved. For younger patients, illicit drugs, e.g., heroin and cocaine, are the main substances involved in drug-related emergencies; for older patients, overdose reactions are most likely to involve "misuse of a psychoactive drug" (LaRue et al., 1985).

The use of psychoactive drugs with older persons brings us into a biobehavioral area different from that of chronic illness and medication. Psychoactive drugs are prescribed to deal with mental and emotional conditions and mental disorders; such drugs do have addictive quality, and psychological and physiological dependency potential needs to be considered. Here, the question of *drug abuse,* both self-generated and iatrogenic, must be raised. It is argued that physical or psychological impairment resulting from psychoactive drug dependency ". . . cannot be classified as substance-abuse disorder by DSM-III criteria" (LaRue et al., 1985). If that is the case, then the definition in the *Diagnostic and Statistical Manual of Mental Disorders* (1980) is inadequate. No one denies that drug dependency can develop among older persons, even when it is qualified as developing primarily ". . . in anxious, depressed, or hypochondriacal older adults" (LaRue et al., 1985). Finlayson (1984) has distinguished appropriate use, unintentional misuse, and purposeful abuse. Of 248 elderly inpatients in a private hospital treatment unit, Finlayson reports 86% to be dependent on alcohol alone, 8% on prescription drugs alone, and 6% on a combination of prescription drugs and alcohol; his observation that for most elderly drug abusers, ". . . stress intensified an established pattern of drug dependence" points to the necessity of obtaining a detailed medical history. Might it be that the majority of elderly psychoactive drug abusers begin such abuse *before* their sixties and a minority are recent-onset abusers? It is apparently true with alcohol abusers and it may also be true with abusers of other substances.

Mental disorders that appear most frequently among older persons include depression, dementia (including Alzheimer's disease), paranoia, hypochondriasis, and iatrogenic drug problems. Alcoholism and schizophrenia are much more frequently the mental disorders of the young and the middle-aged; all diagnostic categories show a drop in first admissions of people 65 and over, except for "brain syndromes" (Kramer et al., 1968). There are several problems in diagnosis. Age norms for most psychodiagnostic instruments are lacking, particularly in diagnosis of milder mental disorders, thereby making age comparison in mental disorder diagnosis uncertain and unreliable. Elderly persons who present with mental illness are also likely to manifest sensory deficits, isolation, poverty, loss of social supports, and chronic illness, which makes the diagnostic picture difficult to interpret. It is postulated that antecedent conditions may combine differently as etiology sources of mental disorder at different life stages (Baltes and Willis, 1977). One hypothesis is that there is close association between physical and psychiatric disorder in the elderly (Verwoerdt, 1981).

A physician's handbook on the use of "psychotherapeutic" drugs with older people (Crook and Cohen, 1981) describes the use of antipsychotic drugs, antidepressants, lithium, antianxiety agents, sedative–hypnotics, and drugs "prescribed to treat cognitive dysfunction.'' One class of the most widely used psychoactive drugs are sedatives and hypnotics; a discussion of these drugs describes the sleep disorders, insomnias due to illness, emotional disorders, life style patterns, and ''. . . decreased physiological need for sleep'' among older people (Greenblatt, 1981). Widespread as insomnia may be among older persons, it is agreed that sleep disorders are not usually life-threatening. Sleep problems may be secondary to medical or psychiatric disorders, in which case treatment of the latter is indicated. Greenblatt (1981) states that insomnia may ''. . . increase feelings of isolation, loneliness and boredom.'' The sleep patterns and problems of older persons need further research development.

Another question of emotional disorder badly in need of research is *depression* among the elderly. Considering the increased amount of chronic illness, changing role and status, personal losses, economics, and attrition of social networks, the remarkable fact is not the high proportion of elderly who are depressed, but the high proportion who express a good deal of life satisfaction! But depression is a major emotional disorder among the elderly, although the criteria for diagnosis are not really agreed upon. Depression appears to be the most common mental illness among those over age 65, with estimated incidence of 10%, and although the incidence may rise in the presence of illness, antidepressant drugs ''. . . are not indicated for all patients'' (Mendels, 1981). There are environmental pressures to be dealt with, and it may be better for the patient to obtain help in dealing with these than to medicate and ignore the environment of the patient.

Caveats about the *diagnosis of depression* among older people need to be observed. Apathy and disorientation may be indicative of brain syndrome as well as of depression. There are problems of circularity: Apathy may lead to malnutrition, which in turn produces confusion (Epstein, 1976). Depression is often accompanied by impairment in memory (Fann and Whelass, 1975). Depression may also go unrecognized when a person presents with apathy, withdrawal, and self-devaluation, regarded by the diagnostician as an appropriate response to aging (Hodkinson, 1975).

National surveys which include the elderly living in the community show high usage of psychoactive drugs. Parry et al. (1973) found 32% of women and 21% of men between 60 and 74 to have used at least one psychoactive drug during the last 12 months. Prentice (1979) comments that older people receive ''. . . disproportionately high percentages'' of psychoactive drug prescriptions, and 50% of older persons who use psychoactive drugs reported that they could not perform their regular daily activities without the medication. A National Institute on Drug Abuse report on aging and psychoactive drug use (1979) has raised the question of *addictive* drug use of psychoactive substances among older people. No question but that it is simpler to write a prescription than to try to modify someone's life situation! Morrant (1983) has suggested that ''the best policy may be to prescribe the fewest drugs in the lowest doses and for as short a time as possible'' (p. 248).

In the United States, there are more persons in *nursing homes* than in all acute hospitals, and some surveys suggest that up to three-quarters of the beds are occupied by persons with behavioral, social, emotional, and mental disorders (DHHS, 1981). Many nursing homes have become institutions for the long-term care of the mentally ill, and multiple drug therapy is common practice (Vestal, 1982). Harper (1985) reports that approximately half of the residents who are given medication receive tranquilizers, and many who receive such medication have not been psychiatrically diagnosed (Levenson, 1981; Ganguli, 1983). It appears that psychoactive medication figures prominently in treatment in nursing homes, and the question may be raised whether a major reason for the use of such medication is minimizing the problem of care and maintenance in these institutions (Waxman et al., 1985). Perhaps nursing homes serve as a variant of hospice and perhaps it can be argued that it is humane to maintain residents on psychoactive drugs. But there are real concerns as to whose interests are best served, patients' or caretakers', and there are concerns about the extent to which such medication *contributes* to the emotional and mental disorders of residents (Cooper, 1986; Cooper, 1988). The problem is not confined to the United States. Overprescribing ". . . in hospitals and nursing homes" exists in Canada, and Morrant has warned that most prescribed drugs and many OTC drugs can cause psychiatric symptoms in older patients (Dobbie, 1977).

Finally, a note on *gender comparison* in use of psychoactive drugs by older persons. Up to age 65, women are more likely to be users of psychoactive drugs than are men (this relates, in part, to the fact that women receive more prescription drugs in general). Early on, an interesting trend appeared in the data about the age group 60–74 (Mellinger et al., 1974): A national survey showed 4% of the men and only 2% of the women in this age group reporting use of an antidepressant during the past year. There is a hypothesis that a triad of disorders appears more frequently among elderly men than elderly women: depression, alcohol problems, and suicide (Gomberg, 1981, 1987). A recent examination of gender differences in national data about psychoactive drug use among older adults showed that in the 65 and older group, men were more likely than women to report use of sedatives, tranquilizers and stimulants during the past year (Robbins and Clayton, submitted for publication). Such a shift might be related to increasing access to medical care and increased use of medical facilities by older men, or it may be related to a hypothesized gender difference in psychiatric disorder among older men and women (Gomberg, unpublished manuscript, 1979).

## 5. BANNED SUBSTANCES

The occasional social use of drugs like marijuana, hashish, and even cocaine probably does occur among older individuals, and there may be users of illicit drugs who began earlier in life and have survived into old age.* The information we have is confined to opiate addicts.

One of the widely held beliefs about opiate addicts was that they did not survive into old age, that they either died or "matured out." However, there are elderly addicts who have survived and who have managed, with more or less success, to conceal their

*Generational differences in experience and experimentation with illegal drugs are consistently found in cross-sectional studies. In a current study of alcoholic women (Gomberg, 1986), for example, a search for predictors of age at onset included an item that asked about the use of marijuana, hashish, and drugs other than alcohol when the respondent was between 13 and 15 years old. Of the alcoholic women interviewed, 41% of the women in their twenties answered affirmatively about use, 9% of the women in their thirties answered affirmatively, and there were no affirmative answers at all among the alcoholic women in their forties.

addiction (Capel et al., 1972); Capel & Peppers, 1978. Glantz (1985) has predicted that the number of such surviving elderly addicts will increase, and Pascarelli (1985) reports that whereas 0.005% of people in the New York City methadone program were 60 and older in 1974, that percentage had risen to approximately 2% in 1985. Nor do we have any idea of what effect the currently later age at onset of heroin addiction will have on survivor rates.

Apparently, heroin addiction does not *begin* when people are 60 and older, and it is an interesting theoretical exercise to try to explain the onset of heroin addiction in adolescence or early adulthood, as opposed to later life initiation, in terms of sensation-seeking theory. Are older persons not likely to experience emotional arousal as a reinforcement?

DesJarlais et al. (1985) examined an older cohort attending methadone clinics in New York City. In 1979, they found 286 patients in methadone maintenance programs who were aged 55–59 and another 262 who were in their sixties. There were also 53 patients in their seventies and five who were between 80 and 86. The patients whose history of addiction was of 20 years' duration and longer were interviewed, and seven factors emerged as major contributors to their longevity: genetic advantage (having parents who were long-lived), living by their wits but avoiding violence, the ability to obtain good supplies of narcotics, a concern for cleanliness of needles, the moderate use of nonopiate drugs (alcohol, in particular), the ability to hold drugs in reserve—moderating and controlling their use of the drug—and, finally, the availability of the methadone treatment program.

Most of the older patients interviewed in the methadone clinics were in good health, and their health problems were similar to those found in that age population. It is ironic to note that more than 90% of these older addicts had been heavy smokers during their lives and that smoking-related health problems were relatively frequent among those who were disabled. Most of the patients, living alone, used the methadone program as a major place for social interaction, as a kind of community or neighborhood center, and many continue to practice concealment successfully into old age. Within the clinics, they are model patients.

The use of banned substances is much more likely to be associated with young persons, as the association of criminal activity and the use of illegal drugs is more prevalent among younger individuals. Within the criminal justice system, elderly substance abusers are much more likely to be alcoholics than addicts, although the number arrested for public intoxication has been decreasing for some years now (Petersen, 1988).

## 6. TOBACCO

As is true throughout the lifespan, men are more likely to be smokers than are women, although the percentage gap between the sexes has narrowed considerably in the last 20 years. The National Center for Health Statistics data for the age group 65 and older show the same narrowing gap. In 1965, 28.5% of older men and 9.6% of older women were current smokers. In 1985, these percentages had become 19.6% and 13.5%, respectively (Smoking, Tobacco and Health, 1987). Not only is the male/female gap narrowed, there is an *increase* in the percentage of older women who are current smokers! This runs contrary to the trend in the other age groups of women: From 1965 to 1985, women from 20 to 64 show a drop in percentage of current smokers. The Public Health Service fact book (Smoking, Tobacco and Health, 1987) notes that there was a marked increase in female smoking during and after World War II and that 20 years after that, lung cancer deaths among women began to rise. By 1985, lung cancer had passed breast cancer as the chief cause of cancer death among women.

An interview study with people over 65 in the state of Massachusetts reported 23% of the respondents to be current smokers (Branch, 1977). Those *less* likely to be current smokers included respondents living alone or with their children, those in the oldest age groups, and those who reported their health as poor or fair.

Although it is true that older people in the United States and Canada are less likely to be current smokers than younger people, it is of interest to note the 1982 per capita consumption of cigarettes by total population (all age groups) in several different countries. Cyprus ranks first, with a per capita consumption of 3117 cigarettes; Canada ranks second, with 2797; and the United States ranks third, with 2678 (Smoking, Tobacco and Health, 1987).

It is difficult to know just what role smoking plays in the health status of older people; a study of drug metabolism among older persons notes that the effects of age, smoking, and drinking alcohol are confounded (Sellers et al., 1982). It is a reasonable certainty that smoking does not play a positive role in the health status of older people.

## 7. ALCOHOL: USE BY OLDER PERSONS

Before we review alcohol abuse among the elderly, it is useful to examine the use of alcoholic beverages by older persons. National surveys of U.S. drinking, primarily quantity and frequency measures, have demonstrated that cross-sectional comparisons show a decrease in the percentage of social and heavy drinkers and an increase in the percentage of abstainers among older people (Clark and Midanik, 1982). In the 1979 survey which Clark and Midanik report, the percentage of drinkers drops, for *women,* from 65% in the 35–39 age group, to 49% in the 50–64 age group, and again drops to 40% in the 65+ group. For *men* in the same age groups, the figures are 73%, 69%, and 59%, respectively. It appears that for women, there is a drop at age 50 and another drop at age 65+, whereas for men, the decrease appears large only at age 65+. The same gender difference appears in the figures for heavy drinkers: For women, there is a significant drop when they reach their fifties, whereas for men, this appears when they are in their sixties.

An interesting fact emerges from *comparison over time:* Clark and Midanik (1982) tabulate the percentage of drinkers in seven earlier surveys and compare these percentages with their own findings. The earlier surveys averaged 48% drinkers for men 65 and over; the 1979 survey showed this to have risen to 59%. The earlier surveys averaged 33% drinkers for women 65 and over; the 1979 survey showed this to have risen to 40%. Since the first of the surveys tabulated was done in 1971, it is clear that the proportion of men and women 65 and older who drink certainly did increase during the 1970s. The percentage of older people who drink remains lower than the percentage for younger people; nonetheless, there are more drinkers in the older age group now than there were a decade ago. Healthier older people, or a shifting view of appropriate behavior for older persons?

The decreasing percentage of drinkers and heavy drinkers as people age does, however, appear to be a stable epidemiological finding. As early as the 1940s, Riley and Marden (1947) reported 64% of people in their twenties, 65% of people 30–50, and 48% of people over 50 to be drinkers. In the 1950s and 1960s, the same decreases appeared in survey studies (Hyman et al., 1980). A 1984 general population survey (Hilton, 1987) shows the same pattern. In Canada, estimates range from 73% to 76% drinkers among those 21–49, but this drops to 61% for those 50 and older (Keller and Guriloi, 1976). The same age trends hold for data from Norway (Keller and Gurioli, 1976) and also from Finland (Mäkelä and Simpura, 1984).

When respondents in a national mental health survey (Veroff et al., 1981) were asked whether they take a drink when they feel worried or tense, ". . . to help handle things," affirmative response was as shown in Table 1.

Drew (1968) has argued that alcoholism is ". . . a self-limiting disease," and it is true that heavier drinkers tend to die early and thereby eliminate themselves from a count of drinkers among the elderly. Nonetheless, the epidemiological evidence over time and in several countries suggests that there are fewer drinkers among older persons than among younger ones.

Although there are few longitudinal studies of drinking behavior, the contention that patterns of drinking, including quantity and frequency, change during a lifetime (Dunham, 1981), but that aging is associated with a ". . . diminished pattern of consumption," (Cohen, 1985) appears to have substantial support. Social drinking by older persons seems to be related to income, health, living arrangements (alone or with others), and social networks. Income is positively related to the use of alcoholic beverages, and drinkers tend to have fewer somatic complaints than older people who do not drink (Guttman, 1977*c*).

The pattern of elderly social drinking appears to be quite different from the drinking of young people: Younger people tend to drink larger quantities less often and older people tend to drink more *frequently* but in *lesser quantities* than the young (Cahalan et al., 1969).

It is important to note that we may be finding a *unique cohort effect,* that the present generation of elders has had particular historical experience (Prohibition, the depression of the 1930s, World War II), and that the lowered proportion of drinkers and lessened

Table 1. Percentage of Men and Women (National Sample) Who Report Taking a Drink ". . . To Help Handle Things" (Veroff et al., 1981)

| Age | Men | Women |
|---|---|---|
| 21–34 | 11.1% | 6.5% |
| 35–54 | 16.5% | 7.4% |
| 55–64 | 10.3% | 1.6% |
| 65 and older | 5.8% | 2.0% |

consumption characterizes the *present* older generation, this age group at this time. There are hazards in inference from cross-sectional data, and the assumption that cross-sectional age differences ". . . necessarily reflect effects of aging" should be cautiously made (Glenn, 1981). There is some support from both cross-sectional and longitudinal data that such a cohort effect exists. Meyers et al. (1981–1982) believe that the data from their cross-sectional study of the Boston elderly support a cohort hypothesis. A longitudinal study of male veterans reports:

> . . . In both 1973 and 1982, older men drank markedly less than younger men. However, there were no significant longitudinal declines in drinking levels. . . . As the men in their fifties moved into their sixties, they did not reduce their alcohol consumption to amounts similar to the amounts consumed by men over 60 in the 1973 survey. (Glynn et al., 1984)

And Glynn et al. (1984) conclude that their data do *not* support the conclusion from earlier cross-sectional studies that aging modifies drinking behaviors. But generalizations must be made cautiously from the data based on a Boston sample of healthy, male veteran volunteers. A community survey of the use of alcohol by healthy, retired adults aged 65–74, living in the San Francisco area, reports almost 90% of the sample to have had at least one drink during the last 6 months (Huffine et al., 1989). National and regional surveys do not necessarily produce the same results and the criteria for inclusion in the sample may differ from study to study. The fact remains that there appears to have been a rise in the percentage of elderly people who drink during the 1970s (Clark and Midanik, 1982).

There is some information about the *characteristics* of elderly social drinkers and nondrinkers. One study with a mixed population of Caucasian, Black, and Latino persons 62 and older found social drinking associated with good health, social contacts, and a sense of well-being (Johnson and Goodrich, 1974). Another survey reported income and life satisfaction related to moderate alcohol use in an elderly sample (Guttmann, 1977*a*). A recent study of 270 adults over 65 found social drinking associated with maleness, income, and amount of education (Goodwin et al., 1987). But the evidence about the social facilitation of moderate drinking is mixed: Elderly persons with more social contacts (Johnson and Goodrich, 1974) and people living with spouse and/or family (Branch, 1977) are more likely to be social drinkers. It is reported that those living *alone* are more likely to be abstainers, and it is also reported that those living alone with limited or nonexistent social networks drink more heavily than people who are socially integrated (Monk et al., 1977). It is quite possible that those who live with other people are more likely to engage in moderate social drinking, and those who live alone are more likely to be abstainers *or* immoderate drinkers. It is also possible that the living-alone abstainers are primarily an elderly *female* population and the living-alone heavy drinkers largely male.

Drinking by older people as sociability versus social isolation has been reviewed in retirement communities (Alexander and Duff, 1988). Social drinking is usually moderate; when isolated and living alone, most older people probably do not drink at all while some drink to assuage feelings of loneliness (Gomberg, 1985).

A sample of older retired people in the San Francisco area was interviewed about use of psychoactive drugs and alcohol and about stress and coping (Huffine, Folkman and Lazarus, 1989). These respondents were more likely to use alcohol than similar age groups in national samples and they showed more heavy use. The investigators attribute the results to the "relatively advantaged status" of the respondents, drinking being associated with income. Results may also be reflecting higher educational achievement levels and geographical/regional differences in alcohol use. As with earlier studies (Johnson and Goodrich, 1974; Guttmann, 1977), social drinking is associated with good health and life satisfaction.

Many explanations have been offered to account for the lessened alcohol consumption associated with aging:

1. *Demographic change,* e.g., lessened income, the relatively high proportion of women in older age groups, or the sizable number of older people living alone.

2. *Health and illness.* People who have more chronic illness and who take medication are probably less likely to engage in social drinking.

3. *The biology of alcohol and aging.* There are differences in experimental reports with human subjects and reports with animal subjects, some investigators reporting heightened blood alcohol concentration with aging (Vestal et al., 1977; Garver, 1984), and others reporting lowered blood alcohol concentration in animal studies (Ott et al., 1985). There is general agreement that older organisms are ". . . more sensitive" to the effects of alcohol as compared with younger, but clearly, questions are unresolved (Wood and Armbrecht, 1982). There is general agreement about the heightened sensitivity of older persons to alcohol (Lamy, 1988).

4. *The behavioral effects of alcohol on older persons.* Intensified behavioral effects of alcohol has been suggested as explanation of lessened alcohol intake among older persons (Vogel-Sprott and Barrett, 1984).

5. *Unique historical experience.* People who are 65 and older at this time have a common historical experience, and it may be that influences of the earlier developmental years have produced attitudes and drinking behaviors that involve less intake than subsequent generations (Gomberg, 1982). There is some evidence to support this explanation.

## 8. BIOLOGICAL EFFECTS OF ALCOHOL

Interest in the biological effects of alcohol on the aging organism has been stimulated by research in the interaction of aging and alcohol abuse (Mishara and Kastenbaum, 1980; Freund and Butters, 1982; Hartford and Samorajski, 1984). Some of the disagreements in the literature may be explained by the use of human subjects in some studies and the use of animal models in others, but there are other methodological problems. Cross-sectional comparison of one group of young subjects and one group of older subjects is inadequate: It cannot be assumed that age differences are linear. Longitudinal research also has problems, primarily the control of cohort effects.

### Blood Alcohol Concentration

With human elderly subjects, adjusted amounts of alcohol (for comparison with younger subjects) yield higher blood alcohol concentrations (Vestal et al., 1977; Garver, 1984; Vogel-Sprott and Barrett, 1984). But Ott et al. (1985) report ". . . significantly lower peak blood ethanol concentration" for their oldest rat subjects.

## Metabolism of Alcohol

Wood and Armbrecht (1982) report slower metabolic rates and others report faster metabolic rates for older animals (Ott et al., 1985). Garver (1984) states that there is no evidence to suggest that there are ". . . age effects on the rate of ethanol metabolism in man."

## Elimination of Alcohol

Ott et al. (1985) report ". . . enhanced ethanol disposition at older ages" of experimental animals. With human subjects, Vogel-Sprott and Barrett (1984) report that alcohol absorption and elimination rates ". . . were not significantly related to age." Garver (1984) concludes that the elimination rates of ethanol ". . . appear to be virtually identical across age groupings."

There is some agreement that older organisms are ". . . more sensitive" to ethanol effects than younger organisms (Wood and Armbrecht, 1982; York, 1982; York, 1983, Lamy, 1987). Age differences and age changes in response to alcohol have been attributed to (1) metabolic rate changes, (2) central nervous system sensitivity changes, and (3) distribution of alcohol in different body compartments, such as body water. The decreased body water in body weight as one ages is preferred as an explanation for age changes by Vogel-Sprott and Barrett (1984) and by Garver (1984), but Garver raises the question of whether there is ". . . true hypersensitivity" of the elderly to alcohol, i.e., changes with aging in the effects of alcohol on receptors, membranes, and neuronal excitability.

## Central Nervous System Effects

There is extensive literature on cerebral and neurological defects in alcoholism (e.g., Carlen, 1982). Neuropsychological correlates of alcohol and aging have been discussed by Blusewicz et al. (1977), and neurotransmitter function in relation to alcoholism and aging has been discussed by Freund (1984). Neuroradiological techniques have suggested relatively frequent cerebral atrophy, ventricular enlargement, reduction in brain density, and cerebellar atrophy among chronic alcoholics (Carlen et al., 1986). Alcohol and aging interact in problems of immune systems (Rice et al., 1983) and in problems of sleep dysregulation and sleep apnea (Issa, 1982).

In spite of an expanding literature on the biology of alcohol effects and the interacting effects of aging and alcohol, it is safe to say that we are at the beginning of knowledge in this area.

# 9. PROBLEM DRINKING AND ALCOHOLISM

Early recognition of alcohol problems in the elderly appeared primarily in case reports (Twigg, 1959; Droller, 1964; Riccitelli, 1967). Interestingly, there were a number of early papers from different parts of the world: Glatt and Rosin (1964) from the United Kingdom, an early issue of *Revue de l'alcoolisme* (1969) in France, Vidojkovic et al. (1970) in Jugoslavia, Ciompi and Eisert (1971) in Switzerland, Wilkinson (1971) from Australia, and Goldstein and Grant (1974) in Canada. In all these reports, discussion and study were of elderly patients in hospitals or other treatment facilities. One early paper, in fact, dealt with diagnostic differences in "psychogeriatric" patients in Toronto, New York, and London and suggested that national differences were probably based on different habits of diagnosis in the different countries; the authors also note that, in part, differences might be attributed to the large number of elderly alcoholics in the Canadian sample (Duckworth and Ross, 1975).

Glatt and Rosin in 1964 were (as far as we can ascertain) first to point out that elderly alcoholics included those who had been drinking for many years and those who developed alcoholism ". . . in later life." This has developed into a classification of sorts of elderly alcoholics, discussed below.

From the beginning of work with elderly alcoholics, the research reports have been dealing with quite different subpopulations within the older age group. Samples have been taken from different kinds of hospitals: state mental hospitals, veterans' medical centers, city hospitals, private hospitals, substance abuse hospitals. Reports about elderly alcoholics are also drawn from arrest records (public intoxication), from outpatient clinics for substance abusers, from services and housing for older people, from surveys of health caretakers, and from survey research, national and regional. It is true of alcoholics in general and it is also true of older alcoholics that there are important differences between elderly alcoholics admitted to expensive private hospitals and those who are seen in public institutions, to say nothing of those elderly alcoholics who exist among the poor, the homeless, and the "street people."

In addition to sampling problems and the comparability of different research samples, there is the very real question of *identification of alcohol abuse* among older persons (Graham, 1985). Clearly, there is a need to define *heavy drinking* among older people, and the definition is not likely to turn out identical with the criteria for heavy drinking among younger people. Are alcohol-related problems the same for different age groups? Can time lost from work or warnings on the job be used as an alcohol-related problem with retired people? Are family objections to the older person's drinking a proper criterion for identifying older problem drinkers? Such objection assumes an intact family. What is needed are relevant criteria for a definition of elderly problem drinking or alcoholism: Such criteria should include falls or accidents, nutritional inadequacy, family problems, increasing social isolation, and—most of all—medical problems associated with heavy alcohol intake (Willenbring and Spring, 1988; Blow et al., forthcoming).

Once diagnosis has been made, there are other methodological problems. Measures of various sorts (psychological tests, standardized interviews, psychophysiological measures) are used with older subjects, frequently without questioning the relevance or norms for older populations.

## 10. SIZE OF THE PROBLEM AND SOME CORRELATES

*Hospital admissions,* earlier the main source of information about older alcoholics, do show high percentages: 20–50% of 540 male admissions to a state hospital (Whittier and Korenyi, 1961); 32% of men and 15% of women among 534 people admitted to a hospital psychiatric ward (Simon et al., 1970); and 44% of 100 admissions to a hospital psychiatric ward (Gaitz and Baer, 1971). These all involve people 60 years of age and older. The percentages are different for admissions to general hospitals (Gomberg, 1980). Goldstein and Grant (1974) in Canada reported that 24% of the men and 7% of the women over 60 in a sample of 179 hospital admissions were diagnosed as manifesting excessive drinking. Zimberg (1974*a*), using 65 as the cutoff stage, reported 17% of 87 patients admitted to a community mental health center as having a drinking problem. In a random survey of patients in a general hospital, Beresford and his collaborators (Beresford et al., 1988) report 6% of patients 60 years of age and older diagnosable as manifesting "alcohol dependence" by Diagnostic and Statistical Manual III-R criteria.

*Surveys*, on the other hand, have shown different results. Two early studies in social psychiatry estimated the percentage of respondents judged to be "alcoholic": The Midtown Manhattan study (Langner and Michael, 1963) estimated 4.6% of their sample, and the Stirling County study (Leighton et al., 1963) estimated 4.3%. Bailey et al. (1965) reported that the percentage of persons, aged 65–74, interviewed in an urban residential area and diagnosed as "probable alcoholics" was 2.2%. Of the 75-and-over age group, the figure was 1.2%, but this study highlighted the possible role of recent loss because 10.5% of elderly widowers were judged to be "probable alcoholics." Rosin and Glatt (1971), in a "field survey" in England, reported 9% of respondents 65 and older to be alcoholic. Barnes (1979) interviewed people in two New York counties but made no diagnoses, limiting her classification to amount drunk: Of some interest is the presence of more heavy drinking among employed older men (22%) than among unemployed older men (13%).

A Baltimore survey of people 55 and over, living in the community and in nursing homes, estimated problem drinkers to constitute 12% of the people interviewed (Rathbone-McCuan et al., 1976). Those with drinking problems tended to report poorer health status, to be unemployed, single, divorced, or separated, and to be more "alienated." A Washington, D.C., survey of people 60 and over living in the community (institutionalized elderly not included) reported 1.1% to have problems related to alcohol use (Guttmann, 1977*a*). Several surveys done in Boston have yielded estimates of 1–2% self-reported problem drinkers in the sample interviewed (Patterson et al., 1974; Meyers et al., 1982). In the 1982 survey, the percentage rises if respondents are asked whether drinking ". . . diminished the quality of their lives"; 4% answered affirmatively.

A Massachusetts study of health practices and mortality among older persons (Branch and Jette, 1984) found that ". . . either few elders are heavy alcohol consumers or very few are willing to admit it." And a recent study of alcohol intake in a healthy elderly sample of 270 persons, 65 and older, reported 1.5% (four persons) who "admitted" to having a problem with alcohol (Goodwin et al., 1987).

After the Bailey et al. study (1965), the estimates of 2–10% of the elderly population surfaced in the gerontology literature frequently; it was not always clear whether it was 2–10% of those who drank or of *all* the elderly. This 2–10% estimate, based on a mixture of populations—psychiatric patients, survey respondents, etc.—has been ". . . uncritically perpetuated" (Whittington, 1988).

The most recent estimates come from the Epidemiological Catchment Area Study, which involves multisite community surveys providing diagnostic assessment of several psychiatric disorders (Holzer et al., 1984). The combined samples of three sites, New Haven, Baltimore, and St. Louis, provide data on 4600 respondents 60 years of age and older. *For men, the 6-month prevalence is between 1.9% and 4.6% and for women, between 0.1% and 0.7%.* The correlates of alcohol abuse were (1) marital status, (2) education, and (3) income.

1. *Marital status.* For men, alcohol abuse is highest among the separated and divorced and next highest for the widowed; for women, it is highest among the married. This raises several questions. For men, it is marital *disruption* which is more associated with alcohol abuse than marital loss, and for women, the question of alcoholism à deux may be raised: elderly women drinking with their husbands?

2. *Education.* For both men and women, alcohol abuse is more prevalent among those who did not finish high school than among those with more education.

3. *Income.* There are higher rates of alcohol abuse among those from the poorest households, regardless of age or sex. Although differences are not statistically significant, *employed* older males report more alcohol abuse than the men in the same age group who are not working. For women, the rate is higher among the nonworking. Race comparisons show very little difference when elderly men are compared, but a higher rate of alcohol abuse among black elderly women than among white elderly women.

Surveys, of course, must deal with the issue, often raised, of *underreporting* (Duffy and Waterton, 1984). There is no empirical evidence that older people do more underreporting than younger people (Herzog and Dielman, 1985; Rodgers and Herzog, 1987). When compared on a number of survey measures (not including alcohol intake, unfortunately), older respondents in their sixties and seventies are sometimes *more* accurate than younger respondents, e.g., in responding to questions about their automobiles, and sometimes *less* accurate than younger respondents, e.g., in describing their neighbors. For many measures, no age differences were detected.

A question of national differences might be noted here. Early studies of alcoholism rates suggested that the prevalence rate for English women was somewhat higher, in relation to male alcoholism, than was true of American women. Male/female ratios are obviously based on estimates of alcoholism rates in the population. However, in discussing elderly people with alcohol problems, it was suggested that women, with their greater longevity, might constitute a larger proportion of the elderly alcoholic population than men (Rosin and Glatt, 1971). While the Epidemiological Catchment Area figures noted earlier show a higher proportion of alcohol problems among elderly men than among elderly women, some of the reports from the United Kingdom continue to emphasize the presence of ". . . alcohol abuse . . . amongst old people, especially old women" (Wattis, 1983) and to report case material about old women alcohol abusers. Of seven cases presented, Wattis (1981) reports on five women and two men. Merry (1980) presents nine cases, all women.

## 11. PSYCHOSOCIAL VARIABLES

The scanty data on alcohol problems among the elderly have been reviewed many times (Schuckit et al., 1978; Gomberg, 1980; Mishara and Kastenbaum, 1980; Petersen and Whittington, 1977; Schuckit, 1977; Wood and Elias, 1982; Sherouse, 1983; Atkinson, 1984*a;* Hartford and Samarajski, 1984; Maddox et al., 1984; Gottheil et al., 1985). The foci of these reviews vary; sometimes the focus is on biomedical issues, sometimes on epidemiology, sometimes on treatment.

What are some of the antecedents, motivations, symptoms, and attitudes toward treatment of older alcoholics?

## Early Onset vs. Recent Onset

One of the most significant issues that has been raised is the *duration* of the elderly person's problematic drinking. Early on, Glatt and Rosin (1964) suggested that there were elderly alcoholics who had been drinking for many years and those who became alcoholic "in later life." These authors thought that psychopathology was more characteristic of the first group and "social pathology" more characteristic of the second group. Wilkinson (1971), reporting from an Australian hospital, estimated that about one-third of elderly alcoholics had begun problem drinking "late in life" and she elaborated the theme of "social pathology," stating that late-life alcoholism was generally precipitated by ". . . severe emotional crises such as bereavement or retirement."

In a review of the literature, Gomberg (1980) distinguished among "survivors," with a long history of problem drinking, "reactive problem drinkers," whose heavy drinking began late in life, and "intermittent problem drinkers," with an intermittent history of heavy drinking. A similar classification was supported by Hubbard et al. (1979), who studied 43 older persons in a mental health outreach program who had alcohol-related problems. Of these 43, long-term alcoholics constituted 46%; recent onset but with sporadic episodes of heavy drinking, "in some cases," constituted 28%; and there was another kind of elderly person with alcohol-related problems: 26% of the sample used alcohol moderately but in combination with medication. The long-term alcoholics lived alone, had many alcohol-related medical problems, and were quite vulnerable to violence inflicted on them. The recent-onset group showed ". . . a lack of meaningful role involvement and positive self-concept," and many of them expressed guilt; family members of recent-onset drinkers were likely to deny the problem. The third group, the alcohol/medication–interaction group, were frequently viewed as "senile" and were characterized by poor nutrition and injuries.

A recent paper has compared early vs. late-onset alcoholism in older persons (Atkinson et al., 1985) and report late onset to be associated with greater psychological stability and less family alcoholism than in the early-onset group. One problem here is the definition of "early" and "late" onset. If late onset is differentiated from early onset by the criterion of alcohol problems after age 40 and alcohol problems before age 40, it means that there are many elderly problem drinkers who would be called recent onset but who would have a problem drinking history of 25 or more years. It has been suggested that we define recent-onset elderly problem drinkers as those whose problem drinking began on or about the age of 60 (Gomberg, 1985).

Do such recent-onset elderly problem drinkers exist at all? Clinical observation is, for many researchers, inadequate evidence. However, in addition to such clinical observation (e.g., Glatt and Rosin, 1964; Wilkinson, 1971; Hubbard et al., 1979), the same phenomenon shows in surveys. Conley's longitudinal research has disclosed a number of persons in a sample, median age 68, who were reported by a spouse to have alcohol problems currently, although no problems were reported in earlier interviews (Gomberg, 1985). Moos and Finney (1984) reported 33.6% of a sample of 440 elderly alcohol abusers to be "late-onset alcohol abusers," and Glynn et al. (1984) found 38% of the men in a veteran study reporting drinking problems in 1982, although the same men had reported no problem in an earlier interview.

Assuming, then, that *the recent-onset elderly problem drinker* does exist, the next question is whether this late onset is associated with *stresses* imposed by the processes of aging. Gomberg (1980) noted retirement and loss of spouse as major stressors. Brody (1982) has suggested that there are at least four: retirement, death among relatives and friends, poor health, and loneliness. There is some evidence that *spouse loss* is a significant stress, although this must be interpreted broadly: Rates of alcohol abuse among older men who are divorced or separated are higher than rates for widowers, which, in turn, are higher than rates for the currently married (Holzer et al., 1984). Marital disruption is more likely to be linked with alcohol abuse than loss of a spouse through death. *Retirement* effects, too, are complicated. Elderly men who are employed are more likely to be heavy drinkers than elderly men who are not working (Barnes, 1979; Holzer et al., 1984). Although survey respondents are not usually asked about the social context of drinking, there is some evidence that drinking with workplace companions is commonplace, and it is sensible to assume that retirement and the termination of such contacts lessens the quantity/frequency of drinking for many older men. The consistent drop in percentage of heavy drinkers among men 65 and older, found in several national surveys, suggests that retirement may produce *less* heavy drinking than workplace participation. On the other hand, in a clinical report describing 224 elderly alcoholic patients at the Mayo Clinic, Finlayson et al. (1985) state that among the ". . . so-called 'crises of aging,' only retirement played a major role in late onset alcoholism." This relates to the difference, perhaps, between white-collar and blue-collar attitudes toward retirement and raises the question whether retirement is not more stressful for retired executives than for retired working-class men.

The problem of stress-as-precipitant is broader than elderly problem drinking (it is, for example, a question that has persisted in the study of female alcoholism). Further research on stress and distress, the coping mechanisms habitually used, and environmental pressures—all acting together—may clarify the problem. It does seem simplistic to explain the onset of problem drinking in late life solely in terms of age-associated problems; this omits family history, biological response to alcohol, changes in social milieu (like moving to a new retirement community), and changes in the social facilitation of drinking. There are, as Moos and Finney have pointed out (1984), drinking-related factors, personal factors, and environmental factors. Risk factors, as listed by Atkinson (1984*b*), include genetics, biological sensitivity, stresses associated with aging, drug interactions, iatrogenic sources, family collusion, and cohort effects.

## Patterns of Drinking

The patterns of drinking and the behavioral effects of alcohol as manifested by elderly problem drinkers have been little discussed. In their national survey, Cahalan et al. (1969) compared problem drinkers who were 60 and older with problem drinkers in their forties. The older problem drinkers reported more interpersonal problems (with spouse, relatives, friends, neighbors), more difficulty with the police, more accidents, more financial worries, and more binge drinking. The younger problem drinkers reported more work-associated problems and more belligerence.

When they appear in hospitals and clinics, elderly alcoholics present with "nonspecific" (Atkinson, 1984*b*) or "more subtle" (Zimberg, 1984) signs than do younger alcohol abusers. These signs may include self-neglect, falls and injuries, confusion, depression, and malnutrition. Most investigators agree that differential diagnosis is more difficult for elderly alcohol abusers. Perhaps because they are relatively few in number in most treatment facilities, little information is gathered about patterns of drinking, history of drinking, and problems associated with drinking of elderly patients.

## Gender and Ethnicity

Information about elderly female alcoholics is sparse. One study compared alcoholic women over 55 with younger alcoholic women, and older alcoholic men with younger alcoholic men (Schuckit et al., 1978). Older women reported *shorter* histories of alcohol abuse before their first hospitalization than did the younger women, but older alcoholic men, on the other hand, reported *longer* histories than the younger men. The older groups were described as "more stable," with fewer alcohol-related problems and a lower incidence of "psychiatric problems." When elderly women alcoholics appear in the literature, it is likely to be in case history presentations (Rathbone-McCuan and Triegaardt, 1979; Glassock, 1982). An investigation of treatment issues with older women (Rathbone-McCuan and Roberds, 1980) involved a sample of 41 women, 25 of them between 45 and 55 years of age (mean 49 years) and 16 of them 55 and older (mean 61.2 years). Among the latter, a larger proportion were married or widowed and a smaller proportion divorced or separated than was true among the middle-aged women. The older women had less education, and a higher proportion were "homemakers" or retired. Older women reported their past histories more positively than did the middle-aged women and were more likely to associate onset with "social roles" and family problems. Drinking styles differed to some extent: The older women reported less morning drinking but more frequently reported seizures and hallucinations. Two-thirds of both age groups were involved with legal prescription drugs as well as alcohol.

A major limitation of gender/age comparisons involving elderly problem drinkers is the absence of parallel comparisons of nonalcoholic samples.

The "emergency room alcohol patient" was described demographically with comparison in terms of ethnicity, age, and sex (Westie and McBride, 1979). Results from a Miami hospital emergency room are shown in Table 2. The female patients were, on the average, 6.8 years younger than the male patients, with patients under the age of 35 much more likely to be female [the emergency room appearance of young women in drug overdoses or in suicide attempts has been discussed by Gomberg (1986)]. Westie and McBride's admissions show an overrepresentation of Hispanics and a higher incidence of alcohol-related emergencies among Black women than among White or Spanish. Apart from ethnicity, male admissions, aged 60 and older, constituted 17.2% of all male admissions, while women in the same age group constituted 7.8% of all female admissions. Disposition of patients varied by age: Those under 25 were likely to be

Table 2. Age, Ethnicity, and Gender of Emergency Room Alcohol Patients (Westie and McBride, 1979)

| Age | Black | Spanish | White |
|---|---|---|---|
| 25–34 | 31.4% | 36.8% | 23.5% |
| 35–59 | 62.4% | 59.6% | 56.1% |
| 60 and older | 6.2% | 3.5% | 20.3% |
| Male:female ratio | 2:1 | 5:1 | 5:1 |

treated and released, and patients admitted to the hospital were primarily between ages 25 and 59. The older emergency room patients, comprising 15.2% of the total, were ". . . surprisingly unlikely to be admitted" to the hospital; almost half of this group of patients was treated and jailed.

## The Chronic Drunkenness Offender

There has been an interesting parallel in the development of research and clinical interest in the *elderly* alcoholic and alcoholism in general: Both began with early focus on the chronic drunkenness offender and homeless men, and rapidly moved away from that group as a focus of interest. The history of the modern alcoholism movement began with interest in the chronic drunkenness offender, as did the most recent history of interest in elderly alcoholism. An early study of Epstein et al., (1970) is indeed titled "Antisocial Behavior of the Elderly" and reported a disproportionately high percentage of arrests for drunkenness and public intoxication among men 60 and older. Bahr and Caplow's book on Skid Row (1974) is titled *Old Men Drunk and Sober*, and Cohen and Sokolovsky (1989) discuss the problems with alcohol of the *Old Men of the Bowery*. The changing nature of the homeless population, which now includes many former mental hospital patients and many female-headed families on welfare, and the gentrification of the Skid Rows of many cities have led to changes in the "homeless man" population. This group, which constituted the Skid Row population, has changed ethnically in the last several decades, with the drift of Blacks and Native Americans to inner-city dilapidated areas. The legal stance has modified so that elderly, homeless alcoholics are more likely to be referred to detoxification centers (Rubington, 1982).

## Social Heterogeneity

Elderly problem drinkers and alcoholics include a large array of subgroups:

1. Homeless derelicts on Skid Row
2. Blue-collar failures, an underclass of people with an irregular work history, likely to appear in emergency rooms, city hospitals, and veterans' hospitals
3. Working-class men and women; if employed, may be reached by employee assistance programs
4. Middle-class people, professional people
5. Upper-income people, including retired executives

These subgroups include the widowed, the married, the divorced, and the separated; people who have been drinking heavily for decades and those who began heavy drinking recently; elderly husbands and wives drinking together; those who live alone and those who are living with others; and people who have been socially integrated most of their lives and people who have been isolated. It is a population as heterogeneous as problem drinkers of any age group: mixed in social status, mixed in temperament, mixed in history. Generalizations should be made with caution and each investigator should define carefully the population of elderly problem drinkers about whom he/she is writing.

### Psychological Characteristics

Older problem drinkers report that they drink to alleviate depression and feelings of isolation (Carruth et al., 1973; Rathbone-McCuan et al., 1976). Some of the dynamics that appear with consistency among younger drinkers, e.g., impulsivity, sensation seeking, unconventionality, do not appear to be appropriate, and these terms have been little used in descriptions of the older problem drinker. When the older alcoholic is described as being in poorer health than his/her age peers or more alienated from society, it is unclear whether poor health and alienation *antecede* the drinking or are the *consequence*, or whether poor health and alienation are both cause *and* effect. A generalization about the empty lives "of most retirees and widows," leading to boredom, loneliness, depression, low self-esteem, and eventually, to alcoholism (Sherouse, 1983), is supported by little empirical data. There is so little information, it is difficult to say anything about the personality characteristics that distinguish elderly problem drinkers from their age peers.

## 12. HEALTH, COGNITIVE IMPAIRMENT, AND THE OLDER PROBLEM DRINKER

The negative effects of both acute and chronic heavy drinking on morbidity have been well documented, and heavy alcohol intake has been linked to cirrhosis, cardiovascular disease, cancer, endocrine disorders, nutritional deficiency diseases, and more. While the *role of ill health* as *etiology* has been posited but not verified, the *consequences* of heavy alcohol intake in negative health effects are clearly seen in facilities that include older problem drinkers (Gambert et al., 1984).

A medical issue that has received recent research attention is neuropsychological impairment. An early summary of the available evidence (Tarter, 1976) described psychological deficits; this summary also noted that "significant recovery" does occur after detoxification and maintenance of sobriety. The literature on the cognitive status of alcoholics has expanded rapidly (Brandt et al., 1983; Tamkin, 1983; Shelton et al., 1984; Grant et al., 1984; Flinn et al., and Ferris, 1984; Noonberg et al., 1985; Pishkin et al., 1985; Tarter and Edwards, 1986; Burger et al., 1987). The methodologies have included those of neuropathology, neuroradiology, electrophysiology, neuroendocrinology, and neuropsychology. Neuropsychological methods have included the Reitan test, the Halstead–Reitan test, the Luria–Nebraska Neuropsychological Battery, tests of learning of paired associates, tests of memory (immediate and delayed), and more.

By and large, few differences have been found in *overall* intelligence test results when alcoholics and matched controls are compared. What has emerged are differences in specific functions: short-term memory, nonverbal abstracting, complex memory tasks, visual–spatial relationships, and the ability to process new information (Flinn et al., 1984; Eckhardt and Martin, 1986). The question of cognitive impairment, temporary or permanent, which accompanies heavy drinking, is still open, and new evidence about particular abilities and losses continues to appear. Furthermore, the cognitive impairment that has been reported may not be simply the *result* of the heavy drinking:

> . . . cognitive impairments exhibited by alcoholics reflect the culmination and interaction of numerous factors that preceded drinking onset, are concurrent with a lifestyle of abusive drinking, and are the consequences of multisystem pathology induced by prolonged and excessive alcoholic beverage consumption. (Tarter and Edwards, 1986, page 133).

Inevitably, the observations about neuropsychological deficits associated with alcoholism and the effects of aging on intellectual abilities came together in the hypothesis that ". . . one effect of alcoholism is premature senescence of intellectual and psychological processes" (Kleinknecht and Goldstein, 1972). The *premature aging* hypothesis has been supported by some studies (e.g., Blusewicz et al., 1977) but support evidence is ambiguous. Grant et al. (1984) concluded that aging, not alcoholism, was related to psychomotor slowing, and ". . . there were no age–alcohol interactions for any neuropsychological test." A recent report by Burger et al. (1987) tested the premature aging hypothesis but did not obtain the expected interaction effects, and the investigators concluded that different mechanisms are probably associated with age-related psychological deficits and psychological deficits associated with alcoholism. Interestingly, the study of premature aging has not involved many elderly alcoholics. Eckhardt and Martin (1986) observe that most of the present knowledge about alcoholism and associated cognitive impairment is based on ". . . middle-aged alcoholics who have been abusers for some time." It would be useful to study *elderly* alcoholics, both those with long drinking histories and those with recent onset.

Relevant to the question of treatment is the issue of reversibility of the neuropsychological impairments (Goldman, 1986) and the implications of such impairments for the recovery process (Wilkinson and Sanchez-Craig, 1981; McCrady and Smith, 1986). Clearly, the timing of treatment interventions needs to take into account the period of detoxification and the regaining of function. Since it is a reasonable hypothesis that this recovery period may be more prolonged with older persons, it would make for more effective treatment programs if more was known and applied to the timing of rehabilitation and therapy programs for the elderly problem drinker.

## 13. TREATMENT AND REHABILITATION

A great deal has been written about treating the elderly problem drinker (Van De Vyvere et al., 1976; Saunders, 1976; Rathbone-McCuan and Triegaardt, 1979; Gross and Capuzzi, 1981; Sherouse, 1983; James, 1983; Janik and Dunham, 1983; Wells-Parker et al., 1983; Atkinson, 1984*a;* Blazer et al., 1984; Gottheil et al., 1985; Saunders et al., 1985; Graham and Tinney, 1986; Kofoed et al., 1987). In addition, the National Institute on Alcohol Abuse and Alcoholism's Information and Feature Service issued a special report (Alcohol and the Elderly, 1982), and the Hazelden Foundation has published an Alcoholics Anonymous appeal to older alcoholics (Carle, 1980).

Two major areas of research need definition and exploration. First, how do elderly alcohol abusers who do get into treatment arrive there? Second, what kinds of special problems, if any, in diagnosis, management, and treatment do these persons present?

*How do older alcoholics come to the attention of caretakers?* A major resource seems to be significant others: spouse, family, friends, neighbors, and other network members (Gomberg, 1982). Other sources of referral are emergency rooms (usually because of accidents, falls, or alcohol-related health problems), the police, physicians, and social agencies. Families are likely to be concerned (Corrigan, 1974), but only if there is an intact family and relationships are maintained, and this is not so likely with long-term alcoholic men who have survived past the age of 60. It is interesting to examine two reports from Minnesota. One is from a state hospital: Hoffman (1976) compared referral sources of patients 65 and older with those of younger patients and noted that older patients were more likely to be referred by physicians, other family members, and law enforcement agencies. Younger patients were more likely to be court-referred. In a description of the same age group, admitted to a private hospital treatment unit, Finlayson et al. (1985) note that ". . . medical problems were the most common factor leading to hospitalization."

If the facility to which the old alcoholic is referred is an outpatient clinic, the basis for referral may be less likely to be medical and more likely to be familial, social, or legal problems. In an evaluation of a Toronto outpatient program, Graham and Tinney (1986) comment that clients ". . . typically enter the program for help with other problems (e.g., accommodation) and not for addictions treatment." A health agency usually refers these clients to the program.

A report of an outpatient program for elderly substance abusers in a veterans' medical center (Kofoed et al., 1984) shows the largest group of referrals to be from the legal system (57%) and about equal referrals from the health care system (19%) or self and family (17%). A case has been made for gender differences in referral, with elderly alcoholic men more likely to be referred by the legal system and referral of elderly alcoholic women more likely to come from "medical or personal" sources (Dunham, 1986). This suggests that older persons, men or women, are likely to come to treatment facilities from the same referral sources as other age groups.

The implication for any outreach program seems to be that the program needs to be geared to the *group one is trying to reach:* higher or lower income, those with medical problems and/or those in trouble with the law, those with families intact and those living alone.

*Are there special problems in diagnosis, management, and treatment?* Zimberg (1984) has a scale of alcohol abuse severity which ranges from "minimal" to "extreme." This has relevance in planning a treatment program, although it is not clear why the description of "severe" (daily drinking, medical consequences, disrupted family relationships, unemployment, arrests, and hospitalizations) is specific to elderly patients.

There is an unresolved question as to whether specific programs for older alcoholics are indicated. Janik and Dunham (1983) concluded that since ". . . there are only a few age-related differences among alcoholics in treatment," there is little need for specialized alcoholism treatment programs. Kofoed et al. (1987) report that older alcoholics treated in "special elderly peer groups" remain in treatment significantly longer than those treated in mixed-age groups. The point about mixed-age groups is dealt with in Carle's work on Alcoholics Anonymous for the elderly (1980), addressed to the "senior citizen" who says: "I'll never be able to relate to all those children."

The observations of Kofoed et al. (1984) of a group therapy program for older alcoholic veterans are useful: first, the rapid development of "a strong attachment among group members." This is consistent with practitioners' reports that older problem drinkers frequently form strong attachments in individual therapy. Second, Kofoed et al. note that the older alcoholics respond ". . . at least as well as younger patients, but the tempo is much slower." Discussions of marriages or of death and dying are rare, and reminiscence about the past, particularly shared military experience, is common. This suggests that discussion of the common experience of this age cohort facilitates social bonding. This may relate to the practitioners' observation that older patients do well with "social therapies." Finally, Kofoed et al. note that the therapist's role and the group interaction are steadfastly supportive rather than confrontive.

Janik and Dunham (1983) found few age-related differences in outcome of treatment. However, it does not follow that age-specific programs should not be encouraged for elderly problem drinkers. The same conclusion can be drawn for this age group as has often been stated for women alcoholics: Specialized *facilities* may be economically unfeasible and have not demonstrated that they are more effective than mixed facilities, but that is not to say that specialized *programs* are also ruled out.

On particular treatment questions—primary focus on the substance abuse itself or on the life situation of the client, group vs. individual therapy, caveats about chemotherapy, and the triagelike resistances of treatment agencies to elderly clients—data are lacking. There have been clinical observations; e.g., prognosis for older alcoholics is good and social therapies are good, but data are lacking. The same treatment questions may be raised about alcohol abusers in all age groups.

## 14. A NOTE ON MISUSE OF MEDICATION

Problems due to the use and misuse of prescribed and over-the-counter medications have been discussed. It is questionable to speak of "therapy" or "treatment" because the problems that arise from polypharmacy or noncompliance are not usually psychological problems. Here the issue seems primarily one of *education:* education directed toward prescribing physicians, toward pharmacists, toward health caretakers, and, above all, toward the consumer. The American Association of Retired Persons' survey of consumer use, attitudes, and behavior in relation to prescription drugs (1984) shows that even with a reasonably well-educated, middle-class group of older persons, consumers are ". . . often passive in asking questions" and have high expectations that physicians and pharmacists will voluntarily provide needed information. When the respondents show noncompliance, their major motivation is improvement in health or concern about side effects. For the indigent elderly, the problem of money and the costs of medication is a more primary issue.

## 15. POSTSCRIPT

The "elderly" have here been defined as those 65 and older, some studies using this criterion and others using the definition of 60 and 55 years of age. We may be on the brink of redefining the "elderly." Dr. T. Franklin Williams, director of the U.S. National Institute on Aging, has noted that much is being written about redefining *middle age* as lasting from 55 to 75 (Arden, 1987). Perhaps the next review of elderly use of drugs and medication will discuss those who are 75 and older?

## REFERENCES

Aizenberg, R., and Treas, J., 1985, The family in late life: Psychosocial and demographic considerations, in: *Handbook of the Psychology of Aging* (J. E. Birren and K. W. Schaie, Eds.), pp. 169–189, Van Nostrand Reinhold, New York.

Alcohol and the Elderly: A Special Report, 1982, National Clearinghouse for Alcohol Information of the National Institute on Alcohol Abuse and Alcoholism IFS No. 103, (Dec. 31, 1982), pp. 1–7.

Alexander, F., and Duff, R. W., 1988, Drinking in retirement communities, *Generations,* **XII:**58.

American Association of Retired Persons, 1984, *Prescription Drugs: A Survey of Consumer Use, Attitudes and Behavior,* 64 pp., AARP, Washington, DC.

Arden, E., 1987, Ready, willing, able and retired, *Michigan Alumnus* **93**(6):32.

Atchley, R. C., 1976, Selected social and psychological differences among men and women in later life, *J. Gerontol.* **24:**42.

Atkinson, R. M., ed., 1984*a*, *Alcohol and Drug Abuse in Old Age,* American Psychiatric Press, Washington, DC.

Atkinson, R. M., 1984*b*, Substance use and abuse in late life, in: *Alcohol and Drug Abuse in Old Age,* R. M. Atkinson, ed., pp. 1–22, American Psychiatric Press, Washington, DC.

Atkinson, R. M., Turner, J. A., Kofoed, L. L., and Tolson, R. L., 1985, Early versus late onset alcoholism in older persons: Preliminary findings, *Alcoholism: Clin. Exp. Res.* **9:**513.

Bahr, H. M., and Caplow, T., 1974, *Old Men Drunk and Sober,* New York University Press, New York.

Bailey, M. P., Haberman, P. W., and Alksne, H., 1965, The epidemiology of alcoholism in an urban residential area, *Q. J. Stud. Alcohol* **26:**19.

Baltes, P. B., and Nesselroade, J. R., 1973, The developmental analysis of individual differences on multiple measures, in: *Life-Span Developmental Psychology Methodological Issues* (J. R. Nesselroade and H. W. Reese, eds.), pp. 219–251, Academic Press, New York.

Baltes, P. B., and Schaie, K. W., 1976, On the plasticity of adult and gerontological intelligence: Where Horn and Donaldson fail, *Am. Psychologist* **31:**720.

Baltes, P. B., and Willis, S. I., 1977, Toward psychological theories of aging and development, in: *Handbook of the Psychology of Aging* (J. W. Birren and K. W. Schaie, eds.), pp. 128–154, Van Nostrand Reinhold, New York.

Baltes, P. B., and Willis, S. I., 1981, Enhancement (plasticity) of intellectual functioning: Penn State's Adult Development and Enrichment Project (ADEPT), in: *Aging and Cognitive Processes* (F. I. M. Craik and S. E. Trehub, eds.), Plenum Press, New York.

Barnes, G. M., 1979, Alcohol use among older persons: Findings from a western New York State survey, *J. Am. Geriatr. Soc.* **24:**244.

Berardo, F. M., 1970, Survivorship and social isolation: The case of the aged widower, *Family Coordinator* **19:**11.
Beresford, T. P., Blow, F. C., Brower, K. J., Adams, K. M., and Hall, R. C. W., 1988, Alcoholism and aging in the general hospital. *Psychosomatics,* **29:**61.
Berkman, L. F., 1985, Stress, social networks and aging, in: *The Combined Problems of Alcoholism, Drug Addiction and Aging* (E. Gottheil, K. A. Druley, T. E. Skoloda, and H. M. Waxman, eds.), pp. 14–35, Charles C Thomas, Springfield, IL.
Berkman, L. F., and Syme, S. L., 1979, Social networks, host resistance, and mortality: A nine-year follow-up study of Alameda County residents, *Am. J. Epidemiol.* **109:**186.
Binstock, R. H., Levin, M. A., and Weatherley, R., 1985, Political dilemma of social intervention, in: *Handbook of Aging and the Social Sciences* (R. H. Binstock and E. Shanas, eds.), pp. 589–618, Van Nostrand Reinhold, New York.
Blazer, D., and Williams, C. D., 1980, Epidemiology of dysphoria and depression in the elderly population, *Am. J. Psychiatry* **137:**439.
Blazer, D., George, L. Woodbury, M., Manton, K., and Jordan, K., 1984, The elderly alcoholic: A profile, in: *Nature and Extent of Alcohol Problems among the Elderly* (G. Maddox, L. N. Robins and N. Rosenberg, eds.), pp. 275–297, U.S. Department of Health and Human Services, Washington, DC.
Blow, F. C., Beresford, T. P., Singer, K. M., Brower, K. J., and Stickney, S. K., forthcoming, Screening for alcohol abuse among hospitalized elderly patients.
Blusewicz, M. D., Dustman, R. E., Schenkenberg, T., and Beck, E. C., 1977, Neuropsychological correlates of chronic alcoholism and aging, *J. Nerv. Ment. Dis.* **165:**349.
Botwinick, J., 1977, Intellectual abilities, in: *Handbook of the Psychology of Aging* (J. E. Birren and K. W. Schaie, eds.), pp. 580–605, Van Nostrand Reinhold, New York.
Boyd, E. L., Shimp, L. A., and Hackney, M. J., 1984, *Home Remedies and the Black Elderly,* Institute of Gerontology, University of Michigan, Ann Arbor.
Branch, L. G., 1977, *Understanding the Health and Social Service Needs of People over Age 65,* Center for Survey Research, University of Massachusetts, M.I.T., and Harvard University, Cambridge, MA.
Branch, L. G., and Jette, A. M., 1984, Personal health practices and mortality among the elderly, *Am. J. Public Health* **74:**1126.
Brandt, J., Butters, N., Ryan, C., and Bayog, R., 1983, Cognitive loss and recovery in long-term alcohol abusers, *Arch. Gen. Psychiatry* **40:**435.
Brody, J. A., 1982, Aging and alcohol abuse, *J. Am. Geriatr. Soc.* **30:**123.
Burger, M. C., Botwinick, J., and Storandt, M., 1987, Aging, alcoholism and performance on the Luria–Nebraska Neuropsychological Battery, *J. Gerontol.* **42:**69.
Burrus-Bammel, L. L., and Bammel, G., 1985, Leisure and recreation, in: *Handbook of the Psychology of Aging* (J. E. Birren and K. W. Schaie, eds.), pp. 848–863, Van Nostrand Reinhold, New York.
Cahalan, D., Cisin, I. G., and Crossley, H. M., 1969, *American Drinking Practices,* College and University Press, New Haven, CT.
Cameron, P., 1975, Mood as an indicant of happiness: Age, sex, social class and situational differences, *J. Gerontol.* **30:**216.
Campbell, A., Converse, P. E., and Rodgers, W. L., 1976, *The Quality of American Life,* Russell Sage Foundation, New York.
Capel, W. C., and Peppers, L. G., 1978, The aging addict: A longitudinal study of known abusers, *Addictive Dis.* **3:**289.
Capel, W. C., Goldsmith, B. M., and Waddell, K. J., 1972, The aging narcotic addict: An increasing problem for the next decades. *J. Gerontol.* **27:**102.
Carle, C. E., 1980, *Letters to Elderly Alcoholics,* Hazelden Foundation, Center City, MN.
Carlen, P. L., 1982, Reversible effects of chronic alcoholism in the human nervous system: Possible biological mechanisms, in: *Cerebral Deficits in Alcoholism* (D. A. Wilkinson, ed.), pp. 107–122, Addiction Research Foundation, Toronto.
Carlen, P. L., Penn, R. D., Fornazzi, L., Bennett, J., Wilkinson, D. A., and Wortzman, G., 1986,

Computerized tomographic scan assessment of alcoholic brain damage and its potential reversibility, *Alcoholism: Clin. Exp. Res.* **10**:226.

Carruth, B., Williams, E. P., Mysak, P., and Boudreaux, L., 1973, *Alcoholism and Drinking Problems among Older Persons: Community Care Providers and the Older Problem Drinker,* Rutgers Center of Alcohol Studies, New Brunswick, NJ.

Chevan, A., and Korson, J. H., 1972, The widowed who live alone: An examination of the social and demographic factors, *Social Forces* **51**:45.

Chien, C. P., Townsend, E. J., and Ross-Townsend, A., 1978, Substance use and abuse among the community elderly: The medical aspect, *Addictive Dis.* **3**:357.

Ciompi, L., and Eisert, M., 1971, Etudes catamnestiques de longue durée sur le vieillissement des alcooliques, *Social Psychiatry* **6**:129.

Clark, W., and Midanik, L., 1982, Alcohol use and alcohol problems among U.S. adults: Results of the 1979 national survey, in: *Alcohol Consumption and Related Problems,* National Institute on Alcohol Abuse and Alcoholism, Alcohol and Health Monograph No. 1, ADM 82-1193, pp. 3–54, U.S. Government Printing Office, Washington, DC.

Cohen, C. I., and Sokolovsky, J., 1989, *Old Men of the Bowery.* Guilford Press, New York.

Cohen, S., 1985, The aging social drinker, in: *The Substance Abuse Problems,* Volume 2 (S. Cohen, ed.), pp. 144–148, Haworth Press, New York.

Cooper, J. W., 1986, Drug-related problems in a geriatric long term care facility, *Journal of Geriatric Drug Therapy,* **1**:47.

Cooper, J. W., 1988, Medication misuse in nursing homes, *Generations,* **XII**:56.

Cooperstock, R., 1976, Psychotropic drug use among women, *Can. Med. Assoc. J.* **115**:760.

Corrigan, E. M., 1974, *Problem Drinkers Seeking Treatment,* Monograph No. 8, Rutgers Center of Alcohol Studies, New Brunswick, NJ.

Costa, P. T., Jr., and McCrae, R. R., 1980, Still stable after all these years: Personality as a key to some issues in adulthood and old age, in: *Life-Span Development and Behavior,* Volume 3 (P. B. Baltes and O. G. Brim, eds.) Academic Press, New York.

Crook. T., and Cohen, G. D. (eds.), 1981, *Physicians' Handbook on Psychotherapeutic Drug Use in the Aged,* Mark Powley Associates, New Canaan, CT.

Cumming, E., and Henry, W. E., 1961, *Growing Old: The Process of Disengagement,* Basic Books, New York.

Department of Health and Human Services, 1981, *Toward a National Plan for the Chronically Mentally Ill,* (ADM) 81-1077, Government Printing Office, Washington, DC.

DesJarlais, D. C., Joseph, H., and Courtwright, D. T., 1985, Old age and addiction: A study of elderly patients in methadone maintenance treatment, in: *The Combined Problems of Alcoholism, Drug Addiction and Aging* (E. Gottheil, K. A. Druley, T. E. Skoloda, and H. M. Waxman, eds.), pp. 201–209, Charles C Thomas, Springfield, IL.

*Diagnostic and Statistical Manual of Mental Disorders,* 3rd ed., 1980, American Psychiatric Association, Washington, DC.

*Diagnostic and Statistical Manual of Mental Disorders,* 3rd ed. revised, 1987, American Psychiatric Association, Washington, DC.

Dobbie, J., 1977, *Substance Abuse among the Elderly,* Addiction Research Foundation, Toronto.

Drew, L. R. H., 1968, Alcoholism as a self-limiting disease, *Q. J. Stud. Alcohol* **29**:956.

Droller, H., 1964, Some aspects of alcoholism in the elderly, *Lancet* **2**:137.

Duckworth, G., and Ross, H., 1975, Diagnostic differences in psychogeriatric patients in Toronto, New York, and London, *Can. Med. Assoc. J.* **112**:847.

Duffy, J. C., and Waterton, J. J., 1984, Under-reporting of alcohol consumption in sample surveys: The effect of computer interviewing in fieldwork, *Br. J. Addiction* **79**:303.

Dunham, R. G., 1981, Aging and changing patterns of alcohol use, *J. Psychoactive Drugs* **13**:143.

Dunham, R. G., 1986, Noticing alcoholism in the elderly and women: A nationwide examination of referral behavior, *J. Drug Issues* **16**:397.

Eckhardt, M. J., and Martin, P. R., 1986, Clinical assessment of cognition in alcoholism, *Alcoholism: Clin. Exp. Res.* **10**:123.

Eckian, A. H., 1985, Self-medication with over-the-counter drugs, in: *Geriatric Drug Use—Clinical and Social Perspectives* (S. R. Moore and T. W. Teal, eds.), pp. 39–46, Pergamon Press, New York.

Epstein L. J., 1976, Symposium on age differentiation in depressive illness. Depression in the elderly, *J. Gerontol.* **31**:278.

Epstein, L. J., Mills, C., and Simon, A., 1970, Antisocial behavior of the elderly, *Compr. Psychiatry* **11**:36.

*Exploding the Myths: Caregiving in America*, 1987, Study of the Subcommittee on Human Services of the Select Committee on Aging, House of Representatives, One Hundredth Congress, Pub. No. 99-611.

*Fact Book on Aging in Canada*, 2nd Canadian Conference on Aging, 1983, Minister of Supply and Services Canada.

Fann, W. E., and Whelass, J. C., 1975, Depression in elderly patients, *South. Med. J.* **68**:468.

Finlayson, R. E., 1984, Prescription drug abuse in older persons, in: *Alcohol and Drug Abuse in Old Age* (R. M. Atkinson, ed.), pp. 61–70, American Psychiatric Press, Washington, DC.

Finlayson, R. E., Hurt, R. D., and Morse, R. M., 1985, Clinical and outcome data in 224 elderly alcoholics, Presented at the Research Society on Alcoholism Conference, April 19, 1985.

Flinn, G. A., Reisberg, B., and Ferris, S. H., 1984, neuropsychological models of cerebral dysfunction in chronic alcoholics, in: *Alcoholism in the Elderly: Social and Biomedical issues* (J. T. Hartford and T. Samorajski, eds.), pp. 193–200, Raven Press, New York.

Fox, J. H., 1985, Effects of retirement and former work life on women's adaptation, in: *Normal Aging III* (E. Palmore, E. W. Busse, G. L. Maddox, J. B. Nowlin, and I. G. Siegler, eds.), pp. 404–415, Duke University Press, Durham, NC.

Freund, G., 1984, Neurotransmitter function in relation to aging and alcoholism, in: *Alcoholism in the Elderly: Social and Biomedical Issues* (J. T. Hartford and T. Samorajski, eds.), pp. 65–84, Raven Press, New York.

Freund, G., and Butters, N., 1982, Alcohol and aging: Challenges for the future, *Alcoholism: Clin. Exp. Res.* **6**:1.

Gaeta, M. J., and Gaetano, R. J., 1977, *The Elderly, Their Health and the Drugs in Their Lives*, Kendall/Hunt, Dubuque, IA.

Gaitz, C. M., and Baer, P. E., 1971, Characteristics of elderly patients with alcoholism, *Arch. Gen. Psychiatry* **24**:372.

Gambert, S. R., Newton, M., and Duthrie, E. H. Jr., 1984, Medical issues in alcoholism in the elderly, in: *Alcoholism in the Elderly: Social and Biomedical Issues* (J. T. Hartford and T. Samorajski, eds.), pp. 175–191, Raven Press, New York.

Gaguli, R., 1983, The rational use of psychotropic drugs, *Urban Health* **42.**

Garver, D. L., 1984, Age effects on alcohol metabolism, in: *Alcoholism in the Elderly: Social and Biomedical Issues* (J. T. Hartford and T. Samorajski, eds.), pp. 153–159, Raven Press, New York.

Gelfand, D. E., 1982, *Aging: The Ethnic Factor*, Little, Brown, Boston.

Gelfand, D. E., and Barresi, C. M. (eds.) *Ethnic Dimensions of Aging*, Springer, 1987.

Glantz, M. D., 1985, The detection, identification and differentiation of elderly drug misuse and abuse in a research survey, in:*The Combined Problems of Alcoholism, Drug Addiction and Aging* (E. Gottheil, K. A. Druley, T. E. Skoloda, and H. M. Waxman, eds.), pp. 113–139, Charles C Thomas, Springfield, IL.

Glassock, J. A., 1982, Older alcoholics: An underserved population, *Generations* **VI**:23.

Glatt, M. M., and Rosin, A. J., 1964, Aspects of alcoholism in the elderly, *Lancet* **2**:472.

Glenn, N. D., 1981, Age, birth cohorts, and drinking: An illustration of the hazards of inferring effects from cohort data, *J. Gerontol.* **36**:362.

Glynn, R. J., Bouchard, G. R., LoCastro, J. S., and Hermos, J. A., 1984, Changes in alcohol consumption behaviors among men in the normative aging study, in: *Nature and Extent of Alcohol Problems among the Elderly* (G. Maddox, L. N. Robins, and N. Rosenberg, eds.), pp. 101–116, Monograph 14, National Institute on Alcohol Abuse and Alcoholism Research, Washington, DC.

Goldberg, P. B., and Roberts, J., 1983, Pharmacologic basis for developing rational drug regimens for elderly patients, *Med. Clin. North Am.* **67:**315.

Goldman, M. S., 1986, Neuropsychological recovery in alcoholics: Endogenous and exogenous processes, *Alcoholism: Clin. Exp. Res.* **10:**136.

Goldstein, E., and Grant, A., 1974, The psychogeriatric patient in hospital, *Can. Med. Assoc. J.* **111:** 329.

Goleman, D., 1987, Personality: Major traits found stable through life, *New York Times,* June 9, 1987.

Gomberg, E. S. L., 1979, Psychological survivorship: Sex differences in aging (unpublished manuscript).

Gomberg, E. S. L., 1980, *Drinking and Problem Drinking Among the Elderly,* Institute of Gerontology, University of Michigan, Ann Arbor.

Gomberg, E. S. L., 1981, Women, sex roles, and alcohol problems, *Professional Psychol.* **12:**146.

Gomberg, E. S. L., 1982, *Alcohol Use and Problems among the Elderly,* Alcohol and Health Monograph No. 4, Special Population Issues, National Institute on Alcohol Abuse and Alcoholism, pp. 263–290, DHHS (ADM) 82-1193.

Gomberg, E. S. L., 1985, Gerontology and alcohol studies, in: *The Combined Problems of Alcoholism, Drug Addiction and Aging* (E. Gottheil, K. A. Druley, T. E. Skoloda, and H. M. Waxman, eds.), pp. 51–73, Charles C Thomas, Springfield, IL.

Gomberg, E. S. L., 1986, Women and alcoholism: Psychological issues, in: *Women and Alcohol: Health-Related Issues,* National Institute on Alcohol Abuse and Alcoholism, pp. 78–120, DHHS (ADM) 86-1139.

Gomberg, E. S. L., 1987, Drug and alcohol problems of elderly persons, in: *Developments in the Assessment and Treatment of Addictive Behavior* (T. D. Nirenberg and S. A. Maisto, eds.), pp. 319–337), Ablex Publishing Corp., Norwood, NJ.

Gomberg, E. S. L., Hsieh, G., and Adams, K. M., 1988, Patterns of drug use in a general medical care clinic for veterans: A pilot study. American Medical Association National Symposium on Medicine and Public Policy: Balancing the Response to Prescription Drug Abuse, Washington, DC, Proceedings (forthcoming).

Goodwin, J. S., Sanchez, C. J., Thomas, P., Hunt, C., Garry, P. J., and Goodwin, J. M., 1987, Alcohol intake in a health elderly population, *Am. J. Public health* **77:**173.

Gottheil, E., Druley, K. A., Skoloda, T. E., and Waxman, H. M., 1985, *The Combined Problems of Alcoholism, Drug Addiction and Aging,* Charles C Thomas, Springfield, IL.

Gove, W. C., 1975, Sex, marital status and mortality, *Am. J. Sociol.* **79:**45.

Graham, K., 1985, Identifying and measuring alcohol abuse among the elderly: Serious problems with existing instrumentation, Presented at the Ontario Psychogeriatric Association, Toronto, Oct. 6–8, 1985.

Graham, K., and Timney, C., 1986, Evaluation of the COPA project (unpublished manuscript).

Grant, I., Adams, K. M., and Reed, R., 1984, Aging, abstinence, and medical risk factors in the prediction of neuropsychologic deficit among long-term alcoholics, *Arch. Gen. Psychiatry* **120:** 710.

Green, R. F., 1969, Age–intelligence relationships between ages sixteen and sixty-four: A rising trend, *Dev. Psychol.* **1:**618.

Greenblatt, D. J., 1981, Sedative–hypnotics: Sleep disorders in the elderly, in: *Physicians' Handbook on Psychotherapeutic Drug Use in the Aged* (T. Crook and G. Cohen, eds.), pp. 58–65, Mark Powley Associates, New Canaan, CT.

Gross, D., and Capuzzi, D., 1981, The elderly alcoholic: The Counselor's dilemma, *Counselor Education Supervision* **20:**183.

Guttman, D., 1976, The cross-cultural perspective: Notes toward a comparative psychology of age, in: *Handbook of the Psychology of Aging* (J. E. Birren and K. W. Schaie, eds.), pp. 302–326, Van Nostrand Reinhold, New York.

Guttmann, D., 1977*a, A Study of Legal Drug Use by Older Americans,* National Institute on Drug Abuse, Washington, DC.

Guttman, D., 1977b, *A Survey of Drug-Taking Behavior of the Elderly,* Catholic University of America, Washington, DC.

Guttmann, D., 1978, Patterns of legal drug use by older Americans, *Addictive Dis.* **3:**337.

Hall, M. R. P., 1986, Drug interactions in geriatric patients, in: *Drugs and Aging* (D. Platt, ed.), Springer-Verlag, Berlin.

Harper, M. S., 1985, Survey of drug use and mental disorders in nursing homes, in: *Geriatric Drug Use—Clinical and Social Perspectives* (S. R. Moore and T. W. Teal, eds.), pp. 101–114, Pergamon Press, New York.

Hartford, J. T., and Samorajski, T., eds., 1984, *Alcoholism in the Elderly, Social and Biomedical Issues,* Raven Press, New York.

Herzog, A. R., and Dielman, L., 1985, Age differences in response accuracy for factual survey questions, *J. Gerontol.* **40:**350.

Hilton, M. E., 1987, Drinking patterns and drinking problems in 1984: Results from a general population survey, *Alcoholism: Clin. Exp. Res.* **11:**167.

Hodkinson, H. M., 1975, Psychological medicine—The elderly mind, *Br. Med. J.* **2:**23.

Hoffman, H., 1976, Referral sources, prehospital events, and after-care of young and old alcoholics, Willmar State Hospital, Willmar, MN (unpublished manuscript).

Holzer, C. E., III, Robins, L. N., Myers, J. K., Weissman, M. M., Tischler, G. L., Leaf, P. J., Anthony, J., and Bednarski, P. B., 1984, Antecedents and correlates of alcohol abuse and dependence in the elderly, in: *Nature and Extent of Alcohol Problems among the Elderly* (G. Maddox, L. N. Robins, and N. Rosenberg, eds.), pp. 217–244, National Institute of Alcohol Abuse and Alcoholism, Washington, DC.

Horn, J. L., 1976, Human abilities: A review of research and theory in the early 1970's, *Annu. Rev. Psychol.* **27:**437.

Horn, J. L., and Donaldson, G., 1976, On the myth of intellectual decline in adulthood, *Am. Psychologist* **31:**701.

House, J. S., Robbins, C., and Metzner, H. L., 1982, The association of social relationships and activities with mortality: Prospective evidence from the Tecumseh Community Health Study, *Am. J. Epidemiol.* **116:**123.

Hubbard, R. W., Santos, J. F., and Santos, M. A., 1979, Alcohol and older adults: Overt and covert influences, *Social Casework* **60:**166.

Huffine, C., Folkman, S., and Lazarus, R. S., 1989, Psychoactive drugs, alcohol, and stress and coping processes in older adults. *American Journal of Drug and Alcohol Abuse,* **15:**101.

Hyman, M. M., Zimmerman, M. A., Gurioli, C., and Helrich, A., 1980, *Drinkers, Drinking and Alcohol-Related Mortality and Hospitalizations,*Center of Alcohol Studies, Rutgers University, New Brunswick, NJ.

Issa, F. G., and Sullivan, C. E., 1982, Alcohol, snoring and sleep apnea, *J. Neurol. Neurosurg. Psychiatry* **45:**353.

Jackson, J. J., 1985, Race, national origin, ethnicity, and aging, in: *Handbook of Aging and the Social Sciences,* 2nd ed. (R. H. Binstock and E. Shanas, eds.), pp. 264–303, Van Nostrand Reinhold, New York.

Jacobsohn, D., 1972, Willingness to retire in relation to job strain and type of work, *J. Indust. Geront.* **13:**65.

James, O. F. W., 1983, Alcoholism in the elderly, in: *Alcohol-Related Problems: Room for Maneuver* (N. Krasner, S. Madin, and R. Walker, eds.), pp. 147–157, Wiley, New York.

Janik, S. W., and Dunham, R. G., 1983, A nationwide examination of the need for specific alcoholism treatment programs for the elderly, *J. Stud. Alcohol* **44:**307.

Johnson, L. A., and Goodrich, C. H., 1974, *Use of Alcohol by Persons 65 Years and Over,* Mt. Sinai School of Medicine, City University of New York, New York.

Jones-Witters, P., and Witters, W. L., 1983, *Drugs and Society, a Biological Perspective,* Wadworth Health Sciences, Monterey, CA.

Kasl, S. W., and Berkman, L., 1981, Psychosocial influences on health status of the elderly: The perspective of social epidemiology, in: *Aging: Biology and Behavior* (J. L. McGaugh and S. B. Kiesler, eds.), pp. 345–385, Academic Press, New York.

Keller, M., and Gurioli, C., 1976, Statistics on consumption of alcohol and on alcoholism, 1976 ed., 18 pp., *Journal of Studies on Alcohol,* New Brunswick, NJ.

Kendrick, R., and Bayne, J. R. D., 1982, Compliance with prescribed medication for elderly patients, *Can. Med. Assoc. J.* **127**:961.

Kingston, E. R., Hirshorn, B. A., and Cornman, J. M., 1986, *Ties That Bind, the Interdependence of Generations,* Gerontological Society of America, Seven Locks Press, Washington, DC.

Kleinknecht, R. A., and Goldstein, S. G., 1972, Neuropsychological deficits associated with alcoholism, *Q. J. Stud. Alcohol* **33**:999.

Klerman, G. L., 1976, Age and clinical depression, *J. Gerontol.* **31**:318.

Kofoed, L. L., Tolson, R. L., Atkingson, R. M., Turner, J. A., and Toth, R. F., 1984, Elderly groups in an alcoholism clinic, in: *Alcohol and Drug Abuse in Old Age* (R. M. Atkinson, ed.), pp. 35–48, American Psychiatric Press, Washington, DC.

Kofoed, L. L., Tolson, R. L., Atkinson, R. M., Toth, R. L., and Turner, J. A., 1987, Treatment compliance of older alcoholics: An elderly-specific approach is superior to "mainstreaming," *J. Stud. Alcohol* **48**:47.

Kramer, M., Taube, C., and Starr, S., 1968, Patterns of use of psychiatric facilities by the aged: Current status, trends, and implications, in: *Aging and Modern Society* (A. Simon and L. J. Epstein, eds.), Psychiatric Research Report No. 23, American Psychiatric Association, Washington, DC.

Labouvie-Vief, G., 1985, Intelligence and cognition, in: *Handbook of the Psychology of Aging* (J. E. Birren and K. W. Schaie, eds.), pp. 500–530, Van Nostrand Reinhold, New York.

Lampe, K. L., 1985, Physician instructions to the patient, in: *Geriatric Drug Use—Clinical and Social Perspectives* (S. R. Moore and T. W. Teal, eds.), pp. 34—38, Pergamon Press, New York.

Lamy, P. P., 1988, Actions of alcohol and drugs in older people, *Generations,***XII**:9.

Lamy, P. P., 1987, Introduction to the aging process, in:*Therapeutics in the Elderly* (J. C. Delafuente and R. B. Steward, eds.), Baltimore: Williams and Wilkins.

Langner, T. S., and Michael, W. T., 1963, *Life Stress and Mental Health,* Free Press, New York.

LaRue, A., Dessonville, C., and Jarvik, L. F., 1985, Aging and mental disorders, in: *Handbook of the Psychology of Aging* (J. E. Birren and K. W. Schaie, eds.), pp. 664–702, Van Nostrand Reinhold, New York.

Leighton, D. C., Harding, J. S., Macklin, D. B., Macmillan, A. M., and Leighton, A. N., 1963, *The Character of Danger: Psychiatric Symptoms in Selected Communities, The Stirling County Study of Psychiatric Disorder and Sociocultural Environment,* Basic Books, New York.

Lesage, J. and Zwygart-Stauffacher, M., 1988, Detection of medication misuse in elders, *Generations* **XII**:32.

Levenson, A. J., 1981, Psychotropic drug use in the elderly: An overview, *Am. Family Physician* **24**: 194.

Maddox, G., Robins, L. N., and Rosenberg, N., eds., 1984, *Nature and Extent of Alcohol Problems among the Elderly,* Research Monograph No. 14, National Institute on Alcohol Abuse and Alcoholism, DHHS (ADM) 84-1321, Washington, DC.

Mäkelä, K., and Simpura, J., 1984, *Experiences Related to Drinking in Finland as a Function of Annual Intake of Alcohol by Sex and Age,* Presented at the meeting of the Epidemiology Section of the International Council of Addictions and Alcoholism, Edinburgh.

McCormack, P., and O'Malley, K., 1986, Biological and medical aspects of drug treatment in the elderly, in: *Food, Drugs and Aging* (R. E. Dunkle, G. J. Petot, and A. B. Ford, eds.), pp. 19–27, Springer, New York.

McCrady, B. S., and Smith, D. E., 1986, Implications of cognitive impairment for the treatment of alcoholism, *Alcoholism: Clin. Exp. Res.* **10**:145.

Mellinger, G. D., Balter, M. B., Parry, H. R., Manheimer, D. I., and Cisin, I. H., 1974, An overview of psychotherapeutic drug use in the United States, in: *Drug Use: Epidemiological and Sociological Approaches* (E. Josephson and E. E. Carroll, eds.), pp. 340–359, Hemisphere, New York.

Mendels, J., 1981, Antidepressants, in: *Physicians' Handbook on Psychotherapeutic Drug Use in the Aged* (T. Crook and G. Cohen, eds.), pp. 26–37, Mark Powley Associates, New Canaan, CT.

Merry, J., 1980, Alcoholism in the aged, *Br. J. Alcohol Alcoholism* **15:**56.

Meyers, A., Goldman, E., Hingson, R., and Scotch, N., 1981–1982, Evidence for cohort or generational differences in the drinking behavior of older adults, *Int. J. Aging Hum. Dev.* **14:**31.

Meyers, A. R., Hingson, R., Mucatel, M., and Goldman, E., 1982, Social and psychological correlates of problem drinking in old age, *J. Am. Geriatr. Soc.* **30:**452.

Minkler, M., 1985, Social support and health of the elderly, in: *Social Support and Health* (S. Cohen and S. L. Syme, eds.), pp. 199–216, Academic Press, New York.

Mishara, B. L., and Kastenbaum, R., 1980, *Alcohol and Old Age,* Grune & Stratton, New York.

Monk, A., Cryns, A. G., and Cabral, R., 1977, Alcohol consumption and alcoholism as a function of adult age, *Gerontologist* **17:**101.

Moos, R., and Finney, J. W., 1984, A systems perspective on problem drinking among older adults, in: *Nature and Extent of Alcohol Problems among the Elderly* (G. Maddox, L. N. Robins, and N. Rosenberg, eds.), pp. 151–172, National Institute on Alcohol Abuse and Alcoholism, Washington DC.

Morrant, J. C. A., 1983, Use and abuse of psychoactive drugs in the elderly, *Can. Med. Assoc. J.* **129:** 245.

National Institute on Drug Abuse, 1979, *The Aging Process and Psychoactive Drug Use,* DHEW 79-815, U.S. Government Printing Office, Washington, DC.

Noonberg, A., Goldstein, G., and Page, H. A. 1985, Premature aging in male alcoholics: "Accelerated aging" or "increased vulnerability"? *Alcoholism: Clin. Exp. Res.* **9:**334.

*Old, Alone and Poor: A Plan for Reducing Poverty among Elderly People Living Alone,* 1987, The Commonwealth Fund Commission on Elderly People Living Alone, Baltimore, MD.

O'Malley, K., Judge, T. G., and Crooks, J., 1980, Geriatric clinical pharmacology and therapeutics, in: *Drug Treatment,* 2nd ed. (G. Avery, ed.), pp. 158–181, Adis Press, Sydney and New York.

Ott, J. F., Hunter, B. E., and Walker, D. W., 1985, The effect of age on ethanol metabolism and on the hypothermic and hypnotic responses to ethanol in the Fischer 344 rat, *Alcoholism: Clin. Exp. Res.* **9:**59.

Ouslander, J. G., 1986, Polypharmacy and the elderly, in: *Food, Drugs, and Aging* (R. E. Dunkle, G. J. Petot, and A. B. Ford, eds.), pp. 29–40, Springer, New York.

Parry, J. H., Balter, M. B., Mellinger, G. D., Cisin, I. H., and Manheimer, D. I., 1973, National patterns of psychotherapeutic drug use, *Arch. Gen. Psychiatry* **28:**769.

Pascarelli, E. F., 1985, The elderly in methadone maintenance, in: *The Combined Problems of Alcoholism, Drug Addiction and Aging* (E. Gottheil, K. A. Druley, T. E. Skoloda, and H. M. Waxman, eds.), pp. 210–214, Charles C Thomas, Springfield, IL.

Patterson, R. D., Abrahams, R., and Baker, F., 1974, Preventing self-destructive behavior, *Geriatrics* **29:**115.

Peplau, L. A., and Perlman, D., 1982, *Loneliness: A Sourcebook of Current Theory, Research, and Therapy,* Wiley, New York.

Petersen, D. M., 1988, Substance Abuse, criminal behavior and older people. *Generations,* **XII:**63.

Petersen, D. M., and Whittington, F. J., 1977, Drug use among the elderly: A review, *J. Psychodelic Drugs* **9:**25.

Pishkin, V., Lovallo, W. R., and Bourne, L. E., 1985, Chronic alcoholism in males: Cognitive deficit as a function of age at onset, age, and duration, *Alcoholism: Clin. Exp. Res.* **9:**400.

Poon, L. W., 1985, Differences in human memory with aging: Nature, causes and clinical implications, in: *Handbook of the Psychology of Aging* (J. E. Birren and K. W. Schaie, eds.), pp. 427–462, Van Nostrand Reinhold, New York.

*A Profile of Older Americans,* 1986, Program Resources Department, American Association of Retired Persons and the Administration on Aging, U.S. Department of Health and Human Services. PF3049(1086) D996, 14 pp.

Prentice, R., 1979, Patterns of psychotherapeutic drug use among the elderly, in: *The Aging Process and*

*Psychoactive Drug Use,* National Institute of Drug Abuse, pp. 17–41, Government Printing Office, Washington, DC.

Raffoul, P. R., Cooper, J. K., and Love, D. W., 1981, Drug misuse in older people, *Gerontologist* **21:** 146.

Rathbone-McCuan, E., and Roberds, L. A., 1980, Treatment of the older female alcoholic, *Focus on Women* **1:**104.

Rathbone-McCuan, E., and Triegaardt, J., 1979, The older alcoholic and the family, *Alcohol Health Res. World* **3:**7.

Rathbone-McCuan, E., Lohn, H., Levenson, J., and Hsu, J., 1976, *Community Survey of Aged Alcoholics and Problem Drinker,* National Institute on Alcohol Abuse and Alcoholism, Levine Geriatric Research Center, Baltimore, MD.

*Revue de l'alcoolisme,* 1969, **15** (Gaillard and Perrin, Pequignot et al., Fresneau, etc.).

Riccitelli, M. L., 1967, Alcoholism in the aged—Modern concepts, *J. Am. Geriatr. Soc.* **15:**142.

Rice, C., Hudig, D., Lod, P. et al., 1983, Ethanol activation of human natural cytotoxicity, *Immunopharmacology* **6:**303.

Riley, J. W., Jr., and Marden, C. F., 1947, The social pattern of alcoholic drinking, *Q. J. Stud. Alcohol* **8:**265.

Robbins, C., and Clayton, R. R., submitted for publication, Gender-related difference in psychoactive drug use among older adults.

Robinson, P. K., Coberly, S., and Paul, C. E., 1985, Work and retirement, in: *Handbook of Aging and the Social Sciences* (R. H. Binstock and E. Shanas, eds.), pp. 503–527, Van Nostran Reinhold, New York.

Rodgers, W. L., and Herzog, A. R., 1987, Interviewing older adults: The accuracy of factual information, *J. Gerontol.* **42:**387.

Rosin, A. J., and Glatt, M. M., 1971, Alcohol excess in the elderly, *Q. J. Stud. Alcohol* **32:**53.

Rosow, I., 1985, Status and role change through the life cycle, in: *Handbook of Aging and the Social Sciences* (R. H. Binstock and E. Shanas, eds.), pp. 62–93, Van Nostrand Reinhold, New York.

Rowe, J. W., and Kahn, R. L., 1987, Human aging: Usual and successful, *Science* **237:**143.

Rubington, D., 1982, The chronic drunkenness offender on Skid Row, in: *Alcohol, Science and Society Revisited* (E. L. Gomberg, H. R. White, and J. A. Carpenter, eds.), pp. 332–336, University of Michigan Press, Ann Arbor.

Russell, J., 1987, Art born in the fullness of age, *New York Times,* Aug. 23, 1987.

Salthouse, T. A., 1985, Speed of behavior and its implications for cognition, in: *Handbook of the Psychology of Aging* (J. E. Birren and K. W. Schaie, eds.), pp. 400–426, Van Nostrand Reinhold, New York.

Sandoz Pharmaceuticals, 1977, Medication and the elderly, *Care* **2:**5.

Saunders, S. J., 1976, Second annual report re reducing drinking problems in a home for the aged, Substudy 745, Addiction Research Foundation, Toronto.

Saunders, S. J., Graham, K., Flower, M. C., and Shea, J. P., 1985, Community older personal alcohol project: Assessment form, ARF Internal Document 58, Addiction Research Foundation, Toronto.

Schaie, K. W., and Willis, S. I., 1986, Can decline in adult intellectual functioning be reversed? *Dev. Psychol.* **22:**223.

Schmucker, D. L., 1984, Drug disposition in the elderly: A review of critical factors, *J. Am. Geriatr. Soc.* **32:**144.

Schuckit, M. A., 1977, Geriatric alcoholism and drug abuse, *Gerontologist* **17:**168.

Schuckit, M. A., Morrissey, E. R., and O'Leary, M. R., 1978, Alcohol problems in elderly men and women, *Addictive Dis.* **3:**405.

Schultz, R., 1985, Emotion and affect, in: *Handbook of the Psychology of Aging* (J. E. Birren and K. W. Schaie, eds.), pp. 531–543, Van Nostrand Reinhold, New York.

Sellers, E. M., Frecker, R. C., and Romach, M. L., 1982, Drug metabolism in the elderly: Confounding of age, smoking and ethanol effects, Substudy 1219, Addiction Research Foundation, Toronto.

Shanas, E., and Maddox, G. L., 1985, Health, health resources, and the utilization of care, in:

*Handbook of Aging and the Social Sciences* (R. H. Binstock and E. Shanas, eds.), pp. 697–726, Van Nostrand Reinhold, New York.
Shelton, M. D., Parson, O. A., and Leber, W. R., 1984, Verbal and visuospatial performance in male alcoholics: A test of the premature-aging hypothesis, *J. Consult. Clin. Psychol.* **52**:200.
Sheppard, H. L., 1976, Work and retirement, in: *Handbook of Aging and the Social Sciences* (R. H. Binstock and E. Shanas, eds., pp. 286–309, Van Nostrand Reinhold, New York.
Sherouse, D. L., 1983, *Professional's Handbook on Geriatric Alcoholism,* Charles C Thomas, Springfield, IL.
Siegel, G. B., 1982, Drugs and the aging, *Regulatory Toxicol. Pharmacol.* **2**:287.
Simmons-Tropea, D., Osborn, R. W., and Schwenger, C. W., 1986, Health status and health services for elderly Canadians, Research Paper 8, Programme in Gerontology, University of Toronto.
Simon, A., Lowenthal, M. F., and Epstein, L., 1970, *Crisis Intervention: The Fate of the Elderly Mental Patient,* Jossey-Bass, San Francisco.
Simonson, W., 1984, *Medications and the Elderly: A Guide for Promoting Proper Use,* Aspen Systems Corporation, Rockville, MD.
*Smoking, Tobacco and Health,* 1987, Public Health Service, DHHS Publication (CDC) 87-8397.
*A Socio-Demographic Profile of the Elderly*, 1984, Metropolitan Toronto District Health Council (February 1984), 46 pp.
Solomon, D. K., Baumgartner, R. P., Weissman, A. M., Briscoe, M. E., Smith, R. M., and McCormick, W. C., 1978, Pharmaceutical services to improve drug therapy for home health care patients, *Am. J. Hosp. Pharm.* **35**:553.
Special report, access to health care in the United States: Results of a 1986 survey, 1987, 11 pp., Robert Wood Johnson Foundation, Princeton, NJ.
Stone, L. O., and Fletcher, S., 1981, *Aspects of Population Aging in Canada, a Chartbook,* National Advisory Council on Aging, Ministry of Supply and Services, Ottawa, Canada.
Sussman, M. B., 1985, The family life of old people, in: *Handbook of Aging and the Social Sciences* (R. H. Binstock and E. Shanas, eds.), pp. 218–243, Van Nostrand Reinhold, New York.
Tamkin, A. S., 1983, Impairment of cognitive functioning in alcoholics, *Military Med.* **148**:793.
Tarter, R., 1976, Empirical investigations of psychological deficit, in: *Alcoholism, Interdisciplinary Approaches to an Enduring Problem* (R. E. Tarter and A. A. Sugerman, eds.), pp. 359–394, Addison-Wesley, Reading, MA.
Tarter, R. E., and Edwards, K. L., 1986, Multifactorial etiology of neuropsychological impairment in alcoholics, *Alcoholism: Clin. Exp. Res.* **10**:128.
Terman, L. M., and Merrill, M. A., 1937, *Measuring Intelligence,* Houghton Mifflin, Boston.
Twigg, W. C., 1959, Alcoholism in a home for the aged, *Geriatrics* **14**:391.
Van De Vyvere, B., Hughes, M., and Fish, D. G., 1976, Elderly chronic alcoholics: A practical approach, *Can. Welfare* **52**:9.
Verbrugge, L., 1979, Marital status and health, *J. Marriage Family* **41**:267.
Veroff, J., Douvan, E., and Kulka, R., 1981, *The Inner American and Mental Health in America,* Basic Books, New York.
Verwoerdt, A., 1981, *Clinical Geropsychiatry,* 2nd ed., Williams & Wilkins, Baltimore, MD.
Vestal, R. F., 1982, Pharmacology and aging, *J. Am. Geriatr. Soc.* **30**:191.
Vestal, R. E., and Dawson, G. W., 1985, Pharmacology and aging, in: *Handbook of the Biology of Aging* (C. E. Finch and E. L. Schneider, eds.), pp. 744–819, Van Nostrand Reinhold, New York.
Vestal, R. E., McGuire, E. A., Tobin, J. D., Andres, R., Norris, A. H., and Mezey, E., 1977, Aging and ethanol metabolism, *Clin. Pharmacol. Ther.* **31**:343.
Vidojkovic, P., Grbesa, B., Miljkovic, S., and Sreckovic, M., 1970, Alcoholism in the aged, *Alkoholizam (Belgrad)* **10**:52.
Vinick, B. H., 1983, Loneliness among elderly widowers, Presented at the Gerontological Society of America meeting, San Francisco, 1983.
Vogel-Sprott, M., and Barrett, B., 1984, Age, drinking habits and the effects of alcohol, *J. Stud. Alcohol* **45**:517.

Warheit, G. J., Arey, S. A., and Swanson, E., 1976, Patterns of drug use: An epidemiologic overview, *J. Drug Issues* **6:**223.

Wattis, J. P., 1981, Alcohol problems in the elderly, *J. Am. Geriatr. Soc.* **29:**131.

Wattis, J. P., 1983, Alcohol and old people, *Br. J. Psychiatry* **143:**306.

Waxman, H. M., Klein, M., Kennedy, R., Randels, P., and Carner, E. A., 1985, Institutional drug abuse: The overprescribing of psychoactive medications in nursing homes, in: *The Combined Problems of Alcoholism, Drug Addiction and Aging* (E. Gottheil, K. A. Druley, T. E. Skoloda, and H. M. Waxman, eds.), pp. 179–190, Charles C Thomas, Springfield, IL.

Wechsler, D., 1958, *The Measurement and Appraisal of Adult Intelligence,* 4th ed., Williams & Wilkins, Baltimore, MD.

Weinstein, W. S., and Khanna, P., 1986, *Depression in the Elderly,* Philosophical Library, New York.

Wells-Parker, E., Miles, S., and Spencer, B., 1983, Stress experiences and drinking histories of elderly drunken-driving offenders, *J. Stud. Alcohol* **44:**429.

Westie, K. S., and McBride, D. C., 1979, The effects of ethnicity, age and sex upon processing through an emergency alcohol health care delivery system, *Br. J. Addictions* **74:**21.

Whittier, J. R., and Korenyi, C., 1961, Selected characteristics of aged patients: A study of mental hospital admissions, *Compr. Psychiatry* **2:**113.

Whittington, F. J., 1988, Making it better: drinking and drugging in old age. *Generations,* **XII:**5.

Wilkinson, D. A., and Sanchez-Craig, M., 1981, Relevance of brain dysfunction to treatment objectives: Should alcohol-related cognitive deficits influence the way we think about treatment? *Addictive Behav.* **6:**253.

Wilkinson, P., 1971, Alcoholism in the aged, *J. Geriatr.* **34:**59.

Willenbring, M., and Spring, W. D., Jr. 1988, Evaluating alcohol use in elders, *Generations,* **XII:**27.

Wilsnack, R. W., and Cheloha, R., 1987, Women's roles and problem drinking across the lifespan, *Social Problems* **34:**231.

Wood, W. G., and Armbrecht, H. J., 1982, Behavioral effects of ethanol in animals: Age differences and age changes, *Alcoholism: Clin. Exp. Res.* **6:**3.

Woods, R. T., and Britton, P. G., 1985, *Clinical Psychology with the Elderly,* Aspen, Rockville, MD.

Woolley, B. H., 1983, Personal communication (Bad medicine—An American Habit, *Los Angeles Times,* Los Angeles, CA, April 10, 1983).

York, J. L., 1982, The influence of age upon the physiological response to ethanol, in: *Alcoholism & Aging: Advances in Research* (W. G. Wood and M. F. Elias, eds.), pp. 99–113, CRC Press, Boca Raton, Fl.

York, J. L., 1983, Increased responsiveness to ethanol with advancing age in rats, *Pharmacol. Biochem. Behav.* **19:**687.

Zborowski, M., 1962, Aging and recreation, *J. Gerontol.* **7:**302.

Zimberg, S., 1974*a,* The elderly alcoholic, *Gerontologist* **14:**221.

Zimberg, S., 1974*b,* Two types of problem drinkers: Both can be managed, *Geriatrics* **29:**135.

Zimberg, S., 1984, Diagnosis and management of the elderly alcoholic, in: *Alcohol and Drug Abuse in Old Age* (R. M. Atkinson, ed.), pp. 23–33, American Psychiatric Press, Washington, DC.

# 7

# Stress and Coping Factors in the Epidemiology of Substance Use

THOMAS ASHBY WILLS

## 1. INTRODUCTION

The purpose of this chapter is to provide a systematic review of the role of stress and coping factors in substance use. In recent years, accumulating evidence from epidemiological studies has shown relationships between life stressors and substance use for each of the major phases of use: initiation, maintenance, and relapse. This research extends a line of investigation beginning with the tension reduction model of alcohol use (Conger, 1956; Cappell and Herman, 1972) and encompasses new studies of stress-related predictors of cigarette smoking, tranquilizers, and opiate use. Here I consider findings from field studies that provide evidence of stress–substance use relationships for each of the three phases. After detailed review of the field evidence, a final section discusses implications for theoretical models of substance use and abuse.

This chapter considers epidemiological research, studying factors that relate to substance use behavior as it occurs in the natural environment of the respondents. The question addressed is whether life stressors are consistently and causally related to higher levels of tobacco, alcohol, and opiate use. Findings from animal models and laboratory experiments with human subjects have shown evidence that stress affects substance use in several paradigms (e.g., Abrams, 1983; Alexander and Hadaway, 1982; Hull and Van Treuren, 1986; Leventhal and Cleary, 1980). From human studies, it is known that many persons try cigarettes and alcohol but relatively few become regular or heavy users (e.g., Cleary et al., 1988). Among regular smokers it is widely perceived that cigarette smoking provides stress-reducing functions (U.S.D.H.H.S., 1988), and similar expectancies about alcohol use have been found both among adolescents (Brown et al., 1980; Christiansen et al., 1982) and among adults (Cahalan et al., 1969; Deardorff et al., 1975; Farber et al., 1980; McCarty and Kaye, 1984). If sub-

THOMAS ASHBY WILLS • Department of Epidemiology and Social Medicine, Albert Einstein College of Medicine, Bronx, New York 10461.

stance use does provide affect-regulation functions for a significant proportion of users, then linkages between stress and substance use should be observed in epidemiological research. Thus, I address the evidence on stress–substance use relationships to determine whether there are notable commonalities in predictive patterns across different stages and types of substance use.

This chapter focuses on the proposition that substance use increases under stress because it is perceived by the user to have an affect-regulation function. Substance use is a multifactorial process: It may be promoted by social pressure or social modeling cues (e.g., Biglan and Lichtenstein, 1984); long-term dependence may be maintained by avoidance of physical withdrawal symptoms (Shiffman, 1979; Jaffe, 1980); and learning processes may be involved in stimuli associated with drug use (Pomerleau, 1981; Siegel, 1979). I do not aim to minimize the importance of these processes in substance use. Rather, the stress-related aspects of drug use seem to present an additional burden for the dependent user, and understanding these aspects may improve understanding of substance use initiation and relapse (Labouvie, 1986b; Wills and Shiffman, 1985).

## Stress

Stress originates with demands from the environment and culminates in changes in subjective well-being. Perceived stress is presumed to depend on an appraisal in which demands from the environment are perceived by an individual as exceeding the available coping resources (Cohen et al., 1983; Lazarus and Folkman, 1984). Life stress may be acute, such as a sudden illness in the family, or may represent chronic life strains that are not quickly resolved and persist over considerable periods of time (Pearlin et al., 1981). At the physiological level, acute stress produces increases in sympathetic nervous system arousal, and chronic stress is linked to changes in endocrine systems and reactivity to challenge (Baum et al., 1982; Grunberg and Baum, 1985). Perceived stress can cause symptoms of general anxiety, tension, or depression; and subjective well-being is influenced independently by increased negative affect and decreased positive affect (Diener, 1984; Wills and Shiffman, 1985). In literature discussed here, objective measures of stress have usually been based on checklists of major life events or chronic life strains, and subjective distress has been indexed with questionnaire measures of anxiety, depression, or general psychological symptomatology. This chapter is not critical of the stress measures used, except for some theoretical issues discussed in the final section (for detailed discussion see Baum et al., 1982).

The stress-coping process is presumed to be guided by ongoing appraisal of current stressors in relation to current coping resources. As coping resources increase, the perceived threat value of life stressors should decrease, but lack of effectiveness at initial coping efforts should increase the current level of perceived stress (Cohen and Williamson, 1988). The coping process is assumed to continue until major stressors are eventually resolved; if further coping attempts are considered unlikely to be effective, chronic stress would ensue.

In the context of overall coping processes, substance use may be construed as an emotion-focused strategy, oriented toward reduction of emotional distress rather than change of environmental conditions (Moos and Billings, 1982). A stress-coping model posits that substance use is more likely when level of life stress is high, and when alternative coping resources are impoverished. Determining whether substance use is an *effective* coping mechanism is a complex issue and has not been generally addressed in the literature (see Caplan et al., 1984; Stone et al., 1987). It can be presumed that although substance use may provide temporary alleviation of distress, reliance on substances as a coping mechanism can prevent the development of alternative coping mechanisms, lead to interpersonal or legal problems, and in the long run cause impairments in health and role performance.

The following sections consider epidemiological evidence on the role of stress and coping factors for initiation, maintenance, and relapse of substance use. Because a good part of the literature is correlational, this chapter gives detailed attention to methodological issues that bear on causal interpretations of field data (Cohen, 1986; Vaillant, 1984). Other issues, such as sampling, completion, and measures of substance use, are comparable in most studies and are not discussed in detail.

## 2. STRESS FACTORS IN THE INITIATION OF SUBSTANCE USE

Prevalence studies based on representative national samples show that initiation of cigarette smoking and alcohol use occurs largely between 12 and 16 years of age (Fishburne et al., 1980; Green, 1979). Hence epidemiological research has concentrated on the early adolescent period to investigate predictors of substance use onset. The greater part of adolescent research has been conducted with school samples, which make it feasible to collect data on substantial numbers of participants and to follow them over time. School samples are not totally representative of the population because drug-using students tend more often to be truant from school and to drop out of longitudinal panels (Kandel, 1978). For research on predictors of substance use, though, school samples are regarded as valid because the samples are reasonably representative, and predicted effects are found even though typical sample biases work against demonstration of these effects.

Three methodological issues are relevant for research on stress factors in adolescent substance use. First, cross-sectional data are generally ambiguous because it is unclear whether some variables (e.g., family conflict, adolescent depression) are antecedents or consequences of substance use (Gorsuch and Butler, 1976; Kandel, 1978). For this reason, prospective studies are more desirable because it is possible to investigate predictor variables related to increases in substance use over time. A second issue concerns the measurement of life stress among adolescents. Although there has been relatively little basic research on adolescent stressors, measures of life events are available that have been adapted for adolescent populations (Johnson and McCutcheon, 1980; Newcomb et al., 1981). The convergence of results from measures at several levels (major life events, daily hassles, and subjective stress) suggests that the assessment methodologies are valid, although additional research on adolescent stressors is needed (see Compas, 1987; Depue and Monroe, 1986; Wills, 1986). Another issue concerns the validity of self-reported substance use on questionnaire measures. The available evidence suggests that self-reports of smoking and alcohol use are basically valid (e.g., Alanko, 1984; Bauman and Koch, 1983; Chassin et al., 1981*a;* Murray et al., 1987).

## Cigarette Smoking

A retrospective study by Hirschman et al. (1984) was based on direct interviews with a sample of 386 public school students in grades 2–10 in Milwaukee, Wisconsin. Subjects were asked about the time of their first smoking experience (if any) and then were asked about second and third smoking experiences (if any) and current smoking status. Measures of stress and coping were based on interview questions about recent change of school, overall life stress, helplessness (not trying to cope), and inadequate coping; these indices were entered simultaneously in multivariate analyses with measures of peer smoking, risk taking, and attitudes toward cigarettes. The results showed that stress factors were not related to trying a first cigarette; initial experimentation was predicted only by age, peer smoking, and risk taking. Helplessness and school change, however, were related to continuation to second and third cigarettes and to short latency (from second to third). Measures of reactions to the first smoking experience showed that strong physiological reactions predicted continuation; dizziness was related to trying a second cigarette, and coughing positively related to current use. These data suggest that greater physiological reactivity may make individuals more susceptible to smoking (cf. Silverstein et al., 1982).

Concurrent data on subjective stress and smoking were obtained from a random sample of 1684 public school students in grades 7–12 in Halifax, Nova Scotia (Mitic et al., 1985). The stress measure was based on items asking the extent to which the respondent had felt "nervous, anxious, or worried" during the past month as a result of 12 potential problem areas. Responses were on a five-point Likert scale, with anchor points Never to Always, and the stress score was based on the number of Often or Always responses. Subjects were classified as nonsmokers vs. light vs. medium vs. heavy smokers on the basis of self-reports. Analysis of variance indicated that for males, nonsmokers scored lower on stress compared with all other smoking categories, and heavy smokers scored higher than all other categories. For females, regular/heavy smokers scored higher than either nonsmokers or occasional users. Data on sources of stress indicated "money" and "parents" to be predictors of smoking for males and females. "Schoolwork" was a unique predictor for males, and "appearance" a unique predictor for females.

A quasiprospective study by Seltzer and Oechsli (1985) was based on a sample of 1217 white adolescents in Oakland, California, initially assessed during a clinic visit at 9–11 years of age and classified for smoking status at 15–17 years of age. Predictor variables were derived from a 100-item behavior questionnaire using mothers' reports of their children's behavior and two cognitive measures, the Peabody Vocabulary Test and the Raven Progressive Matrices. Psychosocial variables were obtained *post facto* through a procedure in which the questionnaire items were classified by expert judges into several scales. Analyses controlling for parental socioeconomic status indicated that at age 10, eventual smokers scored significantly higher on Type A personality, extraversion, anger, "psychoticism," and restless sleep and scored lower on the cognitive measures. No differences were noted for indices of depression and anxiety. The measures of Type A, anger, and restless sleep may index negative affect or physical tension. Although the measures of depression or anxiety were not significant predictors, these were based on mothers' reports, which have relatively low reliability for assessing intrapsychic states of children as compared to observable behaviors.

A prospective study by Wills (1986) was based on two cohorts of public school students in New York City ($n$ = 675 and 901), surveyed in a four-wave design from the beginning through end of their 7th to 8th-grade years (ages 13–15). Predictor variables included a 14-item scale of subjective stress and a 12-item scale of recent negative events, both with a 1-week time frame, and a 15-item scale of major negative life events with a 1-year time frame. Self-reported cigarette smoking (biochemically validated with measures of saliva thiocyanate and cotinine) was indexed through a Guttman score based on dichotomous items asking whether the respondent had smoked ever, more than four times, in the past month, and in the past week. Hypotheses in this study were tested through multivariate analyses in which the smoking score was predicted with controls for sex, race, and other psychosocial variables (self-esteem, self-efficacy, health locus of control, and assertiveness). Prospective analytical models were utilized in which measures at one time point (e.g., beginning of 7th grade) were employed as predictors of smoking at a subsequent time point (e.g., end of 7th grade), with control for smoking score at the point of prediction. In both concurrent and prospective models, it was found that subjective stress and negative events were related to cigarette smoking. Tests of net effects indicated that major negative events showed a unique contribution for predicting cigarette smoking, when entered with recent negative events. Data on coping with general life problems, measured by two different methods, indicated that behavioral coping, cognitive coping, and adult social support were inversely related to smoking and/or alcohol use. Coping strategies of aggression, distraction, and peer social activity were positively related to substance use.

A multivariate analysis by Castro et al. (1987) tested correlates of regular smoking in a multiethnic sample of 810 adolescents in Los Angeles, California, surveyed in 10th–12th grades. A measure of life events was based on items, with a 6-month time frame, concerning events in the areas of family events, relocation, and accident/illness events. A measure of perceived stressfulness was obtained separately for each of the three domains by having subjects rate the stressfulness of each event on a five-point scale; apparently the subjects provided a rating for every event in the checklist, irrespective of whether or not the event had occurred to them. Other predictor variables were a measure of social conformity based on scales for law abidance, liberalism, and religiosity, and a measure of peer smoking. The measure of smoking was based on a mixture of items concerning intentions to smoke in the future plus items on current quantity/frequency of cigarette smoking. Structural modeling analyses for the total sample indicated a significant direct effect of family events on smoking, plus an indirect path of family events mediated through peer smoking, suggesting that negative family events increased the tendency to affiliate with deviant peers. Puzzling results occurred for the measure of perceived stressfulness, which showed a positive direct effect on smoking but was inversely related to family events and showed an indirect inverse effect on smoking, mediated through increased social conformity. The contradictory results for this measure suggest a problem with the construct validity of the scale.

## Stress and Initiation of Alcohol Use

Specific data on initiation of alcohol use are minimal because indices of alcohol use are typically combined with measures of other drug use (discussed in the following section). In the Wills (1986) study, a Guttman score for overall involvement in alcohol use, plus a separate item on heavy drinking during the past month, was analyzed separately from data on smoking; the smoking and alcohol scores were positively correlated ($r$ = 0.50–0.60), reflecting the typical intercorrelation of substance use in adolescent populations. Concurrent and prospective analyses indicated that all stress measures were positively related to alcohol use. The subjective stress measure showed unique contributions for alcohol use when entered with recent negative events, particularly for heavy drinking. This finding was interpreted as indicating that alcohol use is more related to current level of subjective distress, whereas smoking initiation is more related to long-term stress levels.

Similar results were found in a cross-sectional study by Baer et al. (1987) with a sample of 425 junior high-school students. These data showed that measures of negative life events and family conflict were related to an index of the intensity of alcohol use. Data from two high-school samples (Chassin et al., 1988) also showed negative life events related to indices of intensity and consequences of alcohol use. These investigators found that family history of alcoholism showed an independent relationship to alcohol use, but family history and negative life events did not interact in predicting alcohol use.

Kandel et al. (1978) reported data on transitions to hard liquor use among students who had already smoked or drunk beer/wine. Questionnaires were initially administered to a random sample of public high-school students in New York State ($n$ = 8206), and the baseline sample was resurveyed with a 5- to 6-month follow-up interval. Results for hard liquor, based on a panel of 1936 cases, indicated initiation to be related to less closeness to parents and to greater peer social activity, as well as to typical predictors of alcohol use (i.e., parental drinking, peer drinking, attitudes toward alcohol, prior smoking or beer/wine use). For brief scales indexing depression and self-image, no significant effects were observed.

Several studies have been conducted to test problem behavior theory. Studies by Jessor and Jessor (1977) were based on regional samples of high-school students ($n$ = 589) and college students ($n$ = 276), and data from a representative national sample of 13,122 adolescents in grades 7–12 were analyzed by Donovan and Jessor (1978) and Jessor et al. (1980). In these studies, variables such as rebelliousness and independence, lack of closeness to parents, generally positive attitudes toward deviant behavior, low perceived control, and low academic achievement were shown in concurrent and prospective analyses to relate to alcohol and marijuana use. Subsequent replications of these findings have been obtained in several studies (Chassin et al., 1985; Hays et al., 1987; Hull et al., 1986). Although these studies do not measure affective variables *per se*, the relationship of problem behavior constructs to affective factors is discussed subsequently.

## Initiation of Other Drug Use

Two studies of high-school students have related life stress measures to composite indices of drug use. Bruns and Geist (1984) obtained cross-sectional data from a sample (not otherwise characterized) of 566 high-school students from suburban Chicago, combined with a sample of 55 teenagers in residential treatment for drug abuse. An ascending score for drug use (apparently based on self-report) had scale points of abstainer, tobacco only, alcohol only, marijuana user, and other drug use; the treated subjects were arbitrarily given a separate score at the top of the scale. Analyses using data from the Coddington Life Events Scale showed a linear increase in life events across the drug use groups.

A concurrent study by Murray and Perry (1984) is the only one to specifically relate the perceived coping functions of drugs to measures of current substance use. These investigators surveyed a population of 7762 students in 9th–10th grades in schools in Minneapolis, Minnesota, and correlated scores for various functions with indices of 30-day use of a substance. Functional motives were assessed by questions asking the extent to which substance use would help the student respond to a particular need; the six functions were labeled Relief from Boredom, Indicator of Adulthood, Have Fun, Make Friends, Maintain Personal Energy, and Reduce Stress. Results indicated that tobacco, alcohol, and marijuana had somewhat different functional value. While there was commonality in predictive patterns (i.e., high correlations of most functional dimensions with use of all substances), marijuana and tobacco showed largest correlations for Stress Reduction, Boredom Relief, and Having Fun, whereas for alcohol, the Have Fun dimension showed the strongest correlations with recent use. In this study, individual motive dimensions were assessed on different subsamples from the large cohort, so it was not possible to test the unique contributions of dimensions to substance use.

A retrospective study of 424 college students aged 18–19 years in Boston (Deykin et al., 1987) is considered in this section because a lifetime history of substance use was obtained. Subjects were directly interviewed using the Diagnostic Interview Schedule and diagnoses of current psychiatric disorder were made using DSM-III criteria; if a positive indication of diagnosable disorder was evident, age of onset for the disorder(s) was determined in the interview. Results indicated that lifetime diagnoses of alcohol abuse/dependence were strongly associated with diagnoses of major depressive disorder (MDD); the association was stronger for females than for males but was significant in both groups. Diagnoses of other substance abuse (prescription drugs, marijuana, cocaine) also were significantly associated with lifetime diagnosis of MDD; here the association was stronger for males. Alcohol abuse was specifically associated with depressive disorder, whereas drug abuse diagnosis was associated with other psychiatric diagnoses besides depression (although the numbers of cases for the latter were small). Reports based on the eight subjects with a history of depressive disorder suggested that alcohol abuse tended to follow the onset of psychiatric disturbance, and a similar pattern was noted by the authors for the 19 subjects with drug abuse and another diagnosis; but no statistical tests were presented to support these conclusions.

Concurrent and longitudinal analyses were performed by Newcomb and Harlow (1986) on data from two adolescent samples. The concurrent analysis was based on a stratified sample of 376 students aged 12–18 years, living in New Jersey and surveyed by telephone. Predictor variables were negative life events in the domains of family, relocation, and accident/illness (cf. Castro et al., 1987) and three-item scales indexing perceived loss of control and sense of meaninglessness in life. A score for overall drug use was based on subscales for alcohol, marijuana, and other drugs (cocaine, heroin, psychedelics). Structural modeling analyses for concurrent data indicated a good fit for a "quasi-simplex" model, with an effect of life events on perceived control and an effect of control on meaninglessness, which showed the only direct effect on the drug use measure.

Longitudinal analyses were based on the Los Angeles subject pool used by Castro et al. (1987), employing data collected from 640 subjects surveyed during high school and resurveyed 4 years later. These analyses employed life events (assessed during high school) as predictors of perceived control, meaninglessness, and drug use assessed at follow-up; i.e., only the life events measure was a prospective predictor. These analyses showed best fit for a model in which life events had a direct effect on substance use, not mediated through control. From this mixed prospective–concurrent model it can be concluded that stressful events are temporally antecedent to a high level of drug use. In this study the mixed temporal ordering of the variables and the lack of a true prospective analysis of drug use present some qualifications on interpretation of the data. The authors tested several models using the available data and concluded that low perceived control and high meaninglessness were not consequences of drug involvement, but enough support was found for alternative models that the authors suggested, "readers may choose that [model] which is most theoretically appealing and interpretable to them" (Newcomb and Harlow, 1986, p. 573).

Similar findings were obtained by Labouvie (1986) in a study of an age-stratified sample of 1234 adolescents, all of whom had engaged in some substance use during the previous year. The dependent variable was a classification of substance use (alcohol, marijuana, and illicit drugs) based on intensity and reasons for use. Predictor variables included indices of subjective stress based on the extent to which respondents reported they were bothered by various hassles and overall life stress (meaninglessness and powerlessness). Results indicated that persons who were high on reactive drug use reported higher levels of social stress and overall life problems, and lower levels of overall life satisfaction.

In a study described previously, Kandel et al. (1978) analyzed predictors of transitions to marijuana and illicit drug use in a high-school panel. The database for these analyses was (1) students who had smoked and/or used hard liquor but not marijuana ($n = 1947$), and (2) students who had used one legal drug (cigarettes or alcohol) and marijuana, but no other illicit drug ($n = 523$). Predictors of marijuana use onset were similar to those for hard liquor, including peer use and lack of closeness to parents. Unique predictors for marijuana were desire to experience effects of the drug and previous alcohol use motivated by the desire for "pleasure." For onset of other drug use, unique predictors were poor family decision making, lack of close friendships among peers, depression, and previous marijuana use motivated by the desire to decrease depression. Of the three specific drugs measured by Kandel et al. (1978), initiation of illicit drug use seems more related to negative affective states and poor interpersonal relations.

The only long-term analysis of marijuana use is based on a panel of 2158 students in Houston, Texas, originally surveyed during 7th grade and followed up 10 years subsequently (Kaplan et al., 1986). A variety of psychosocial measures were obtained at the baseline and follow-up surveys, and at follow-up the respondent was asked whether he/she had ever used marijuana almost daily for at least a month. This item was used by the investigators as the criterion of escalated marijuana use. Analyses based only on respondents who had not tried marijuana at Time 1 indicated direct effects for earlier age at first use, avoidant coping style, psychological distress at time of first use, *absence* of social pressure at first use, and belief that marijuana use caused aggravation to significant others (e.g., parents). The Time 1 variables of rejection by family and failure at school had indirect effects on escalated marijuana use, mediated through increased psychological distress at first use.

These findings are generally consistent with prospective analyses of composite indices of drug use from this data set (Kaplan et al., 1982, 1984). These analyses used panel data from measurements made in the 7th, 8th, and 9th grades. Increases in overall drug use were related to rejection by family and school and endorsement of socially deviant attitudes. In these analyses a measure of self-derogation (not included in the preceding analyses) showed a number of direct and indirect effects on drug use during the junior-high-school period. Evidence was also found for a social modeling process, in that peer use at one time point was prospectively related to increased drug use at subsequent time points. Some evidence was also found for a reciprocal process, in which early substance use increased rejection by family and school, which in turn was a risk factor for increased substance use subsequently. These data underscore the multifactorial determination of substance use.

Specific analyses of cocaine use were performed by Newcomb and Bentler (1986) using data from the Los Angeles study (cf. Castro et al., 1987; Newcomb and Harlow, 1986). The data analyzed were from Years 4–5 of the study; the longitudinal panel was 847 students. In a true prospective analysis, variables from Year 4 were utilized as predictors of cocaine use at Year 5, with control for level of cocaine use at Year 4. Analyses of eight scales of psychopathology showed that a measure of depression was prospectively related to cocaine use. Analyses of related drug use indicated that prior marijuana, but not alcohol, use predicted increased cocaine use over the 1-year period.

A long-term analysis by Lerner and Vicary (1984) utilized data from early childhood to predict drug use in young adulthood. A sample of 133 children was initially assessed at 1, 3, and 5 years of age and classified on temperamental variables (Thomas et al., 1977). The syndrome of difficult temperament was indicated by presence of low adaptability, frequent negative mood, and high intensity of reactions to stimuli. Subjects were followed into late adolescence/young adulthood, and direct interview data were coded for use of three substances (tobacco, alcohol, and marijuana). Results showed that difficult temperament in childhood was related to substance use at all points in follow-up. The strength of relationships was greater for illicit drugs (marijuana) than for licit ones (tobacco), and strength of relationships generally increased as the subjects grew older. Somewhat similar results occurred in a study by Kellam et al. (1982), who obtained teacher and parent ratings of children during 1st grade and related these to a composite index of licit/illicit substance use obtained from subjects 10 years subsequently. These data indicated that early aggressiveness (for males) and psychological distress (for females) showed significant prospective relationships to substance use.

## Summary

The recent research on adolescents indicates a consistent relationship between stress factors and initiation of substance use. As a general conclusion, it can be stated that adolescents who are experiencing a high level of psychological distress are more likely to initiate tobacco or alcohol use and more likely to make subsequent transitions to marijuana or illicit drug use. Although the literature is quite variable with respect to the stage of initiation that is studied, some supportive evidence is available for tobacco (Hirschman et al., 1984), alcohol (Wills, 1986), and other illicit drugs (Kandel et al., 1978; Newcomb and Bentler, 1986). The prospective study by Seltzer and Oechsli (1985) also indicates that personality measures linked to negative affectivity relate to substance use from a point of prediction at age 10 years.

Several major methodological issues have been addressed by the recent research. The possibility that high stress is a consequence, rather than an antecedent, of initiation of substance use has been ruled out in several true prospective studies (Newcomb and Bentler, 1986; Seltzer and Oechsli, 1985; Wills, 1986). The findings from prospective research are consistent with results from concurrent and retrospective studies supporting the conclusion that stress is a predisposing factor for substance use.

An issue less clearly resolved is whether life stressors operate through a direct-effect mechanism or whether stress has an indirect effect mediated through other factors. Studies of initial adoption have tended to show a direct effect independent of other variables such as risk taking, self-esteem, and social skills (Hirschman et al., 1984; Wills, 1986). Studies conducted with somewhat older groups (10th–12th grades) provide mixed results, typically showing a mixture of direct and indirect effects mediated through variables such as peer smoking or perceived control (Castro et al., 1987; Newcomb and Harlow, 1986). Since the latter data are mostly derived from the same subject panel and mix different age groups within the same analysis, there is a need for further research with detailed study of age–predictor interactions.

There are considerable gaps in the literature. Stressors may well have different impact for students of different ages and at different points in the smoking/alcohol initiation process, but there has been no systematic study of different age groups (cf. Mittelmark et al., 1987). The sources of stress, and the perceived functional value of tobacco, alcohol, and marijuana for coping, may differ considerably for various cultural and gender groups, but these demographic variables have rarely been tested in general population studies. Physiological differences in reactivity to stress or to nicotine are plausibly related to initiation, but have received little attention (cf. Abrams et al., 1987; Silverstein et al., 1982), and how physiological factors relate to perceptions of the functional effects of drug use is unknown. All of these issues need to receive systematic investigation.

## 3. LIFE STRESS AND ONGOING SUBSTANCE USE

A number of studies of adults have analyzed data on life stressors in relation to indices of current smoking or alcohol use. The nature of the samples varies considerably, with some studies employing representative national or regional samples; other studies are based on more specialized populations, such as occupational groups. Methodological issues are more troublesome in this area. Although the goal of the research is to test a relationship between life stress and increased substance use, the available studies are generally cross-sectional or retrospective in design; hence, from most of these data it is not possible to rule out the suggestion that higher stress/anxiety is a consequence of substance use. In this area, laboratory research has investigated short-term relationships between stress and substance use. This research shows manipulated stressors related to increases in smoking (see U.S.D.H.H.S., 1988) and alcohol use (see Hull and Bond, 1986), thus strengthening causal interpretation of other findings.

In addition to issues deriving from interpretation of correlational data, two other methodological issues are salient in this area. First, the study designs have typically measured life stressors over a considerable period (usually a 1-year or 6-month time frame) but have employed criterion variables of current smoking/alcohol use. In theory, these designs would be statistically sensitive only to the extent that life events act to increase long-term levels of substance use. If current substance use were more closely linked to recent happenings (e.g., in the past day or week), then measures of typical consumption would be relatively insensitive for detecting significant relationships that might exist. Unfortunately, there is almost no field research that has examined short-term covariation of stress and substance use in the natural environment of the subjects.

Second, a considerable body of literature on personality correlates has shown trait measures of anxiety/depression related to smoking and alcohol use (see Cox, 1979; Kozlowski, 1979). While this literature has its own interpretational difficulties, it raises the issue of whether persons who are high on trait anxiety/depression are more likely to perceive a given level of events as more stressful, or possibly to cause more negative life events. This issue remains ambiguous in field studies because there have been few attempts to include personality control variables in the study designs.

## Cigarette Smoking

Two retrospective studies have examined relationships between life events and smoking in community samples. Lindenthal et al. (1972) surveyed a metropolitan probability sample of 938 adults in New Haven, Connecticut. Measures included a 20-item scale of psychological symptomatology and a 62-item checklist of events occurring during the previous year. A four-point index of current smoking frequency was marginally related to the psychological distress measure, with control for demographic characteristics. Among smokers, a high level of undesirable life events was related to increase in smoking (retrospectively reported), this effect occurring primarily among persons classified as "Very Impaired" on the psychological distress measure. Billings and Moos (1983*b*) obtained data from a representative community sample of 608 adults in the San Francisco area, including a 15-item checklist of negative life events experienced during the previous year. Comparisons of self-reported nonsmokers vs. light smokers vs. heavy smokers showed the latter group to be higher on psychological distress, negative life events, and work strain. Among smokers, measures of negative events, psychological distress, and low self-confidence showed small to moderate correlations with current amount of smoking. In both studies the data suggested that life stress was related to increased smoking through increases in psychological distress, but no path analyses were performed.

A concurrent study by Burr (1984) was based on a worksite sample of 505 Navy enlisted men deployed on ships in the Western Pacific. Measures of perceived stress were obtained through five-item scales covering the areas of job stress, organizational stress, and family stress, and a locus-of-control scale (Levenson, 1973) was also included. Multiple discriminant analysis comparing smokers vs. nonsmokers indicated that family strain and job-related role conflict showed independent effects for discriminating the smoker group. Smokers also scored lower on the internal subscale of the locus-of-control measure, but not on the other two subscales.

Tagliacozzo and Vaughn (1982) surveyed a worksite sample of 448 hospital staff nurses with a questionnaire including a 26-item measure of job stress with scales related to job overload, role ambiguity, and role conflict. For each item, respondents rated on a 1–5 scale how often they were bothered by the situation that the item described. (This presents some confounding of objective stress with reactivity to stress.) Analysis of these scales showed that smokers scored higher on overall stress. This effect was contributed by two subscales specific to job stress (emotional stress and dissatisfaction with rewards); scales concerned with role-related stress were not significant discriminators. An interaction between stress and marital status indicated the stress-smoking relationship to obtain primarily among single respondents.

Cohen and Williamson (1988) analyzed data obtained from a national probability sample of 2387 U.S. adults, interviewed by telephone. Predictor variables included a 14-item scale of subjective stress with a 1-month time frame (Cohen et al., 1983); a 16-item life events scale with a 1-year time frame; and a measure of job stress. Data were obtained on current smoking status and for a quantity/frequency index of alcoholic beverage consumption. Descriptive analyses indicated that subjective stress was related strongly to negative life events, and also to job responsibilities and perceptions of poor health. Perceived stress was higher for current smokers, compared with nonsmokers or exsmokers; however, there was no significant correlation between perceived stress and amount smoked in packs per day. (This may be an insensitive measure.)

For alcohol, among the sample of drinkers the number of drinks per day was positively related to perceived stress. There was a marginal inverse association between stress and number of days alcohol was consumed, suggesting that stress-related drinking occurred on a relatively small number of days. Usage of prescription drugs was also correlated with perceived stress; relationships were significant for both prescription and nonprescription drugs and for three major categories of licit drugs (depressant/ gastrointestinal/other). The analyses performed were all for zero-order relationships and did not include demographic controls.

The only repeated-measures study in the literature (Conway et al., 1981) was conducted with a sample of 34 U.S. Navy petty officers during an officer training program. Data were collected on 14 study days over a 9-month period. Measures of subjective stress and mood were collected on each study day, together with self-reports of number of cigarettes per day during the previous week. In addition to the subjective measures, the investigators used an *a priori* classification scheme to classify the observation days as high vs. low in stress. A repeated-measures ANOVA using the stress categorization showed greater amounts of smoking on high-stress days, compared with low-stress days. Within-subject correlational analyses using the subjective stress measures indicated that global ratings of daily stress and work load were both significantly correlated with amount of smoking; the mood rating of anger was also significantly correlated with smoking, but a rating of depression was not significant. Aggregated analyses suggested that stress–smoking relationships were contributed primarily by a few individuals with chronic tendency to perceive high stress; however, no personality measures were obtained in this study, so there is no way of discriminating more reactive individuals from others.

## Alcohol Use

Several cross-sectional studies of life stress and alcohol use have been based on community samples. Pearlin and Radabaugh (1976) analyzed data from a representative community sample of 2300 adults from metropolitan Chicago. Respondents (if not abstainers) were asked about their reasons for alcohol use based on eight potential categories, and a score for distress control was created based on endorsement of items indicating that alcohol "helps me forget my worries" or "cheers me up when in a bad mood" (from Cahalan et al., 1969). Measures were obtained of life strains from the areas of work, finances, marriage, and child rearing, and scales indexing anxiety and perceived control were also obtained. It was found that irrespective of life stress, persons who scored high on the functional measure showed significantly higher levels of heavy drinking during the previous month. In turn, the tendency to use alcohol for distress control was significantly related to current anxiety level. The relationship between anxiety and drinking was strongest among persons who were low on perceived control. In this sample, anxiety and lack of control were strongly related to life strains from low income and inadequate finances.

A series of reports on life events and drinking patterns (Neff and Husaini, 1982, 1985) was based on a representative sample of 713 rural residents in Tennessee. Life stress was indexed with a 50-item checklist of negative events with a 1-year time frame, and a measure of depressive symptomatology (CES-D) with a 1-week time frame was also obtained. Alcohol use was indexed with a quantity/frequency measure that was not time-referenced. Analyses showed a strong relationship between life events and drinking pattern, with heavy drinkers overrepresented among persons with a high level of negative events. Life events and depression were also related in the usual manner, but drinking pattern was not related to the depression measure. The authors performed *post hoc* interaction tests (life events–drinking pattern) and found that the relationship between life events and depression obtained primarily among abstainers, not among moderate or heavy drinkers. Interpretation of this analysis is qualified by small cell sizes for some of the categories, but was interpreted by the authors as indicating a stress-buffering effect of alcohol consumption.

A survey by Cooke and Allan (1984) was restricted to women in the midlife period (mean age = 51 years). A sample was drawn from electoral rolls in Glasgow, Scotland, and respondents were directly interviewed with a semistructured assessment of life events during the previous year and an assessment of alcohol consumption with a 1-week time frame. Subjects were classified as occasional drinkers if they were not abstainers but had not consumed alcohol during the previous week; subjects were classified as heavy drinkers if they were more than 1 SD above the mean alcohol consumption for the sample. Correlational analyses, apparently using total alcohol consumption (g absolute alcohol equivalent), showed correlations with life stress in the 0.20–0.30 range for regular and heavy drinkers. These analyses were reported by the authors as nonsignificant, but this is probably attributable to small sample size ($n$ = 28 and 29 for the above analyses) rather than lack of a relationship.

A cross-sectional study by Timmer et al. (1985) was based on household interviews conducted with a representative U.S. national sample ($n = 2264$). Measures of life stress from the economic, marital, and job domains were obtained, together with measures of social support, coping styles, and physical and psychological symptomatology. The index of alcohol use was a question asking whether the respondent drank alcoholic beverages to "help you handle things" when worried or nervous, i.e., alcohol use as a coping mechanism. Multivariate analyses showed that economic stress, feelings of vulnerability, marital stress, job stress, and poor physical health all showed significant relationships with alcohol use. Persons with low social support were more likely to use alcohol for coping, and persons who used prayer as a coping strategy were less likely to drink. Interaction effects indicated that alcohol use to cope was more likely among women with economic stress who were younger and unmarried; men with marital problems; women with marital problems who were older and felt more helpless; and younger women with job problems.

Several repeated-measures studies of alcohol use have been conducted. Conway et al. (1981), in the study previously described, analyzed correlations of daily stress with both smoking and alcohol use. In contrast to results on smoking, no significant relationships were observed for alcohol use. This was attributed by the authors to environmental constraints: The high-stress days were those on which participants were heavily involved in training activities and were unable to gain access to alcohol. Stone, Lennox, and Neale (1985) classified a self-selected sample of 79 community adults as light, moderate, or heavy drinkers on the basis of typical-consumption reports and then examined relationships of drinking status with measures of negative life events in the previous year and daily negative events aggregated over an observation period of approximately 84 days. In analyses of variance, no significant differences in previous life events or aggregated daily events were found across the drinking groups. Aggregated data on coping indicated that heavier drinkers tended to use less social support as a coping mechanism. Classification of open-ended responses indicated that when subjects listed alcohol use as a daily coping response, they viewed it as a means of achieving the coping goal of relaxation.

Rohsenow (1982) conducted a repeated-measures study of a sample of 36 college students who were classified as heavy drinkers. (It is not clear how this sample was obtained from the larger college population.) After baseline testing, subjects recorded mood reports and alcohol consumption on the evening of each day over a period of 4 months. Daily drinking data were not correlated with daily mood measures of anxiety, depression, or anger. Baseline measures of trait anxiety and depression were not related to total drinking behavior. Heavy drinking was related to higher levels of social support, and a baseline measure of social anxiety was inversely related to total drinking over the study period. These results appear to derive from a sample where drinking behavior was more socially based.

Two prospective studies have examined alcohol use in community samples over 1-year study periods. Aneshensel and Huba (1983) analyzed data from a probability sample of the Los Angeles metropolitan area (panel $n = 742$). Two direct interviews were conducted over a 1-year interval, obtaining measures of depression (CES-D) with a 1-week time frame and alcohol use (quantity/frequency) with a 2-month time frame. Between the two household interviews, telephone probes for depressive symptomatology were conducted at the 4- and 8-month points. While no significant concurrent relationships of depression and alcohol use were found, a moderate longitudinal effect of depression for increased alcohol use was found with a 4-month lag. Alcohol use at baseline was related to somewhat *decreased* levels of depression at the 4- and 8-month points, but was related to *increased* depression at the 1-year follow-up. These data suggest that alcohol use may have a depression-reduction effect in the short term, but not in the long term.

Cronkite and Moos (1984) obtained data from the San Francisco community sample at two points with a 1-year follow-up period (panel $n = 242$). Measures of depressive mood and physical symptomatology were obtained from scales with 7 and 11 items, respectively, and life events were indexed by a 15-item checklist with a 1-year time frame (assessed retrospectively at the second wave). Measures of social support and coping responses were also obtained at Time 2. Alcohol consumption was indexed as the ounces of alcohol consumed on a typical drinking day.

The data from this study were rather complex. Zero-order correlations indicated that alcohol use was concurrently related to negative life events, avoidance coping, lower family support, and spouse's alcohol consumption. There were some data suggesting that spouse's baseline alcohol use contributed to undesirable events between Time 1 and Time 2, i.e., reverse causation, but this analysis was not prospective. True prospective analyses (measures available at both waves) showed no evidence that Time 1 depression was related to increased alcohol use at follow-up, nor was there evidence that Time 1 alcohol use was related to depression at follow-up (contrary to Aneshensel and Huba). Mixed concurrent and prospective analyses showed that for husbands, *low* self-esteem of wives was related to increased alcohol use, whereas for wives, husband's depressed mood and *high* self-esteem related to increased alcohol use. Interaction tests indicated that for wives, relationships between avoidance coping and alcohol use were stronger when the husband was high on depressive or physical symptoms. The authors concluded that their measure of typical alcohol use was only weakly related to depressive or physical symptomatology and could be regarded as reflecting a normative behavioral response, influenced more by cultural factors than by ongoing life experiences. The stress measures used in this study were related to relapse (discussed in the next section), so there is reason to question the alcohol measures, but not the sample.

## Tranquilizers

Research on life stress and tranquilizer use may be less informative theoretically because these are not exclusively self-administered. (Tranquilizers are commonly prescribed by physicians for psychological distress.) Several well-designed epidemiological studies have obtained accurate data on prescription drug use among community samples. Mellinger et al. (1978) conducted direct household interviews with a national probability sample of 2552 adult respondents. Life stress was indexed with the Holmes and Rahe checklist, and psychological distress with the Hopkins Symptom Checklist, both with a 1-year time frame. Data on psychological distress replicated the usual findings from psychiatric epidemiology, with higher prevalence among persons who were younger, female, minority, of lower socioeconomic status, divorced/separated, and with no religious affiliation. Tranquilizer use was greater overall among women, alcohol use greater among men. Indices of drug use were related to psychological distress; use was associated with either anxiety or depression, but rates were highest among persons who scored high on both anxiety and depression. Zero-order associations suggested that tranquilizer use was more strongly related to psychological distress than to the life events measure; in contrast, heavy drinking was more strongly associated with the life events measure than with the psychological distress measure. The measures of distress used were global and did not differentiate physical illness problems from other types of life events. A related regional study conducted in Oakland, California (Uhlenhuth et al., 1978) found that physical illness in combination with psychological distress accounted for more drug use than did psychological distress alone. No path analyses of the data were performed in either case.

In the study by Timmer et al. (1985) previously described, use of "medicine or drugs" as a coping mechanism was also assessed. These data indicated that drug use was related to feelings of vulnerability, poor health, economic stress, and marital stress. Data on coping indicated that social support tended to be positively related to drug use (among men only), whereas coping through prayer was inversely related to drug use under high stress. In general, correlations between coping and drug use were found less frequently than for alcohol use.

A related study by Radelet (1981) was based on a random sample ($n$ = 166) and a clinic sample of tranquilizer users ($n$ = 15), both drawn from a college student health service. Respondents answered a variety of items about health perceptions and social network composition and responded to two items indexing prescription and usage of minor tranquilizers (e.g., Valium, Librium) during the previous 2 years. Discriminant analyses indicated that tranquilizer use was related to higher anxiety, lower symptom tolerance, and belief that other students were in poor health. Also, tranquilizer users were more likely to define anxiety as a physical rather than a social problem.

Cafferata et al. (1983) analyzed data from the National Medical Care Expenditure Survey, conducted with a national probability sample of 11,083 households. A scale of family stressors consisted of eight specific items. In this study, the drug use index was based on a question asking whether the respondent had obtained a psychotropic drug; actual usage was not determined, and apparently there was no time frame specified for the question. A strong sex difference was found, with women twice as likely as men to report drug use. Use was higher in households with unemployment and in nonintact households. Of the family stressors measured, three (death in family, spouse in poor health, and child in poor health) related to increased drug use; one (birth of child) was related to lower drug use; and one (hospitalization in family) was related to increased drug use for women but decreased drug use for men. In this study the measures of life stressors apparently are confounded with physical health problems, so interpretation of relationships is somewhat problematic.

Finally, a detailed study of Valium use (Caplan et al., 1984) was based on a sample of respondents obtained through pharmacies ($n$ = 367 users, $n$ = 308 nonusers). The focus of the study was on whether tranquilizer use had a consistent effect on well-being over time. Respondents in both panels were interviewed on four occasions at 6-week intervals; at each interview, respondents provided data on stress, subjective well-being, and other psychosocial variables during the previous 6-week period. Concurrent analyses generally replicated previous findings, showing tranquilizers used for reasons related to anxiety disorders, and showing correlations with indices of high stress and low life quality. Longitudinal analyses generally indicated no consistent main effects of tranquilizer use on subjective well-being, but there was some indication that drug use produced buffering of the effects of stressors on psychological distress, with Valium use reducing the impact of current stressors on anxiety and other indices of distress. In the area of role performance, however, drug use tended to have reverse effects; i.e., when drug use was high, stress was more strongly related to worse performance. The high stability of life stressors and health problems over time was shown to have a strong influence on the patterning of the zero-order relationships.

Data on subjects' motivations for tranquilizer use were somewhat confusing. Self-report data on physical health indicated a high level of health problems in the sample, with 92% of respondents reporting having some physical problem at baseline. The most common complaints were back or musculoskeletal problems, with hypertension next most frequent; only 14% of respondents mentioned tension/anxiety as their primary complaint. However, subjects' reports about their reasons for taking Valium showed that the most common decision rule was to take Valium when tense or anxious; taking it to fall asleep was second, and taking it to relax or keep calm was third. Reasons involving physical illness constituted the remaining reports, with sore muscles (6%) most frequently mentioned, followed by a variety of idiosyncratic reports. It was found that Valium users consumed less alcohol than nonusers. Whether this was due to compliance with medical admonitions (not to drink when taking tranquilizers), or to substitute mood-modifying effects, is not known.

## Summary

Studies of life stress and current substance use have been strong from the standpoint of sampling, and results are fairly consistent in showing relationships between stress measures and indices of substance use. However, almost all the available literature is cross-sectional and the studies provide little information about causal ordering. When multivariate data are available, path analyses typically have not been performed, so causal models remain untested. Laboratory studies of stress–smoking and stress–alcohol use effects help to alleviate this difficulty, however, and the consistency of results is striking. Some studies have shown that perceived stress is related concurrently to several types of substance use, including smoking, alcohol, and tranquilizers (Cohen and Williamson, 1988). Further, some studies have shown quite specific relationships between stressors and smoking, including instances in which the stress measure is unlikely to be a consequence of use (Burr, 1984; Tagliacozzo and Vaughn, 1982).

A noteworthy aspect in this literature are some clear differential relationships. First, there is a clear sex difference in alcohol vs. tranquilizer use, with males favoring alcohol and females favoring tranquilizers. Whether these correspond to sex differences in desired functional aspects of drug use is not known and should be investigated. Second, it is apparent that alcohol use as a coping mechanism is relevant only for a minority of the population (Pearlin and Radabaugh, 1976; Timmer et al., 1985), lending support to the need for research that concentrates on population subgroups for whom substance use is salient as a coping mechanism. The connection between substance use and indices of poor physical health (Caplan et al., 1984; Cohen and Williamson, 1988;

Mellinger et al., 1978) also is noteworthy and has not been emphasized in previous research.

The prospective studies in this area deserve special discussion. Employing a straightforward prospective design and a measure of recent alcohol use, Aneshensel and Huba (1983) found evidence for a lagged relationship between depression and alcohol use over a 4-month period, and these data are supplemented by concurrent studies using time-referenced measures for perceived stress (Cohen and Williamson, 1988), chronic life strain (Pearlin and Radabaugh, 1976), and negative life events (Cooke and Allan, 1984). Cronkite and Moos (1984), employing an index of typical (not time-referenced) alcohol use, observed no prospective relationships of depression to alcohol use, nor did Neff and Husaini (1982) find significant main effects in concurrent data. A plausible resolution of these divergent findings is that only time-referenced alcohol use measures are sensitive to current life stressors. Measures of "typical consumption" may, as Cronkite and Moos suggested, be more reflective of prevailing cultural patterns than of ongoing rates of substance use.

## 4. STRESS AND RELAPSE

A considerable body of research has indicated a link between life stressors and relapse among persons who had achieved cessation of smoking, alcoholism, or opiate use. The literature is consistent in showing negative affective states to be a major predictor of relapse. This research differs in some respects from studies previously discussed, because relapse typically occurs in a discrete episode, rather than as a slow or changeable process. Thus, research on relapse has focused on identifying particular situations associated with relapse and attempting to determine physical and emotional states that occur in these situations. Also, research on relapse has been based largely on treated samples, with few studies of success or failure in self-initiated quitting (cf. Curry and Marlatt, 1985; DiClemente and Prochaska, 1985).

In this area a major methodological issue derives from the retrospective nature of most of the studies. Since measures of relapse-provoking situations are typically obtained some time after the actual relapse, there is the possibility that subjects' reports are influenced by recall bias or self-enhancement processes (e.g., guilt, cognitive dissonance) that could color reports about relapse. This issue is best dealt with by prospective studies that assess psychological variables prior to the relapse episode. There is, in fact, considerable convergence of results from retrospective and prospective studies, strengthening confidence in the basic findings.

A more subtle issue concerns the salience and labeling of affective variables by subjects. When data on relapse situations are obtained from subjects' self-report, the resultant data are strongly dependent on the salience of different cues to the respondent. For example, if physical discomfort were labeled by subjects as psychological stress when there were environmental factors present, then the contribution of physiological factors to relapse might be underestimated (cf. Kozlowski and Wilkinson, 1987; Schachter and Singer, 1962). Similarly, if the operation of social influence processes were relatively nonsalient to subjects, then the role of environmental or physical factors might be overemphasized relative to the role of social factors. Currently there is controversy concerning the relative contributions of internally based physical cravings vs. externally based affective states as determinants of relapse (Shiffman et al., 1986). At present, stress-related factors are believed to play an important role in relapse.

## Cigarette Smoking

Two studies were based on clinic samples. Gunn (1983) surveyed a sample of 231 smokers attending an American Cancer Society smoking cessation program. Before program implementation, subjects completed a 14-item life events scale, scored through a median split as low vs. high stress. Smoking status was indexed at end of treatment by self-report, and all dropouts were considered treatment failures. Analyses indicated that high life stress was a predictor of noncessation and treatment dropout for men; for women, no significant relationships were found. Analysis of individual items suggested that social exits, legal problems, illness, and accidents were independent predictors of treatment failure.

An index of motive functions was obtained by Pomerleau et al. (1978), who followed a group of 100 consecutive admissions to a smoking cessation program. Smoking status was determined at end of treatment and follow-up through self-report, supplemented by urinary nicotine analysis for a subgroup. Data obtained through 1-year follow-up indicated that relapse was more likely among persons who described themselves as "negative affect smokers"; i.e., they smoked when frustrated, tense, or anxious. Although smoking type did not predict cessation at end of treatment, it was consistently related to relapse at each of the follow-up points.

Gordon and Cleary (1986) analyzed epidemiological data on self-quitting in a national probability sample of U.S. adults aged 20–64. Data were obtained in the National Survey of Health Practices, in which respondents were interviewed two times by telephone, with a 1-year follow-up interval (panel $n = 863$, based on persons who were current smokers at Time 1). Analyses of quitting attempts and outcome showed that women were more likely to make a quit attempt during the year, but less likely to be successful; hence overall quitting rates were 12% for both sexes. Measures of stress were based on single items, scored dichotomously; since the predictor variables were all single items, statistical reliability is relatively low. Prospective analyses showed that job stress predicted fewer quit attempts and lower success rates for men; for women there were no consistent prospective relationships. Concurrent analyses using data obtained at Time 2 replicated the prospective findings for men and showed concurrent "emotional problems" related to lower success rates for women. A measure of perceived control over health showed that men with low perceived control were less likely to make a quit attempt, but women with high control were less likely to quit. Results reported are all zero-order relationships; no multivariate analyses were performed.

Several papers have reported findings on stress and smoking cessation using data from the MRFIT program. Ockene et al. (1982) followed a group of 169 smokers, all males aged 35–57 who participated in a broad-spectrum smoking cessation intervention. Subjects were assessed at baseline and followed at 4-month intervals after end of treatment, with smoking status assessed through self-report and serum thiocyanate. Life stress was measured with a major events inventory, and measures of self-esteem and perceived control were also obtained. Based on data obtained through 2-year follow-up, multiple discriminant analysis yielded two significant functions. The first function discriminated long-term successful quitters from continuing smokers and relapsers. This function was loaded by low stress, high expectation of success, and high personal security (essentially a measure of psychological adjustment). On this function successful quitters were high, relapsers intermediate, and continuing smokers low. The second function, which discriminated relapsers from the other two groups, was loaded by low personal security and low change during treatment. On this function relapsers were high, continuing smokers and quitters intermediate. Thus, in this study the stress measure primarily predicted long-term success, not relapse (cf. Benfari et al., 1982).

Cummings et al. (1985) followed a sample of 107 smokers attending a hospital-based smoking cessation clinic. Information on relapse episodes was obtained at end of treatment and at 1-month and 1-year follow-up, through telephone interviews. Data on mood at time of relapse were obtained with an eight-item adjective checklist, used to classify the situation as positive vs. negative affect. The majority (83%) of relapses occurred when the subject was experiencing negative affect, and 52% of subjects attributed their relapse to a specific emotional crisis situation, usually family- or work-related. Of the relapses not associated with a crisis situation, the reasons for relapse were predominantly presence of smoking/alcohol/food cues, withdrawal symptoms, and boredom. Analysis of reasons for relapse by time since cessation showed that relapses occurring within 1 week were more often attributed to withdrawal symptoms, whereas relapses occurring later were attributed more frequently to emotional crisis situations. However, emotional crisis variables represented a substantial proportion of relapses at all stages.

Prospective studies investigating perceived stress as a predictor of smoking cessation/relapse have been conducted by Cohen and colleagues (Cohen et al., 1983; Mermelstein et al., 1986). The first report was based on a sample of 64 participants in a university-based smoking cessation program. During a pretreatment assessment, subjects completed the Perceived Stress Scale (PSS) and a 71-item checklist of negative events with a 6-month time frame. The PSS was repeated at end of treatment and at 1- and 3-month follow-ups. Smoking status was assessed through self-report with carbon monoxide verification. Neither life events nor perceived stress was related to status at end of treatment. However, perceived stress was related to higher smoking rates at the 1- and 3-month follow-up points.

The second report included data from 1-year follow-up. Results indicated a patterning of stress measures in which never-quitters were higher than relapsers, who were higher than successful long-term quitters. Stress measures obtained after treatment indicated that relapsers reported more stress at follow-up points, compared with abstainers. Also, subjects who successfully quit after a lapse scored lower on perceived stress, and life events measured from end of treatment to the 6-month point predicted increased smoking at the 1-year point. Data from interviews with subjects who had relapsed indicated that the majority of stress-related relapses occurred after the 1-month follow-up, whereas early relapses were more related to other causes (e.g., smoking cues, habit).

Replication of these data was reported by Glasgow et al. (1985) in a study of 134 participants in a community-wide stop-smoking contest. Prospective analyses based on data obtained before quit date and at 1-month follow-up indicated that perceived stress was the only variable that significantly predicted success at self-quitting. Coping measures, reported retrospectively at the follow-up, indicated that one behavioral coping strategy (self-reward) and one cognitive coping strategy (positive self-statements) were significant discriminators of successful quitters. Strategies of stimulus control and reliance on "willpower" were inversely related to success.

Shiffman (1982, 1984*a,b*, 1985) obtained data at the time of relapse from 264 exsmokers who called a telephone hotline for relapse prevention. Interviews lasting 20–30 min were recorded and subsequently coded on a number of variables. The majority of the calls occurred on the same day as the relapse crisis and took place a mean of 36 days after quitting. Results indicated that approximately 70% of relapse crises occurred in the presence of negative affect, with anxiety being most common, and frustration and depression also represented. Subjects were asked about whether they were experiencing withdrawal symptoms (craving excluded). The majority of subjects (54%) reported no withdrawal symptoms. Of the remainder, symptoms labeled as physical (headache, nausea), psychological (irritability, anxiety), arousal (drowsiness, sleep disturbances), and appetite increase were about equally represented. Shiffman classified reports of coping in the crisis situation into several types of behavioral coping (e.g., distracting activity, relaxation) and cognitive coping (e.g., think of consequences, intent to delay). Results indicated that almost every one of the coping responses was effective, and no significant difference was found between cognitive and behavioral coping. However, subjects who employed both cognitive and behavioral coping were less likely to relapse than those who used only one coping mechanism.

An almost exact replication of Shiffman's findings was obtained in a study by Curry and Marlatt (1985) in which a sample of 118 self-quitters was followed from the time of their quit attempt. Basic descriptive information was obtained at a baseline assessment. Subjects were interviewed subsequently by telephone at 1 month and 4 months after the quit date to determine whether they had experienced a relapse temptation and, if so, what the outcome had been. The interviews included probes to elicit data about cognitive and behavioral coping responses employed in the high-risk situations. The characteristics of high-risk situations were consistent with findings from Shiffman (1982) and Marlatt and Gordon (1980), with intrapersonal negative affect and interpersonal conflict comprising the majority of relapse episodes. Results on coping indicated that either cognitive or behavioral coping reduced the probability of relapse, compared with no coping; the combination of cognitive and behavioral coping was superior to either type of coping employed alone. As in the Shiffman (1984*a,b*) study, it was found that among subjects who made no coping response, virtually every one relapsed.

The only laboratory study in this area (Abrams et al., 1987) compared stress reactivity and coping responses of 22 recent relapsers and a matched sample of successful recent quitters with a mean abstinence of 22 months. Coping skills and reactivity, indexed by heart rate and self-report, were measured with situational assessments for general social competence, high-demand social anxiety, and two types of relapse temptations (intrapersonal and interpersonal negative affect). In four of the five assessments, relapsers were more reactive than quitters; only in high-demand social anxiety were there no differences. Coping data indicated that relapsers scored lower than quitters in smoking-specific situations, but not in situations related to general social competence. Differences between the groups during a relaxation period suggested that successful quitters had better relaxation skills than the relapsers, consistent with data from Shiffman (1984*a,b*) and Wills (1986). Correlational analyses indicated that reactivity and coping skills tended to be inversely correlated; also, self-report anxiety was related to stronger urges to smoke. This study provides the only evidence that individual differences in reactivity to stress are related to relapse.

## Alcohol Relapse

In this area there is a mixture of retrospective and prospective studies. Rosenberg (1983) obtained retrospective data from a sample of patients in a Veterans Administration alcohol treatment program ($n$ = 25 relapsers, $n$ = 25 nonrelapsers). Psychosocial measures indicated that the relapsers experienced more negative life events during the previous year, whereas the nonrelapsers experienced more positive events. Indices of social support showed that the relapsers had lower levels of family/friend support, emotional support, and perceived support from their overall network. Measures of coping skills using the Situational Competence Test (Chaney et al., 1978) indicated that the relapsers scored lower on two types of coping, noncompliance and saying they would not drink in a problem situation; but they did not differ on latency, duration, or specificity of responses.

Data on relapse precipitants and coping were obtained by Litman and colleagues (Litman et al., 1979, 1983, 1984) in studies of alcoholics in treatment. Initially a retrospective study suggested that recent relapsers showed a greater number of relapse precipitants and lower levels of cognitive coping. Litman et al. (1983) then obtained prospective data for 256 consecutive admissions to inpatient treatment, initially surveyed while in hospital and followed up 6–12 months later. At follow-up, subjects were classified as abstainers ($n$ = 77) vs. light/moderate drinkers ($n$ = 27) vs. heavy drinkers ($n$ = 89). Follow-up data indicated that relapsers scored higher on number of "dangerous situations" encountered. Of three dimensions of relapse precipitants, Unpleasant Mood States was the strongest discriminator and External Situations was also significant. This analysis did not relate relapse to specific dangerous situations, but showed that relapsers had experienced more such situations.

Litman et al. (1984) subsequently reported data on the relationship between coping behaviors and relapse. Shortly after hospital admission, subjects completed a 36-item inventory to indicate what they did at times when they wanted to start drinking (coping behavior) and how effective each response was perceived to be (coping effectiveness). Factor analysis indicated four dimensions of coping, termed Positive Thinking, Negative Thinking, Distraction/Avoidance, and Seeking Social Support. Prospective analyses indicated that the baseline measures of coping behavior did not discriminate the subsequent relapsers vs. survivors, but the measures of coping effectiveness for Positive Thinking and Distraction were significant discriminators. Ambiguities in these data are that the amount of coping may be correlated with the severity of temptation (in relapse crises occurring before hospital admission). The questions on perceived coping effectiveness may be indexing general self-efficacy, but these were highly correlated with the behavioral measures, so they are not a completely independent dimension of measurement.

Moos and colleagues have investigated stress and coping behavior as predictors of relapse in a sample of 124 treated alcoholics followed up approximately 18 months after discharge (Billings and Moos, 1983*a;* Cronkite and Moos, 1980; Finney and Moos, 1981; Finney et al., 1980; Moos et al., 1981). Data were obtained from a comprehensive inventory administered at the follow-up measurement (so these reports are concurrent or retrospective). The stress measure included 13 negative events with a 1-year time frame, and the coping inventory assessed the use of 29 possible responses to a single recent problem, i.e., general stress-coping responses. Analyses that controlled for initial symptom levels indicated that posttreatment stress and coping were related to relapse; persons who relapsed had experienced more negative events and scored lower on a global index of coping. Work stress and family stress situations were independently related to relapse. Recovered alcoholics scored higher on active–cognitive coping and behavioral coping, whereas relapsers used more avoidance and aggressive coping (taking out emotions on other people). A supportive family environment was related concurrently to lower levels of life stress and more productive coping patterns, but did not have either a direct effect or an indirect effect on outcome.

A retrospective study by Marlatt and Gordon (1980) is the only one to obtain comparable data on relapse for different types of substance use. Detailed accounts of relapse episodes were obtained from samples of persons who had relapsed after alcohol treatment ($n$ = 70), smoking cessation ($n$ = 35), and heroin treatment ($n$ = 32). Because all subjects were interviewed within 90 days posttreatment, these would be classified as early to intermediate-stage relapses. Classification of the relapse situations by a hierarchical system, with only one code allowed per subject, indicated that the characteristics of relapse episodes were similar across the three substance use groups. The majority of episodes were characterized as involving negative emotional states, either intrapersonal (37% of all relapses) or from interpersonal conflict (15% of all relapses). The remaining categories were social pressure (24%), positive emotional states (9%), and urges and temptations (7%). Negative physical states, i.e., withdrawal symptoms, were identified in only a small proportion of episodes (4%). There were some differences in characteristics of relapse episodes for particular substances, but the pattern of results was comparable for each; negative emotional states accounted for the majority of relapses for smoking, alcohol, and opiates.

The personality variable of self-consciousness was investigated by Hull et al. (1986) with a sample of 35 alcoholic subjects surveyed before discharge from a treatment unit and followed up at 3 and 6 months. A measure of life events with a 1-year time frame was obtained before discharge, and events were classified as either self-relevant (primarily individual failure) or other (primarily habit changes, personal health, and events occurring to others). Analyses indicated that the rated impact of self-relevant life events was related to relapse, but primarily among subjects high on self-consciousness. No other personality data were obtained in this study.

## Opiate Relapse

Several studies have examined the predictors of relapse among addicts who have been treated for opiate dependence, either in methadone maintenance programs or in drug-free therapeutic communities. Krueger (1981) conducted a retrospective study of life events and return to heroin use among a sample of 48 clients in methadone maintenance. Among persons who relapsed, scores on the Social Readjustment Rating Scale (SRRS) were significantly higher both in comparison to a control group of patients and compared to their own previous scores during a period of heroin-free stabilization. Events such as social exits, depression, or exacerbation of intense affect were all found to be associated with the return to heroin use.

A longitudinal study was conducted by Rhoads (1983) with a sample of 49 clients recently discharged from heroin detoxification programs. Direct interviews were conducted 1, 2, and 3 months postdischarge. The criterion variable in this study was a composite score based on quantity/frequency of use of 11 commonly abused drugs. Results indicated that for females, negative life events during the past month measured by the Life Events Schedule (LES) led both to increased depression and to increases in drug use over 1-month time lags. An interactive relationship with social support was noted, with drug use disproportionately elevated among clients having a high level of negative events and a low level of emotional support (cf. Cohen and Wills, 1985). A similar patterning of variables was noted among males, but life stress and low social support did not appear to lead to drug use. In these analyses, some evidence was found that drug and alcohol use led to an increased number of negative events over 1-month lags. Having close friends who were heroin users also led to increases in drug use over time. In this study there was still some retrospective element because events and drug use were both measured over a 1-month period, so precise temporal relationships between events and drug use are uncertain.

Kosten et al. (1983) used a longitudinal design over a 6-month period in a sample of 123 patients in a multimodal opiate treatment program. Negative life events, measured retrospectively at the follow-up measurement, were related both to depression and to greater illicit drug use during the follow-up period. Drug use, poor occupational functioning, and psychological symptoms were most strongly related to interpersonal conflict, but social exits were also significantly related both to drug use and to depressive symptomatology. The authors suggested that drug use may serve as form of self-medication for coping with the depressive affect caused by interpersonal conflict or loss of a support system, but the retrospective design places some qualification on interpretation of the temporal ordering of the variables.

Chaney and Roszell (1985) conducted a prospective study with a sample of 50 patients enrolled in a multimodal treatment program. Measures were based on a previous study with a sample of relapsers who indicated the characteristics of situations in which they relapsed. Multidimensional scaling indicated that these comprised one general domain of negative-affect events (depression, pain, insomnia) and one domain of positive-affect/social pressure events (think about chipping, friends using). Withdrawal symptoms represented an isolated, minor category not included in the above. The researchers developed a situational competency test, an analog measure of coping with eight relapse temptation situations (based on Chaney et al., 1978), and administered this test to clients shortly after intake. Subjects' predicted coping responses did not relate to illicit drug use during the program, as indicated by periodic urinalyses, but their perceived efficacy for terminating a relapse crisis was in the predicted direction: Clients with lowest drug use had the highest efficacy expectations.

In a 22-month follow-up, Chaney examined the predictors of two relapse episodes as defined through urinalysis data: one that followed the longest interval of abstinence from illicit drug use, and one that occurred after the longest time in treatment. Subjects' reports indicated that in 78% of the episodes they perceived the drug use as an attempt to cope with a problematic situation, and in 91% of the episodes they had contemplated drug use well in advance of the actual relapse situation. The affect-related relapses were reported as related to negative emotional states, physical discomfort (pain), and interpersonal conflict. In only a minority of episodes (38%) was coping of any kind attempted, and virtually all of these attempts were unsuccessful. The low use of coping in this population was suggested by the authors as deriving from the generally low efficacy expectations of the clients. In absolute terms, subjects' efficacy was rather low, with the majority of clients at baseline expecting that they would eventually relapse.

## Summary

Consistent with evidence previously discussed on initiation and maintenance of substance use, studies of relapse have shown that stress factors are of considerable importance for relapse episodes. Negative life events, perceived stress, and stress-related patterns of substance use have all been shown to be predisposing factors for relapse to substance use. In discussing this relationship it is important to distinguish between factors that predict treatment outcome and factors that predict posttreatment success. Typically, stress factors measured pretreatment do not predict treatment outcome (i.e., cessation), but they do relate strongly to maintenance of cessation. There are some exceptions to this pattern, mainly for self-quitting, where it appears that life stress may affect either the number or success of quitting attempts (Glasgow et al., 1985; Gordon and Cleary, 1986).

There is also evidence that predictors of relapse are temporally linked. Relapses that occur shortly after cessation seem to be attributable more to physical withdrawal symptoms, whereas relapses occurring at later stages (1 month or more postcessation) seem predominantly linked to emotional distress. There remains some ambiguity in knowing the extent to which persons may be labeling withdrawal symptoms as deriving from environmental stress, or the converse (labeling emotional distress as withdrawal symptoms). Taking subjects' reports at face value, however, does provide a model of the cessation process that is consistent with physiological theory, since withdrawal symptoms for smoking, for example, usually subside within 2 weeks after cessation (Shiffman, 1979).

In addressing the question of whether increased life stress may be primarily a consequence of relapse, the evidence suggests a qualified "no." Several studies based on direct interviews have elicited reports from subjects indicating that emotional distress preceded the relapse episode and was, in fact, perceived by respondents as a causative factor in provoking the relapse (Chaney et al., 1985; Curry and Marlatt, 1985; Shiffman, 1982, 1984*a,b*). Studies with repeated measures of the subject panel do suggest that a full relapse episode may create prolonged stress because it exacerbates tension in interpersonal relationships and probably creates more psychological distress for the relapser through feelings of failure and low efficacy. However, the evidence from direct interviews and prospective studies of subjective stress seems to clearly indicate a causal relationship. Unfortunately, there is no direct statistical evidence in the literature, namely, a multivariate model showing that negative environmental events increase anxiety/depression, which is the proximal factor for increasing risk of relapse. Such analyses would provide more detailed understanding of the causation of relapse episodes.

The role of coping responses is more clear in this area, and it is evident that either behavioral or cognitive coping responses, employed during a relapse crisis, markedly influence the probability of successful maintenance. The literature is less clear on whether coping assessments can prospectively predict successful maintenance. The studies by Moos and colleagues (see Billings and Moos, 1983) did find evidence that general stress-coping responses were related to relapse among alcoholic subjects, but these data are not truly prospective. The few prospective studies using analog coping assessments (Chaney and Rozell, 1985; Litman et al., 1984) have not found significant relationships for subjects' predictions of their relapse-specific coping responses, but this may be a reflection of the validity of analog procedures (for discussion see Biglan et al., 1985). Abrams et al. (1987) did find that reactivity and coping responses differentiated quitters from recent relapsers.

Another replicated finding is that subjects' perceived efficacy for terminating a relapse crisis (Chaney and Rozell, 1985) or the perceived effectiveness of coping strategies (Litman et al., 1984) has significant predictive value. There is still much confounding in these data, analytically because specific coping measures are sometimes entered in the same analysis with measures of coping effectiveness, or conceptually because efficacy measures may simply be indexing current substance use status (Baer et al., 1986). Considering the paucity of data on coping and efficacy in the literature, this is a priority for further investigation of coping and relapse.

## 5. GENERAL DISCUSSION

Two major points have been discussed in the preceding sections. First, empirical relationships between stress and substance use are observed consistently across the major phases of substance use. Measures of life stressors and subjective stress predict initiation of smoking, alcohol, and illicit drug use during the adolescent period; measures of life strains are correlated with rates of substance use among regular users (although results are more variable in this area); and negative affect is found to figure prominently in the process of relapse to smoking, alcohol, and opiate use. This evidence indicates that stress-related factors have considerable generality for research on substance use and abuse. For some types of research it is possible to suggest that the perceived stress-related aspects of drug use are accounted for by alleviation of withdrawal symptoms (e.g., Schachter et al., 1977). Given the generality of stress–substance use relationships across different phases, however, these models lose some explanatory force. The present evidence suggests that the relationship between stress and substance use is not attributable simply to withdrawal effects.

The second issue is the temporal ordering of stress–substance use relationships. From the available evidence it can reasonably be concluded that high stress is temporally antecedent to the substance use phenomena observed (initiation, ongoing use, relapse) and is not primarily a consequence of substance use. This is not to say that substance use behavior may not create problems for the user, either with significant others or with the larger society; but the crucial theoretical point is whether life stress can plausibly be advanced as a causative factor in substance use. Subject to some theoretical issues discussed following, the convergence of results from concurrent and prospective studies provides, I think, evidence of a causative role.

One issue not well resolved is the extent to which stress factors are a common process in different types of substance use. Evidence on this issue is limited because studies typically have taken a piecemeal approach, focusing on one type of drug use (e.g., alcohol) while not considering other types of drug use that are concurrently pursued (e.g., smoking). Epidemiological studies do show that there is a high degree of correlation among different types of drug use (e.g., Istvan and Matarazzo, 1984; Kandel, 1978), so research that focuses on one type of use may miss confounding factors associated with other types of use. Whether multiple use is attributable more to physiological factors, affective factors, or normative factors is not well understood at present.

In the present case, by summarizing across the results of different studies, it could be said that relationships with stress have been observed for three major drugs of abuse. Correlations are most consistent for smoking and tranquilizer use. Evidence for opiates is minimal, but studies of opiate relapse are consistent in showing life stress as a provoking factor. Evidence for alcohol is more erratic, particularly in studies of ongoing alcohol use, where a number of null results have been reported (although these may be attributable to methodological factors). Finally, a few studies comparing predictors of alcohol use and another drug have found commonality in stress–substance use relationships, both for adolescents and for adults.

Although there has been ample research showing increased substance use under stress, virtually no research is designed to study the effect of substance use on stress among respondents surveyed in their natural environment. Of all the studies discussed, only *one* (Caplan et al., 1984) was specifically designed to determine whether substance use (in this case, Valium) had an effect on subjective well-being. The consequences of smoking, alcohol, or other drug use on subjective well-being may be very different over short-, intermediate-, or long-term periods, but there is virtually no theory or research to suggest how these effects might vary over time (cf. Abrams, 1983; Alexander and Hadaway, 1982; Hull and Bond, 1986; U.S.D.H.H.S., 1988).

## External Stressors vs. Underlying Psychopathology

There have been few direct tests of theoretical models of affective factors in substance use. In the following I discuss two general issues for further research and suggest methodological approaches to these issues.

In field research on life stress, a troublesome issue lies in determining the causation of negative life events. To the extent that individuals' levels of negative events or subjective stress are quite stable over time, and the events in question could be caused by the individual, then it is not clear whether observed results are primarily attributable to externally caused stress or to underlying psychopathology of the individual. The latter argument (Depue and Monroe, 1986) suggests that the kinds of negative events measured in typical life events inventories (e.g., unemployment, divorce, interpersonal conflict) may be self-caused by the individual and hence may represent consequences of underlying psychopathology, such as depressive disorder or personality disorder. Measures of subjective stress do not necessarily eliminate this concern because level of subjective stress is highly correlated with level of negative life events both among adults (Cohen and Williamson, 1988) and among adolescents (Wills, 1986).

This issue breaks down into two separate questions. First is the question of whether negative life events are self-caused. In principle, this could be tested by *a priori* classification of events as those which could be self-caused (e.g., unemployment) versus those which are unlikely to be self-caused by the respondent (e.g., illness of a family member). Alternatively, causation of events could be indexed directly through self-reports by the respondent, through independent reports provided by significant others, or through clinical judgment of trained raters, based on detailed protocols of the circumstances surrounding each life event. None of these methods is infallible. For example, unemployment could be due to large-scale economic changes rather than to poor job performance by the individual, and self-reports of event causation could be colored by the self-enhancing biases that have been found prevalent in many areas of social psychology. At least, investigators can attempt to obtain some data on event causation and test whether the effects of life stress are primarily attributable to self-caused or externally caused events.

A strict test of the above question would only indicate whether substance use is more closely linked to chronic emotional distress or to current distress that is linked to negative environmental events. The following question is whether substance use is causally related to negative affect at all, but may actually be caused by a third variable that happens to be correlated with both life events and distress. The main version of the third-variable argument, derived from problem-behavior theory (Jessor and Jessor, 1977), is that smoking, drinking, and other forms of substance use are causally related to identification with a deviant life style in which substance use is considered normative. The causal role in this model is attributed to affiliation with deviant (hence drug-using) peers and to social pressure from these peers to conform with group norms. In this sociological model, affective variables are presumed to be an epiphenomenon that may be correlated with other problem-behavior variables (e.g., alienated attitudes, poor relationships with parents or school) but have no direct causal role in drug use. Because of the continuity of drug use and antisocial behavior over time among groups of adolescent drug abusers (e.g., Kandel, 1986), this issue is relevant for substance use in adulthood, as well as in adolescence.

Testing these alternative models would, in principle, require longitudinal studies that obtained data over time on objective/subjective stress measures and on indices of deviant attitudes, behavior, and social affiliations. Such research would indicate whether high levels of substance use over a specific age range (e.g., 12–18 years or 20–28 years) are primarily attributable to direct effects of stress factors or to indirect effects that are mediated through alienated attitudes and delinquent peer-group affiliations.

## Affect Regulation vs. Self-Control Ability

Assuming that the relationship between stress and substance use is not spurious, it is possible to propose two models of stress effects that involve, respectively, affective vs. nonaffective factors.

Affect Regulation Effect. This model assumes that there are coping functions provided by tobacco, alcohol, or opiate use that provide an actual stress-reduction effect and, hence, motivate increased use under stressful conditions. The operative physiological mechanism may vary somewhat across different drugs, but there is some evidence that nicotine can reduce anxiety and provide antinociceptive effects (U.S. Surgeon General, 1988), that alcohol can reduce responses to sympathetic nervous system (SNS) arousal and increase positive affect under appropriate conditions (Hull and Bond, 1986; Marlatt, 1976), and that opiates have both analgesic and positive mood effects (Stewart, De Wit, and Eikelboom, 1984; Grunberg and Baum, 1985). The involvement of catecholamine mechanisms and endogeneous opioid systems has been suggested as a common physiological basis for stress-related substance use (Grunberg and Baum, 1985; Pomerleau and Pomerleau, 1984). Physiological effects of substances on cognitive systems, such as to distract attention from stressors or interfere with self-related information processing, have also been suggested as a stress-coping mechanism (Hull and Van Treuven, 1986). The possibility that substance use may both reduce negative affect and increase positive affect, combined with some biphasic effects on SNS arousal, has been proposed as a factor in the coping functions of tobacco and alcohol use (Wills and Shiffman, 1985). This model would have considerable generality: Adolescents under stress may initiate substance use in order to obtain perceived affect-regulation functions; regular users may show increased use under stress as part of their attempts to cope with the stressors; and for persons who have ceased regular use, the remembered coping functions of prior use may be an important factor for relapse temptations when levels of emotional distress are high.

Self-Control Effects. It is known that stress has both immediate effects and aftereffects on task performance (e.g., Cohen, 1980). It is possible that a similar mechanism produces decrements in self-control ability under stress because of increased cognitive load and interference of emotional distress with efficacy systems that are relevant for self-control and resistance to temptation (cf. Carver and Scheier, 1983; Marlatt and Gordon, 1980). This model assumes that substance use is perceived to have a mixture of desirable and undesirable properties and that under ordinary circumstances, persons are able to exert sufficient self-control to avoid use (or high level of use) of the substance. A breakdown in self-control ability, however, would increase the salience of positive aspects of substance use and decrease resistance to negative aspects. Life stressors may exert an influence on self-control because of a generalized lowering of perceived personal efficacy (Curry and Marlatt, 1985) or because of decrements in specific regulatory systems necessary for effective self-control. This kind of model would suggest that adolescents under stress are more likely to adopt substance use because their ability to cope with social pressure or other influences for drug use is reduced; that regular users would be less restrained in their use when stress level was high; and that exsmokers or exdrinkers relapse under stress because their perceived ability to regulate their own emotions is reduced.

How might these alternative models be tested? In the laboratory, studies could pursue controlled investigations of how stressors affect aspects of the self-control process and how affective states may provoke urges or temptations for substance use. In field studies, studies could investigate how measures of efficacy and self-control vary with life stress and whether measures of self-control show significant unique contributions in accounting for substance use onset or relapse. Comparative studies, then, would attempt to measure consequences of stress on affective systems (anxiety, depression, subjective stress) and self-regulatory systems (perceived efficacy, social competence, risk-taking tendency) and test the unique contributions of each system as predictors of substance use outcomes.

ACKNOWLEDGMENTS

This work derives from a collaborative effort carried on over the past several years with Sheldon Cohen, Neil Grunberg, and Saul Shiffman. David Abrams, Allan Goldstein, and Arthur Stone have also contributed to this work at various points. Any errors, omissions, or distortions are the responsibility of the author.

## REFERENCES

Abrams, D. B., 1983, Psychosocial assessment of alcohol and stress interactions, in: *Stress and Alcohol Use* (L. A. Pohorecky and J. Brick, eds.), Elsevier, New York.

Abrams, D. B., Monti, P. M., Pinto, R. P., Elder, J. P., Brown, R. A., and Jacobus, S. I., 1987, Psychosocial stress and coping in smokers who relapse or quit, *Health Psychol.* **6**:289–303.

Alanko, T., 1984, An overview of techniques and problems in the measurement of alcohol consumption, in: *Research Advances in Alcohol and Drug Problems,* Volume 8 (R. G. Smart et al., eds.), Plenum Press, New York.

Alexander, B. K., and Hadaway, P. F., 1982, Opiate addiction: The case for an adaptive orientation, *Psychol. Bull.* **92**:367–381.

Aneshensel, C. S., and Huba, G. J., 1983, Depression, alcohol use, and smoking over one year: A four-wave longitudinal model, *J. Abnormal Psychol.* **92**:134–150.

Baer, P. E., Garmezy, L. B., McLaughlin, R. J., Pokorny, A. D., and Wernick, M. J., 1987, Stress, coping, family conflict, and adolescent alcohol use, *J. Behav. Med.* **10**:449–466.

Baer, J. S., Holt, C. S., and Lichtenstein, E., 1986, Self-efficacy and smoking reexamined, *J. Consult. Clin. Psychol.* **54**:846–852.

Baum, A., Grunberg, N. E., and Singer, J. E., 1982, Psychological and neuroendocrinological measurements in the study of stress, *Health Psychol.* **1**:217–236.

Bauman, K. E., and Koch, G. C., 1983, Validity of self-reports and descriptive and analytical conclusions: The case of cigarette smoking by adolescents and their mothers, *Am. J. Epidemiol.* **118**:90–98.

Benfari, R. C., Eaker, E. D., Ockene, J., and McIntyre, K. M., 1982, Hyperstress and outcomes in a long-term smoking intervention program, *Psychosom. Med.* **44**:227–235.

Biglan, A., and Lichtenstein, E., 1984, A behavior-analytic approach to smoking acquisition, *J. Appl. Soc. Psychol.* **14**:207–223.

Biglan, A., Weissman, W., and Severson, H., 1985, Coping with social influences to smoke, in: *Coping and Substance Use* (S. Shiffman and T. A. Wills, eds.), Academic Press, New York.

Billings, A. G., and Moos, R. H., 1983*a*, Psychosocial processes of recovery among alcoholics and their families, *Addict. Behav.* **8**:205–218.

Billings, A. G., and Moos, R. H., 1983*b*, Social-environmental factors among light and heavy cigarette smokers: A controlled comparison with nonsmokers, *Addict. Behav.* **8**:381–391.

Brown, S. A., Goldman, M. S., Inn, A., and Anderson, L. R., 1980, Expectations of reinforcement from alcohol: Their domain and relation to drinking patterns, *J. Consult. Clin. Psychol.* **48**:419–426.

Bruns, C., and Geist, C. S., 1984, Stressful life events and drug use among adolescents, *J. Hum. Stress,* **10**:135–139.

Burr, R. G., 1984, Smoking among U.S. Navy enlisted men, *Psychol. Rep.* **54**:287–294.

Cafferata, G. L., Kasper, J., and Bernstein, A., 1983, Family roles and stressors in relation to sex differences in obtaining psychotropic drugs, *J. Health Soc. Behav.* **24**:132–143.

Cahalan, D., Cisin, I. H., and Crossley, H. M., 1969, *American Drinking Practices: A National Study of Drinking Behavior and Attitudes,* Rutgers University Center of Alcohol Studies, New Brunswick, NJ.

Caplan, R. D., Abbey, A., Abramis, D. J., Andrews, F. M., Conway, T. L., and French, J. R. P., Jr., 1984, *Tranquilizer Use and Well-Being: A Longitudinal Study of Social and Psychological Effects,* Institute for Social Research, Ann Arbor, MI.

Cappell, H., and Herman, C. P., 1972, Alcohol and tension reduction: A review, *Q. J. Stud. Alcohol* **33**:33–64.

Carver, C. S., and Scheier, M. F., 1983, A control-theory approach to human behavior, and implications for problems in self-management, in: *Advances in Cognitive-behavioral Research and Theory,* Volume 2 (P. Kendall, ed.), Academic Press, New York.

Castro, F. G., Maddahian, E., Newcomb, M. D., and Bentler, P. M., 1987, A multivariate model of the determinants of cigarette smoking among adolescents, *J. Health Soc. Behav.* **28**:273–289.

Chaney, E. F., and Roszell, D. K., 1985, Coping in opiate addicts maintained on methadone, in: *Coping and Substance Use* (S. Shiffman and T. A. Wills, eds.), Academic Press, New York.

Chaney, E. F., O'Leary, M. R., and Marlatt, G. A., 1978, Skill training with alcoholics, *J. Consult. Clin. Psychol.* **46**:1092–1104.

Chassin, L., Presson, C., Bensenberg, M., Corty, E., Olshavsky, R., and Sherman, S. L., 1981, Predicting adolescents' intentions to smoke cigarettes, *J. Health Soc. Behav.* **22**:445–455.

Chassin, L. A., Presson, C. C., and Sherman, S. J., 1985, An acquisition-oriented approach to primary prevention, *J. Consult. Clin. Psychol.* **53**:612–622.

Chassin, L., Mann, L. M., and Sher, K. J., 1988, Self-awareness theory, family history of alcoholism, and adolescent alcohol involvement, *J. Abnormal Psychol.* **97**:206–217.

Christiansen, B. A., Goldman, M. S., and Inn, A., 1982, Development of alcohol-related expectancies in adolescents, *J. Consult. Clin. Psychol.* **50**:336–344.

Cleary, P. D., Hitchcock, J., Semmer, N., Flinchabaugh, L. J., and Pinney, J. M. 1988, Adolescent smoking: Research and health policy, *The Milbank Quarterly,* **66**:137–171.

Cohen, S., 1980, Aftereffects of stress on human performance and social behavior: A review of research and theory, *Psychol. Bull.* **88**:82–108.

Cohen, S., 1986, Correlational field methodology in the study of stress, in: *Behavior, Health, and Environmental Stress* (S. Cohen, G. Evans, D. Stokols, and D. Krantz), Plenum Press, New York.

Cohen, S., and Williamson, G. M., 1988, Perceived stress in a probability sample of the United States, in: *The Social Psychology of Health: Claremont Symposium on Applied Social Psychology* (S. Spacapan and S. Oskamp, eds.), Sage, Newbury Park, CA.

Cohen, S., and Wills, T. A., 1985, Stress, social support, and the buffering hypothesis, *Psychol. Bull.* **98**:310–357.

Cohen, S., Kamarck, T., and Mermelstein, R., 1983, A global measure of perceived stress, *J. Health Soc. Behav.* **24**:385–396.

Compas, B. E., 1987, Coping with stress during childhood and adolescence, *Psychol. Bull* **101**:393–403.

Conger, J. J., 1956, Alcoholism: Theory, problem and challenge. II. Reinforcement theory and the dynamics of alcoholism, *Q. J. Stud. Alcohol* **17**:296–305.

Conway, T. L., Vickers, R. R., Jr., Ward, H. W., and Rahe, R. H., 1981, Occupational stress and variation in cigarette, coffee, and alcohol consumption, *J. Health Soc. Behav.* **22**:155–165.

Cooke, D. J., and Allan, C. A., 1984, Stressful life events and alcohol abuse in women: A general population study, *Br. J. Addict.* **79**:425–430.

Cox, W. M., 1979, The alcoholic personality: A review of the evidence, in: *Progress in Experimental Personality Research,* Volume 9 (B. H. Maher, ed.), Academic Press, New York.

Cronkite, R. C., and Moos, R. H., 1980, Determinants of the posttreatment functioning of alcoholic patients: A conceptual framework. *J. Consult. Clin. Psychol.* **48**:305–316.

Cronkite, R. C., and Moos, R. H., 1984, The role of predisposing and moderating factors in the stress–illness relationship, *J. Health Soc. Behav.* **25**:372–393.

Cummings, K. M., Jaen, C. R., and Giovino, G., 1985, Circumstances surrounding relapse in a group of recent exsmokers, *Prev. Med.* **14**:195–202.

Curry, S. G., and Marlatt, G. A., 1985, Unaided quitters' strategies for coping with temptations to smoke, in: *Coping and Substance Use* (S. Shiffman and T. A. Wills, eds.), Academic Press, Orlando, FL.

Deardorff, C. M., Melges, F. T., Hout, C. N., and Savage, D. J., 1975, Situations related to drinking alcohol: A factor analysis of questionnaire responses, *J. Stud. Alcohol* **36**:1184–1195.

Depue, R. A., and Monroe, S. M., 1986, Conceptualization and measurement of human disorder in life stress research, *Psychol. Bull.* **99**:36–51.

Deykin, E. Y., Levy, J. C., and Wells, V., 1987, Adolescent depression, alcohol and drug abuse, *Am. J. Public Health* **76**:178–182.

DiClemente, C. C., and Prochaska, J. O., 1985, Processes and stages of self-change: Coping and competence in smoking behavior change, in: *Coping and Substance Use* (S. Shiffman and T. A. Wills, eds.), Academic Press, New York.

Diener, E., 1984, Subjective well-being, *Psychol. Bull.* **95**:542–575.

Donovan, J. E., and Jessor, R., 1978, Adolescent problem drinking: Psychosocial correlates in a national-sample study, *J. Stud. Alcohol* **39**:1506–1524.

Farber, P. D., Khavari, K. A., and Douglas, F. M., 1980, A factor analytic study of reasons for drinking, *J. Consult. Clin. Psychol.* **48**:780–781.

Finney, J. W., and Moos, R. H., 1981, Characteristics and prognoses of alcoholics who became moderate drinkers and abstainers after treatment, *J. Stud. Alcohol* **42**:94–105.

Finney, J. W., Moos, R. H., and Mewborn, C. R., 1980, Posttreatment experiences and treatment outcome of alcoholic patients six months and two years after hospitalization, *J. Consult. Clin. Psychol.* **48**:17–29.

Fishburne, P. M., Abelson, H. I., and Cisin, I., 1980, *National Survey on Drug Abuse, 1979,* National Institute on Drug Abuse, Washington, DC.

Gilbert, D. G., 1979, Paradoxical tranquilizing and emotion-reducing effects of nicotine, *Psychol. Bull.* **86**:643–661.

Glasgow, R. E., Klesges, R. C., Mizes, J. S., and Pechacek, T. F., 1985, Quitting smoking: Strategies used and variables associated with success in a stop-smoking contest, *J. Consult. Clin. Psychol.* **53**: 905–912.

Golding, J., and Mangan, G. L., 1982, Arousing and de-arousing effects of cigarette smoking under conditions of stress and mild sensory isolation, *Psychophysiology* **19**:449–456.

Gordon, N. P., and Cleary, P. D., 1986, *Smoking cessation in a national probability sample cohort, 1979–1980,* Discussion paper, Harvard University Institute for the Study of Smoking Behavior and Policy, Cambridge, MA.

Gorsuch, R. L., and Butler, M. C., 1976, Initial drug abuse: A review of predisposing social-psychological factors, *Psychol. Bull.* **83**:120–137.

Green, D. E., 1979, *Teenage smoking: Immediate and Long-Term Patterns,* National Institute of Education, Washington, DC.

Grunberg, N. E., and Baum, A., 1985, Biological commonalities in stress and substance abuse, in: *Coping and Substance Use* (S. Shiffman and T. A. Wills, eds.), Academic Press, New York.

Gunn, R. C., 1983, Smoking clinic failures and recent life stress, *Addict. Behav.* **8**:83–87.

Hays, R. D., Stacy, A. W., and DiMatteo, M. R., 1987, Problem behavior theory and adolescent alcohol use, *Addict. Behav.* **12**:189–193.

Hirschman, R. S., Leventhal, H., and Glynn, K., 1984, The development of smoking behavior: Cross-sectional survey data, *J. Appl. Soc. Psychol.* **14**:184–206.

Hull, J. G., and Bond, C. F., Jr., 1986, Social and behavioral consequences of alcohol consumption and expectancy, *Psychol. Bull.* **99**:347–360.

Hull, J. G., and Van Treuren, R. R., 1986, Experimental social psychology and the causes and effects of alcohol consumption, in: *Research Advances in Alcohol and Drug Problems,* Volume 9 (H. D. Cappell et al., eds.), Plenum Press, New York.

Hull, J. G., Young, R. D., and Jouriles, E., 1986, Applications of the self-awareness model of alcohol consumption: Predicting patterns of use and abuse, *J. Pers. Soc. Psychol.* **51**:790–796.

Istvan, J., and Matarazzo, J. D., 1984, Tobacco, alcohol, and caffeine use: A review of their interrelationships, *Psychol. Bull.* **95**:301–326.

Jaffe, J. H., 1980, Drug addiction and drug abuse, in: *The Pharmacological Basis of Therapeutics,* 6th ed. (A. G. Gilman, L. S. Goodman, and A. Gilman, eds.), Macmillan, New York.

Jessor, R., and Jessor, S., 1977, *Problem Behavior and Psychosocial Development,* Academic Press, New York.

Jessor, R., Chase, J. A., and Donovan, J. E., 1980, Psychosocial correlates of marijuana use and problem drinking in a national sample of adolescents, *Am. J. Public Health* **70**:604–613.

Johnson, J. H., and McCutcheon, S., 1980, Assessing life stress in older children and adolescents, in: *Stress and Anxiety,* Volume 7 (I. G. Sarason and C. D. Spielberger, eds.), Hemisphere, Washington, DC.

Kandel, D., 1978, Convergences in longitudinal studies of drug use in normal populations, in: *Longitudinal Research on Drug Use* (D. B. Kandel, ed.), Wiley, New York.

Kandel, D., 1984, Marijuana users in young adulthood, *Arch. Gen. Psychiatry* **41**:200–209.

Kandel, D., Kessler, R. C., and Margulies, R. Z., 1978, Antecedents of adolescent initiation into stages of drug use, in: *Longitudinal Research on Drug Use* (D. B. Kandel, ed.), Wiley, New York.

Kaplan, H. B., Martin, S. S., and Robbins, C., 1982, Application of a general theory of deviant behavior: Self-derogation and adolescent drug use, *J. Health Soc. Behav.* **23**:274–294.

Kaplan, H. B., Martin, S., S., and Robbins, C., 1984, Pathways to adolescent drug use: Self-derogation, peer influence, weakening of social controls, and early substance use, *J. Health Soc. Behav.* **25**:270–289.

Kaplan, H. B., Martin, S. S., Johnson, R. J., and Robbins, C. A., 1986, Escalation of marijuana use, *J. Health Soc. Behav.* **27**:44–61.

Kellam, S. G., Brown, C. H., and Fleming, J. P., 1982, Social adaptation to first grade and teenage drug, alcohol and cigarette use, *J. School Health* **52**:301–306.

Kosten, T. R., Rounsaville, B. J., and Kleber, N. D., 1983, Relationship of depression to psychosocial stressors in heroin addicts, *J. Nerv. Ment. Dis.* **171**:97–104.

Kozlowski, L. T., 1979, Psychosocial influences on cigarette smoking, in: *The Behavioral Aspects of Smoking* (N. A. Krasnegor, ed.), National Institute on Drug Abuse, Rockville, MD.

Kozlowski, L. T., and Harford, M. R., 1976, On the significance of never using a drug: An example from cigarette smoking, *J. Abnormal Psychol.* **85**:433–434.

Kozlowski, L. T., and Wilkinson, D. A., 1987, Use and misuse of the concept of craving by alcohol, tobacco, and drug researchers, *Br. J. Addict.* **82**:31–36.

Krueger, D. W., 1981, Stressful life events and return to heroin use, *J. Hum. Stress* **7**(2):3–8.

Labouvie, E. W., 1986a, Alcohol and marijuana use in relation to adolescent stress, *Int. J. Addict.* **21**:333–345.

Labouvie, E. W., 1986b, The coping function of adolescent alcohol and drug use, in: *Development as Action in Context* (R. K. Silbereisen, K. Eyferth, and G. Rudinger, eds.), Springer, New York.

Lazarus, R. S., and Folkman, S., 1984, *Stress, Appraisal, and Coping,* Springer, New York.

Lerner, J. V., and Vicary, J. R., 1984, Difficult temperament and drug use, *J. Drug Educ.* **14**:1–8.

Levenson, H., 1973, Multidimensional locus of control in psychiatric patients, *J. Consult. Clin. Psychol.* **41**:397–404.

Leventhal, H., and Cleary, P. D., 1980, The smoking problem: A review of research and theory, *Psychol. Bull* **88**:370–405.

Lindenthal, J. J., Myers, J. K., and Pepper, M. P., 1972, Smoking, psychological status, and stress, *Soc. Sci. Med.* **6**:583–591.

Litman, G. K., Eiser, J. R., Rawson, N. S. B., and Oppenheim, A. N., 1979, Differences in relapse precipitants and coping behaviour between alcohol relapsers and survivors, *Behav. Res. Ther.* **17**: 89–94.

Litman, G. K., Stapleton, J., Oppenheim, A. N., Peleg, M., and Jackson, P., 1983, Situations related to alcoholism relapse, *Br. J. Addict.* **78**:381–389.

Litman, G. K., Stapleton, J., Oppenheim, A. N., Peleg, M., and Jackson, P., 1984, The relationship between coping behaviours, their effectiveness, and alcoholism relapse and survival, *Br. J. Addict.* **79**:283–291.

Marlatt, G. A., 1976, Alcohol, stress, and cognitive control, in: *Stress and Anxiety,* Volume 3 (I. G. Sarason and C. D. Spielberger, eds.), Hemisphere, Washington, DC.

Marlatt, G. A., and Gordon, J. R., 1980, Determinants of relapse, in: *Behavioral Medicine: Changing Health Lifestyles* (P. O. Davidson and S. M. Davidson, eds.), Brunner/Mazel, New York.

McCarty, D., and Kaye, M. 1984, Motivational patterns and alcohol use among college students, *Addict. Behav.* **9**:185–188.

Mellinger, G. D., Balter, M. B., Manheimer, D. I., Cisin, I. H., and Parry, H. J., 1978, Psychic distress, life crisis, and use of psychotherapeutic medications, *Arch. Gen. Psychiatry* **35**:1045–1052.

Mermelstein, R., Cohen, S., Lichtenstein, E., and Kamarck, T., 1986, Social support and smoking cessation and maintenance, *J. Consult. Clin. Psychol.* **54**:447–453.

Mitic, W. R., McGuire, D. P., and Neumann, B., 1985, Perceived stress and adolescents' cigarette use, *Psychol. Rep.* **57**:1043–1048.

Mittelmark, M. B., Murray, D. M., Luepker, R. V., Pechacek, T. F., Pirie, P. L., and Pallonen, U. E., 1987, Predicting experimentation with cigarettes, *Am. J. Public Health* **77**:206–208.

Moos, R. H., and Billings, A. G., 1982, Conceptualizing and measuring coping resources and processes, in: *Handbook of Stress* (L. Goldberger and S. Bresnitz, eds.), Macmillan, New York.

Moos, R. H., Finney, J. W., and Chan, D. A., 1981, The process of recovery from alcoholism: I. Comparing alcoholic patients and matched community controls, *J. Stud. Alcohol* **42**:383–402.

Murray, D. M., and Perry, C. L. (1984, August). The functional meaning of adolescent drug use, Presented at the meeting of the American Psychological Association, Toronto.

Murray, D. M., O'Connell, C. M., Schmid, L. A., and Perry, C. L., 1987, The validity of smoking self-reports by adolescents, *Addict. Behav.* **12**:7–15.

Neff, J. A., and Husaini, B. A., 1982, Life events, drinking patterns, and depressive symptomatology, *J. Stud. Alcohol* **43**:301–318.

Neff, J. A., and Husaini, B. A., 1985, Stress-buffer properties of alcohol consumption: The role of urbanicity and religious identification, *J. Health Soc. Behav.* **26**:207–222.

Newcomb, M. D., and Bentler, P. M., 1986, Cocaine use among adolescents: Longitudinal associations with social context, psychopathology, and use of other substances, *Addict. Behav.* **11**:263–273.

Newcomb, M. D., and Harlow, L. L., 1986, Life events and substance use among adolescents, *J. Pers. Soc. Psychol.* **51**:564–577.

Newcomb, M. D., Huba, G. J., and Bentler, P. M., 1981, Multidimensional assessment of stressful life events among adolescents, *J. Health Soc. Behav.* **22**:400–415.

Ockene, J. K., Benfari, R. C., Nuttall, R. L., Hurwitz, I., and Ockene, I. S., 1982, Relationship of psychosocial factors to smoking behavior change in an intervention program, *Prev. Med.* **11**: 13–28.

Pearlin, L. I., Menaghan, E. G., Lieberman, M. A., and Mullan, J., 1981, The stress process, *J. Health Soc. Behav.* **22**:337–356.

Pearlin, L. I., and Radabaugh, C. W., 1976, Economic strains and the coping functions of alcohol, *Am. J. Sociol.* **82**:652–663.

Pomerleau, O. F., 1981, Underlying mechanisms in substance abuse: Examples from research on smoking, *Addict. Behav.* **6**:187–196.

Pomerleau, O. F., and Pomerleau, C. S., 1984, Neuroregulators and the reinforcement of smoking, *Neurosci. Biobehav. Rev.* **8**:503–513.

Pomerleau, O. F., Adkins, D., and Pertschuck, M., 1978, Predictors of outcome and recidivism in smoking cessation treatment, *Addict. Behav.* **3**:65–70.

Radelet, M. L., 1981, Health beliefs, social networks, and tranquilizer use, *J. Health Soc. Behav.* **22**: 165–173.

Rhoads, D. L., 1983, A longitudinal study of life stress and social support among drug abusers, *Int. J. Addict.* **18**:195–222.

Rohsenow, D. J., 1982, Social anxiety, daily moods, and alcohol use over time among heavy social drinking men, *Addict. Behav.* **7**:311–315.

Rosenberg, H. S., 1983, Relapsed vs. nonrelapsed alcohol abusers: Coping skills, life events, and social support, *Addict. Behav.* **8**:183–186.

Schachter, S., Silverstein, B., and Perlick, D., 1977, Psychological and pharmacological explanations of smoking under stress, *J. Exp. Psychol.: General* **106**:31–40.

Schachter, S., and Singer, J. E., 1962, Cognitive, social, and physiological determinants of emotional state, *Psychol. Rev.* **69**:379–399.

Seltzer, C. C., and Oechsli, F. W., 1985, Psychosocial characteristics of adolescent smokers before they started smoking, *J. Chronic Dis.* **38**:17–26.

Shiffman, S., 1979, The tobacco withdrawal syndrome, in: *Cigarette Smoking as a Dependence Process* (N. A. Krasnegor, ed.), National Institute on Drug Abuse, Rockville, MD.

Shiffman, S., 1982, Relapse following smoking cessation: A situational analysis, *J. Consult. Clin. Psychol.* **50**:71–86.

Shiffman, S., 1984*a*, Cognitive antecedents and sequelae of smoking relapse crises, *J. Appl. Soc. Psychol.* **14**:296–309.

Shiffman, S., 1984*b*, Coping with temptations to smoke, *J. Consult. Clin. Psychol.* **52**:261–267.

Shiffman, S., 1985, Processes of coping with temptation to smoke, in: *Coping and Substance Use* (S. Shiffman and T. A. Wills, eds.), Academic Press, Orlando, FL.

Shiffman, S., Shumaker, S. A., Abrams, D. B., Cohen, S., Garvey, A., Grunberg, N. E., and Swan, G. E., 1986, Models of smoking relapse, *Health Psychol.* **5**(Suppl.):13–27.

Siegel, S., 1979, The role of conditioning in drug tolerance and addiction, in: *Psychopathology in Animals: Research and Clinical Applications* (J. D. Keehn, ed.), Academic Press, New York.

Silverstein, B., Kelly, E., Swan, J., and Kozlowski, L. T., 1982, Physiological predisposition toward becoming a cigarette smoker: Evidence for a sex difference, *Addict. Behav.* **7**:83–86.

Stewart, J., de Wit, H., and Eikelboom, R., 1984, Role of unconditioned and conditioned drug effects in the self-administration of opiates and stimulants, *Psychol. Rev.* **91**:251–268.

Stone, A., Lennox, S., and Neale, J. M., 1985, Daily coping and alcohol use in a sample of community adults, in: *Coping and Substance Use* (S. Shiffman and T. A. Wills, eds.), Academic Press, Orlando, FL.

Stone, A. A., Helder, L., and Schneider, M. S., 1987, Coping with stressful events: Coping dimensions and issues, in: *Stressful Life Events: Theoretical and Methodological Issues* (L. Cohen, ed.), Sage, Beverly Hills, CA.

Tagliacozzo, R., and Vaughn, S., 1982, Stress and smoking in hospital nurses. *Am. J. Public Health* **72**: 441–448.

Timmer, S. G., Veroff, J., and Colten, M. E., 1985, Life stress, helplessness, and use of alcohol and drugs to cope: An analysis of national survey data, in: *Coping and Substance Use* (S. Shiffman and T. A. Wills, eds.), Academic Press, Orlando, FL.

Uhlenhuth, E. H., Balter, M., and Lipman, R., 1978, Minor tranquilizers: Clinical correlates of use in an urban population, *Arch. Gen. psychiatry* **35**:650–655.

U.S. Department of Health and Human Services, 1988, *The Health Consequences of Smoking: Nicotine Addiction. A Report of the Surgeon General,* Public Health Service, DHHS Publication No. (CDC) 88-8406, U.S. Department of Health and Human Services, Washington, DC.

Vaillant, G. E., 1984, The contribution of prospective studies to the understanding of etiological factors in alcoholism, in: *Research Advances in Alcohol and Drug Problems,* Volume 8 (R. G. Smart et al., eds.), Plenum Press, New York.

Wills, T. A., 1986, Stress and coping in early adolescence: Relationships to smoking and alcohol use in urban school samples, *Health Psychol.* **5**:503–529.

Wills, T. A., and Shiffman, S., 1985, Coping and substance use: A conceptual framework, in: *Coping and Substance Use* (S. Shiffman and T. A. Wills, eds.), Academic Press, Orlando, FL.

8

# Women, Illicit Drugs, and Crime

PATRICIA G. ERICKSON and VALERIE A. WATSON

## 1. INTRODUCTION

Illicit drug use is, by definition, a crime. That simple observation thrusts illicit drug use into the realm of law-breaking behaviors long dominated by men. Thus, the question of women's patterns of illicit drug use and their relation to criminal activities must be addressed within the broader context of gender differences in criminal and delinquent behavior. The literature reviewed in this chapter is unequivocal on two points; that research on women has been neglected in the fields of both criminology and addictions (Miller, 1983; Prather and Fidell, 1978; Adelberg and Currie, 1987), and that male and female patterns of both crime and substance use are very different (Provine, 1987; Ferrence and Whitehead, 1980).

The focus of this chapter is women's criminal behavior related to drug use. This includes the woman's role as a consumer of illicit drugs, as a potential distributor (seller, dealer) in the illegal market, and as an offender if she is arrested for drug possession or trafficking. The first area of investigation considers women primarily as experimenters or recreational users of illicit drugs.

Also considered are the crimes, mainly prostitution, that addicted women are thought to commit in order to obtain drugs. Indeed, the limitations of available research are highlighted in Adler and Simon's comment that "what research has been done on females and drugs has been largely within the purview of the literature on prostitution" (1979, p. 99). Therefore, this second group of studies is centered on female addiction as a cause or consequence of other criminal activities.

By way of introduction, we want to explore why the issue of legality, as opposed to illegality, is central to understanding female substance use. At the turn of the century, in

---

PATRICIA G. ERICKSON and VALERIE A. WATSON • Drug Policy Research Program, Prevention Studies Department, Addiction Research Foundation, Toronto, Ontario M5S 2S1, Canada. The views expressed in this publication are those of the authors and do not necessarily reflect those of the Addiction Research Foundation.

the United States, twice as many women as men were addicted to opiate narcotics (Cuskey et al., 1972). The Harrison Act of 1914, which made narcotics illegal, shifted that ratio, and from approximately 1920 onward, male addicts outnumbered females by nearly two to one (Ferrence and Whitehead, 1980). What had been acceptable, or at least tolerated, quasimedical use became a forbidden activity.

A further example comes from Britain, where the medical model of addiction remained dominant until the 1960s (Trebach, 1982). Prior to 1962, the majority of British opiate addicts were women; since then, with increased emphasis on repression and control (i.e., heroin use has become a more deviant activity), male addicts have outnumbered females (d'Orban, 1970). Currently, in most Western countries, men are the heaviest users of cocaine, heroin, phencyclidine (PCP), cannabis, and other prohibited substances (Colten and Marsh, 1984; Ferrence, 1984). Men are also more likely than women to use alcohol and tobacco and to use them more frequently (Ferrence, 1984). Female drug use exceeds male use only for the medicinal and legal mood-modifying drugs, i.e., tranquilizers, barbiturates, and over-the-counter drugs (Cooperstock, 1976), and then only when obtained by prescription. Men dominate in illicit consumption, but *overall* drug consumption may not be very different for men and women (Kalant, 1980).

Female illicit drug users are doubly deviant. Not only do they break the law, they also participate in a predominantly male activity (Ferrence and Whitehead, 1980). It is instructive to examine the parallel course in the explanation of female deviance in the criminology literature. Female criminals have been variously described over the past 80 years as "devious, deceitful and emotional . . . intellectually dull and passive . . . closer to animals in evolution . . . immoral . . . lonely and dependent . . .[and] a pathetic lot" (Klein and Kress, 1976, p. 35). The deviant behavior of males and females was assumed to reflect different underlying processes and motivations (Smith and Paternoster, 1987). While men have been viewed as seeking monetary success, status, or peer acceptance through criminal pursuits, their female counterparts have been portrayed as personally or socially maladjusted or as the victims of biological imbalance (Smith and Paternoster, 1987). The current trend is away from gender-specific theories of deviance, toward more comprehensive explanations of deviant behavior in both males and females (see Hagan et al., 1985).

Men far outnumber women as perpetrators of crime and especially as committers of more serious and violent offences (Silverman, 1982). In the 1970s, a renewed interest in female crime provoked a flood of studies which assessed the convergence hypothesis—the notion that women were becoming more like men in the frequency and nature of offending. Adler's *Sisters in Crime* (1975) promoted the image of a new violent female criminal. Simon's (1979) assessment of arrest statistics for the period 1953–1974 indicated, however, that increases in female crime were concentrated in the category of property offenses. A more recent analysis (Steffensmeier, 1987) showed that this trend continued to 1985 (i.e., of increased female involvement in larceny, fraud, embezzlement, and forgery but not in violent, personal crime). The assessment of sex differences in crime occupies many researchers and is reviewed elsewhere (Adler and Simon, 1979). We turn now to our main topic—sex differences in illicit drug use—and consider recent evidence from surveys and community studies.

## 2. WOMEN IN THE ILLICIT RECREATIONAL DRUG MILIEU

### Women as Consumers

While the convergence hypothesis was assumed by some authors to apply to both criminality and illicit drug use (e.g., Wechsler and McFadden, 1976), proper assessment of its validity had to await the accumulation of survey evidence. By 1980, a very comprehensive review of Canadian and American studies provided evidence for the conclusion that "there are major sex differences in the use of most drugs and that these differences persist over time. . . . there is also no evidence that patterns of drug use are converging" (Ferrence and Whitehead, 1980, p. 185). The one exception was marijuana use. That review noted that marijuana rates were closing between men and women; moreover, young people displayed less pronounced sex differences in drug use than adults. For illicit drugs, the sex differences in use were greatest for cocaine and heroin, followed by hallucinogens and inhalants, and then marijuana. A later review (Ferrence, 1984) projected no dramatic reversals in these pronounced sex differences in illicit drug use.

Most recent surveys support the above conclusion. Among Canadian high-school students, Smart and Adlaf (1987*a*) found that cannabis use declined steadily for both males and females between 1981 and 1987. Levels of cannabis use remained higher in 1987 among males than females (18.7% compared to 13.2%) a pattern paralleled at much lower levels of use (under 10%) for heroin, cocaine, lysergic acid diethylamide (LSD), PCP, and other hallucinogens (Smart and Adlaf, 1987*a*). Since female rates declined slightly more than male rates, these data actually showed some divergence in rates of use between the sexes.

Among adults, Smart and Adlaf (1987*b*) found that cannabis and cocaine continued to be more widely used by men than by women. For example, in 1987, 12.3% of men, compared to 6.8% of women, reported using cannabis in the past 12 months; for cocaine, the comparable figures were 7.2% for men and 4.7% for women (Smart and Adlaf, 1987*b*). Closer examination of these data by age indicated that declines in reported cannabis use occurred for *both* males and females in the 18- to 29-year age group, and increased for both sexes among 30- to 49-year-olds (Smart and Adlaf, 1987*b*, p. 29). Again, these data indicate an absence of further convergence in cannabis use. For cocaine, Smart and Adlaf (1987*b*) found that between 1984 and 1987, use had risen more sharply for the younger (18–29) cohort than the older (30–49) cohort, and most disproportionately among younger women. Ferrence and Whitehead (1980, p. 177) cautioned that few data were available on cocaine; nevertheless, they argued that a new drug tends to be taken up more quickly by men than by women. Thus, it might be expected that cocaine would follow a pattern similar to that of cannabis, namely, a gradual decrease in sex differences as use became more widespread.

With respect to trends in sex differences in drug use in the United States, Johnston et al. (1987) observed the following patterns among high-school seniors, young adults, and college students between 1975 and 1986. Males were most likely to use illicit drugs, and the differences between males and females were largest at the higher levels of use. For example, daily marijuana use among high-school seniors in 1986 was reported by

5.7% of males vs. 2.3% of females; among young adults, the proportions were similar: 5.3% vs. 2.9%; and among college students, 2.8% of males compared to 1.5% of females. As part of the overall downward trend in the use of illicit drugs since 1979, Johnston et al. (1987) noted that some convergence had resulted from a more rapid drop in use by males than by females. In other words, what has been witnessed in the United States is a greater similarity in younger male and female illicit drug use, but for opposite reasons than those proffered in the early 1970s: Men's behavior is approximating women's, rather than vice versa. The Canadian pattern is somewhat different in showing continuing divergence despite declining use by both sexes.

Surveys provide an important perspective, but cannot readily pinpoint the reasons for these sex differences, such as motives and patterns of use that may vary between the sexes. For instance, the only population surveyed that showed nearly identical rates of cannabis use among men and women—14% and 15%, respectively—was the Canadian Armed Forces (Lanphier and McCauley, 1985), but no explanations can be offered beyond the obvious workforce and job stress similarities. Ferrence and Whitehead (1980) also drew attention to the lack of information linking drug use to variables where the sexes differ markedly, such as employment status and income. Others have noted that the social meaning of drug use, for instance in courtship/seduction rituals, can be different for males and females (Bowker, 1978*b*).

Most studies of heroin use that include women concentrate on addicted users or do not analyze data separately by sex (e.g., Johnson et al., 1985). When patterns of nondependent heroin use were examined in samples containing men and women, the motivation, perceived benefits, and methods of regulating intake did not appear to be expressed differently by men and women (Blackwell, 1983). Similarly with cocaine, recreational use patterns and practices did not seem to vary by sex (Erickson and Murray, 1989; Murphy et al., 1986). Erickson et al. (1987) found that the major appeal of cocaine for women was to make them feel more sociable and confident during social interactions, while for men, physical energy was its most appealing aspect (Erickson et al., 1987, p. 84). More generally, Bell (1980) asserted men's and women's similarity in seeking "the pleasure of a high" from drug use. In contrast, Bowker (1978*a*) found that women report *more* satisfaction from drug use, and he speculated that because cultural norms disapprove of female drug use, only those females who experience particular satisfaction from illicit drugs will persevere.

Multivariate studies that have examined problems related to onset of cocaine use (Newcomb and Bentler, 1986) and persistence of cannabis use (Kaplan et al., 1986) are similar in the lack of significance placed on the sex variable, other than the expected correlation of being male with heavier levels of use. Erickson and Murray (1989) found no sex differences in acute or chronic effects of cocaine use in a sample of predominantly recreational users. The somewhat greater tendency of women to perceive that drug use poses health risks (Ferrence and Whitehead, 1980; Erickson, 1989), particularly with respect to pregnancy (Yamaguchi and Kandel, 1985), has also been documented. Smith and Paternoster (1987) found that both the prevalence and frequency of marijuana use were explained by much the same set of factors among males and females, leading them to conclude that seeking gender-specific explanations of drug use was unwarranted.

The studies just cited lend support to more gender-neutral explanations of drug use.

While males clearly have a greater propensity to engage in illicit drug use than females, among those who do (at least at the recreational level), the content of the experience seems more similar than dissimilar for both sexes. A fuller explanation of sex differences in illicit drug use awaits the more comprehensive testing of theories to explain the fundamental differences in criminal behavior between men and women.

## Women as Distributors

As in crime generally, men dominate the upper and middle echelons of the traffic in drugs (Anglin et al., 1987). Adler and Simon (1979, p. 99) offer this summary: "There are no studies of women as 'pushers' or managers or entrepreneurs in the illicit drug world. Perhaps there are no data because women do not play such roles and have not gained admittance into the criminal hierarchy of the buying and distribution of illicit drugs." There are a few recent case studies—the exceptions to the rule. Simpson (1987) reported on the activities of an American woman involved in a multi-million-dollar cocaine-selling network. Nicholl (1985), in a journalistic exposé of the cocaine trade in Colombia, provided a similar account of a high-level businesswoman who used her contacts to expand into cocaine trafficking. Most accounts of women as sellers, however, have been at the retail, street-level end of the business and have usually been detailed within studies of prostitution (see Inciardi, 1986).

Even at the more informal levels of distribution, e.g., first introductions to drugs within friendship networks, it is clear that women have been more likely to receive than to give (Bowker, 1978*b;* Ferrence, 1984; Hser et al., 1987*b*). Illicit drugs are first used by males in the company of other males; females are almost never initiated into drug use by other females. This appears to be true whether the setting has been college (Bowker, 1978b), high school (Nielson and Hirabayashi, 1975), or the street (Rosenbaum, 1981 *b*). While cocaine has been hailed as the latest "gateway" drug for seduction-minded males, this may just be the most recent expression of the popular stereotype of women's loss of control after the ingestion of psychoactive substances (Fillmore, 1984; Erickson and Murray, 1989). The female role in drug distribution activities has been summarized as follows: "Women are no more big-time drug dealers than they are finance capitalists' (Klein and Kress, 1976, p. 41).

## Women as Offenders

As befits their lesser role as committers of crimes, women have also been largely overlooked players in the criminal justice system until recently (Klein and Kress, 1976; Provine, 1987). There is now a large literature examining bias in enforcement and sentencing patterns of female offenders (see Nagel and Hagan, 1982, for a review). Criminal justice practices in relation to female drug offenders in Canada are fairly typical of the situation in other countries (see Adler and Simon, 1979).

Male offenders outnumbered female offenders in all drug categories between 1980 and 1985 (Table 1). For every 10 women convicted of cannabis offenses, about 111 men were convicted. For LSD, about 90 men were convicted for every 10 women. For every 10 women convicted of cocaine offenses, the number of men convicted was 67 in 1980, jumped to 111 in 1981, and then dropped to 72 in 1985. The patterns with heroin have

Table 1. Convictions by Gender for Various Drugs, Canada, 1980–1985[a]

| Drug | Year | Total convictions | Males *N* | Males % | Females *N* | Females % | M/F ratio[b] |
|---|---|---|---|---|---|---|---|
| Cocaine | 1980 | 850 | 740 | 87.1 | 110 | 12.9 | 67 |
| | 1981 | 1,255 | 1,151 | 91.7 | 104 | 8.3 | 111 |
| | 1982 | 1,334 | 1,187 | 89.0 | 147 | 11.0 | 81 |
| | 1983 | 1,592 | 1,410 | 88.6 | 182 | 11.4 | 77 |
| | 1984 | 2,234 | 1,995 | 89.3 | 239 | 10.7 | 83 |
| | 1985 | 2,218 | 1,949 | 87.9 | 269 | 12.1 | 72 |
| Cannabis | 1980 | 40,781 | 37,477 | 91.9 | 3,304 | 8.1 | 113 |
| | 1981 | 43,880 | 40,264 | 91.8 | 3,616 | 8.2 | 111 |
| | 1982 | 34,886 | 32,015 | 91.8 | 2,871 | 8.2 | 112 |
| | 1983 | 28,955 | 26,444 | 91.3 | 2,511 | 8.7 | 105 |
| | 1984 | 26,193 | 24,044 | 91.8 | 2,149 | 8.2 | 112 |
| | 1985 | 22,510 | 20,654 | 91.8 | 1,856 | 8.2 | 111 |
| Heroin | 1980 | 309 | 239 | 77.3 | 70 | 22.7 | 34 |
| | 1981 | 261 | 201 | 77.0 | 60 | 23.0 | 34 |
| | 1982 | 286 | 213 | 74.5 | 73 | 25.5 | 29 |
| | 1983 | 295 | 224 | 75.9 | 71 | 24.1 | 32 |
| | 1984 | 302 | 221 | 73.2 | 81 | 26.8 | 27 |
| | 1985 | 256 | 214 | 83.6 | 42 | 16.4 | 51 |
| LSD | 1980 | 2,076 | 1,900 | 91.5 | 176 | 8.5 | 108 |
| | 1981 | 2,232 | 1,960 | 87.8 | 272 | 12.2 | 73 |
| | 1982 | 1,774 | 1,595 | 89.9 | 179 | 10.1 | 89 |
| | 1983 | 1,423 | 1,281 | 90.0 | 142 | 10.0 | 90 |
| | 1984 | 1,083 | 981 | 90.6 | 102 | 9.4 | 96 |
| | 1985 | 710 | 645 | 90.8 | 65 | 9.2 | 99 |

[a]From *Annual Reports*, Bureau of Dangerous Drugs, Health Protection Branch, Health and Welfare Canada, Ottawa.
[b]Shows number of male convictions for every ten female convictions.

been more steady than those with cocaine, hovering around 30 convictions of men for every 10 convictions of women until 1985, when about 50 men were convicted for every 10 women. Numerically, cannabis accounts for the greatest number of offenders, and heroin the fewest. The proportion of female offenders fluctuated very little for most of the drugs over the 6-year period from 1980 to 1985.

In Table 2, sentences under the Narcotic Control Act for males and females are compared for two different years, 1980 and 1985. For all age and sex groups, there is a decline in the awarding of the most lenient option—the discharge. Women are slightly less likely than men to receive the shorter jail sentence in both time periods, but are more likely to get probation. However, the patterns are not that dissimilar and would need to be examined in more detail by type of offense to determine whether women receive significantly different sentences than men.

By virtue of detection of their illicit drug use and selling, at least some women become criminal offenders and serve sentences for these crimes. The more than 2500 women processed under the Narcotic Control Act in 1985 is a relatively small proportion (3.5%) of the 71,437 female criminals recorded in that year (Johnson, 1987).

Table 2. Sentences under the Narcotic Control Act by Sex and Age, Canada, 1980 and 1985[a]

| | Under 20 | | 20–29 | | 30 and older | |
|---|---|---|---|---|---|---|
| Sentences | Males | Females | Males | Females | Males | Females |
| 1980 | | | | | | |
| Fine | 54.0 | 43.6 | 59.4 | 50.2 | 55.9 | 44.2 |
| Probation | 7.3 | 12.7 | 3.2 | 7.6 | 4.1 | 11.5 |
| Discharge | 29.4 | 37.9 | 20.2 | 28.9 | 16.2 | 26.6 |
| Jail ≤ 6 mos. | 7.9 | 5.4 | 12.7 | 9.3 | 14.6 | 13.7 |
| Jail > 6 mos. | 1.4 | 0.4 | 4.5 | 4.0 | 9.2 | 4.0 |
| Total | 100.0 | 100.0 | 100.0 | 100.0 | 100.0 | 100.0 |
| *N* | 13,228 | 1203 | 22,045 | 1935 | 3298 | 373 |
| 1985 | | | | | | |
| Fine | 55.2 | 45.9 | 61.4 | 55.0 | 55.9 | 43.5 |
| Probation | 12.4 | 19.8 | 3.7 | 12.3 | 3.4 | 23.0 |
| Discharge | 19.0 | 23.3 | 12.2 | 17.5 | 10.4 | 12.5 |
| Jail ≤ 6 mos. | 11.4 | 8.9 | 17.0 | 10.2 | 17.9 | 14.7 |
| Jail > 6 mos. | 2.0 | 2.1 | 5.7 | 5.0 | 12.4 | 6.3 |
| Total | 100.0 | 100.0 | 100.0 | 100.0 | 100.0 | 100.0 |
| *N* | 4527 | 429 | 14,434 | 1525 | 4682 | 687 |

[a]From *Annual Reports*, Bureau of Dangerous Drugs, Health Protection Branch, Health and Welfare Canada, Ottawa.

In summary, this first area of studies has concentrated on women as recreational illicit drug users, sellers, and offenders. Women play a role in all these aspects of criminal behavior related to drug use, but are predominantly consumers. More studies are needed that include drug use as one of a range of deviant activities for which criminological theories can be tested for both sexes. More case studies and community studies would illuminate the subtle variations in practices that may account for different patterns of use. Little attention has been paid to the role of economic, occupation, and availability factors in relation to sex differences in illicit drug use (Ferrence, 1984). Any tendency toward convergence—whether the result of females using more or males using less—should continue to be monitored.

## 3. ADDICTED WOMEN: DRUGS AND PROSTITUTION

> Female addiction has been most often linked with crime in the form of prostitution, which typically has been regarded as the female equivalent of crime. (Datesman, 1981, p. 88)

The close association between female drug use and prostitution has been the major topic in the literature concerning women and illicit drug use. Much past work has accepted the historical assumption that there is a simple connection between addiction and prostitution. These two forms of deviance have been intertwined, whether women were thought to become prostitutes in order to support their drug habit or to take drugs regularly in order to cope with their work (Adler and Simon, 1979; Inciardi, 1986). More recent studies have broadened this scope by depicting the wide range of criminal behavior engaged in by addicted women and by exploring the variety of motivations for involvement in both prostitution and drug use.

In this section, a number of studies—most done in the United States—are examined, and major issues explored in the drugs and prostitution literature are discussed. Considerably more research is needed before these complex social problems can be clearly understood. Because the focus of this chapter is women's criminal behavior related to drug use, we have chosen to examine the literature on women, illicit drugs, and prostitution, rather than the more general literature on women and drugs. Space does not permit the exploration of literature that examines broader aspects of women and substance use (i.e., female addiction to tranquilizers and other prescription medication; substance use by women in various occupations).

## Criminal Activities of Drug-Using Women

Research examining women, illicit drug use, and prostitution has focused primarily on criminality. Reports in American literature of the proportion of female drug users who are also involved in prostitution range from 23% (Hser et al., 1987*a*) to 71% (Datesman and Inciardi, 1979). Goldstein (1979) has reported that the proportion of prostitutes who also use drugs ranges from approximately 40 to 85%. Silbert et al. (1982) found that 59% of their prostitute sample were using drugs at the time of the study and an additional 36% had used them in the past. Although no Canadian statistics on drug use among prostitutes are available, reports submitted to the Special Committee on Pornography and Prostitution (1985, p. 354) indicated that the use of drugs by prostitutes is "much higher than for the population as a whole." The Special Committee, on the other hand, also reported that while "some prostitutes use drugs and alcohol to help them endure their work . . . the majority do not because the dangers of their job require that they be constantly alert."

Drug use and prostitution, however, are not generally the only criminal behaviors engaged in by drug users, prostitutes, and drug-using prostitutes. Table 3 highlights the wide range of criminal activity of women drug users. The reviewed studies consistently report, contrary to the stereotype (i.e., that prostitution is the most common criminal activity among drug-using women), that the most common criminal activities among these women are drug offenses (primarily drug dealing) and not prostitution. However, as Rosenbaum (1981*b*, p. 71) has cautioned in referring to her study of 100 women addicted to heroin, "although slightly more women . . . had used dealing than prostitution to earn their money, . . . their dealing was quite sporadic and spouse-related." James et al. (1979), in their study of 268 women offenders, found that only 37% of addict prostitutes ranked drug sales as their most important source of illegal support, while 54% ranked prostitution as most important. While the proportion of women who engaged in drug offenses may be higher than the proportion who engage in prostitution, it seems that prostitution provides slightly more economic support to the women who regularly use drugs.

File et al. (1974) have proposed an either/or model of criminality. They concluded,

Table 3. Criminal Activities of Women Drug Users (Self-Reported Involvement of Sample)

| Researcher(s) | Criminal offense | | | | | | |
|---|---|---|---|---|---|---|---|
| | Prostitution (%) | Drug offenses (%) | Forgery (%) | Shoplifting (%) | Robbery (%) | Theft (%) | Burglary (%) |
| Anglin and Hser, 1987 | 37 | — | 45 | — | 13 | 70 | 46 |
| Datesman and Inciardi, 1979 | 71 | 80 | 30 | 73 | 18 | — | 22 |
| File et al., 1974[a] | 41 | 81 | 9 | — | 13 | 45 | 21 |
| Hser et al., 1987*a* | 23 | — | 32 | — | 9 | 45 | 27 |
| Inciardi and Pottieger, 1986 | 54 | 56 | — | 31 | 17 | — | 34 |
| James et al., 1979 | 35 | — | 13 | 26 | — | 19 | — |
| Rosenbaum, 1981*a* | 26 | 63 | 38 | — | 6 | 43 | — |
| Rosenbaum, 1981*b* | 60 | 61 | 21 | 28 | — | — | 18 |
| Weissman and File, 1976[a] | 33 | 88 | 14 | — | — | 65 | 24 |

[a]Percent ever arrested for specified offense.

through their study of 227 women arrested in Philadelphia, that "a female addict will either choose to engage in prostitution almost exclusively, or she will engage in a wide variety of other (non-prostitute) criminal hustles; she will almost never engage in both" (File et al., 1974, p. 178). File et al. (1974), Goldstein (1979), and James (1976), among others, have distinguished addicts, prostitutes, and addict prostitutes. There certainly are women who regularly use drugs and who never or rarely act as prostitutes, and vice versa, and each group of women clearly distinguishes itself from the other. James (1976, p. 616), in her study of 100 prostitutes, addicts, and addict prostitutes, found that it would be unlikely for a professional prostitute to become an addict, and d'Orban (1970, 1973), in his original and 4-year follow-up studies of 66 British female narcotic addicts, found that the addicts did not take up prostitution.

Because few longitudinal studies of prostitutes and drug addicts have been carried out, it is difficult to determine the proportion of women who continue to engage in prostitution and regular drug use. In fact, women's descriptions of their work and criminal behavior may vary over time. According to File (1976, p. 267), "female roles are defined by which role is primary at the time of data collection, not by which role describes an exclusive career condition." Because most existing research provides a perspective at only one point in time, it would be misleading to generalize such findings to women's life experiences with drugs and prostitution.

Few studies present information about the proportion of drug-using women involved in crime. Datesman (1981), in her study of 153 Florida female heroin users, found that only 4% of the active female users were involved exclusively in prostitution. The largest percentage of the women (67%) were involved in both prostitution and other serious crimes (person and/or property crimes). Similarly, Inciardi et al. (1982), in their study of the drug use and criminal involvement of 63 black female heroin users, found that, although 64% of the respondents had engaged in prostitution in the last 12 months, prostitution had accounted for only about one-quarter of all offenses during this time. Moreover, their analyses determined that prostitution accounted for the majority of the criminal activities of only 18% of the women. In fact, over 90% of these offenses were prostitution. These findings suggest that prostitution is a primary criminal activity for only a small proportion of drug-using women, particularly narcotics addicts. Most women who regularly use drugs engage in a diversity of criminal behaviors.

In a study of 328 addicted women, Anglin and Hser (1987) found that addicted women engage in three major types of crime: prostitution; reselling narcotics or assisting male drug dealers; and property crimes (larceny, forgery, shoplifting, burglary, and robbery). They concluded that "although the traditional characterization of the woman addict is as a prostitute, the data indicate that prostitution is but one of a number of alternative activities by which those women support themselves and their drug use" (Anglin and Hser, 1987, p. 362). These sentiments have been repeated in numerous studies, including Weissman and File's (1976) study of 380 addicted female arrestees, Inciardi et al.'s (1982) study of 63 black female heroin users, Datesman and Inciardi's (1979) study of 153 active female heroin users, and James et al.'s (1979) study of 268 addicts, prostitute addicts, prostitutes, and other female offenders. The latter study concluded that the offenses women commit are related to various factors: ". . . female offenders gravitate to those activities which are easily available, provide a satisfactory return, are within their skills and opportunities, and carry the lowest risk of arrest"

(James et al., 1979, p. 229). According to Sheehy (1971, p. 16), prostitutes are becoming more and more involved in violent crime: "The bulk of their business is not the dispensation of pleasure. It is to swindle, mug, rob, knife and possibly even murder their patrons." More recent literature discounts the view that prostitutes are becoming increasingly violent.

Although the traditional association between drug use and prostitution seems to have been discredited in the literature, a relationship does exist which should not be minimized. While prostitution may not be the most common criminal activity engaged in by most regular drug users, it is, nevertheless, widespread and it provides women with financial support.

The findings of Inciardi and Pottieger (1986), in their study of two cohorts of women heroin users, suggest a renewed need for study of the illicit drug use–prostitution relationship. They reported that the proportion of women involved in prostitution increased from 38% in the 1977/1978 cohort (of 153 women) to 54% in the 1983/1984 cohort (of 133 women). Unlike the earlier cohort, the later cohort had a marked preference for prostitution and drug sales over property offenses. Such changes in criminal behavior could be related to myriad factors, including changes in drug availability, criminal fads in the drug cultures, legislation, law enforcement practices, and historical circumstances.

## Drug Use among Prostitutes

The few studies that have asked prostitutes about their drug use have found variations among different categories of prostitutes. Certain forms of drug use are a detriment to entry into prostitution (Goldstein, 1979). Women addicted to any illicit substances are reportedly shunned by madams and massage parlor managers, while women addicted to heroin are rejected by street pimps. Heroin use, however, is the substance typically reported by street prostitutes in the United States (File et al., 1974; Goldstein, 1979; James, 1976; James et al., 1979; Marshall and Hendtlass, 1986). Goldstein (1979) found that cocaine and other stimulant use is also common among street prostitutes and call girls (33% in his study used cocaine).

In Canada, the drugs typically used by prostitutes may be changing. A report on prostitution in Vancouver in 1975 (as cited in Lowman, 1986) suggested "an almost inevitable convergence of street prostitution and drug addiction." This was not evident in the 1980s, when two newer street prostitution areas of that city were examined. Heroin-using prostitutes likely confine their work to certain areas or "tracks." The Special Committee described a pattern of drug use that did not typically include heroin: "the use of soft, as opposed to hard, drugs is characteristic of prostitutes" (Special Committee on Pornography and Prostitution, 1985, p. 375). Almost all of the prostitutes interviewed in an Ontario study reported use of "intoxicants" (including alcohol) (Fleischman, 1984).

The most accurate picture of North American prostitutes' drug-using behavior is probably one of multiple drug use. Lautt (1984) found that different drugs were used for different reasons. Among women who used drugs socially, most used alcohol, cocaine (when they could afford it), and cannabis. Those who used drugs while working predominantly used whatever combination of prescription and nonprescription drugs they could obtain. Street prostitutes in San Francisco reported that they used a combination of drugs: cannabis (53%); heroin (41%); stimulants/amphetamines/uppers/speed (38%); sedatives, barbiturates, downers (34%); and cocaine (20%) (Silbert et al., 1982).

Very little is known about the frequency and duration of drug use among prostitutes. One of the few studies (Fleischman, 1984) to explore frequency of drug use found that 50% of the prostitutes used drugs every day. Silbert et al. (1982) also found that the frequency of use was very high, with 58% reporting use all the time, 20% reporting use almost every day, 19% reporting occasional use, and only 3% reporting infrequent and rare use. The average duration of use was 5.25 years. These women were very involved with drugs.

Miller (1986) found that the pattern of drug use among the prostitutes she studied was not typically a progression from intermittent to daily and dependent use. Rather, she found that there was no distinctive pattern: Sometimes use was intermittent, sometimes it was heavy, and sometimes it was light; different drugs were used at different times; and use was sometimes of lengthy and sometimes of brief duration. Patterns of use were reportedly influenced by a range of factors, including income; expenses; availability of drugs; patterns of arrest and confinement; psychological state; whim; and the tempo and drug use patterns of the street life.

Patterns of drug use among family members of prostitutes have rarely been studied. Silbert et al. (1982) found that approximately 90% of the families of 200 juvenile and adult prostitutes had members who were "excessively" involved in drug and alcohol use.

## Reasons for Prostitution among Drug Users

Economic motives for prostitution are frequently reported in the literature. Goldstein (1979), for example, found that these motives were among those most frequently reported among drug-using women. This finding appears to lend credence to the popular belief that women are thought to engage in prostitution in order to support expensive drug habits. With as many as 51% of one American sample of prostitutes reporting that they were addicted to drugs (Silbert et al., 1982), this economic–drug motive may be very common.

In Ontario, Fleischman (1984) found that 71% of his sample of 48 female prostitutes became involved in prostitution for economic reasons. For a large proportion of this sample (42%), prostitution was the only source of income. Only 8% of the sample, however, described money for drugs as the primary reason for becoming a prostitute. On the other hand, drugs were among the most significant budget items of one sample of 36 prostitutes in the Prairie Provinces (Lautt, 1984).

The Special Committee on Pornography and Prostitution (1985, p. 397) has challenged the assumed economic–drug motive. The Committee found that the majority of prostitutes are primarily involved in prostitution to support themselves and not their drug purchases. "The notion that prostitutes are on the street in order to earn the large amounts of money necessary to support a serious drug habit, does not find significant support from the research. There are some prostitutes who are in this position but they appear to be a very small part of the business and not at all typical." Lowman (1987) also reported that drug dependency is uncommon among reasons for entry into prostitution.

Among addicted women, however, the economic–drug motive seems to play the largest role in prostitution. Regular illicit use of addictive drugs, unlike recreational use, requires a constant, substantial income which few women can earn from legal jobs (James et al., 1979, p. 216). Most investigators report very low legitimate employment rates among their samples of addicted women (Hser et al., 1987*a;* Inciardi and Pottieger, 1986; Rosenbaum, 1981*a;* Suffet and Brotman, 1976). Employment rates in legitimate occupations in one sample were reportedly as low as 3% (Rosenbaum, 1981*a,* p. 869). In her study of heroin addicts, however, Rosenbaum found that employment in "quasi-legitimate spheres" could allow working addicts to use heroin. "While it is generally not sanctioned, addicts employed in sex occupations such as topless dancing, massage parlors, and the pornographic industry are able to both maintain a heroin habit and work" (Rosenbaum, 1981*b,* p. 65). Legal employment with flexible schedules, such as taxi driving, could also enable a regular drug user to retain her employment.

Sex role socialization and associated gender role expectations have been proposed as additional forces for prostitution among drug-using women. Prostitution has traditionally been assumed to be women's "hustle of choice." This assumption is strongly linked to female gender roles in North American society which define women in sexual terms from an early age. Women's behavior has been described as counting "only in the sexual sphere" (Klein, 1973, p. 27). Women's sexually oriented socialization, role expectations, and gender role-determined criminal opportunities have ultimately resulted in a predominance of sexually oriented criminal behaviors among women (Hoffman-Bustamante, 1973; Klein, 1973). Being female in American society has been described as "prescrib(ing) an automatic loss of respect and reputation congruent with promiscuity and addiction" (James, 1976, p. 615).

## Reasons for Drug Use among Prostitutes

Preliminary research on reasons for drug use among prostitutes has revealed differing motivations. Goldstein (1979, p. 146) found that drugs were used by prostitutes *functionally,* to facilitate work performance, and *subculturally,* as expected activities of the drug-using subculture (i.e., both drug use and prostitution are expected behaviors). James (1976, p. 607) found that narcotic drug use increased with involvement of addict prostitutes in prostitution because the drugs, "1) made it easier to work, 2) increased their ability to withstand emotional and physical stress, 3) were available in their working environment, 4) helped them to relax after work, 5) could be easily purchased with their earnings, and 6) gave them a lot of pleasure."

The most commonly reported motive of drug use for prostitutes is functional—as an aid to socializing with clients (Goldstein, 1979). Certain types of nonnarcotic drugs, such as amphetamines, other stimulants, and alcohol, are used to facilitate work performance of prostitutes by combatting the physically and emotionally stressful aspects of their job (James et al., 1979, p. 216; Goldstein, 1979, p. 147). Narcotics can have functional occupational benefits among prostitutes and other people whose jobs require contact with the public. Heroin, for example, has been described as a drug which, in some occupations, could facilitate retaining the job: "in those work situations where the woman must endure constant haranguing by customers, heroin use can make the job more bearable" Rosenbaum (1981*b,* p. 65). While some prostitutes use alcohol and drugs in order to assist them in coping with their work, the Special Committee on

Pornography and Prostitution (1985) found that many do not use these substances while working because they want to be as alert as possible in what can often be a very dangerous job.

## Direction of the Relationship between Drug Use and Prostitution

Many researchers have examined the direction of the relationship between drug use and prostitution. While some women are engaged in either regular drug use or prostitution, others do both simultaneously. Most studies consider the temporal sequence of these two activities. Because no studies have fully explored these relationships (e.g., exploring *all* possible related variables and their interrelationships and using adequately defined and sized samples), tentative patterns rather than causal relationships can be reported. The three general theoretical patterns are as follows: (1) Prostitution precedes regular drug use; (2) regular drug use precedes prostitution; and (3) prostitution and regular drug use begin at the same time. Support for the first pattern is reported by Miller (1986). The overwhelming majority of women in her study who reported serious substance abuse problems developed these problems only after becoming prostitutes.

The second pattern is supported by Goldstein (1979), Silbert et al. (1982), and James (1976) (Fig. 1). Goldstein (1979) reported that among the 27 women in his study

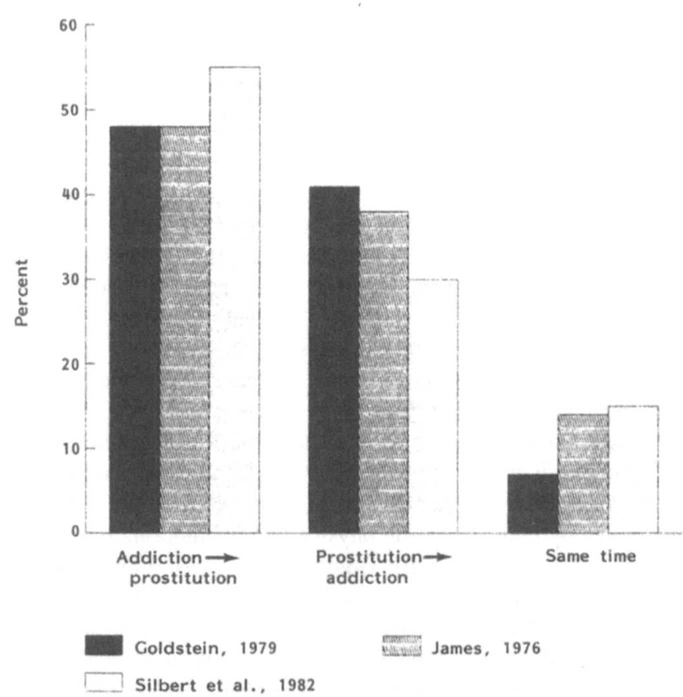


Figure 1. Sequence of initiation into drug addiction and prostitution in three subsamples of addict/prostitutes.

who were both addicts and prostitutes, addiction was only slightly more likely to predate prostitution (48%) than vice versa (41%). James (1976), in her study of 100 prostitutes, addicts, and addict prostitutes, found similar patterns between the onset of addiction and entrance into prostitution. An almost equal proportion of women reported addiction before (48%) and after (38%) prostitution. The time span between prostitution and onset of addiction was longer than that between addiction and subsequent prostitution. These patterns were essentially replicated in Silbert et al.'s (1982) study, with 55% of the women reporting addiction before prostitution and 30% reporting the reverse. Although no clear pattern has been established, women seem to be slightly more likely to be regular drug users prior to engaging in prostitution.

Other studies, in contrast, have indicated that criminal behavior, including prostitution, among female regular drug users emerges far earlier than their narcotic use. Inciardi et al. (1982), for example, found that prostitution was the first crime committed by 11% of the 63 black female heroin users studied. Clearly, prostitution is not, in all cases, entered into simply as a means of supporting drug use.

Other research has found that for some drug-using prostitutes, regular drug use and prostitution begin at the same time. Adler's assertion that addiction and prostitution can be simultaneously occurring elements of a deviant lifestyle is supported in some research. Addiction and prostitution began at the same time among 14% of James's (1976), and 15% of Silbert et al.'s (1982), and 7% of Goldstein's (1979) samples. Experimental drug use and criminal activity also began at similar ages among Inciardi and Pottieger's (1986) sample. The findings of these studies suggest that, for some women, drug use and criminal activity (including prostitution) are less likely to be causally related than to be the results of other factors. To assume such a cause–effect relationship is too simplistic, as many other factors influence this relationship.

Age could mediate the prostitution–drug use relationship. James (1976), for example, found that younger women get involved in regular drug use first and turn to prostitution as a support system, whereas women who enter prostitution at an older age are less likely to become regular drug users. The typical initiation of young women into prostitution has been described as a welcome by other street members, followed by a 2-week period of "partying" in which friendship, lodging, alcohol, and drugs are provided, after which a "payback" of a decision to work the street is expected (Fleischman, 1984). This pattern of initiation has been challenged by Bagley (1985), who found that among preteen and teenage women, entry into prostitution is not, by and large, strictly voluntary, but is coerced by the realities of poverty, homelessness, and relationships with street figures, including pimps.

Possible additional factors mediating or causing the prostitution–drug use relationship include type of drug used and willingness to engage in other criminal behaviors. Research suggests that regular use of illicit and particularly narcotic drugs may be more likely to lead to prostitution than vice versa. Goldstein (1979) found that narcotic addicts were almost twice as likely to become prostitutes as prostitutes were likely to become addicts. One explanation may be that entrance into prostitution among addict women can be an economic necessity for some women, whereas the step into addiction among prostitutes actually adds expense. At the same time, however, many prostitutes who use drugs supplement their incomes through drug dealing. Since some drug-using women may not be willing to engage in either drug sale or prostitution, escalation of otherwise unaffordable drug use may be effectively limited.

The level of drug use is another mediating factor. Although most studies report a high incidence of drug use among prostitutes, many describe an incompatibility between the social world of the addict who engages in street prostitution and the social world of the street prostitute who may or may not use drugs (see Miller, 1986). The lives of addicts are reportedly chaotic, focusing almost exclusively on obtaining the needed "score," which makes them undesirable members of cooperative prostitution networks. "[W]hen the addict most needs the deviant street network, she has the least to give it and is, in fact, perceived as a threat to it" (Miller, 1986, p. 111).

When interpreting these data, it is important to keep in mind that although many studies examine initiation patterns into both prostitution and drug use, temporal sequence alone does not sufficiently imply causality. One may conclude from the literature only that drug use and prostitution are interrelated. Although drug addiction may lead to prostitution in some instances, other factors are likely more important.

## Cultural Differences in Involvement in Drug Use and Prostitution

The cultural component of women's criminality has been found to be significant, yet has not been sufficiently examined in the literature. Studies consistently report large differences between prostitution and drug-using patterns of women from different cultural groups, yet few attempt to explain these differences. American studies generally find that among women who regularly use drugs, black women are involved in prostitution and other criminal activities to a much greater extent than are Hispanic or white women (File et al., 1974; Miller, 1986; Rosenbaum, 1981*a;* Weissman and File, 1976). One study (Silbert et al., 1982), however, reports much higher proportional involvement of white women than other cultural groups in prostitution. Inconsistent findings are reported about the relative patterns of criminal involvement of white and Hispanic women. Some studies report less involvement in prostitution among Hispanic women (Anglin and Hser, 1987; Hser et al., 1987*a*), but some report more (for example, Rosenbaum, 1981*a*) or the same (for example, Weissman and File, 1976) levels of involvement. Hispanic and white women are reportedly more likely than black women to become involved in prostitution because of a need for drugs (Miller, 1986).

In Canada, the cultural background of prostitutes is somewhat different than in the United States. In the Prairie Provinces, most prostitutes are young Native women. In large metropolitan areas, Native, as well as other visible minority women, are the majority of prostitutes (Special Committee on Pornography and Prostitution, 1985, p. 347).

Determining the etiology of women's drug abuse is currently constrained because the different causes, patterns, and consequences of racial and ethnic subgroups of women drug users have not been sufficiently explored. Until recently, when racial differences have been explored, the focus has been on white and black groups only. The important Native groups in Canada and Hispanic groups in the United States have virtually been ignored (Hser et al., 1987*b*). In addition, studies that do explore cultural differences generally ignore sex differences within the cultures (Hser et al., 1987*a*).

This section has provided some information about the relationship between regular drug use and prostitution among women. The literature presents findings which are inconsistent and which provide an incomplete understanding of the relationship. Possible explanations for the conflictual findings include the following: The use of small and/or atypical samples; different methods of recruiting and interviewing; and social, political, economic, legal, and geographical variations. Despite the weaknesses in the literature, it leaves no doubt that a complex relationship exists. While sex role socialization and functional assistance in the work of prostitution seem to contribute to the likelihood of drug users engaging in prostitution, economic motives were generally found to be most compelling. Because the forms of prostitution are so diverse, few generalizations about prostitutes' experiences, including their drug-using experiences, can be made in the areas explored. Most studies focus on street prostitutes (or streetwalkers), whose drug and prostitution experiences may be quite different from those of other prostitutes. Many of the relationships between drug use and prostitution that have been explored here are not unique to prostitution. As Goldstein concluded, "the use of drugs by prostitutes may constitute only a specific case or example of a more general relationship between drug use and certain types of work" (1979, p. 151). Clearly, more research is needed.

While little research on women, drug use, and prostitution has been carried out in Canada, future research can be guided by that which has been done in the United States and Britain. Perhaps the most compelling reason for such research was articulated in the City of Regina's submission to the Special Committee on Pornography and Prostitution (1985, p. 350):

> National figures show that instances of drug use and addiction are inordinately high among street prostitutes, so much so that between violent death and drug overdose their mortality rate may be forty times the national average.

Many important research questions have been raised throughout this chapter, including the following:

- What is the prevalence of drug use among women employed in quasilegitimate and legitimate occupations?
- What are the occupations in which women run a relatively high risk of becoming regular drug users?
- What are the functional and dysfunctional aspects of drug use among women as they relate to specific occupations and associated tasks?
- What role does the need for money to buy drugs play in motivating regular drug users to engage in prostitution?
- What are the functional and dysfunctional aspects of drug use among the various types of drug-using prostitutes?
- What factors lead to maturation from or discontinuation of both regular drug use and prostitution? Does maturation/discontinuation of both drug use and prostitution occur at the same time?
- What are the criminal behavior patterns of women addicts, prostitutes, and addict prostitutes over time?
- What are the criminal behavior patterns of different types of prostitutes over time?
- What are the social, political, economic, and cultural factors influencing changes

in the criminal behaviors of drug-using women? What role do these factors play in influencing the behaviors?

- What are the cultural differences in patterns of regular drug use and prostitution? What factors explain these cultural differences?

In summary, the traditional assumptions, that addiction explains the entry of most women into a career of prostitution or that taking drugs is essential to cope with the nature of the work, have been dismissed as overly simplistic. The more recent literature reviewed in this section portrays a dynamic and complex relationship between drug use and prostitution. For many drug-using prostitutes, their range of choices is circumscribed by poverty and lack of education. Prostitution may, in many instances, simply be the most lucrative profession open. But this is somewhat different than viewing prostitutes as helpless victims of an enslaving habit. Like male criminals, women can make rational choices that serve a narrow range of self-interests. It is also important to recognize that while most prostitutes use illicit drugs, not all are addicted to them.

## 4. CONCLUDING REMARKS

It is evident, when studying the use of illicit drugs by women within the larger framework of criminal behavior, that many of the stereotypes of female drug users have their roots in more general assumptions about female deviance. Thus, female addicts and female criminals have been viewed as more "abnormal" than their male counterparts. And indeed, the past depictions of the lives of female addicts were almost synonymous with lives of prostitutes. Female drug use, like female criminality, had been underresearched, at least until the 1970s when the imbalance began to be rectified.

Surveys of illicit drug use in the population which include women demonstrate that, like men, women are capable of experimenting with a variety of illicit substances and, for the most part, use them infrequently without developing dependence. The surveys also document that recreational illicit drug use is clearly more common for men than women, and men are also more likely to be heavier users of all illicit substances. Earlier predictions of convergence of male and female patterns of illicit drug use (i.e., during the first rapid increases of this behavior in the late 1960s and early 1970s) assumed that women's use levels would rise to approximate levels of use among men. In fact, the opposite occurred, through a leveling off and decline in drug use in the 1980s. The resulting convergence in the United States, although slight, reflects a more rapid dropoff by men than women in the use of several illicit drugs. It is not clear to what extent these patterns will be mirrored in Canada. In both countries, an exception to watch closely is cocaine, a new arrival on the illicit drug scene, for which certain age–sex groups may be registering increased use.

The literature on prostitution, drug use, and other criminality has enjoyed an upsurge in recent years which has challenged earlier simplistic assumptions about a cause–effect relationship. Female addicts tend to commit more crimes than their nonaddicted sisters; however, female addicts are less criminally involved than male addicts. Nevertheless, female addicts engage in less prostitution and in a greater variety of independent criminal activities than is commonly believed. Conversely, not all prostitutes are addicted, though their rates of illicit drug use are higher than in the general population. Moreover, many display patterns of very little or no recreational drug use. A more recent trend in the literature has been to recognize the role of autonomy and choice in the lives of prostitutes, in contrast to the earlier portrayals of enslaved victims.

What is the future of female illicit drug use? We concur with Ferrence (1984) in the view that dramatic increases in this behavior by women are unlikely. It is important in future research to assess opportunity factors (e.g., income, access) and the possible risk factors associated with specific occupations.

Drug use by women also may be more sensitive to fluctuations in the life cycle such as marriage, childbearing, and aging. The growing appreciation of volition in studies of female criminality is a healthy counterbalance to the excessively passive image of women in earlier criminological theories and a necessary prerequisite to the testing of gender-neutral explanations of crime and deviance. We have, for purposes of convenience, divided this chapter into the two sections of women in the illicit recreational drug milieu and addicted women. Like men's drug use, women's drug use falls along a continuum. The challenge for researchers is to explain the reasons for variation in levels of drug use and related problems and to suggest the most appropriate prevention strategies for both sexes.

### Acknowledgments

The authors thank Joan Moreau and Sharon Rutter for their assistance with this chapter. They also thank Yuet-Wah Cheung, Reginald Smart, and anonymous reviewers for their helpful comments and suggestions.

## REFERENCES

Adleberg, E., and Currie, C., eds., 1987, *Too Few to Count: Canadian Women in Conflict with the Law*, Press Gang Publishers, Vancouver.

Adler, F., 1975, *Sisters in Crime*, McGraw-Hill, New York.

Adler, F. and Simon, R. J., 1979, *The Criminology of Deviant Women*, Houghton Mifflin, Boston.

Anglin, M. D., and Hser, Y-I., 1987, Addicted women and crime, *Criminology* **25**:359–397.

Anglin, M. D., Hser, Y-I., and McGlothlin, W., 1987, Sex differences in addict careers. 2. Becoming addicted, *Am. J. Drug Alcohol Abuse* **13**:59–71.

Bagley, C., 1985, Child sexual abuse and juvenile prostitution: A comment on the Badgley Report On Sexual Offences against Children and Youth, *Can. J. Public Health* **76**:65–66.

Bell, D. S., 1980, Dependence on psychotropic drugs and analgesics in men and women, in: *Alcohol and Drug Problems in Women* (O. J. Kalant, ed.), pp. 423–463, Plenum Press, New York.

Blackwell, J., 1983, Drifting, controlling and overcoming: Opiate users who avoid becoming chronically dependent, *J. Drug Issues* **13**:219–235.

Bowker, L. H., 1978*a*, Women and drugs; Beyond the hippie subculture, in: *Women, Crime and the Criminal Justice System* (L. H. Bowker, ed.), pp. 57–99, Lexington Books, Lexington, MA.

Bowker, L. H., 1978*b*, The relationship between sex, drugs, and sexual behavior on a college campus, *Drug Forum* **7**:69–80.

Bureau of Dangerous Drugs, Health Protection Branch, 1981–1986, *Annual Reports*, Health and Welfare Canada, Ottawa.

Colten, M. E., and Marsh, J. C., 1984, A sex-roles perspective on drug and alcohol use by women, in: *Sex Roles and Psychopathology* (C. S. Widom, ed.), pp. 217–248, Plenum Press, New York.

Cooperstock, R., 1976, Psychotropic drug use among women, *Can. Med. Assoc. J.* **115:**760–763.

Cuskey, W. R., Premkumar, T., and Sigel, L., 1972, Survey of opiate addiction among females in the Untied States between 1850 and 1970, *Public Health Rev.* **1:**5–39.

Datesman, S. K., 1981, Women, crime, and drugs, in: *The Drugs–Crime Connection* (J. A. Inciardi, ed.), pp. 85–104, Sage Publications, Beverly Hills, CA.

Datesman, S. K., and Inciardi, J. A., 1979, Female heroin use, criminality, and prostitution, *Contemp. Drug Problems* **8:**455–473.

d'Orban, P. T., 1970, Heroin dependence and delinquency in women—A study of heroin addicts in Holloway Prison, *Br. J. Addiction* **65:**67–78.

d'Orban, P. T., 1973, Female narcotic addicts: A follow-up study of criminal and addiction careers, *Br. Med. J.* **4:**345–347.

Erickson, P. G., 1989, Living with prohibition: Regular cannabis users, legal sanctions and informal controls, *Int. J. Addictions* **24:**175–188.

Erickson, P. G. and Murray, G. F., 1989, Sex differences in cocaine use and experiences: A double standard revived? *Am. J. Drug Alcohol Abuse,* **15:**135–152.

Erickson, P. G., Adlaf, E. M., Murray, G. F., and Smart, R. G., 1987, *The Steel Drug: Cocaine in Perspective,* D. C. Heath, Lexington, MA.

Ferrence, R. G., 1984, Preventing substance abuse: Implications of sex differences in patterns of use, *Contemp. Drug Problems* **12:**439–458.

Ferrence, R. G., and Whitehead, P. C., 1980, Sex differences in psychoactive drug use: Recent epidemiology, in: *Alcohol and Drug Problems in Women* (O. J. Kalant, ed.), pp. 125–201, Plenum Press, New York.

File, K. N., 1976, Sex roles and street roles, *Int. J. Addictions* **11:**263–268.

File, K. N., McCahill, T. W., and Savitz, L. D., 1974, Narcotics involvement and female criminality, *Addictive Dis.: Int. J.* **1:**177–188.

Fillmore, K. M., 1984, "When angels fall": Women's drinking as cultural preoccupation and as reality, in: *Alcohol Problems in Women* (S. C. Wilsnack and L. J. Beckman, eds.), pp. 7–35, Guilford Press, New York.

Fleischman, J., 1984, *A Report on Prostitution in Ontario,* Working Papers on Pornography and Prostitution Report #10. Department of justice, Ottawa.

Goldstein, P. J., 1979, *Prostitution and Drugs,* D. C. Heath, Lexington, MA.

Hagan, J., Gillis, A. R., and Simpson, J., 1985, The class structure of gender and delinquency: Toward a power–control theory of common delinquent behavior, *Am. J. Sociol.* **90:**1151–1178.

Hoffman-Bustamante, D., 1973, The nature of female criminality, *Issues Criminol.* **8:**117–136.

Hser, Y-I., Anglin, M. D., and Booth, M. W., 1987*a,* Sex differences in addict careers. 3. Addiction, *Am. J. Drug Alcohol Abuse* **13:**231–251.

Hser, Y-I., Anglin, M. D., and McGlothlin, W., 1987*b,* Sex differences in addict careers. 1. Initiation of use, *Am. J. Drug Alcohol Abuse* **13:**33–57.

Inciardi, J. A., 1986, *The War on Drugs: Heroin, Cocaine, Crime, and Public Policy,* Mayfield, Palo Alto, CA.

Inciardi, J. A., and Pottieger, A. E., 1986, Drug use and crime among two cohorts of women narcotics users: An empirical assessment, *J. Drug Issues* **16:**91–106.

Inciardi, J. A., Pottieger, A. E., and Faupel, C. E., 1982, Black women, heroin and crime: Some empirical notes, *J. Drug Issues* **12:**241–250.

James, J., 1976, Prostitution and addiction: An interdisciplinary approach, *Addictive Dis.: Int. J.* **2:**601–618.

James, J., Gosho, C., and Wohl, R. W., 1979, The relationship between female criminality and drug use, *Int. J. Addictions* **14:**215–229.

Johnson, B. D., Goldstein, P. J., Preble, E., Schmeider, J., Lipton, D. S., Sprunt, B., and Miller, T., 1985, *Taking Care of Business; The Economics of Crime by Heroin Abusers,* D. C. Heath, Lexington, MA.

Johnson, H., 1987, Getting the facts straight: A statistical overview, in: *Too Few to Count: Canadian Women in Conflict with the Law* (E. Adelberg and C. Currie, eds.), pp. 23–46, Press Gang, Vancouver, BC.

Johnston, L. D., O'Malley, P. M., and Bachman, J. G., 1987, *National Trends in Drug Use and Related Factors among American High School Students and Young Adults, 1975–1986*, National Institute on Drug Abuse, Rockville, MD.

Kalant, O. J., 1980, Sex differences in alcohol and drug problems—Some highlights, in: *Alcohol and Drug Problems in Women* (O. J. Kalant, ed.), pp. 1–24, Plenum Press, New York.

Kaplan, H. B., Martin, S. S., Johnson, R. J., and Robins, C. A., 1986, Escalation of marijuana use: Application of a general theory of deviant behavior, *J. Health Social Behav.* **27**:44–61.

Klein, D., 1973, The etiology of female crime: A review of the literature, *Issues Criminol.* **8**:3–30.

Klein, D. and Kress, J., 1976, Any woman's blues: A critical overview of women, crime and the criminal justice system, *Crime Social Justice* **5**:34–49.

Lanphier, C. M., and McCauley, G. F., 1985, Prevalence and consequences of non-medical use of drugs among Canadian Forces personnel: 1982, *Am. J. Drug Alcohol Abuse* **11**:231–247.

Lautt, M., 1984, *A Report on Prostitution in the Prairie Provinces*, Working Paper on Pornography and Prostitution Report #9, Department of Justice, Ottawa.

Lowman, J., 1986, Prostitution in Vancouver: Some notes on the genesis of social problem, *Can. J. Criminol.* **28**:1–16.

Lowman, J., 1987, Taking young prostitutes seriously, *Can. Rev. Sociol. Anthropol.* **24**:99–116.

Marshall, N., and Hendtlass, J., 1986, Drugs and prostitution, *J. Drug Issues* **16**:237–248.

Miller, E. M., 1983, International trends in the study of female criminality: An essay review, *Contemp. Crises* **7**:59–70.

Miller, E. M., 1986, *Street Woman*, Temple University Press, Philadelphia.

Murphy, S. B., Reinarman, C., and Waldorf, D., 1986, *An 11-Year Follow-up of a Network of 27 Cocaine Users*, Presented at the annual meeting of the Society for the Study of Social Problems, New York, August.

Nagel, I., and Hagan, J., 1982, Gender and crime: Offense patterns and criminal court sanction, in: *Crime and Justice* (N. Morris and M. Tonry, eds.), pp. 91–144, University of Chicago Press, Chicago.

Newcomb, M. D., and Bentler, P. M., 1986, Cocaine use among adolescents: Longitudinal associations with social context, psychopathology, and use of other substances, *Addictive Behav.* **11**:263–273.

Nicholl, C., 1985, *The Fruit Palace*, St. Martin's Press, New York.

Nielson, M., and Hirabayashi, G., 1975, *Women and Soft Drug Use: The Changing Adolescent Scene*, Non-Medical use of Drugs Directorate, Health and Welfare Canada, Ottawa.

Nurco, D. N., Wagner, N., and Stephenson, P., 1982, Female narcotic addicts; Changing profiles, *J. Addictions Health* **3**:62–105.

Prather, J. E., and Fidell, L. S., 1978, Drug use and abuse among women: An overview, *Int. J. Addictions* **13**:863–885.

Provine, D. M., 1987, Gender, crime, and criminal justice: Edwards' *Women on Trial, Am. Bar Foundation Res. J.* **3**:571–583.

Rosenbaum, M., 1981*a*, Sex roles among deviants; The woman addict, *Int. J. Addictions* **16**:859–877.

Rosenbaum, M., 1981*b*, *Women on Heroin*, Rutgers University Press, New Brunswick, NJ.

Sheehy, G., 1971, *Hustling: Prostitution in Our Wide Open Society*, Delacorte Press, New York.

Silbert, M. H., Pines, A. M., and Lynch, T., 1982, Substance abuse and prostitution, *J. Psychoactive Drugs* **14**:193–197.

Silverman, I. J., 1982, Women, crime and drugs, *J. Drug Issues* **12**:167–183.

Simon, R. J., 1979, Arrest statistics, in: *The Criminology of Deviant Women* (F. Adler and R. J. Simon, eds.), pp. 101–113, Houghton Mifflin, Boston.

Simpson, S. S., 1987, *Women in Elite Deviance: A Grounded Theory*, Presented at the 39th annual meeting of the American Society of Criminology, Montreal, November.

Smart, R. G., and Adlaf, E. M., 1987*a*, *Alcohol and Other Drug Use Among Ontario Students in 1987, and Trends since 1977*, Addiction Research Foundation, Toronto.

Smart, R. G., and Adlaf, E. M., 1987*b*, *Alcohol and Other Drug Use Among Ontario Adults: 1977–1987*, Addiction Research Foundation, Toronto.

Smith, D. A., and Paternoster, R., 1987, The gender gap in theories of deviance: Issues and evidence, *J. Res. Crime Delinquency* **24:**140–172.

Special Committee on Pornography and Prostitution, 1985, *Pornography and Prostitution in Canada*, Department of Supply and Services, Ottawa.

Steffensmeier, D. J., 1987, *Contemporary Patterns of Female Criminality*, Presented at the 39th annual meeting of the American Society of Criminology, Montreal, November.

Suffet, F., and Brotman, R., 1976, Female drug use: Some observations, *Int. J. Addictions* **11:**19–33.

Trebach, A., 1982, *The Heroin Solution*, Yale University Press, New Haven, CT.

Wechsler, H., and McFadden, M., 1976, Sex differences in adolescent alcohol and drug use: A disappearing phenomenon, *J. Stud. Alcohol* **37:**1291–1301.

Weissman, J. C., and File, K. N., 1976, Criminal behavior patterns of female addicts: A comparison of findings in two cities, *Int. J. Addictions* **11:**1063–1077.

Yamaguchi, K., and Kandel, D. B., 1985, On the resolution of role incompatibility: A life event history analysis of family roles and marijuana use, *Am. J. Sociol.* **90:**1284–1325.

# 9

# The Inverse Relationship between Tobacco Use and Body Weight

NEIL E. GRUNBERG

## 1. INTRODUCTION

Cigarette smoking in the United States is responsible for one-third of cardiovascular diseases, one-third of cancer deaths, a large number of respiratory diseases, and a substantial proportion of deaths by fire (USDHEW, 1979; USDHHS, 1982, 1983, 1984). Other forms of tobacco use (e.g., smokeless tobacco) are responsible for additional cases of neck and head cancer (USDHHS, 1986; NIH Consensus Conference, 1986). In fact, more than twice as many deaths are caused by tobacco products in this country than by all other addictive drugs combined, including alcohol (USDHHS, 1988). Despite the well-known and extensively documented health risks of cigarette smoking and tobacco use, 51.1 million Americans smoke cigarettes and additional millions consume other forms of tobacco (USDHHS, 1988). Improved understanding of why people use tobacco products and are reluctant to give them up is important in order to design more effective cessation and prevention strategies.

Many smokers report that control of body weight is a major reason why they smoke and refuse to quit (Charlton, 1984; Klesges and Klesges, 1988; Page, 1983). This chapter reviews evidence that there is an inverse relationship between cigarette smoking and body weight and discusses the role of nicotine in this relationship. Possible reasons for the inverse relationships between smoking and body weight, and nicotine and body weight, are presented, and studies that examine each of these reasons are reviewed. Mechanisms that may underlie the reasons for the nicotine/body weight relationship are discussed. Finally, the data and postulates linking nicotine and body weight are considered with respect to other pharmacological agents of addiction.

NEIL E. GRUNBERG • Medical Psychology Department, Uniformed Services University of the Health Sciences, Bethesda, Maryland 20814-4799. The opinions or assertions contained herein are the private ones of the author and are not to be construed as official or reflecting the views of the Department of Defense or the Uniformed Services University of the Health Sciences.

## 2. CIGARETTE SMOKING AND BODY WEIGHT

The generalization that cigarette smoking helps to control body weight is supported by two types of data: (1) cross-sectional between-subjects comparisons of the body weights of smokers and nonsmokers; and (2) longitudinal within-subject assessment of the body weights of smokers who quit smoking compared to nonsmokers. These two data bases are reviewed.

### Between-Subjects Comparisons of the Body Weights of Smokers, Nonsmokers, and Ex-smokers

Studies comparing the body weights of smokers and nonsmokers date back 100 years. There are several reports published in the 19th century that tobacco use stunts growth (Otis, 1884; Kitchen, 1889; Seaver, 1897). Between 1900 and 1970, many studies reported that tobacco use was associated with lower body weights (Anderson, 1914; Ashford et al., 1961; Blackburn et al., 1960; Bogen, 1929; Fink, 1921; Heath, 1958; Higgins and Kjelsberg, 1967; Holt, 1921; Jenkins et al., 1968; Lickint, 1933; Pemberton and Macleod, 1956; Taylor, 1910). However, some studies conducted during this period reported no significant weight differences between smokers and nonsmokers (Anderson, 1914; Diehl, 1929; Hadley, 1941; Holt, 1922–1923; Peters and Ferris, 1967; Shah et al., 1959; Short et al., 1939; Turley and Harrison, 1932).

Grunberg (1980, 1986*a*) pointed out that most of the null findings regarding smoking and body weight were based on studies of adolescents and young adult males. He suggested that the limited exposure of these subjects to tobacco may be partially responsible for the lack of a smoking/body weight relationship. Also, the high metabolic rates that naturally occur for young people may have masked or offset any effects of tobacco on body weight. Possibly, the sex of the subjects contributed to the weak findings as well.

Studies that included a large age range of subjects report a consistent inverse relationship between cigarette smoking and body weight. Moreover, examination of subjects by age group supports Grunberg's (1980, 1986*a*) suggestion that the null findings reported by some investigators are attributable to the youth of their subjects. For example, Higgins and Kjelsberg (1967) compared the body weights of 5020 smokers and nonsmokers who ranged in age from 16 to 79 years. Over all ages smokers weighed significantly less (roughly 8 lb less) than did nonsmokers. However, the 16- to 19-year-old smokers had body weights similar to their nonsmoking counterparts. Kopczynski (1972) studied 1245 smokers and 1814 nonsmokers and similarly reported that, except for 19- to 20-year-old males, smokers weighed less than comparably aged nonsmokers.

A recent review (USDHHS, 1988) of cross-sectional studies on smoking and body weight published between 1971 and 1987 revealed the following (see Table 1): (1) 25 of the 28 (i.e., 89%) studies found that smokers weighed less than nonsmokers; (2) one study reported this relationship for women but not for men (Sutherland et al., 1980); (3) one study reported this relationship for 45- to 49-year-old men but not for 40- to 44-year-old men (Hjermann et al., 1976); (4) one study did not find a body weight difference (Waller and Brooks, 1972).

Table 1. Cross-Sectional Evaluations of Smoking and Body Weight[a]

| Study | Design and sample | Major results | Moderator variables | Limitations |
|---|---|---|---|---|
| Albanes et al. (1987) | 12,103 men and women, NHANES II Survey | Smokers weighed 5.95 lb less than nonsmokers, controlled for age, sex; smokers taller and leaner than nonsmokers, based on skinfold | Age: current smokers gained less after age 25 than either nonsmokers or ex-smokers<br>Smoking duration: body mass index decreased with smoking duration increase<br>Smoking rate: moderate smokers leaner than low or high rate smokers | Smoking self-report |
| Andrews and McGarry (1972) | All 18,631 pregnant women, Cardiff, Wales, 1965–1968 | Across all heights, smoking mothers lighter than nonsmokers | | Pregnant women only; birth survey record data; actual weight changes not presented |
| Biener (1981) | 274 (174 men, 100 women) ex-smokers, worksite setting | 49% women, 39% men gained weight following cessation; quitter approximate average gain: women 11 lb, men 15 lb | | Retrospective postcessation gain self-report; no nonsmoker control group |
| Blair et al. (1980) | 183 white male, 284 white female insurance company employees; average age 34 | Smokers 2.64–7.5 lb lighter than nonsmokers, 0.88–15.21 lb lighter than ex-smokers; smaller skinfolds for smokers of both sexes than nonsmokers | | Small sample size; white office workers only |
| Bjelke (1971) | 8,638 male, 10,331 female respondents, mail survey. Norway general population "systematic sample" | Used "bulk index" (weight/height$^2$); both sexes current smokers less bulky than quitters and never smokers | Smoking rate: not related to weight<br>Age: older respondents greater smoker/nonsmoker bulk differences<br>Sex: women greater smoker/nonsmoker bulk differences | Self-report by mail; no weights, no statistical analyses presented |

*(continued)*

Table 1. *(Continued)*

| Study | Design and sample | Major results | Moderator variables | Limitations |
|---|---|---|---|---|
| Fehily et al. (1984) | 211 nonsmoking, 282 smoking men, aged 45–59, heart disease study | Smokers weighed 7.5–10.3 lb less than nonsmokers, 6.6–9.4 lb less than ex-smokers; pipe/cigar smokers weighed 2.4 lb more than nonsmokers; weight/height$^2$ index results similar | | Small, all white, restricted sample; smoking self-report |
| Fisher and Gordon (1985) | 15% random sample, 10 U.S., Canadian clinics; 2269 male, 2105 female whites, aged 20–59, LRC Prevalence Study | Men: smoking nondrinkers weighed 6.6 lb less than nonsmoking nondrinkers; smoking drinkers weighed 2.2 lb less than nonsmoking drinkers<br>Women: smoking nondrinkers weighed 2.2 lb less than nonsmoking nondrinkers; smoking drinkers weighed 4.4 lb less than nonsmoking drinkers | | All white population; smoking self-report |
| Friedman et al. (1981) | 38 smoking-discordant monozygotic twin pairs, average age 40 years | Smokers weighed 5.07 lb less than nonsmokers | | Self-report by mail; small restricted sample |
| Garn et al. (1978) | 17,649 pregnant women, national health survey | Smoking mothers prepregnancy weight less than nonsmoking mothers; difference: whites 2.43 lb, blacks 3.53 lb | SES and race: no smoking/weight relationship influence | Pregnant women only; self-reports |
| Garrison et al. (1983) | Framingham study participants; assessed 1949–1952 | Nonsmokers 55% of highest weight group; smokers 80% of lowest weight group | | Sample size, weights not given; no statistical evaluation |
| Goldbourt and Medalie (1977) | 10,059 male government workers, aged 40–65 | Current smokers 1/4 inch taller, 2.36 lb less than nonsmokers; ex-smokers in between; leaner skinfolds for smokers than ex-smokers and nonsmokers | | Limited age range, employment group; smoking self-report |
| Gyntelberg and | 5249 employed men, aged 40– | Nondrinking smokers 1.5 per- | | All-male sample, one city; |

| | | | | |
|---|---|---|---|---|
| Meyer (1974) | 59, Denmark | centile points lighter than nondrinking nonsmokers; light drinking smokers 2.9 percentile points lighter; heavy drinking smokers 5.9 percentile points lighter than drinking nonsmokers | | smoking self-report |
| Hjermann et al. (1976) | Approximately 18,000 male participants, aged 40–49, coronary risk factor screening, Oslo | Aged 45–49 smokers body weight 3.09 lb less than nonsmokers; aged 40–44 difference not significant; no group weight/height$^2$ index differences | Smoking rate: heavy smoker (>20/day) body weights higher than lighter smoker<br>Age: older smokers (45–49) weighed less than nonsmokers; younger smokers (40–44) no effect | Smoking self-report; limited age range; one city; all men |
| Holcomb and Meigs (1972) | 226 manufacturing company male hourly employees, aged 55–59 | Mild to moderate smokers 14 lb lighter than never-smokers, ex-smokers, and heavy smokers | Smoking rate: heavy smokers (> 1 pack/day) heavier than lighter smokers, equivalent to nonsmokers | Smoking self-report; limited age, incomes; all men |
| Huston and Stenson (1974) | 184 men, British field regiment | $\leq$10 mm subscapular skinfold men averaged 22 cigarettes/day; $\geq$15 mm subscapular skinfold men averaged 12 cigarettes/day | | Limited male sample; smoking self-report; no separate smoker/nonsmoker data |
| Jacobs and Gottenborg (1981) | 3291 white men and women, aged 20–59, no cardiovascular disease or elevated risk factors; randomly selected middle-class suburb census tract blacks | Smokers lighter than never smokers and quitters | Smoking rate: male moderate smokers (14–29 cigarettes/day) 6.39 lb lighter than nonsmokers, 2.65–9.93 lb lighter than light and heavy smokers; female moderate smokers 5.07 lb lighter than never smokers, 1.54–8.38 lb lighter than heavy smokers<br>Age: moderate/never-smoker weight difference increased with age | Smoking self-report; restricted population |

(*continued*)

Table 1. *(Continued)*

| Study | Design and sample | Major results | Moderator variables | Limitations |
|---|---|---|---|---|
| Khosla and Lowe (1971) | 10,482 male steel workers, Wales | Per weight/height$^2$ index, smokers lighter than nonsmokers | Smoking rate: heavy smokers (>35 cigarettes/day) heavier than moderate smokers (15–34)<br>Age: group weight differences increased after age 35 | Smoking self-report; restricted population |
| Kittel et al. (1978) | 8284 male factory workers, Belgium | Relative weights significantly lower for cigarette smokers than never-smokers, ex-smokers, and pipe/cigar smokers | | Limited population, risk factor treatment program |
| Kopczynski (1972) | 3059 random selectees, pulmonary disease study, Poland | Nonsmokers heavier than smokers, except 20-year-old men | Sex, age, smoking rate: no smoking/weight relationship influence | Smoking self-report; weights not reported |
| Lincoln (1970) | 3220 male household heads, aged 41–70, across United States | Smokers weighed 3–14 lb less than nonsmokers | SES: smoker/nonsmoker weight difference increased as income decreased<br>Smoking rate: heavy smokers (≥21 cigarettes/day) weighed 4 lb more, moderate smokers (11–20) 4 lb less than all-smoker average | Restricted population; men |
| Matsuya (1982) | 90 telephone employees, Japan | Ex-smokers weighed 5.29 lb more than nonsmokers; light smokers 2.87 lb less, heavy smokers 0.44 lb less than ex-smokers | | Small, nonrepresentative sample; data self-report |
| Nemery et al. (1983) | 210 steelworkers, aged 45–55, ≥10 years service, Belgium | Smokers weighed 12.13 lb less than never-smokers, 14.33 lb less than ex-smokers | | Restricted population; smoking self-report |

| | | | | |
|---|---|---|---|---|
| Stamford et al. (1984*a*) | 164 (56 smokers, 108 nonsmokers) premenopausal women; smokers: ≥20 cigarettes/day, ≥5 years, inhale | Smokers weighed 11.96 lb less, had lower average Quetelet Index than nonsmokers | | Small sample size; premenopausal women only; data self-report |
| Stamford et al. (1984*b*) | 269 adult men, fitness center screened; smokers: ≥20 cigarettes/day, ≥5 years, inhale | Smokers weighed 14.99 lb less, had 12% less body fat than nonsmokers | | Select sample, exercising men; smoking self-report; heavy smokers |
| Stephens and Pederson (1983) | 15,518 persons aged >10; questionnaire, anthropometry | Smokers weighed less than nonsmokers; female smokers weighed 1.32 lb more to 5.73 lb less than female nonsmokers; men weighed 3.09–7.7 lb less; smokers averaged 3.445 lb less than nonsmokers | | White women self-report, smoking self-report; no statistical significance tests |
| Sutherland et al. (1980) | Random sample, 175 men and women, rural town, New Zealand | Weight/height$^2$ index and skinfolds significantly higher in nonsmoking than smoking women; higher for nonsmoking men, but not significant | Sex: male smokers not significantly leaner than nonsmokers; smoking women lighter than nonsmoking women | Smoking self-report; small sample size |
| Waller and Brooks (1972) | 2169 health exhibit visitors | "Little weight difference" among current smokers, nonsmokers, and ex-smokers | | Smoking self-report; bathroom scale weight; health-conscious population; high % cigar/pipe smokers; no statistical evaluations |
| Zeiner-Henriksen (1976) | Approximately 15,000 randomly selected Norwegians | Current smokers average and relative weight lower than nonsmokers or ex-smokers | | Smoking and weight self-report, questionnaire |

[a]From USDHHS, 1988.

Several cross-sectional studies of smoking and body weight have broadly classified daily cigarette consumption (e.g., <15, 15–24, 25–34, 35+) and have compared these self-reported estimates to body weight (Albanes et al., 1987; Hjermann et al., 1976; Holcomb and Meigs, 1972; Jacobs and Gottenborg, 1981; Khosla and Lowe, 1971; Lincoln, 1970; Schoenborn and Benson, 1988; Stephens and Pederson, 1983). Overall, these analyses have yielded inverse relationships between smoking and body weight and clear inverse relationships exist from 0 to a pack or so of cigarettes a day. However, many of these analyses report curvilinear functions, with a trough in body weight at about 20 cigarettes per day.

The fact that, in these studies, body weight does not continue to decline with cigarette consumption greater than a pack a day can follow from several different factors. Most conservatively, this curvilinear function potentially raises qualifications on the inverse smoking/body weight relationship. Perhaps "heavy smokers" is a meaningful *double entendre* that identifies a group of smokers who, like "chippers" (people who do not appear to be addicted to tobacco), are less responsive to the effects of nicotine than are most smokers. This interesting possibility deserves careful consideration. Alternatively, there are no qualifications necessary. It is important to remember that these cigarette consumption analyses are cross-sectional and, therefore, compare different people. People who smoke more are usually older, are a smaller percentage of the population and are a less representative subsample, are more likely to be male, tend to consume more alcohol, and are different individuals. Moreover, differences in self-reported amounts of cigarettes consumed per day are questionably related to nicotine intake. Some of these differences could be controlled statistically, but few studies have reported the results with sophisticated multivariate analyses of these variables. Even when they are controlled statistically, the analyses are still cross-sectional and therefore compare different people. To determine the effects of smoking on body weight, therefore, it is important to examine body weight as smoking behavior changes.

In general, cross-sectional studies indicate that smokers weigh less than comparably aged, same-sex nonsmokers. It is likely that tobacco use is responsible for the body weight differences between smokers and nonsmokers. However, between-subjects comparisons are open to several interpretations. Based on these data alone, it remains possible that people who choose to consume cigarettes and other forms of tobacco may weigh less than nonsmokers for some reason other than tobacco consumption. If tobacco use is not the culprit, then cessation of tobacco use should not lead to weight gains. If tobacco use is the key reason for the difference in body weight between smokers and nonsmokers, then cessation of tobacco consumption should be accompanied by weight gains.

## Within-Subject Comparisons of Body Weight with Changes in Smoking

Longitudinal studies of body weights of smokers before and after they quit smoking began appearing in the research literature in the late 1960s (e.g., Peterson et al., 1968, reported that smokers who quit smoking gain weight). Some of these studies compared smokers who quit with smokers who kept smoking; some studies included nonsmokers as a control group to allow for changes in body weight with age; and some studies included ex-smokers who were not smoking over the period of the time studied. A recent review of the 43 longitudinal studies of this type published between 1970 and 1980 (USDHHS, 1988) revealed that 37 of 43 (86%) found that cessation of smoking resulted in weight gains that exceeded weight gains by nonsmokers, and that people who began smoking lost weight compared to nonsmokers who did not begin smoking (see Table 2). Of the six studies that did not report these findings, (1) three studies examined pregnant women (Gormican et al., 1980; Haworth et al., 1980; Rantakallio and Hartikainen-Sorri, 1981); (2) two studies compared subjects who were making broad life-style changes because they were at high risk for cardiovascular diseases (Hickey and Mulcahy, 1973; Holme et al., 1985); and (3) one study reported too little information to clearly conclude what differences occurred (Kramer, 1982).

Based on cross-sectional and longitudinal studies, smokers generally weigh less than nonsmokers and many smokers who quit smoking gain weight. There are individuals, of course, who do not show these effects, possibly because they intentionally diet or exercise to avoid unwanted weight gains. Overall, the inverse relationship between cigarette smoking and weight gain is clear.

## 3. DRAWING CAUSAL CONCLUSIONS ABOUT SMOKING AND BODY WEIGHT: THE ROLE OF NICOTINE

Despite the clarity and consistency of the cross-sectional evidence, this type of data does not allow causal conclusions to be unequivocally drawn. Longitudinal evidence increases confidence in inferring causality, but nothing is as convincing as a true experiment. With respect to the effects of tobacco or its constituents on body weight, experiments with human subjects randomly assigned to smoking or no-smoking conditions for days, months, or years are considered unethical and, therefore, are impossible. Animal experiments allow direct manipulation of exposure to tobacco or nicotine and measurement of body weight and consummatory behavior before, during, and after drug administration.

In general, animal experiments using different species (guinea pig, dog, hamster, mouse, rabbit, rat) indicate that tobacco or nicotine administration decreases body weight. In the dog, tobacco consumption decreases body weight to the point of complete emaciation (Wright, 1846). Nicotine consumption also reduces body weight of dogs substantially (Favarger, 1906), but subcutaneous (s.c.) injection of nicotine tartrate does not (Esser, 1903). In the guinea pig, exposure to tobacco dust decreases body weight (Kardasevitch and Khais, 1940) and s.c. nicotine decreases body weight (Leschtschinskaja, 1926). One study reported that chronic nicotine intoxication does not decrease body weight of guinea pigs (Kim, 1936).

In the hamster, tobacco smoke reduces body weight (Passey et al., 1959, 1961; Wehner et al., 1976). In the mouse and rabbit, tobacco or nicotine administration reduces body weight (see Larson et al., 1961, for detailed discussions of 33 experiments). In the rat, tobacco smoke or nicotine inhibits growth (see Larson et al., 1961, for a discussion of 12 rat studies published before 1961). More recently, it has been reported that nicotine administration to rats decreases body weight in a dose-dependent manner and that, in addition, cessation of nicotine results in body weight gains (Grun-

Table 2. Longitudinal Evaluations of Smoking and Body Weight[a]

| Study | Design and sample | Major results | Moderator variables | Limitations |
|---|---|---|---|---|
| Blitzer et al. (1977) | 57,032 women, aged 20–59, self-help weight loss groups | Quitters gained 7.0–10.2 lb more than continuing smokers | Smoking rate: weight gain/previous smoking rate proportional | Smoking and weight self-reports; all women trying to lose weight |
| Bosse et al. (1980) | 1749 adult men, Normative Aging Study, assessed over 5 years | Average 5-year gains: never smokers 1.81 lb; former smokers 1.87 lb; current smokers 2.00 lb; ex-smokers who quit 6.34 lb | Age: younger quitters gained more<br>Adiposity: fatter quitters gained more<br>Tar rate: higher pretest tar rate smokers gained most<br>Anxiety: high related to higher gain | Smoking self-reports; all men; actual weights not presented |
| Burse et al. (1982) | 4 paid volunteers; 11-day baseline, 21-day quit period, 20-day resumption period | 3 of 4 gained weight; 1.98 lb increase during cessation; 1.76 lb loss on resumption | | Very small sample, paid volunteers; short-term evaluation |
| Cambien et al. (1982) | 1097 Paris civil servants, aged 25–35, screened, randomly assigned, cardiovascular risk factor reduction intervention or control groups; 2-year followup evaluation | Treatment group quitters gained 4.85 lb, control group quitters 7.50 lb; nonsmokers and no-change smokers gained 1.54 lb in treatment group, 2.2 lb in control | | Smoking self-report; risk factor reduction program participants |
| Carney and Goldberg (1984) | 13 women, 5 men, aged 28–67, smoked ≥20 cigarettes/day, ≥5 years; 12 male controls; 15 smokers abstained 2 weeks | Quitters weight change range: −3.09 to +9.0 lb | Smoking rate/duration: no weight change relationship<br>Biological variables: weight gain positively related to lipoprotein lipase activity in adipose tissue | Smoking self-report; controls weight changes not reported; short-term evaluation |
| Coates and Li (1983) | 373 male asbestos-exposed smokers, aged ≥42; 87% white, mean education 12.8 years, 12 months assessment after cessation effort | Continuous quitters gained 5.15 lb; continuous smokers gained 0.35 lb | | Smoking self-report; all male, nonrandom sample |

| | | | | |
|---|---|---|---|---|
| Comstock and Stone (1972) | 502 male telephone workers, aged 40–59, mostly white; 2 assessments 5 years apart | 5-year followup average gains: never-smokers 2.43 lb, ex-smokers 5.07 lb, continuing smokers 2.42 lb; quitters 11.24 lb and showed greatest skinfold increases | Smoking rate: increasing quitter weight gain with heavier prequit smoking | Smoking self-report; men only |
| Dallosso and James (1984) | 16 (8 men, 8 women) antismoking clinic participants; mean age, men 47.1, women 35.4; assessed before and 6 weeks after clinic | 10 quitters gained 3.00 lb; 5 continuing smokers lost 0.99 lb | | Small sample size; smoking self-report; limited followup |
| Emont and Cummings (1987) | 125 stop-smoking clinic participants; pretreatment and 1-month followup assessments | 76% quitters and slippers (≤5 cigarettes/day) averaged 5.8 lb gain | Nicotine gum: gain/gum use reliable negative correlation for heavy smokers; gain not related to age, sex, marital status, baseline body weight | Weight gain, smoking self-report, confounded by gum use; limited followup; incomplete data |
| Fagerstrom (1987) | 28 nicotine gum users; abstinent at 6 months | Infrequent gum users gained 6.83 lb, frequent users 1.98 lb | Nicotine gum: frequent users gained less weight | Small sample size; measures unclear |
| Friedman and Siegelaub (1980*a*) | Multiphasic health checkup patients; smoked, then quit 12–18 months later (N = 3825) or continued (N = 9392) | Quitters gained 2–3 lb more than continuing smokers | Smoking rate: higher initial smoking rate related to greater weight gain after cessation | Smoking self-report; whites only data |
| Garn et al. (1978) | 6979 women followed through ≥2 pregnancies | Higher prepregnancy weights for habitual nonsmokers than habitual smokers: whites 3.4 lb, blacks 4.1 lb; lower habitual smoker gains between pregnancies for both races | Race: no weight/smoking relationship influence | Smoking self-reports; restricted population |
| Garvey et al. (1974) | 870 white male veterans, aging study, assessed 4–7 years after initial assessment | Smoking/weight change significantly related; recent quitters (≤5 years) gained 4.19 lb more than smokers, nonsmokers, former smokers | Age: 40–54 quitter weight increase greatest | Smoking self-report; exact quit date unknown |

*(continued)*

Table 2. *(Continued)*

| Study | Design and sample | Major results | Moderator variables | Limitations |
|---|---|---|---|---|
| Glauser et al. (1970) | 7 male smokers, cessation program; assessed preprogram, 1 month postprogram | At 1-month followup, participants gained 6.4 lb | | Smoking self-report; exact quit date unknown |
| Gordon et al. (1975) | 4798 Framingham study participants: 1498 male smokers, 492 male nonsmokers, 1634 female nonsmokers, 1174 female smokers; examined short-term changes after biennial exam 1, long-term effects between biennial exams 4, 10 | At entry, male smokers weighed 8.0 lb less than nonsmokers; short-term male quitters gained 3.8 lb, nonsmokers 0.5 lb, continuing smokers 0.3 lb; new smokers lost 9 lb; too few female quitters to evaluate | | Smoking self-report; change analysis, men only |
| Gormican et al. (1980) | 301 pregnancy obstetrics records, women, aged 17–35 | Smoker, nonsmoker prepregnancy weight similar; no last 2 trimester weight gain difference (nonsmokers 24.6 lb, smokers 22.6 lb) | | Clinic record data; pregnancy weight gain data only |
| Grinstead (1981) | 45 subjects (38 women, 7 men), average age 40; evaluated 6 months after cessation treatment; saliva thiocyanate verification | During program, 63% subjects averaged 2.88 lb increase, 34% averaged 2.46 lb decrease; at followup, 37% averaged 6.97 lb gain, 43% averaged 3.27 lb loss | | Questionnaire, phone interview data |
| Gritz et al. (in press) | 554 self-quitters (245 men, 309 women), mean age 41.4, 85% Caucasian, 9% black, 4% Asian, 1% Asian-American, 1% Native American; 1-year followup | 35% previous quitters gained, 3% lost; at 1 year, abstainers averaged 6.1 lb gain; relapsers gained 2.71 lb while abstinent, lost 1.3 lb upon relapse; continuous smokers gained 0.3 lb | | Questionnaire, phone interview data |
| Grossarth-Maticek et al. (1983) | 1353 subjects, Yugoslavian village of 14,000; every 2d household oldest member; evaluated 1965–1966, 1969 | Smoking reduction/weight increase relationship (regression coefficient −0.30) | | Smoking self-report; weights, weight changes not reported |

| | | | | |
|---|---|---|---|---|
| Gunn and Shapiro (1985) | 89 cessation clinic participants; all quit at initial evaluation; 3-month followup assessment | 43 of 54 (80%) quitters gained 2–30 lb | | Smoking, height, weight self-report; inadequate statistical evaluation |
| Hall et al. (1986) | 255 smoker participants (122 men, 133 women), 2 smoking treatment trials; 6-, 12-month followups; biochemical verification | Abstainers gained more than smokers at 1 year | Smoking rate: pretest smoking level/postcessation weight gain positively related<br>Chronic dieting: chronic diet subjects gained most | Multiple treatment (e.g., nicotine gum) participant data included |
| Hatsukami et al. (1984) | 27 smokers hospitalized 7 days; 20 subjects smoked 3 days, then quit 4 days; 7 control group subjects smoked throughout | Quitters gained 1.76 lb in 4 days | | Small sample size; inpatient environment |
| Haworth et al. (1980) | 536 women (234 nonsmokers, 302 smokers) interviewed last prenatal visit (18%) or within day after delivery (82%) | No smoker/nonsmoker pregnancy weight gain difference | | Smoking self-report; pregnancy weight gain data only |
| Hickey and Mulcahy (1973) | 150 men (124 smokers); 6-month, 2-year followups after myocardial infarction | Quitter, reducer, continuing smoker differences not significant | | Smoking self-report; postmyocardial infarction may motivate healthy behavior |
| Holme et al. (1985) | 16,202 Oslo men, aged 40–49, screening program; 1232 (elevated cholesterol or upper quartile coronary risk score) randomly assigned diet/smoking intervention or control; 5-year followup | 17% controls, 24% intervention quit; 1- to 2-year-quitter weight increased more than controls, then decreased to below prequit level | | Smoking self-report; confounded by high cardiovascular disease risk health intervention; weights not reported |
| Howell (1971) | Retrospective, 1121 men, aged 40–54; 15- to 20-year weight gain examinations | Light smokers (<20 cigarettes/day) gained 1.9 lb less than heavy smokers, 3.1 lb less than ex-smokers, 3.6 lb less than never-smokers | Smoking rate: lower rate related to less weight gain | Retrospective report |
| Hughes and Hutchinson (1983) | 37 smokers and 19 ex-smokers with pulmonary emphysema followed ≥3 years | Smokers lost 0.32 lb/yr, ex-smokers gained 1.17 lb/yr; significant difference | | Smoking self-report; pulmonary emphysema population |

(*continued*)

Table 2. *(Continued)*

| Study | Design and sample | Major results | Moderator variables | Limitations |
|---|---|---|---|---|
| Jenkins et al. (1973) | 2318 men (546 never smokers, 359 previous quitters, 547 light smokers, 866 heavy smokers), aged 39–49, 11 California corporations in Western Collaborative Group Study; changes assessed since age 25; 1960–1969 study | Weight loss more likely for light and heavy smokers than never smokers and quitters | | Smoking self-report; weights not presented |
| Kramer (1982) | 175 subjects, commercial cessation program (41 nonparticipants or nonlocated, 59 quitters, 75 continuing smokers) ≥1-year followup | 76% nonsmokers, 56% smokers gained weight; these smokers mean gain 1.7 lb, these nonsmokers mean gain 3.0 lb | | All data self-report; high attrition, data loss; presentation incomplete |
| Lund-Larsen and Tretli (1982) | 12,329 men and women, aged 20–49, cardiovascular disease project; 2 screenings 3 years apart | Smokers mean and relative weight less than nonsmokers; female quitters gained 5.95 lb, male quitters 7.84 lb; smoking-starter men lost 1.98 lb, women 5.5 lb; smokers, nonsmokers little/no change | Sex: men, women weight change/smoking cessation and initiation similar | Self-report |
| Manley and Boland (1983) | 39 male, 55 female smokers, cessation program; randomly assigned, 1 of 3 4-week treatments or attention placebo control; 3-month followup; CO verification | 31% abstinent at followup: abstainers averaged 10.93 lb gain, relapsers 6.92 lb | | Relapser definition unclear |
| Noppa and Bengtsson (1980) | 1302 Swedish women, aged 38–60 | Current smokers leaner than nonsmokers; At 6 years, quitters gained 7.72 lb; smoking-starters lost 1.54 lb, nonchangers gained 3.09 lb | | Smoking self-report |

| | | | | |
|---|---|---|---|---|
| Pincherle (1971) | 222 upper-class male quitters; followup ≥1 year after first visit | 28% gained weight; 22% lost | | Smoking self-report; limited population; incomplete report; no weights presented |
| Powell and Mc-Cann (1981) | 29 women, 22 men, 5-day cessation project; 2- and 6-month followup | At 2 months, 54% gained weight, range 3–20 lb, mean 8.96 lb; all subjects mean 4.69 lb | | Smoking self-report; no separate abstainer, smoker data; small sample size |
| Puddey et al. (1985) | 66 cessation program volunteers, pair-matched by age, sex, body mass index; randomly assigned experimental, control groups; 2-week baseline, 6-week treatment, 6-week followup; thiocyanate, CO verification | 14 quitters gained 3.97 lb; controls 0.44 lb | | Small sample size |
| Rabkin (1984) | 40 male, 67 female smokers, assigned to 3 cessation groups; followup 3 weeks post-completion; biochemical verification | 67.3% gained weight, average 1.76 lb; skinfold increase 6.6 mm | No age, age at smoking start, rate, relative weight, anxiety correlation to male or female weight change | Small sample size; weight self-report |
| Rantakallio and Hartikainen-Sorn (1981) | 12,068 pregnant women, n. Finland, 1966; 15% smokers (smoked after 2 months pregnant); nonsmoking controls matched for age, parity, place of residence, marital status | No smoking/nonsmoking pregnancy weight gain difference | | Pregnant women only; smoking self-report; pregnancy weight gain data only |
| Rush (1974) | 162 low-income urban pregnant women, no known medical problems, <140 lb preconception weight; had borne low birthweight infant; randomized controlled nutritional supplementation trial | Mean pregnancy weight gain lower for smokers (0.73 lb/wk) than nonsmokers (0.90 lb/wk) | Smoking rate: higher rate related to lower pregnancy weight gain | Pregnant women only; smoking self-report; pregnancy weight gain data only |

(*continued*)

Table 2. *(Continued)*

| Study | Design and sample | Major results | Moderator variables | Limitations |
|---|---|---|---|---|
| Schoenenberger (1982) | 4421 male MRFIT volunteers, aged 35–57, good health but upper 10–15% coronary risk factor score; randomly assigned intervention or control groups; followup 3 annual visits | With MRFIT intervention, significant body weight decrease in smokers (mean 4.6 lb), nonsmokers (mean 5.8 lb), reducers (mean 3.75 lb); quitters average weight change minimal (mean 0.55 lb) | | Smoking self-report; confounded by risk factor reduction program participation; restricted population |
| Seltzer (1974) | 794 adult white male veterans, average age 45, Normative Aging Study; screened for "high" health level, geographic stability; 214 screened at 5 years | At admission, ex-smokers 5.9 lb heavier than nonsmokers, 8.1 lb heavier than current smokers; at 5 years, quitters gained 8.0 lb, continuing smokers 3.5 lb | | White veterans; smoking self-report |
| Stamford et al. (1986) | 13 sedentary women, 48-day successful quitters; 1-year followup | At 48 days; weight increased 4.85 lb; at 1 year, quitter increased 18.07 lb; 3 relapsers reduced weight to baseline levels; per hydrostatic weighing, gain was 96% fat | | Small female sample; smoking self-report |
| Tuomilehto et al. (1985) | 10,940 cardiovascular disease prevention program participants, aged 25–59, random sample, e. Finland; selectees with high blood pressure or hypertensive medicine assessed 5 years apart; smoking data from 2264 | Quitters body mass increased 2.31 $lb/m^2$; starting smokers decreased 1.46 $lb/m^2$ | | Smoking self-report; hypertensives |
| Vandenbroucke et al. (1984) | 3091 Netherlands civil servants, spouses (1583 men, 1508 women), aged 40–65, general health exam; 25-year followup | 76.6% lean, 65.1% obese men smoked; 22.1% lean, 11.3% obese women smoked | | Smoking self-report; restricted population |

[a]From USDHHS, 1988.

berg, 1982; Grunberg et al., 1984, 1986, 1987, 1988*a;* Grunberg and Bowen, 1985; Levin et al., 1987; McNair and Bryson, 1983; Morgan and Ellison, 1987; Schechter and Cook, 1976; Wellman et al., 1986).

Recent human studies with nicotine polacrilex chewing gum are consistent with the animal findings. Fagerstrom (1987) reported that smokers who quit smoking and chewed nicotine gum are less likely to gain weight than are exsmokers who did not chew nicotine gum. Emont and Cummings (1987) reported an inverse relationship between number of pieces of nicotine gum chewed and body weight gain by heavy smokers (26 cigarettes/day) who quit smoking. Stitzer and Gross (1988) also found that ex-smokers who chewed gum gain less weight than do exsmokers who do not consume nicotine in any form.

The animal experiments indicate that smoking and nicotine decrease body weight compared to controls. Animal experiments also indicate that cessation of nicotine increases body weight. These effects are dose-dependent; i.e., the greater the dose of nicotine, the greater are the effects. Therefore, nicotine affects body weight and probably is the component of tobacco responsible for body weight changes that accompany changes in tobacco use. The results of the nicotine gum studies are consistent with the interpretation that nicotine is responsible for the changes in body weight in human smokers.

## 4. EXPLANATIONS FOR THE INVERSE RELATIONSHIP BETWEEN TOBACCO USE AND BODY WEIGHT

The inverse relationship between tobacco use and body weight may result from changes in energy intake, changes in energy expenditure, or both. Energy intake involves consumption of foods from all available taste categories (including sweet, salty, and bland) and nutrient classes (including carbohydrates, proteins, and fats). Energy expenditure involves behavioral factors (physical activity) and biological factors (e.g., resting metabolic rate, thermogenesis). The evidence for each of these factors is discussed in the following sections.

### Energy Intake

Energy intake is affected by changes in consumption of all foods or changes in consumption of specific foods. Food consumption changes are frequently interpreted to be synonymous with changes in appetite (i.e., hunger for food). However, this assumption may or may not be true, especially in humans. Decreased food consumption, for example, can reflect (1) decreased general hunger or appetite; (2) dieting or purposeful restraint; (3) dislike for the food that is available; (4) physical illness that makes it difficult or impossible to eat (e.g., ulcers in the mouth; sore throat; nausea); or (5) mental illness that is accompanied by disinterest in food (e.g., depression). Increased food consumption can reflect (1) increased general hunger or appetite; (2) purposeful overconsumption (e.g., carbohydrate load by athletes before a competitive event; excessive consumption to "please" the food preparer); (3) particular preference for the available food; or (4) psychopathological eating pattern, such as bingeing.

With regard to the relationship between tobacco use and body weight, one possible explanation is that smokers eat less than do nonsmokers and that ex-smokers increase their food consumption and thereby gain weight (Birch, 1975). This straightforward explanation for the tobacco/body weight relationship, if true, could reflect (1) effects of tobacco or nicotine on general appetite; (2) a substitution of habits involving the hands and mouth; or (3) a replacement of stimuli for oral gratification (as suggested by McArthur et al., 1958). Alternatively, tobacco use could affect consumption of some (e.g., sweets), but not all, food. If the latter explanation is correct, then studies that do not differentiate among specific foods consumed may obtain different results depending on what foods are available.

Energy Intake: Human Studies. Before the 1980s few human studies evaluated the relationship between tobacco and food consumption and these studies reached different conclusions. Lincoln (1969) evaluated retrospective self-reports of food consumption by 885 male smokers and nonsmokers and reported (in a "letter to the editor") that male smokers consume roughly 350 calories per day more than do nonsmokers. In contrast, Gaudet and Hugli (1969) collected retrospective self-reports from 645 people (including 223 who had changed their smoking habits) and reported no significant changes in eating behavior with changes in smoking habits. S. Schachter and P. D. Nesbitt (personal communication) examined food consumption of smokers in the laboratory during two 8-hr periods: They were allowed to smoke freely on one day and abstained on the other day. Overall, caloric intake was roughly 33% greater during the no-smoking day. In a short-term laboratory setting, Perlick (1977) found that smokers who were deprived of nicotine (by complete smoking abstinence or by smoking low-nicotine cigarettes) ate twice as many gumdrops as did nondeprived smokers and nonsmokers. Based on these studies, smoking either increases food consumption, decreases food consumption, or has no effect on food consumption.

Perrin et al. (1961) wrote: "There is a belief that smokers do prefer more savoury foods, and that, with abstinence from smoking, sweeter foods are preferred, and this possibility accounts for the subsequent increase in weight that has been reported" (p. 387). The studies performed before 1979 did not carefully examine the possibility that smoking may have decreased consumption of some (e.g., sweet), but not all, foods. The Perlick (1977) study clearly reported increased sweet food consumption (i.e., gumdrops) with nicotine deprivation. Because only gumdrops were available in this study, the increased consumption may also reflect changes in general hunger. Grunberg (1980, 1982) reanalyzed the Schachter and Nesbitt data by taste class and found that consumption of sweet and salty foods doubled on the no-smoking days and that consumption of all other foods did not change. These findings suggest that smoking or abstinence from smoking results in changes in consumption of some, but not all, foods. Caution must be exercised in interpreting these results because the sweet and salty foods in this study were all easily accessible snack foods while the other foods required some preparation (e.g., making sandwiches). Also, without nonsmokers as control subjects, it is unclear whether smoking decreased consumption of specific foods, whether abstinence increased consumption of specific foods, or both.

In a study of quitting smoking, Gilbert and Pope (1982) studied 19 smokers for 2 days; 1 day subjects could smoke and 1 day they could not. On the nonsmoking day subjects ate significantly more. A closer examination of food consumption revealed that on the nonsmoking days subjects ate significantly more snacks (candies and peanuts) but significantly less at mealtimes. Caloric consumption of snack foods as a proportion of total daily caloric intake increased significantly on the nonsmoking days, suggesting that abstinence from smoking increased consumption of specific foods. Unfortunately, as in the Perlick (1977) study, the sweet and salty snack foods were readily accessible, which may have contributed to their increased consumption. In addition, there were no nonsmokers as control subjects. Therefore, it is impossible to conclude from this study that smoking affects specific or general food consumption.

In order to compare the effects of cigarette smoking and abstinence on general and specific food consumption without the ambiguity of these previous studies, Grunberg (1982) conducted a human laboratory experiment. Male and female smokers ($N = 28$) and nonsmokers ($N = 14$) were recruited to participate in a food-tasting study that was run around lunchtime. Smokers were divided into two experimental groups: Half of the subjects were allowed to smoke two cigarettes during a baseline period before tasting the foods; half of the subjects were not allowed to smoke at this time. All subjects filled out questionnaires during this baseline period, and the smoking manipulation was done in such a way to avoid suspicion by subjects of the importance of smoking or not smoking in this experiment. After the baseline period, subjects were escorted to a food-tasting room. Nine foods (three sweet, three salty, three bland) were set out in bite-size pieces in individual bowls. Subjects were instructed to taste each food and to rate each food on a series of taste judgment scales. Almost as an afterthought, the experimenter explained to subjects that after they rated the foods they could feel free to eat whatever they wanted. The bowls of food were weighed before and after the session to determine exactly how much was eaten of each food. In addition to this measure of food consumption, subjects were asked to select three foods to eat again in another part of the study. This selection provided a second index of food preferences.

Smokers who were allowed to smoke ate less sweet food than did nonsmokers and than did smokers who abstained from smoking. There were no differences in consumption of the nonsweet foods among the three groups. In addition, smokers allowed to smoke were less likely to choose sweet foods to eat again than were the other two groups. These results indicate that smoking decreases preference for and consumption of sweet foods in particular (Grunberg, 1982). These results are consistent with those of Schachter and Nesbitt (personal communication) and Perlick (1977).

In an attempt to determine whether these findings generalize to the world, Grunberg and Morse (1984) compared per capita cigarette consumption in the United States between 1964 and 1977 with per capita consumption of every major foodstuff. These years were chosen for analysis because U.S. per capita consumption of cigarettes during this period was a U-shaped function (a trough occurred from 1969 to 1972 following the federal government's intensive and highly publicized antismoking campaign). In effect, this curvilinear function of cigarette consumption acted as an experimental manipulation. Although per capita food consumption data could not, of course, be separated for smokers and nonsmokers, Grunberg and Morse (1984) reasoned that if the relationship between specific food consumption and tobacco consumption is a robust phenomenon, then analysis of national food consumption should be consistent with the laboratory findings. As predicted, there was a significant inverse correlation between cigarette and sugar consumption, in particular.

More recently, several investigators have conducted prospective studies of eating behavior in smokers who quit smoking. Hatsukami et al. (1984) carefully measured dietary intake in 27 smokers in a hospital setting. Eating behavior was monitored for 3 days and then 20 of 27 smokers quit smoking for 7 days, during which daily eating behavior was measured for all 27 subjects. The smokers who quit smoking showed significant increases in caloric intake and gained an average of 1.8 lb. Stamford et al. (1986) and Robinson and York (1986) also monitored dietary intake carefully and reported that caloric intake increased in smokers who quite smoking. Dallosso and James (1984) reported an increase in dietary intake after smoking cessation (6.5%), but it was not statistically significant. Unfortunately, these studies did not report food consumption separately by taste classes. Rodin (1987) performed a prospective study and reported changes in consumption by food categories: Smokers who gained weight after quitting smoking increased their sugar consumption. These results supported the conclusions of Grunberg (1982) and Grunberg and Morse (1984) that the inverse relationship between smoking and sweet food consumption may partially determine the inverse relationship between smoking and body weight.

Taken together, these studies suggest that smoking decreases food consumption, especially of sweet foods, and that cessation of smoking increases food consumption, especially of sweet foods (compared to smokers who keep smoking). These changes in energy intake probably contribute to the body weight changes. Although the results of the human laboratory experiments and prospective human studies are consistent, cross-sectional surveys report conflicting findings. Based on self-report data, some studies hold that there is no difference in food consumption between smokers and nonsmokers (Albanes et al., 1987; Fehily et al., 1984; Fisher and Gordon, 1985; Matsuya, 1982). Other studies indicate that smokers report eating more than do nonsmokers (Picone et al., 1982; Stamford et al., 1984*a,b*). These inconsistent findings may reflect the invalidity of self-report dietary data. Alternatively, these findings may reflect the fact that these studies do not separate foodstuffs into different categories or types. In addition, it is important to consider that most people alter their eating behavior to help control their body weight. A recent cross-sectional study of smoking and eating that partially broke down responses by food types and that evaluated dietary habits by smoking, social class, age, and sex found that smokers were significantly less likely to eat fruits frequently (sweet foods), to eat breakfast, or to eat brown bread. The smokers were more likely to eat fried foods (Whichelow et al., 1988). This cross-sectional study still relied on self-report data, but it considered important variables (e.g., specific food, age, sex) in the evaluation of the results and reported findings consistent with the laboratory and short-term prospective studies, i.e., smokers and nonsmokers differ in consumption of specific foods, including sweet-tasting foods and carbohydrates.

The effects of cigarette smoking on eating behavior may be clearly revealed in the laboratory and in short-term prospective studies, whereas some summary data report no food consumption differences between smokers and nonsmokers because nonsmokers and ex-smokers exert self-control to avoid getting fat. Without objective measures of food consumption, separation by food categories, or measures of dietary restraint, it is difficult to interpret most of the survey data. [The Whichelow et al. (1988) study is an exception.] Moreover, because the laboratory and short-term prospective studies of food intake by smokers do not randomly manipulate smoking and do not report nicotine levels in the body, based on these studies alone, it is impossible to reach causal conclusions about the effects of cigarette smoking or nicotine on eating behavior.

Energy Intake: Animal Studies. Animal experiments that administer tobacco smoke or nicotine to subjects and measure food consumption provide complementary data to the human studies of smoking and eating. Several experiments conducted before 1980 reported that cigarette smoke or nicotine injection decrease food consumption in rats, humans, and guinea pigs (Averett, 1962; Becker and King, 1966; Munster and Battig, 1975; Evans et al., 1967; Passey et al., 1959, 1961; Hughes et al., 1970). Other studies reported that there were no changes or that the decreases were not significant (Kerschbaum et al., 1965; Schechter and Cook, 1976). Most of these studies also reported that there were body weight decreases that could not be explained by the decreased food consumption, either because the time course of the changes did not match or because the food intake changes were too small (Evans et al., 1967; Schechter and Cook, 1976; Passey et al., 1959, 1961; Hughes et al., 1970).

These studies do not conclusively establish whether or not changes in energy intake are involved in the effects of nicotine on body weight. When food intake decreased, so did body weight. But body weight also decreased at times when food intake did not change. Either something is going on in addition to energy intake or instead of energy intake to account for the inverse relationship between nicotine and body weight.

A closer look at these studies also reveals several methodological limitations: (1) None of these studies examined eating behavior or body weight after cessation of nicotine or tobacco smoke; (2) many of the studies that reported decreased food intake measured it for a short period of time immediately after nicotine or tobacco smoke administration; (3) all of these studies provided only one food (a bland laboratory chow). Therefore, the finding of some studies that nicotine or tobacco smoke decreases food intake is unconvincing because the decreased food intake usually occurred immediately after a bolus injection of nicotine or acute exposure to tobacco smoke. It is hardly surprising that immediately after a jolt of nicotine (an extremely toxic substance), food intake may decrease for a short time. In contrast, human smokers chronically self-administer nicotine and can eat whenever they choose. The conclusion of other studies that food intake does not change much is also open to question because only bland foods were available. In human studies, smoking decreases consumption of sweet foods (see "Energy Intake: Human Studies"). In addition, none of the animal studies cited here examined food intake after cessation of nicotine. One cannot simply assume that if nicotine decreases general or specific food intake, cessation of nicotine will have the exact opposite effect.

With the limitations of previous animal studies in mind, Grunberg (1982) examined the effects of nicotine on body weight and consummatory behavior of rats. Unlike the previous animal experiments, subjects in this study had continuous access to laboratory chow, water, and three different sugar solutions (10%, 25%, and 35% w/v *d*-glucose). Because nicotine injections might cause decreased food intake by making subjects sick or uncomfortable, Grunberg (1982) administered nicotine via Alzet osmotic minipumps that were implanted subcutaneously between the withers (shoulder blades) of the rats. These devices provide a slow, constant release (roughly 0.5 μl/hr) of their contents for weeks (Theeuwes and Yum, 1977). Body weight and food consumption were measured daily for 2-week periods before, during, and after drug administration. Animals received either 0 (i.e., physiological saline), 2.5, 5.0, or 10.0 mg nicotine per kg body weight per day during the drug administration period. Nicotine dihydrochloride was dissolved in physiological saline to make the solutions. Dosages (expressed as nicotine base) were determined from previous research and pilot work to produce body weight effects comparable to those reported for human smokers but to avoid making the rats sick. This paradigm was designed to allow daily measures before, during, and after nicotine administration and to avoid the behavioral and biological stress of daily nicotine injections. Also, this paradigm was designed to allow both between-subjects and within-subject analyses. This precaution was meant to avoid the interpretative difficulties of studies that lacked control groups for time, exposure to experimental procedures, and individual differences.

Before receiving saline or nicotine, all experimental groups had similar body weights and consumed similar amounts of the sweet and nonsweet foods. During drug administration, there was an inverse dose–effect relationship between nicotine and body weight: Animals receiving nicotine gained significantly less weight than did the control animals. After cessation of nicotine, animals gained weight at greater rates than did controls. All treatment groups consumed similar amounts of the bland laboratory chow before, during, and after nicotine or saline administration. In contrast, nicotine administration significantly decreased sugar solution consumption. Cessation of nicotine was accompanied by significant increases in sugar solution consumption. These effects were greatest for the highest nicotine group. Moreover, the animals receiving nicotine decreased consumption of the sweetest solutions during drug administration and increased consumption of the water and lowest concentration sugar solution during drug administration. After cessation of nicotine, they did just the opposite. There were no differences in total liquid consumption among groups. This experiment clearly found that nicotine affected body weight and sweet food consumption (Grunberg, 1982).

In this experiment the decreased caloric intake (from sweet foods) was similar across all nicotine groups, whereas the body weight changes were dose-dependent. Therefore, decrease in caloric intake from sweet foods contributes to the effects of nicotine on body weight, but some additional factor is involved. This interpretation is consistent with the previous animal studies but clarifies that nicotine does decrease energy intake from sweet foods (consistent with the human experiments). In contrast, the increased caloric intake from sweet foods after cessation of nicotine was dose-related in a fashion that could fully explain the dose-related body weight increases after cessation. To summarize the findings of Grunberg's (1982) rat experiment: (1) nicotine decreases sweet food consumption; (2) the effect of nicotine on energy intake contributes to decreased body weight during nicotine administration; (3) cessation of nicotine results in increased sweet food consumption; and (4) the increased energy intake after cessation of nicotine accounts for increased body weight after cessation of nicotine.

The human and animal experiments reported by Grunberg (1982) suggest that if only nonsweet foods are available: (1) food intake should not change with nicotine administration or cessation; (2) effects of nicotine on body weight should be reduced; (3) effects of cessation of nicotine on body weight should be reduced or eliminated. Grunberg et al. (1984) used the animal paradigm of Grunberg (1982) to empirically examine the effects of nicotine on body weight and food intake when only bland laboratory chow and water were available (i.e., no sweet foods). Animals were monitored for roughly 2-

week periods before, during, and after administration of saline or nicotine (4, 8, or 12 mg/kg per day). As predicted, there were no effects of nicotine or cessation of nicotine on food consumption when no sweet foods were available. Body weights were similar before drug administration. Nicotine administration was inversely related to body weight in a dose–response fashion, but the effect of nicotine on body weight was less than when sweet foods were available and food intake changed. After cessation of nicotine, all groups of animals gained weight at similar rates. That is, when no sweet foods were available, there was no effect of nicotine cessation on body weight or food intake. The lack of excessive weight gain after cessation of nicotine when bland food was available was in marked contrast to the increased weight gain following cessation of nicotine when sweet food was available.

Grunberg et al. (1984) performed a second experiment that administered nicotine for 3 weeks while only bland food was available. The results were virtually identical to the first experiment. With only bland food available, there were no differences among groups in food intake, body weight was inversely related to nicotine in a dose–effect relationship, and there was no effect of cessation of nicotine on body weight.

Because the effects of nicotine on body weight were attenuated when type of food was restricted, changes in consumption of sweet foods must contribute to decreased body weight during nicotine administration. However, because nicotine significantly affected body weight without affecting bland food consumption, nicotine must also affect energy expenditure. Because nicotine cessation did not cause body weight gains when bland food was available but did cause increased body weight and food consumption when sweet foods were available, changes in energy intake are critical to excessive weight gains following cessation of nicotine (Grunberg, 1982; Grunberg et al., 1984).

The sweet foods in Grunberg's (1982) human and animal experiments covaried sweet taste and carbohydrate content. To determine whether nicotine affects consumption of sweet-tasting foods regardless of nutrient or caloric content, and to determine whether nicotine affects consumption of carbohydrates that are not sweet-tasting, Grunberg et al. (1985) conducted two rat experiments. All animals had continuous access to two foods. In both experiments one food was a low-calorie, nonsweet laboratory chow. In one experiment, the second food was a low-calorie, saccharin-sweetened laboratory chow. In the other experiment, the second food was a nonsweet laboratory chow with carbohydrate (maltose dextrin) added. Body weight and food intake were measured daily for roughly 2-week periods before, during, and after saline or nicotine (6 or 12 mg/kg per day) administration.

In both experiments, there was an inverse dose–effect relationship between nicotine and body weight. After cessation of nicotine, animals gained weight at greater rates than did control animals. Nicotine administration decreased consumption of the sweet, low-carbohydrate food and cessation of nicotine markedly increased consumption of this food compared to controls. It is clear that nicotine administration and cessation alters sweet food consumption; sweet taste is important. Nicotine administration and cessation had smaller, but similar effects on carbohydrate consumption. Therefore, carbohydrate content also is involved in nicotine's effects on energy intake. Not surprisingly, the effects of nicotine on body weight were less in the experiment that provided sweet, low-calorie foods. This result further supports the previous conclusion that changes in energy intake contribute to the effects of nicotine on body weight.

However, as indicated earlier, administration of nicotine and tobacco smoke also can decrease body weight when food intake does not change. This fact has been reported in the 1980s in other laboratories in addition to that of Grunberg and co-workers (e.g., Wellman et al., 1986; Wager-Srdar et al., 1984). Therefore, administration of nicotine must somehow alter energy expenditure.

Grunberg et al. (1986) pointed out that virtually all of the previous animal studies of nicotine, energy intake, and body weight used male subjects. Women are more likely than men to report concerns about body weight and to report that they smoke to control body weight (Feldman et al., 1985; Page, 1983; Klesges and Klesges, 1988). This difference between men and women may reflect sociocultural pressures and biases that create different concerns about body weight. Alternatively, there may be a sex difference in the effects of nicotine on body weight. To test this possibility, Grunberg et al. (1986) examined the effects of nicotine or saline on body weight and consummatory behavior of female rats that had access only to bland laboratory chow and water. This food was provided because the studies of male rats using this paradigm found no changes in bland food intake, body weight changes during nicotine administration, and no effects on body weight gain after cessation of nicotine (Grunberg et al., 1984). Therefore, any sex difference should become obvious in comparison to these results. In female rats, nicotine administration was inversely related to food intake and body weight, and cessation of nicotine was positively related to food intake and body weight. These pronounced changes were statistically significant and were greater than the effects of nicotine on body weight and food consumption by male rats (Grunberg et al., 1986). Grunberg et al. (1987) replicated and extended these findings by measuring body weight for 4 months after cessation of nicotine. Again, the effects of nicotine on body weight and food intake were greater in female rats than in male rats. The greater body weight gains by female rats after cessation of nicotine persisted throughout the entire experiment (i.e., 4 months after cessation). Levin et al. (1987) reported similar effects of nicotine on body weight and food intake of female rats. If these sex differences observed in animals generalize to humans, then the greater concerns reported by many women about weight gains after smoking cessation may reflect a biological difference in nicotine's effects. This possibility requires empirical evaluation.

Overall, the studies on energy intake indicate that nicotine administration to animals and smoking by humans decrease energy intake and cessation of nicotine or smoking increases energy intake. These effects are particularly pronounced when the foods are sweets and carbohydrates. The effects of nicotine on food intake seem to be greater in females than in males. Changes in energy intake contribute to the effects of nicotine and tobacco on body weight. However, energy expenditure also must be involved in the body weight changes during nicotine administration.

## Energy Expenditure

Energy expenditure involves behavioral and biological factors. Physical activity uses up energy and burns calories. If physical activity increases without changing energy intake, then some weight may be lost. Based on energy utilization equations, substantial increases in physical activity are required to lose weight (Powers, 1980). In addition to changes in physical activity, energy expenditure involves the rate at which the body utilizes energy (i.e., metabolism). If nicotine administration or cessation changes spontaneous physical activity or metabolism, then body weight could change. Some human and animal studies have addressed these possibilities, although not to the extent or in the detail of the energy intake experiments.

Energy Expenditure: Physical Activity. Cross-sectional human studies comparing physical activity in smokers and nonsmokers report a weak negative relationship with smoking (Blair et al., 1985; Kannas, 1981) or no relationship at all (Gyntelberg and Meyer, 1974; Stamford et al., 1984*a,b;* Stephens and Pederson, 1983). Prospective human studies have reported no changes in physical activity accompanying smoking abstinence (Hatsukami et al., 1984; Hofstetter et al., 1986; Klesges et al., 1987; Rodin, 1987; Stamford et al., 1986).

Animal studies of acute nicotine injection and short-term physical activity changes have reported increases (Bryson et al., 1981; Schlatter and Battig, 1979, 1981) and decreases (Hatchell and Collins, 1980; Rodgers, 1979) in physical activity. These studies did not examine chronic nicotine administration, did not measure body weight changes, did not examine physical activity for more than 45-min periods, and did not examine effects of nicotine cessation. Therefore, it is impossible to extrapolate from any of these studies to the human condition. Two recent animal experiments used the Grunberg (1982) paradigm and measured physical activity for 24-hr periods from the 2-week periods before, during, and after nicotine or saline administration. Grunberg and Bowen (1985) reported that nicotine increased physical activity in male rats, but these increases were small and occurred after body weight decreases had already shown up. After cessation of nicotine, physical activity decreased and preceded the weight gains. In contrast, Bowen et al. (1986) reported that nicotine administration or cessation did not alter physical activity in female rats, although body weight changes clearly occurred.

It appears that physical activity does not contribute to the effects of nicotine or smoking to decrease body weight. Similarly, there is no evidence that physical activity contributes to body weight increases after cessation of smoking, but one study indicates that it may contribute to body weight gains in male rats after cessation of nicotine. Too few animal data are available to reach unequivocal conclusions about chronic nicotine, physical activity, and body weight. The human studies suggest strongly that physical activity is not involved in the effects of smoking or abstinence on body weight. It may be that smokers who quit smoking intentionally increase physical activity to help offset weight gains. If this is occurring against a backdrop of naturally decreased activity, then it is likely that no changes will be detected. Based on the available human and animal evidence, there is little reason to presume that physical activity is an important factor in the smoking/body weight relationship. However, intentional increased physical activity may be a useful tool to help reduce unwanted weight gains after cessation of smoking.

Energy Expenditure: Metabolism. Human and animal studies have examined effects of nicotine and tobacco smoke on metabolism. Several studies comparing smokers and nonsmokers report that, in general, smokers have a higher basal metabolic rate (BMR) and respiratory quotient (RQ) (Schlumm, 1930, 1932; Hadley, 1941–1942; Brozek et al., 1958). Some studies report that BMR and RQ increase immediately after smoking (Hiestand et al., 1940; Baroni and Mandrioli, 1952; Haggard and Greenberg, 1934), but other studies report no effects of smoking on these measures (Dill et al., 1934; Larson et al., 1961). More recent studies report that acute nicotine administration increases metabolism (Ghanem, 1973; Ilebekk et al., 1975; Robinson and York, 1986; Schievelbein et al., 1978; Wennmalm, 1982). None of these studies establish whether these effects of nicotine and tobacco smoke alter body weight in smokers or ex-smokers because most of these studies measured metabolism for short periods of time after smoking, did not measure body weight, and did not monitor either variable after cessation of smoking.

A few studies have measured metabolic rate after cessation of smoking. Schlumm (1932) reported that, for many smokers, after cessation of smoking, BMR decreased and weight gain occurred. Unfortunately, the data provided are sketchy and food intake is not reported. Glauser et al. (1970) reported decreases in oxygen consumption 1 month after smoking cessation. Dallosso and James (1984) reported a small drop in metabolic rate 6 weeks after smoking cessation. Hofstetter et al. (1986) found that the total energy expenditure of smokers was higher during 1 day when they were allowed to smoke versus 1 day that they were not allowed to smoke; there were no differences in resting metabolic rate. In contrast, Silbert and Friedlander (1931) reported no changes in metabolism after cessation of tobacco use. Burse and co-workers (1975, 1982) reported no changes in resting metabolic rate 3 weeks after smoking cessation. Robinson and York (1986) reported no changes in total energy expenditure 7 days after smoking cessation. Stamford et al. (1986) reported no changes in oxygen consumption 2 days after smoking cessation.

Schmitthenner et al. (1957) reported that nicotine increased total body oxygen consumption in dogs. Bizzi et al. (1972) found that nicotine increases lipolysis of adipose tissue in rats. Ilebekk et al. (1975) reported that cigarette smoke increases total body oxygen consumption in dogs. Wellman et al. (1986) reported that nicotine alone did not alter thermogenesis in rats, but that nicotine plus caffeine increased brown adipose tissue thermogenesis markedly.

The effects of nicotine and tobacco smoke on metabolism are not clear. Because nicotine can decrease body weight without significantly changing energy intake (see "Energy Intake") and without significantly changing physical activity (see "Energy Expenditure: Physical Activity"), there must be biological changes in energy expenditure that contribute to the effects of nicotine on body weight. Yet the human and animal studies of nicotine and metabolism do not provide consistent, robust findings. A recent review of this topic suggested that the small sample sizes of the human studies of smoking and energy expenditure may not allow sufficient statistical power to detect any small, but important changes in resting metabolic rate (USDHHS, 1988). Perhaps nicotine and tobacco increase energy expenditure of some sources of energy (e.g., fats, carbohydrates), but not all sources of energy. If so, then studies may report different findings depending on the measures of metabolism used and the macronutrient content of the foods consumed. At this point, it is logical to conclude that energy expenditure is involved in the nicotine/body weight relationship, but it is not clear exactly how.

## 5. POTENTIAL MECHANISMS UNDERLYING THE EFFECTS OF NICOTINE ON ENERGY INTAKE AND EXPENDITURE

Based on the available empirical evidence: (1) smoking acts to keep body weight down; (2) smoking cessation results in increased body weight; (3) nicotine is responsible for the effects of smoking on body weight; (4) smoking and nicotine administration decrease food intake, especially of sweets and carbohydrates; (5) cessation of smoking or nicotine increases food intake, especially of sweets and carbohydrates; (6) the decreased food intake during smoking or nicotine administration partially contributes to the decreased body weight; (7) the increased food intake after cessation of smoking or nicotine largely explains the increased body weight; (8) changes in physical activity play a small or no role in the smoking/body weight or nicotine/body weight relationship; (9) increased biological energy expenditure (e.g., metabolism) during smoking and nicotine administration seems to be involved in decreasing body weight; and (10) decreased biological energy expenditure after cessation of smoking or nicotine may contribute to increased body weight. The effects of smoking and nicotine on energy intake have been extensively studied, and this database allows consideration of the next level of analysis, i.e., mechanisms that may underlie changes in energy intake and specific food consumption. The energy expenditure literature is not as clear and mechanisms are only beginning to be explored.

Although the scientific world has only recently convinced itself that smoking is inversely related to body weight, the tobacco industry made use of this well-accepted "fact" in advertisements for Lucky Strikes in the 1920s and, implicitly, in advertisements for Virginia Slims in the 1970s. Similarly, while scientists bicker about energy intake and expenditure, everyone "knows" that smokers who quit smoking get fat because they eat more cakes and candies and their metabolism slows down. In the 1920s the Lucky Strike people told us to "Reach for a Lucky instead of a sweet." The empirical evidence now supports what our grandparents assumed to be true. When we turn to the next level of analysis, however, commonly held beliefs give way as careful laboratory analyses reveal important distinctions. Potential mechanisms involved in the smoking/body weight relationship are presented next.

## Potential Mechanisms Underlying Changes in Energy Intake

Taste Perception. It is widely held that increased food consumption, especially of sweets, after cessation of smoking results from changes in taste perception. It seems reasonable that if cigarette smoking blunts the ability to taste foods, then food consumption might decrease. Conversely, if smoking cessation is accompanied by improved ability to taste foods, then increased food consumption would be a reasonable accompaniment. Many studies have examined the effects of smoking on taste acuity.

Pangborn and Trabue (1973) reviewed studies performed between 1935 and 1970 on smoking and taste sensitivity. Typically, smokers and nonsmokers tasted low-concentration flavored solutions (e.g., sweet, salty, bitter) that were close to the lower limits of taste detectability: 11 studies reported that heavy smoking impaired taste acuity; five studies reported no differences between groups. Even the studies that reported that smokers had impaired taste sensitivity were not consistent across taste classes. For example, Krut et al. (1961) reported that smokers had higher thresholds for bitter, but that smokers and nonsmokers did not differ for sweet, sour, or salt. Kaplan and colleagues (Fischer et al., 1963; Kaplan and Glanville, 1964; Kaplan et al., 1965) also reported that smoking is related to higher thresholds for bitter. Peterson et al. (1968) reported that ability to perceive bitter taste improved in smokers who quit smoking, but the ex-smokers' ability was similar to that of a group of smokers who kept smoking.

Pursell et al. (1973) questioned the results of these previous studies because they did not consider the subjects' response criteria. Using two measures of sensitivity based on signal detection theory (area under ROC curve and $d_s$), Pursell et al. (1973) found that smokers were significantly *more* sensitive to near threshold solutions and were somewhat more sensitive to suprathreshold solutions. Based on the percent of correct responses, there were no differences in taste sensitivity between smokers and nonsmokers. McBurney and Moskat (1975) also used more careful psychophysical methods (including up–down–transformed–response method) to study taste thresholds in smokers and nonsmokers. Smokers were slightly less sensitive to bitter and slightly more sensitive to sweet, but the effects were small, inconsistent, and not significant. It is unlikely that the small or nonexistent changes in taste threshold accompanying smoking would result in significant changes in sweet food intake.

The smoking and taste threshold studies indicate that smoking may slightly reduce ability to taste bitter foods, but that's about it for smoking and taste sensitivity. Adaptation to bitter potentiates the taste of sweet foods and makes water taste sweet (McBurney and Moskat, 1975). Therefore, the effects of smoking on ability to taste bitter may affect the perception of sweet foods, but the effect is not documented and would be minimal or nonexistent. Further, there is no evidence that *nicotine* affects bitter or any other taste sensitivity, yet animal studies with nicotine similarly show altered preference for sweet foods. The effects of smoking and nicotine on consumption of sweet foods cannot be explained by altered taste perception. This conclusion is consistent with the generalization that taste sensitivity accounts for little variance in food selection (Rozin, 1984).

Intentional Food Restriction or Choice. General and specific food consumption change when foods are intentionally sought or rejected to purposely manipulate a healthful, restricted, or philosophically based diet. Such intentional changes in food consumption are unlikely to explain the inverse relationship between nicotine and sweet food consumption. It seems reasonable to conclude that laboratory rats did not intentionally change specific food consumption to control their weight or diet. Moreover, if intentional manipulation of diet explained the human results, one would expect people to purposely avoid sweet, high-caloric foods after cessation of smoking to avoid weight gains. They certainly would not purposely seek fattening foods as their weight crept up. If anything, restraint in consumption of high-caloric foods should act (and may have in the longitudinal studies) to attenuate the increased sweet food consumption after cessation of smoking.

Food Preferences. A third possible explanation for changes in energy intake is that preference for and enjoyment of specific foods change with nicotine administration and cessation. As discussed earlier, Grunberg (1982) found that human smokers allowed to smoke ate less sweet food and were less likely to choose sweet foods to eat later in the experimental session. Smokers not allowed to smoke ate more sweets and, compared to smokers smoking and nonsmokers, were most likely to choose sweet foods to eat again. Further, Grunberg (1980, 1982) found that all three experimental groups rated the foods similarly on taste perception scales. The smokers and nonsmokers judged the intensity of food tastes similarly, but expressed significant differences in food preferences that paralleled the actual food intake. Unlike the taste threshold studies discussed earlier, Grunberg (1982) used foods rather than near-threshold solutions. As a result, these results may reflect a combination of suprathreshold tastes.

To further compare the effects of smoking on taste perception versus taste preferences, as distinguished by Grunberg (1982), Redington (1984) had smokers and nonsmokers rate intensity and pleasantness of near-threshold solutions before and after a glucose load. Smokers reported decreased hedonic judgment of sweet solutions after a glucose load; the intensity ratings were similar for all subjects. More recently, Rodin (1987) tested the pleasantness/intensity distinction in a prospective study of smoking cessation. Again, preference for sweets increased after smoking cessation, but judgments of taste intensity did not change.

Based on these studies, it seems that smoking decreases the pleasantness of sweet foods and that smoking cessation increases this variable. The increased sweet preference after cessation of smoking overshoots the preference expressed by nonsmokers (Grunberg, 1982). These changes in preference for specific tastes parallel the changes in specific food intake. The fact that animals during nicotine administration and cessation show similar changes in sweet food consumption suggests that nicotine acts to alter preference for sweets which translates into changed consumption, unless an individual (e.g., an ex-smoker trying to avoid weight gains) purposely self-restrains to control sweet food consumption.

This discussion of nicotine and food preferences can be cast in the broader context of food selection or specific appetites. Differences in food selection involve biological and cultural factors (Rozin, 1984). In the case of nicotine and specific food consumption, the rapidity of the changed preferences revealed in human and animal laboratory studies strongly suggests that biological factors underlie these behavioral changes. Learning and expectations certainly may be involved in changes in sweet food preferences with smoking and after cessation. However, the increased consumption of sweet foods by smokers hours after cessation and the marked changes in sweet food consumption by animals soon after nicotine administration or cessation strongly suggest a biological basis for these effects.

To understand why nicotine affects specific food preferences requires a digression to the food selection literature. The careful animal experiments by Curt Richter (1939, 1943) clearly established that changes in nutrient and electrolyte levels in the body affect food selection. The notion that specific appetites are a mechanism by which the body maintains intake of necessary foodstuffs and makes adjustments based on needs grew largely out of Richter's work and a study by Clara Davis (1928) of human infants and food selection. Basically, the idea is that humans and animals consume the nutrients they need to maintain a functioning body. Specific appetites develop in response to these needs. Because certain tastes are associated with intake of particular needs (e.g., salt for sodium), tastes are reinforced after consumption of the necessary foodstuff and the organism learns to choose that foodstuff.

P. T. Young went beyond stimulus–response (S-R) theory in interpreting Richter's findings about biologically based drives for specific food selection. According to Young (1955), biological need results in an altered hedonic or affective tone such that a specific food may be craved or taste particularly good. Therefore, a specific appetite results from a biological need giving rise to altered hedonic response to specific tastes or foodstuffs, which, in turn, translates into altered food choice and consumption. Young's (1936) "hedonic theory" was the basis for this reinterpretation of Richter's work. At first glance, the differences in interpretation may seem subtle, but they are not. At a time when S-R theory reigned supreme, Young (1936) applied "hedonic theory" to the results of animal as well as human experiments. Young's (1955) argument for an affective component to specific appetites is convincing as he points out the limitations of a strict S-R interpretation of motivation. In the present context, Young's point again becomes relevant because the time course of altered food preferences with nicotine administration and cessation is short or immediate and humans report clear changes in preferences for which foods taste better.

Also relevant to understand nicotine's effects on specific food preferences is Cabanac's (1971, 1979) notion of "alliesthesia" or "changed sensation." Basically, this term refers to the phenomenon in which a particular food is perceived as pleasant or unpleasant depending on the internal state ("milieu intérieur") of the body. Cabanac's (1971) "alliesthesia" is similar to Young's (1955) reinterpretation of Richter's (1943) experiments. However, whereas Richter studied rats and (mostly) salt selection, Cabanac studied humans and sweet selection. For example, after ingestion of glucose, humans report that formerly pleasant sweet solutions become unpleasant (Cabanac, 1971).

The work of Richter, Young, and Cabanac may apply to the case of nicotine and specific food preferences. Following from Richter and Young, nicotine may act to alter levels or availability of specific nutrients that translate into altered preferences for sweet carbohydrates. Following from Cabanac, the change in preferences for sweet taste may involve a change in glucose availability. Consistent with this possibility, Larson et al. (1961) noted that 27 of 30 animal studies reviewed reported transient, but significant, increases in blood sugar after nicotine injection. However, with respect to humans and smoking, Larson et al. (1961) wrote: "In contrast to the near unanimity of results following the injection of controlled doses of nicotine into animals, the effect of smoking on the blood-sugar level in man is notably inconsistent" (p. 325). Based on these studies, effects of nicotine on glucose may or may not underlie changes in preference for sweet foods.

A related possibility is that nicotine alters insulin levels in the body and thereby alters preference for sweet foods (possibly by altering glucose transport). Jacobs (1958) reported that insulin injections to rats resulted in increased preference for sweet foods. Briese and Quijada (1979) reported similar results in humans. Kanarek et al. (1980) reported that insulin injections to rats increased carbohydrate consumption.

With these studies and theories as background, Grunberg et al. (1988*b*) examined the effects of nicotine administration on blood levels of glucose and insulin in rats. Unlike the previous animal studies of nicotine and glucose that examined the effects of acute nicotine injections, Grunberg et al. (1988*b*) administered nicotine or saline continuously for 2 weeks via osmotic minipump. As in previous studies, nicotine administration was accompanied by a short-lived increase in blood glucose. This rise in blood glucose disappeared within a day or so *before* body weight was affected by nicotine. In contrast, nicotine decreased blood levels of insulin, and this decreased level persisted throughout the experiment. Grunberg et al. (1988*b*) suggested that these changes in blood insulin may underlie the effects of nicotine on sweet food preferences.

Nicotine also changes consumption of carbohydrates even when they are not sweet-tasting (Grunberg et al., 1985). Again, if Richter's "we eat what we need" and Young's "what we need tastes good" principles apply, then there must be an effect of nicotine that alters need for carbohydrates. Because carbohydrates break down in the body by glycolysis to provide glucose and in light of Kanarek et al.'s (1980) finding that insulin injections increase carbohydrate intake, Grunberg et al.'s (1988*b*) findings for nicotine and insulin also may underlie carbohydrate craving. However, there is another potential mechanism. It has been suggested that increased carbohydrate consumption results in increased levels of the neurotransmitter serotonin in the body (Fernstrom and Wurtman, 1971*a,b,* 1972, 1973; Wurtman, 1982; Wurtman et al., 1981). In animals, nicotine administration reduces serotonin turnover, resulting in increased central levels (Balfour et al., 1975; Fuxe et al., 1987). Therefore, it may be that nicotine's effects on serotonin result in altered preference for carbohydrates. This idea is consistent with reports that drugs that enhance serotonin transmission decrease carbohydrate consumption (Wurtman and Wurtman, 1979). Interestingly, there seem to be effects of insulin on serotonin availability (Wurtman, 1987). Therefore, it is reasonable to postulate that both insulin and serotonin are involved in the effects of nicotine on specific food preferences and that these biochemicals may act via a common mechanism. If this postulate is correct, then Richter's notion of selective appetites now can be extended to the level of food selection to modulate levels of specific neurotransmitters.

P. T. Young should not be forgotten in this context either, although he is rarely cited in recent discussions of foods and mood. Based on Fernstrom, R. Wurtman, and J. Wurtman's work on carbohydrates and serotonin, there have been human studies of the effects of food on mood and performance (Spring, 1984; Spring et al., 1982/1983, 1984). Basically, these studies report that carbohydrate consumption is followed by feelings of calm or sleepiness (Spring et al., 1984). Grunberg (1986*b*) applied these findings to nicotine and specific appetites by suggesting that cessation of nicotine (or smoking) is accompanied by increased carbohydrate consumption to alleviate the unpleasantness induced by nicotine abstinence. In effect, carbohydrate consumption might be viewed as a form of self-medication to offset the undesired pharmacological actions of nicotine abstinence. Based on Wurtman's animal studies, Spring's human studies, and Grunberg's (1986*b*) reasoning for smoking following from the work of Fernstrom, R. Wurtman, J. Wurtman, and Spring, Bowen et al. (D. J. Bowen, B. Spring, and E. Fox, personal communication) assigned 31 smokers who agreed to quit smoking to two daily diet groups: The experimental group consumed a high-carbohydrate, low-protein diet (7/1 ratio of carbohydrate/protein) plus tryptophan (hypothetically to raise serotonin and attenuate the unpleasantness of withdrawal); the control group consumed a placebo and a low-carbohydrate diet (1/1 carbohydrate/protein ratio). Two weeks after the quit-smoking date, 75% of the high-carbohydrate group were abstinent compared to 47% of the control group. In addition, the high-carbohydrate group reported less anxiety on the Multiple Affect Adjective Checklist (Zuckerman and Lubin, 1965) and less severe withdrawal symptoms as measured by the Smokers Complaint Scale (Schneider and Jarvik, 1984).

To summarize potential mechanisms underlying energy intake, there is evidence that changes in insulin levels may be involved in the changes in specific food preferences for sweets and carbohydrates. In addition, altered preference for carbohydrates may involve effects of these foodstuffs on mood and on serotonin levels. These possibilities are consistent with studies of selective appetites and nutritive needs. Effects of nicotine on other neurotransmitters and biochemicals (e.g., dopamine, norepinephrine, neuropeptide Y) also may be involved in the effects of nicotine on energy intake, but these possibilities have not yet been explored.

### Potential Mechanisms Underlying Changes in Energy Expenditure

In contrast to the extensive consideration of mechanisms underlying nicotine's actions on food intake, there has been minimal attention to potential mechanisms underlying nicotine and energy expenditure. The existing evidence points to an important role for energy expenditure in the nicotine/body weight relationship, but few studies or investigations have gone beyond the "what happens" stage and on to the "why it happens stage." The Grunberg et al. (1988*b*) study described earlier was designed with this limitation in mind. Insulin and catecholamines were measured daily during 2 weeks of nicotine administration to rats. In addition to the postulate concerning insulin and taste preferences, these biochemicals were measured because they affect energy utilization. Nicotine administration was accompanied by increased blood levels of catecholamines, but this increase was greatly attenuated after a week. Increased catecholamines increase energy utilization, so these changes may have contributed to the effects of nicotine on body weight. However, the fact that these biochemical changes did not last makes it unlikely that these effects play an important role in nicotine's effects on body weight. Nicotine administration was also accompanied by decreased blood levels of insulin that persisted throughout the experiment. These changes are consistent with a decrease in lipogenesis. Possibly, the effects of nicotine on insulin are involved in changes in energy expenditure as well as changes in energy intake. This possibility deserves further research attention.

Another mechanism that may underlie effects of nicotine on energy expenditure involves enzymatic activity. Carney and Goldberg (1984) reported a significant, positive correlation between body weight gains in ex-smokers and precessation lipoprotein lipase (LPL) activity in adipose tissue. This finding has generated interest in this enzyme and its role in the smoking/body weight phenomenon. Experiments need to be performed that indicate more than a correlational relationship for LPL and smoking-related body weight changes. Enzymatic changes may be an important mechanism to consider.

## 6. COMMONALITIES WITH OTHER ADDICTIVE DRUGS

If there presently is a *zeitgeist* regarding drugs of addiction, then it is that there are common mechanisms involved in the actions and effects of these drugs. That is not to say, however, that all addictive agents act identically. But there is value in comparing the effects of these drugs on behavior and in exploring mechanisms that may account for some of the actions of these drugs. In this context, it is intriguing that the effects of nicotine on food intake, and on sweet carbohydrate intake in particular, are not unique to nicotine. For example, similar to the effects of nicotine, oral self-administration of morphine by rats is accompanied by decreased carbohydrate consumption; cessation of morphine results in increased carbohydrate consumption (Marks-Kaufman and Lipeles, 1982). Morphine injections to rats also decrease carbohydrate intake while increasing fat intake (Marks-Kaufman, 1982). Conversely, when sugar is consumed, rats addicted to morphine consume less morphine; when sugar is removed, morphine intake increases (Kanarek and Marks-Kaufman, 1988). This finding is consistent with the fact that increased food consumption decreases self-administration of psychoactive drugs and that decreased food consumption increases self-administration of these drugs (Carroll and Meisch, 1984).

It also has been reported that there is an inverse relationship between sucrose and alcohol consumption in rats (Lester and Greenberg, 1952; Samson et al., 1982). Like Bowen et al.'s (personal communication) findings with diet and smoking abstinence, Yung et al. (1983) reported that alcoholics who remained sober for 30 days consumed significantly more sugar and carbohydrates than did individuals who relapsed to alcohol use in this period. Perhaps specific foods should be used in treatment programs to help avoid relapse to addictive drugs.

Comparisons of drugs of addiction and eating behavior may reveal commonalities underlying substances of abuse. Grunberg and Baum (1985) suggested that drugs that are addicting may "short-circuit" neurochemical pathways that underlie control of body weight and food intake. With repeated administration of these drugs, the body may adapt such that the drugs are "misinterpreted" as necessary foodstuffs. Then, the mechanisms of food selection and regulation may come to govern drug self-administration as well. This possibility is consistent with the available literature but clearly requires extensive empirical examination. Kanarek and Marks-Kaufman (1988) similarly point out that the relationship between food intake and drug-seeking behavior reveals important similarities that may help to elucidate biological bases of addiction and food selection.

Future research that addresses food selection and interaction with pharmacological agents must be carefully designed so that interpretation of results is clear. As discussed by Blundell (1983) in a comprehensive review of food selection studies, many methodological concerns must be considered in designing and conducting such studies. In any case, the potential contributions of studies of drugs and body weight to better understand addictive behaviors is vast and deserves substantial research attention.

It is also important to remember that people who use addictive drugs commonly use more than one. In the present context, it is relevant that tobacco and alcohol use are highly correlated and that both of these drugs can affect body weight (Kozlowski et al., 1986; Schoenborn and Benson, 1988; Williamson et al., 1987). Therefore, cross-sectional and longitudinal analyses of the effects of tobacco use on body weight, energy intake, and energy expenditure should carefully consider and partial out effects of alcohol and other drugs on these variables. Moreover, laboratory experiments should examine whether effects of these drugs are additive, interactive, or interchangeable. Such studies might provide a better understanding of similarities and differences in mechanisms of addictive drug actions.

## 7. DIGEST

Cigarette smoking is inversely related to body weight. This relationship results from effects of nicotine on energy intake and energy expenditure. The relative contribution of changes in energy intake in the nicotine/body weight relationship appears to be particularly important in accounting for weight gains after cessation of nicotine administration but also contributes to decreased body weight during nicotine administration. The effects of nicotine on energy intake are most pronounced for sweet foods and carbohydrates. These effects of nicotine on sweet carbohydrates are similar to effects of opiates and alcohol. The effects of these drugs of addiction on specific food selection may reveal biological processes that underlie drug addiction in general and that relate to body weight control.

## REFERENCES

Albanes, D. M., Jones, Y., Micozzi, M. S., and Mattson, M. E., 1987, Associations between smoking and body weight in the US population: Analysis of NHANES II, *Am. J. Public Health* **77** (4):439–444.

Anderson, W. G., 1914, Smoking is detrimental, quoted in *Med. Times* **42:**167–173.

Andrews, J., and McGarry, J. M., 1972, A community study of smoking in pregnancy, *J. Obstet. Gynaecol. Br. Commonw.* **79**(12):1057–1073.

Ashford, J. R., Brown, S., Duffield, D. P., Smith, C. S., and Fay, J. W. J., 1961, The relation between smoking habits and physique, respiratory symptoms, ventilatory function, and radiological pneumoconiosis amongst coal workers at three Scottish collieries, *Br. J. Prev. Soc. Med.* **15:**106–116.

Averett, J. W., 1962, The effects of nicotine on weight increment, activity, food intake, and water intake in weanling albino rats, *Diss. Abst. Int.* **23:**2187.

Balfour, D. J. K., Khuller, A. K., and Longden, A., 1975, Effects of nicotine on plasma corticosterone and brain amines in stressed and unstressed rats, *Pharmacol. Biochem. Behav.* **3**(2):179–184.

Baroni, W., and Mandrioli, C., 1952, Effetti del fumo di sigaretta sul metabolismo di base, *Policlinico* **59:**101–103.

Becker, R. F., and King, J. E., 1966, Effects of nicotine absorption in rats during pregnancy, *Science* **154:**417–418.

Biener, K., 1981, Exraucherinnen [Women who have stopped smoking], *Munchen. Med. Wochenschr.* **123**(25):1035–1038.

Birch, D., 1975, Control: Cigarettes and calories, *Can. Nurse* **71**(3):33–55.

Bizzi, A., Tacconi, M. T., Medea, A., and Garattini, S., 1972, Some aspects of the effect of nicotine in plasma FFA and tissue triglycerides, *Pharmacology* **7:**216–224.

Bjelke, W., 1971, Variation in height and weight in the Norwegian population, *Br. J. Prev. Soc. Med.* **25:**192–202.

Blackburn, H., Brozek, J., and Taylor, H. L., 1960, Common circulatory measurements in smokers and nonsmokers, *Circulation* **22:**1112–1124.

Blair, A., Blair, S. N., Howe, H. G., Pate, R. R., Rosenberg, M., Parker, G. M., and Pickle, L. W., 1980, Physical, psychological, and sociodemographic differences among smokers, exsmokers, and nonsmokers in a working population, *Prev. Med.* **9**(6):747–759.

Blair, S. N., Jacobs, D. R., and Powell, K. E., 1985, Relationships between exercise or physical activity and other health behaviors, *Public Health Rep.* **100**(2):172–180.

Blitzer, P. H., Rimm, A. A., and Giefer, E. E., 1977, The effect of cessation of smoking on body weight in 57,032 women: Cross-sectional and longitudinal analyses, *J. Chronic Dis.* **30**(7):415–429.

Blundell, J. E., 1983, Problems and processes underlying the control of food selection and nutrient intake, in: *Nutrition and Brain*, Volume 6 (R. J. Wurtman and J. J. Wurtman, eds.), pp. 163–221, Raven Press, New York.

Bogen, E., 1929, The composition of cigarettes and cigarette smoke, *JAMA* **93:**1110–1114.

Bosse, R., Garvey, A. J., and Costa, P. T., Jr., 1980, Predictors of weight change following smoking cessation, *Int. J. Addictions* **15**(7):969–991.

Bowen, D. J., Eury, S. E., and Grunberg, N. E., 1986, Nicotine's effects on female rats' body weight: Caloric intake and physical activity, *Pharmacol. Biochem. Behav.* **25**(6):1131–1136.

Briese, E., and Quijada, M., 1979, Positive alliesthesia after insulin, *Experientia* **35:**1058–1059.

Brozek, J., Blackburn, H., Taylor, H. L., and Keys, A., 1958, Pulse rate and blood pressure in male cigarette smokers and non-smokers. Delivered at Third World Congress of Cardiology.

Bryson, R., Biner, O. M., McNair, E., Bergondy, M., and Abrams, O. R., 1981, Effects of nicotine on two types of motor activity in rats, *Psychopharmacology* **73:**168–170.

Burse, R. L., Bynum, G. D., Pandolf, K. B., Goldman, R. F., Simms, E. A. H., and Danforth, E. R., 1975, Increased appetite and unchanged metabolism upon cessation of smoking with diet held constant, *Physiologist* **18:**157.

Burse, R. L., Goldman, R. F., Danforth, E., Horton, E. S., and Sims, E. A. H., 1982, Effects of cigarette smoking on body weight, energy expenditure, appetite, and endocrine function, U.S. Army Medical Research and Development Command, Fort Detrick, Frederick, Maryland, Report #M25/82, NTIS No. AD-A114 213/2.

Cabanac, M., 1971, Physiological role of pleasure, *Science* **173:**1103–1107.

Cabanac, M., 1979, Sensory pleasure, *Q. Rev. Biol.* **54:**1–29.

Cambien, F., Richard, J. L., Ducimetiere, P., Warnet, J. M., and Kahn, J., 1982, The Paris cardiovascular risk factor prevention trial. Effects of two years of intervention in a population of young men, *J. Epidemiol. Commun. Health* **35**(2):91–97.

Carney, R. M., and Goldberg, A. P., 1984, Weight gain after cessation of cigarette smoking. A possible role for adipose-tissue lipoprotein lipase, *N. Engl. J. Med.* **310**(10):614–616.

Carroll, M. E., and Meisch, R. A., 1984, Increased drug-reinforced behavior due to food deprivation, in: *Advances in Behavioral Pharmacology,* Volume 4 (T. Thompson, P. Dews, and J. E. Barrett, eds.), pp. 47–88, Academic Press, New York.

Charlton, A., 1984, The Brigantia Smoking Survey: A general review, in: *Public Education about Cancer. Recent Research and Current Programmes* (P. Hobbs, ed.), pp. 92–102, UICC Technical Report Series—Volume 77.

Coates, T. J., and Li, V., 1983, Does smoking cessation lead to weight gain?: The experience of asbestos-exposed shipyard workers, *Am. J. Public Health* **73:**1303–1304.

Comstock, G. W., and Stone, R. W., 1972, Changes in body weight and subcutaneous fatness related to smoking habits, *Arch. Environ. Health* **24**(4):271–276.

Dallosso, H. M., and James, W. P. T., 1984, The role of smoking in the regulation of energy balance, *Int. J. Obesity* **8**(4):365–375.

Davis, C., 1928, Self-selection of diets by newly-weaned infants, *Am. J. Dis. Children* **36:**651–679.

Diehl, H. S., 1929, The physique of smokers as compared to non-smokers, *Minn. Med.* **12:**424–427.

Dill, D. B., Edwards, H. T., and Forbes, W. H., 1934, Tobacco smoking in relation to blood sugar, blood lactic acid and metabolism, *Am. J. Physiol,* **109:**118–122.

Emont, S. L., and Cummings, K. M., 1987, Weight gain following smoking cessation: A possible role for nicotine replacement in weight management, *Addictive Behav.* **12:**151–155.

Esser, J., 1903, Die Beziehungen des Nervus vagus su Erkrankungen von Herz und Lungen, speziell bei experimenteller chronischer Nikotinvergiftung, *Arch. Exp. Pathol. Berlin* **49:**190–212.

Evans, J. R., Hughes, R. E., and Jones, P. R., 1967, Some effects of cigarette smoke on guinea-pigs, *Proc. Nutr. Soc.* **26:**xxxvi.

Fagerstrom, K. O., 1987, Reducing the weight gain after stopping smoking, *Addictive Behav.* **12:**91–93.

Favarger, H., 1906, Zur frage der chronischen Tabakver-giftung, *Wien. Klin. Wochenschr.* **19:**636–637.

Fehily, A. M., Phillips, K. M., and Yarnell, W. G., 1984, Diet, smoking, social class, and body mass index in the Caerphilly Heart Disease Study, *Am. J. Clin. Nutr.* **40**(4):827–833.

Feldman, W., Hodgson, C., and Corber, S., 1985, Relationship between higher prevalence of smoking and weight concern amongst adolescent girls, *Can. J. Public Health* **76:**205–206.

Fernstrom, J. D., and Wurtman, R. J., 1971*a*, Brain serotonin content: Physiological dependence on plasma tryptophan levels, *Science* **173:**149–152.

Fernstrom, J. D., and Wurtman, R. J., 1971*b*, Brain serotonin content: Increase following injection of carbohydrate diet, *Science* **174:**1023–1025.

Fernstrom, J. D., and Wurtman, R. J., 1972, Brain serotonin content: Physiological regulation by plasma neutral amino acids, *Science* **178:**414–416.

Fernstrom, J. D., and Wurtman, R. J., 1973, Control of brain 5-HT content by dietary carbohydrates, in: *Serotonin and Behavior* (J. Barchas and E. Usdin, eds.), pp. 121–128, Academic Press, New York.

Fink, B., 1921, Smoking and scholarship again, *School Soc.* **14:**87–89.

Fischer, R., Griffen, F., and Kaplan, A. R., 1963, Taste thresholds, cigarette smoking, and food dislikes, *Med. Exp.* **9:**151–169.

Fisher, M., and Gordon, T., 1985, The relation of drinking and smoking habits to diet: The Lipid Research Clinics Prevalence Study, *Am. J. Clin. Nutr.* **41**(3)**:**623–630.

Friedman, G. D., and Siegelaub, A. B., 1980, Changes after quitting cigarette smoking, *Circulation* **61:** 716–723.

Friedman, G. D., King, M-C., Klatsky, A. L., and Hulley, S. B., 1981, Characteristics of smoking-discordant monozygotic twins, in: *Twin Research 3, Part C: Epidemiological and Clinical Studies* (L. Gedda, P. Parisi, and W. E. Nance, eds.), pp. 17–22, Alan R. Liss, New York.

Fuxe, K., Andersson, K., Eneroth, P., Harfstrand, A., Nordberg, A., and Agnati, L. F., 1987, Effects of nicotine and exposure to cigarette smoke on discrete dopamine and noradrenaline nerve terminal systems of the telencephalon and diencephalon of the rat. Relationship to reward mechanisms and distribution of nicotine binding sites in brain, in: *Tobacco Smoking and Nicotine. A Neurobiological Approach* (W. R. Martin, G. R. Van Loon, E. T. Iwamoto, and L. Davis, eds.), pp. 225–262, Plenum Press, New York.

Garn, S. M., Shaw, H. A., and McCabe, K. E., 1978, Effect of maternal smoking on weight and weight gain between pregnancies (Letter), *Am. J. Clin. Nutr.* **31**(8)**:**1302–1303.

Garrison, R. J., Feinleib, M., Castelli, W. P., and McNamara, P. M., 1983, Cigarette smoking as a confounder of the relationship between relative weight and long-term mortality. The Framingham Heart Study, *JAMA* **249**(16)**:**2199–2203.

Garvey, A. J., Bosse, R., and Seltzer, C. C., 1974, Smoking, weight change, and age: A longitudinal analysis, *Arch. Environ. Health* **28**(16)**:**327–329.

Gaudet, F. J., and Hugli, W. C., Jr., 1969, Concomitant habit changes associated with changes in smoking habits, *Med. Times* **97:**195–205.

Ghanem, M. H., 1973, Metabolic effects to tobacco smoking, *Alexandria Med. J.* **19**(3)**:**224–235.

Gilbert, R. M., and Pope, M. A., 1982, Early effects of quitting smoking, *Psychopharmacology* **78:** 121–127.

Glauser, S. C., Glauser, E. M., Reidenberg, M. M., Rusy, B. F., and Tallarida, R. J., 1970, Metabolic changes associated with the cessation of cigarette smoking, *Arch. Environ. Health* **20**(3)**:** 377–381.

Goldbourt, U., and Medalie, J. H., 1977, Characteristics of smokers, nonsmokers, and ex-smokers among 10,000 adult males in Israel, II. Physiologic, biochemical, and genetic characteristics, *Am. J. Epidemiol.* **105**(1)**:**75–86.

Gordon, T., Kannel, W. B., Dawber, T. R., and McGee, D., 1975, Changes associated with quitting cigarette smoking: The Framingham study, *Am. Heart J.* **90**(3)**:**322–328.

Gormican, A., Valentine, J., and Satter, E., 1980, Relationships of maternal weight gain, prepregnancy weight, and infant birthweight, *J. Am. Diet. Assoc.* **77**(6)**:**662–667.

Grinstead, O. A., 1981, Preventing weight gain following smoking cessation: A comparison of behavioral treatment approaches. Doctoral dissertation, University of California, Los Angeles, Thesis No. 82-06024, University Microfilms International, Ann Arbor, MI.

Gritz, E. R., Carr, C. R., and Marcus, A. C., 1988, Unaided smoking cessation: Great American Smokeout and New Year's Day quitters, *J. Psychosoc. Oncol.* **6**(3/4)**:**217–235.

Grossarth-Maticek, R., Kanazier, D. T., Vetter, H., and Jankovic, M., 1983, Smoking as a risk factor for lung cancer and cardiac infarct as mediated by psychosocial variables, *Psychother. Psychosoma.* **39**(2)**:**94–105.

Grunberg, N. E., 1980, The effects of nicotine on food consumption and taste preferences (Doctoral dissertation, Columbia University), *Diss. Abstr. Int.* **41**(2)**:**728-B.

Grunberg, N. E., 1982, The effects of nicotine and cigarette smoking on food consumption and taste preferences, *Addictive Behav.* **7**:317–331.

Grunberg, N. E., 1986*a*, Behavioral and biological factors in the relationship between tobacco use and body weight, in: *Advances in Behavioral Medicine*, Volume 2 (E. S. Katkin and S. B. Manuck, eds.), pp. 97–129, JAI Press, Greenwich, CT.

Grunberg, N.E., 1986*b*, Nicotine as a psychoactive drug: Appetite regulation, *Psychopharmacol. Bull.* **22**(3):875–881.

Grunberg, N. E., and Baum, A., 1985, Biological commonalities of stress and substance abuse, in: *Coping and Substance Use* (S. Shiffman and T. A. Wills, eds.), pp. 25–62, Academic Press, New York.

Grunberg, N. E., and Bowen, D. J., 1985, The role of physical activity in nicotine's effects on body weight, *Pharmacol. Biochem. Behav.* **23**:851–854.

Grunberg, N. E., and Morse, D. E., 1984, Cigarette smoking and food consumption in the United States, *J. Appl. Soc. Psychol.* **14**:310–317.

Grunberg, N. E., Bowen, D. J., and Morse, D. E., 1984, Effects of nicotine on body weight and food consumption in rats, *Psychopharmacology* **83**:93–98.

Grunberg, N. E., Bowen, D. J., Maycock, V. A., and Nespor, S. M., 1985, The importance of sweet taste and caloric content in the effects of nicotine on specific food consumption, *Psychopharmacology* **87**(2):198–203.

Grunberg, N. E., Bowen, D. J., and Winders, S. E., 1986, Effects of nicotine on body weight and food consumption in female rats, *Psychopharmacology* **90**(1):101–105.

Grunberg, N. E., Winders, S. E., and Popp, K. A., 1987, Sex differences in nicotine's effects on consummatory behavior and body weight in rats, Psychopharmacology **91**:221–225.

Grunberg, N. E., Popp, K. A., and Winders, S. E., 1988*a*, Effects of nicotine on body weight in rats with access to "junk" foods, *Psychopharmacology* **94**:536–539.

Grunberg, N. E., Popp, K. A., Bowen, D. J., Nespor, S. M., and Winders, S. E., 1988*b*, Effects of chronic nicotine administration on insulin, glucose, epinephrine, and norepinephrine, *Life Sci.* **42**: 161–170.

Gunn, R. C., and Shapiro, A., 1985, Life stress, weight gain, and resuming smoking after success in a cessation clinic, *Psychol. Rep.* **57**(3, Part 2):1035–1039.

Gyntelberg, F., and Meyer, J., 1974, Relationship between blood pressure and physical fitness, smoking, and alcohol consumption in Copenhagen males aged 40–59, *Acta Med. Scand.* **195**(5):375–380.

Hadley, H. G., 1941, The effect of tobacco upon growth, longevity and metabolism, *Med. Rec.* **153**: 350–352.

Hadley, H. G., 1941–1942, The effect of tobacco upon the basal metabolic rate, *J. Med.* **22**:121–122.

Haggard, H. W., and Greenberg, L. A., 1934, The effects of cigarette smoking upon the blood sugar, *Science* **79**:165–166.

Hall, S. M., Ginsberg, D., and Jones, J. T., 1986, Smoking cessation and weight gain, *J. Consult. Clin. Psychol.* **54**(3):342–346.

Hatchell, P. C., and Collins, A. C., 1980, The influence of genotype and sex on behavioral sensitivity to nicotine in mice, *Psychopharmacology* **71**:45–49.

Hatsukami, D. K., Hughes, J. R., Pickens, R. W., and Svikis, D., 1984, Tobacco withdrawal symptoms: An experimental analysis, *Psychopharmacology* **84**(2):231–236.

Haworth, J. C., Ellestad-Sayed, J. J., King, J., and Dilling, L. A., 1980, Fetal growth retardation in cigarette-smoking mothers is not due to decreased maternal food intake, *Am. J. Obstet. Gynecol.* **137**(6):719–723.

Heath, C. W., 1958, Differences between smokers and non-smokers, *Arch. Intern. Med.* **101**:377–388.

Hickey, N., and Mulcahy, R., 1973, Effect of cessation of smoking on body weight after myocardial infarction, *Am. J. Clin. Nutr.* **26**(4):385–386.

Hiestand, W. A., Ramsey, H. J., and Hale, D. M., 1940, The effects of cigarette smoking on metabolic rate, heart rate, oxygen pulse, and breathing rate, *J. Lab. Clin. Med.* **25**:1013–1017.

Higgins, M. W., and Kjelsberg, M., 1967, Characteristics of smokers and nonsmokers in Tecumseh, Michigan, *Am. J. Epidemiol.* **86**:60–77.

Hjermann, I., Helgeland, A., Holme, I., Lund-Larsen, P. G., and Leren, P., 1976, The intercorrelation of serum cholesterol, cigarette smoking and body weight, *Acta Med. Scand.* **200**:479–485.

Hofstetter, A., Schutz, Y., Jequier, E., and Wahren, J., 1986, Increased 24-hour energy expenditure in cigarette smokers, *N. Engl. J. Med.* **314**(2):79–82.

Holcomb, H. S., and Meigs, J. W., 1972, Medical absenteeism among cigarette and cigar and pipe smokers, *Arch. Environ. Health* **25**(4):295–300.

Holme, I., Hjermann, I., Helgeland, A., and Leren, P., 1985, The Oslo study: Diet and antismoking advice. Additional results from a 5-year primary preventive trial in middle-aged men, *Prev. Med.* **14**(3):279–292.

Holt, W. L., 1921, Educational research and statistics. Apparent effects of smoking among University of Tennessee freshmen, *School Soc.* **14**:136–138.

Holt, W. L., 1922–1923, A statistical study of smokers and nonsmokers at the University of Tennessee, *J. Am. Stat. Assoc.* **18**:766–772.

Howell, R. W., 1971, Obesity and smoking habits (Letter), *Br. Med. J.* **4**(5787):625.

Hughes, J. A., and Hutchinson, D. C. S., 1983, Smoking, lung function, and body weight (Letter), *Br. Med. J.* **286**(6369):977.

Hughes, R. E., Jones, P. R., and Nicholas, P., 1970, Some effects of experimentally-produced cigarette smoke on the growth, vitamin C metabolism and organ weights of guinea-pigs, *J. Pharm. Pharmacol.* **22**:823–827.

Huston, J. J., and Stenson, K., 1974, The development of obesity in fit young men: A regimental survey, *Practitioner* **212**(1271):700–705.

Ilebekk, A., Miller, N. E., and Mjos, O. D., 1975, Effects of nicotine and inhalation of cigarette smoke on total body oxygen consumption in dogs, *Scand. J. Clin. Lab. Inves.* **35**(1):67–72.

Jacobs, D. R., and Gottenborg, S., 1981, Smoking and weight: The Minnesota Lipid Research Clinic, *Am. J. Public Health* **71**(4):391–396.

Jacobs, H. L., 1958, Studies on sugar preference: I. The preference for glucose solutions and its modification by injections of insulin, *J. Comp. Physiol. Psychol.* **51**:304–310.

Jenkins, C. D., Rosenman, R. H., and Zyzanski, S. J., 1968, Cigarette smoking—Its relationship to coronary heart disease and related risk factors in the western collaborative group study, *Circulation* **38**:1140–1155.

Jenkins, C. D., Zyzanski, S. J., & Rosenman, R. H., 1973, Biological, psychological, and social characteristics of men with different smoking habits, *Health Serv. Rep.* **88**(9):834–843.

Kanarek, R. B., and Marks-Kaufman, R., 1988, Animal models of appetitive behavior: Interaction of nutritional factors and drug seeking behavior, in: *Control of Appetite: Current Concepts in Nutrition* (M. Winick, ed.), pp. 1–25, Wiley, New York.

Kanarek, R. B., Marks-Kaufman, R., and Lipeles, B. J., 1980, Increased carbohydrate intake as a function of insulin administration in rats, *Physiol. Behav.* **25**:779–782.

Kannas, L., 1981, The dimensions of health behavior among young men in Finland, *Int. J. Health Educ.* **24**(3):146–155.

Kaplan, A. R., and Glanville, E. V., 1964, Taste thresholds for bitterness and cigarette smoking, *Nature* **202**:1366.

Kaplan, A. R., Glanville, E. V., and Fischer, R., 1965, Cummulative effect of age and smoking on taste sensitivity in males and females, *J. Gerontol.* **20**:334–337.

Kardasevitch, B. I., and Khais, L. M., 1940, The histological changes in the respiratory apparatus of guinea-pigs under the influence of nicotine inhalations in manufacturies, *J. Otol. Rhinol. Laryngol.* **17**:237–241.

Kerschbaum, A., Bellet, S., and Khorsandian, R., 1965, Elevation of serum cholesterol after administration of nicotine, *Am. Heart J.* **69**:206–210.

Khosla, T., and Lowe, C. R., 1971, Obesity and smoking habits, *Br. Med. J.* **4**(5778):10–13.

Kim, S. S., 1936, The influence of continuous subcutaneous injection of nicotine or adrenal gland and anterior lobe of hypophysis. II. Histological studies of the reaction of silver nitric granules of vitamin C. *Chosen Igaku-Kwai Zasshi* **26**:S1.

Kitchen, J. M. W., 1889, On the health-value to man of the so-called divinely beneficent gift, tobacco, *Med. Rec.* **35**:459–460.

Kittel, F., Rustin, R. M., Dramaix, M., DeBacker, G., and Kornitzer, M., 1978, Psycho-socio-biological correlates of moderate overweight in an industrial population, *J. Psychosom. Res.* **22**(3): 145–158.

Klesges, R. C., and Klesges, L. M., 1988, Cigarette smoking as a dietary strategy in a university population, *Int. J. Eating Dis.* **7**:413–419.

Klesges, R. C., Meyers, A. W., Hanson, C. L., and Eck, L., 1987, Smoking cessation and weight gain in males and females, Presented at the Association for the Advancement of Behavior Therapy, Boston.

Kopczynski, J., 1972, Height and weight of adults in Cracow, *Epidemiol. Rev.* **26**(4):452–463.

Kozlowski, L. T., Jelinek, L. C., and Pope, M. A., 1986, Cigarette smoking among alcohol abusers: A continuing and neglected problem, *Can. J. Public Health* **77**:205–207.

Kramer, J. F., 1982, A one-year follow-up of participants in a Smoke Stoppers program, *Patient Counsel. Health Educ.* **4**(2):89–94.

Krut, L. H., Perrin, M. J., and Bronte-Stewart, B., 1961, Taste perception in smokers and non-smokers, *Br. Med. J.* **1**:379–384.

Larson, P. S., Haag, H. B., and Silvette, H., 1961, *Tobacco: Experimental and Clinical Studies* (2 parts), Williams & Wilkins, Baltimore.

Leschtschinskaja, O., 1926, The toxicology of nicotine (In Russian with German Summary), *Bezopasnosti* No. 7–8:26–36.

Lester, D., and Greenberg, L. A., 1952, Nutrition and the etiology of alcoholism. The effect of sucrose, saccharin, and fat on the self-selection of ethyl alcohol by rats, *Q. J. Stud. Alcohol* **13**: 553.

Levin, E. D., Morgan, M. M., Galvez, C., and Ellison, G. D., 1987, Chronic nicotine and withdrawal effects on body weight and food and water consumption in female rats, *Physiol. Behav.* **39**:441–444.

Lickint, F., 1933, Einfluss des Tabaks auf die korperliche und geistige Entwicklung der Schuljugend, *Gesundheit Erzieh* **46**:465–478.

Lincoln, J., 1969, Weight gain after cessation of smoking, *JAMA* **210**:1765.

Lincoln, J. E., 1970, Relation of income to body weight in cigarette smokers and nonsmokers (Letter), *JAMA* **214**(6):1121.

Lund-Larsen, P. G., and Tretli, S., 1982, Changes in smoking habits and body weight after a three-year-period—The cardiovascular disease study in Finnmark, *J. Chronic Dis.* **35**:773–780.

Manley, R. S., and Boland, F. J., 1983, Side-effects and weight gain following a smoking cessation program, *Addictive Behav.* **8**(4):375–380.

Marks-Kaufman, R., 1982, Increased fat consumption induced by morphine administration in rats, *Pharmacol. Biochem. Behav.* **16**:949–955.

Marks-Kaufman, R., and Lipeles, B. J., 1982, Patterns of nutrient selection in rats orally self-administering morphine, *Nutr. Behav.* **1**:33–46.

Matsuya, T., 1982, Alcohol intake and smoking habits of Japanese telephone employees and their effects on the dietary intakes, *J. Formosan Med. Assoc.* **81**(7):857–867.

McArthur, C., Waldron, E., and Dickinson, J., 1958, The psychology of smoking, *J. Abnorm. Soc. Psychol.* **56**:267–275.

McBurney, D. H., and Moskat, L. J., 1975, Taste thresholds in college-age smokers and non-smokers, *Perception Psychophysics* **18**(2):71–73.

McNair, E., and Bryson, R., 1983, Effects of nicotine on weight changes and food consumption in rats, *Pharmacol. Biochem. Behav.* **18**(3):341–344.

Morgan, M. M., and Ellison, G., 1987, Different effects of chronic nicotine treatment regimens on body weight and tolerance in the rat, *Psychopharmacology* **91**(2):236–238.

Munster, G., and Battig, K., 1975, Nicotine-induced hypophagia and hypodipsia in deprived and in hypothalamically stimulated rats, *Psychopharmacologia* **41**:211–217.

Nemery, B., Moavero, N. E., Brasseur, L., and Stanescu, D. C., 1983, Smoking, lung function, and body weight, *Br. Med. J.* **286**(6362):249–251.

NIH Consensus Development Conference on Health Implications of Smokeless Tobacco Use, Jan. 13–15, 1986, National Institutes of Health, Bethesda, MD.

Noppa, H., and Bengtsson, C., 1980, Obesity in relation to smoking: A population study of women in Goteborg, Sweden, *Prev. Med.* **9**(4)**:**534–543.

Otis, E. O., 1884, The use of tobacco by boys, *Boston Med. Surg. J.* **110:**99–103.

Page, R. M., 1983, Assessing gender differences in college cigarette smoking intenders and nonintenders, Doctoral dissertation, Southern Illinois University, Thesis No. 82-21953, University Microfilms International, Ann Arbor, MI.

Pangborn, R. M., and Trabue, I. M., 1973, Gustatory responses during periods of controlled and ad lib cigarette smoking, *Perception Psychophysics* **1:**139–144.

Passey, R. D., Elson, L. A., and Lewis, P. A., 1959, Tobacco smoke and growth rate, *Br. Empire Cancer Campaign, Ann. Rep.* **37:**89.

Passey, R. D., Elson, L. A., and Connors, T. A., 1961, Growth and metabolic effects of cigarette smoking and nicotine inhalation, *Br. Empire Cancer Campaign, Ann. Rep.* **39**(Part II)**:**90.

Pemberton, J., and Macleod, K. I. E., 1956, Rural health survey of men over forty, *Public Health Rep.* **71:**1213–1220.

Perlick, D., 1977, The withdrawal syndrome: Nicotine addiction and the effects of stopping smoking in heavy and light smokers. Unpublished doctoral dissertation, Columbia University, New York, Doctoral dissertation, Columbia University, Thesis No. 77-14, 833, University Microfilms International, Ann Arbor, MI.

Perrin, M. J., Krut, L. H., and Bronte-Stewart, B., 1961, Smoking and food preferences, *Br. Med. J.* **1:** 387–388.

Peters, J. M., and Ferris, B. G., Jr., 1967, Morphological constitution and smoking, *Arch. Environ. Health* **14:**678–681.

Peterson, D. L., Longergan, L. H., and Hardinge, M. G., 1968, Smoking and taste perception, *Arch. Environ. Health* **16:**219.

Picone, T. A., Allen, L. H., Schramm, M. M., and Olsen, P. N., 1982, Pregnancy outcome in North American women. I. Effects of diet, cigarette smoking, and psychological stress on maternal weight gain, *Am. J. Clin. Nutr.* **36**(6)**:**1205–1213.

Pincherle, G., 1971, Obesity and smoking habits (Letter), *Br. Med. J.* **4**(5782)**:**298.

Powell, D. R., and McCann, B. S., 1981, The effects of a multiple treatment program and maintenance procedures on smoking cessation, *Prev. Med.* **10:**94–104.

Powers, P. S., 1980, *Obesity, the Regulation of Weight,* Williams & Wilkins, Baltimore.

Puddey, I. B., Vandongen, R., Beilin, L. J., English, D. R., and Ukich, A. W., 1985, The effect of stopping smoking on blood pressure—A controlled trial, *J. Chronic Dis.* **38**(6)**:**483–493.

Pursell, E. D., Sanders, R. E., and Haude, R. H., 1973, Sensitivity to sucrose in smokers and nonsmokers: A comparison of TSD and percent correct measures, *Psychophysics* **14**(1)**:**34–36.

Rabkin, S., 1984, Relationship between weight change and the reduction or cessation of cigarette smoking, *Int. J. Obesity* **8**(6)**:**665–673.

Rantakallio, P., and Hartikainen-Sorri, A., 1981, The relationship between birth weight, smoking during pregnancy and maternal weight gain, *Am. J. Epidemiol.* **113**(5)**:**590–595.

Redington, K., 1984, Taste differences between cigarette smokers and nonsmokers, *Pharmacol. Biochem. Behav.* **21:**203–208.

Richter, C. P., 1939, Salt taste thresholds of normal and adrenalectomized rats, *Endocrinology* **24:**367–371.

Richter, C. P., 1943, Total self regulatory functions in animals and human beings, *Harvey Lecture Series* **38:**63–103.

Robinson, S., and York, D. A., 1986, The effect of cigarette smoking on the thermic response to feedings, *Int. J. Obesity* **10:**407–417.

Rodgers, R. J., 1979, Effects of nicotine, mecamylamine and hexamethonium on shock-induced fighting, pain reactivity and locomotor behavior in rats, *Psychopharmacology* **66:**93–98.

Rodin, J., 1987, Weight changes following smoking cessation: The role of food intake and exercise, *Addictive Behav.* **12:**303–317.

Rozin, P., 1984, The acquisition of food habits and preferences, in: *Behavioral Health: A Handbook of Health Enhancement and Disease Prevention* (J. D. Matarazzo, S. M. Weiss, J. A. Herd, N. E. Miller, and S. M. Weiss, eds.), pp. 590–607, Wiley, New York.

Rush, D., 1974, Examination of the relationship between birthweight, cigarette smoking during pregnancy and maternal weight gain, *J. Obstet. Gynaecology Br. Commonw.* **81**(10):746–752.

Samson, H. H., Roehrs, T. A., and Tolliver, G. A., 1982, Ethanol reinforced responding in the rat: A concurrent analysis using sucrose as the alternate choice, *Pharmacol. Biochem. Behav.* **17**:333–339.

Schechter, M. D., and Cook, P. G., 1976, Nicotine-induced weight loss in rats without an effect on appetite, *Eur. J. Pharmacol.* **38**(1):63–69.

Schievelbein, H., Heinemann, G., Loeschenkohl, K., Troll, C., and Schlegel, J., 1978, Metabolic aspects of smoking behavior, in: *Smoking Behaviour. Physiological and Psychological Influences* (R. E. Thornton, ed.), Churchill Livingstone, Edinburgh.

Schlatter, J., and Battig, K., 1979, Differential effects of nicotine and amphetamine on locomotor activity and maze exploration in two rat lines, *Psychopharmacology* **64**:155–161.

Schlatter, J., and Battig, K., 1981, The adrenergic role in the manifestation of nicotine effects on maze ambulation in Roman High- and Roman Low-Avoidance rats, *Br. J. Addict.* **76**:199–209.

Schlumm, F., 1930, Nikotinabusus und grundumsatz, *Verh. Deut. Ges. inn. Med.* **42**:151–155.

Schlumm, F., 1932, Tabakmissbrauch und hyperthyreoidismus, *Ztschr. Klin. Med.* **120**:648–653.

Schmitthenner, J. E., Hafkenshiel, J. B., Forte, I., and Riegel, C., 1957, The effects of nicotine on left-ventricular work and coronary blood flow, *Am. J. Med. Sci.* **234**:487–488.

Schneider, N. G., and Jarvik, M. E., 1984, Time course of smoking withdrawal symptoms as a function of nicotine replacement, *Psychopharmacology* **82**:143–144.

Schoenborn, C. A., and Benson, V., 1988, Relationships between smoking and other unhealthy habits: United States, 1985, *NCHS Advancedata* **154**:1–8.

Schoenenberger, J. C., 1982, Smoking change in relation to changes in blood pressure, weight, and cholesterol, *Prev. Med.* **11**(4):441–453.

Seaver, J. W., 1897, The effects of nicotine, *Q. J. Inebriates* **19**:132–141.

Seltzer, C. C., 1974, Effect of smoking on blood pressure, *Am. Heart J.* **87**(5):558–564.

Shah, J. R., Warawadeker, M. D., Deshmukh, P. A., and Phutane, P. N., 1959, Institutional survey of pulmonary tuberculosis with special reference to smoking habits, *Ind. J. Med. Sci.* **13**:381–392.

Short, J. J., Johnson, H. J., and Ley, H. A., 1939, The effects of tobacco smoking on health, *J. Lab. Clin. Med.* **24**:586–589.

Silbert, S., and Friedlander, M., 1931, Studies in thrombo-angiitis obliterans (Buerger). VII. The basal metabolism, *JAMA* **96**:1857–1858.

Spring, B., 1984, Recent research on the behavioral effects of tryptophan and carbohydrate, *Nutr. Health* **3**:55–68.

Spring, B., Maller, O., Wurtman, J., Digman, L., and Cozolino, L., 1982/1983, Effects of protein and carbohydrate meals on mood and performance: Interactions with sex and age, *J. Psychiatr. Res.* **17** (2):155–167.

Spring, B. J., Lieberman, H., Swope, G., and Garfield, G., 1984, Effects of carbohydrates on mood and behavior, Presented at Diet and Behavior: A Multidisciplinary Evaluation, Arlington, VA, Nov. 27–29, 1984.

Stamford, B. A., Matter, S., Fell, R. D., Sady, S., Cresanta, M. K., and Papanek, P., 1984*a*, Cigarette smoking, physical activity, and alcohol consumption: Relationship to blood lipids and lipoproteins in premenopausal females, *Metabolism: Clin. Exp.* **33**:585–590.

Stamford, B. A., Matter, S., Fell, R. D., Sady, S., Papanek, P., and Cresanta, M., 1984*b*, Cigarette smoking, exercise, and high density lipoprotein cholesterol, *Atherosclerosis* **52**(1):73–83.

Stamford, B. A., Matter, S., Fell, R. D., and Papanek, P., 1986, Effects of smoking cessation on weight gain, metabolic rate, caloric consumption, and blood lipids, *Am. J. Clin. Nutr.* **43**(4):486–494.

Stephens, T., and Pederson, L., 1983, Smoking, physical activity and health: Findings from the Canada Fitness Survey, in: *Proceedings of the World Conference on Smoking and Health,* Volume 1 (F. Forbes, R. C. Frecker, and D. Nostbakken, eds.), pp. 217–223, Canadian Council on Smoking and Health, Ottawa.

Stitzer, M. L., and Gross, J., 1988, Nicotine replacement: Effect on post cessation withdrawal symptoms and weight gain, in: *Problems of Drug Dependence,* NIDA Research Monograph No. 81 (L. Harris, ed.), pp. 53–58, U.S. Govt. Printing Office, Washington, DC.

Sutherland, W. H. F., Temple, W. A., Nye, E. R., and Herbison, G. P., 1980, Adiposity, lipids, alcohol consumption, smoking, and gender, *Am. J. Clin. Nutr.* **33**(12):2581–2587.

Taylor, C. K., 1910, The boy and the cigarette, *Psychol. Clin. Philadelphia* **1**:54–55.

Theeuwes, F., and Yum, S. I., 1977, Principles of the design and operation of generic osmotic pumps for the delivery of semisolid or liquid drug formulations, *Ann. Biomed. Eng.* **4**:343–353.

Tuomilehto, J., Jalkanen, L., Salonen, J. T., and Nissinen, A., 1985, Factors associated with changes in body weight during a five-year follow-up of a population with high blood pressure, *Scand. J. Soc. Med.* **13**(4):173–180.

Turley, F. C., and Harrison, T. R., 1932, Respiratory measurements as affected by smoking and by athletics, *Am. J. Med. Sci.* **183**:702–707.

USDHEW, 1979, *Smoking and Health: A Report of the Surgeon General,* Department of Health, Education, and Welfare, Public Health Service, Office on Smoking and Health, DHEW Publ. No. (PHS) 79-50066.

USDHHS, 1982, *The Health Consequences of Smoking: Cancer. A Report of the Surgeon General,* Department of Health and Human Services, Public Health Service, Office on Smoking and Health, DHHS Publ. No. (PHS) 82-50179.

USDHHS, 1983, *The Health Consequences of Smoking: Cardiovascular Disease. A Report of the Surgeon General,* Department of Health and Human Services, Public Health Service, Office on Smoking and Health, DHHS Publ. No. (PHS) 84-50204.

USDHHS, 1984, *The Health Consequences of Smoking: Chronic Obstructive Lung Disease. A Report of the Surgeon General,* Department of Health and Human Services, Public Health Service, Office on Smoking and Health, DHHS Publ. No. 84-50205.

USDHHS, 1986, *The Health Consequences of Using Smokeless Tobacco, A Report of the Advisory Committee to the Surgeon General,* NIH Publ. No. 86-2874.

USDHHS, 1988, *The Health Consequences of Smoking: Nicotine Addiction. A Report of the Surgeon General,* Department of Health and Human Services, Public Health Service, Office on Smoking and Health, DHHS Publ. No. (CDC) 88-8406.

Vandenbroucke, J. P., Mauritz, B. J., DeBruin, A., Verheesen, J. H. H., Van der Heide-Wessel, C., and Vander Heide, R. M., 1984, Weight, smoking, and mortality, *JAMA* **252**:2859–2860.

Wager-Srdar, S. A., Levine, A. S., Morley, J. E., Hoidal, J. R., and Niewoehner, D. E., 1984, Effects of cigarette smoke and nicotine on feeding and energy, *Physiol. Behav.* **32**(3):389–395.

Waller, R. E., and Brooks, A. G. F., 1972, Heights and weights of men visiting a public health exhibition, *Br. J. Prev. Soc. Med.* **26**(3):180–185.

Wehner, A. P., Olson, R. J., and Busch, R. H., 1976, Increased life span and decreased weight in hamsters exposed to cigarette smoke, *Arch. Environ. Health* **31**:146–153.

Wellman, P. J., Marmon, M. M., Reich, S., and Ruddle, J., 1986, Effects of nicotine on body weight, food intake, and brown adipose tissue thermogenesis, *Pharmacol. Biochem. Behav.* **24**(6):1605–1609.

Wennmalm, A., 1982, Effect of cigarette smoking on basal and carbon dioxide stimulated cerebral blood flow in man, *Clin. Physiol.* **2**(6):529–535.

Whichelow, M. J., Golding, J. F., and Treasure, F. P., 1988, Comparison of some dietary habits of smokers and non-smokers, *Br. J. Addiction* **83**:295–304.

Williamson, D. F., Forman, M. R., Binkin, N. J., Gentry, E. M., Remington, P. L., and Trowbridge, F. L., 1987, Alcohol and body weight in United States adults, *Am. J. Public Health* **77**(10):1324–1330.

Wright, S., 1846, Experiments on the physiological action of tobacco, *London M. Gaz. N.S.* **92**:592–593.

Wurtman, J. J., and Wurtman, R. J., 1979, Drugs that enhance central serotoninergic transmission diminish elective carbohydrate consumption by rats, *Life Sci.* **24**:895–904.

Wurtman, R. J., 1982, Nutrients that modify brain function, *Sci. Am.* **246**:50–59.

Wurtman, R. J., 1987, Dietary treatments that affect brain neurotransmitters, *Ann. NY Acad. Sci.* **499**: 179–190.

Wurtman, R. J., Hefti, F., and Melamed, E., 1981, Precursor control of neurotransmitter synthesis, *Pharmacol. Rev.* **32**:315–335.

Young, P. T., 1936, *Motivation of Behavior,* Wiley, New York.

Young, P. T., 1955, The role of hedonic processes in motivation, in: *Nebraska Symposium on Motivation* (M. R. Jones, ed.), pp. 193–238, University of Nebraska Press, Lincoln.

Yung, L., Gordis, E., and Holt, J., 1983, Dietary choices and likelihood of abstinence among alcoholic patients in an out-patient clinic, *Drug Alcohol Dependence* **12:**355.

Zeiner-Henriksen, T., 1976, Rokevaner i den Norske befolking [Smoking habits of the Norwegian population], *Tiddskr. Norske Laegeforening* **96**(11):617–620.

Zuckerman, M., and Lubin, B., 1965, *Manual for the Multiple Affect Adjective Checklist,* Educational and Industrial Testing Service, San Diego, CA.

# 10

# Effects of Abstinence from Tobacco

## A Critical Review

JOHN R. HUGHES, STEPHEN T. HIGGINS, and DOROTHY HATSUKAMI

## 1. INTRODUCTION

Many smokers, ex-smokers, and scientists have strong opinions about the effects of abstinence from tobacco. Some believe the effects are mild, are not true withdrawal phenomena, and have little to do with the inability of smokers to stop. Others believe abstinence effects can produce significant distress, are similar to the classical withdrawal syndromes of opiates and sedatives, and account for much of the inability of smokers to stop.

Over the last 40–50 years, the withdrawal syndromes from opiates (e.g., Martin, 1977; Katz and Valentino, 1986), alcohol (e.g., Mello and Mendelson, 1977), sedatives/hypnotics (Woods et al., 1987), and benzodiazepines have been well characterized (Fig. 1) and determinants of withdrawal, such as dose and duration of drug use, have been well delineated (e.g., Kalant et al., 1971; Martin, 1977). Finally, the role of withdrawal in the maintenance and cessation of such drugs has been empirically studied (Cappell and Leblanc, 1971).

In contrast, well-designed, systematic studies of abstinence from tobacco have been completed only in the last 5 years. Of the several possibilities to explain the lag in studying tobacco withdrawal, two appear salient. First, consensus that smoking is a drug dependence is a new phenomenon, only appearing in the 1980s (American Psychiatric Association, 1980; National Institute on Drug Abuse, 1983). Second, with a few exceptions (e.g., Grunberg, 1985), animal models of withdrawal so helpful with opiates and alcohol have not been well developed.

Recent interest in tobacco withdrawal may be due to several factors. One pos-

JOHN R. HUGHES and STEPHEN T. HIGGINS • Departments of Psychiatry, Psychology, and Family Practice, University of Vermont, Burlington, Vermont 05405. DOROTHY HATSUKAMI • Departments of Psychiatry and Psychology, University of Minnesota, Minneapolis, Minnesota 55455.

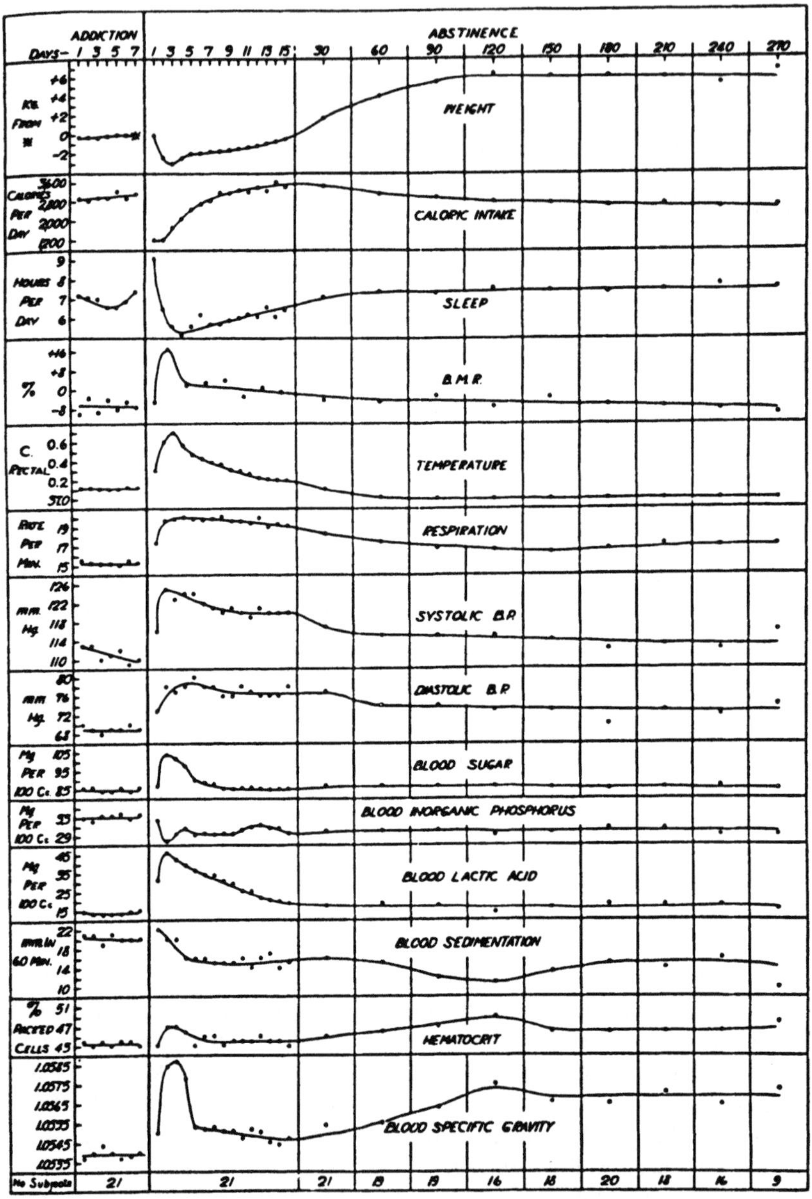


Figure 1. Opiate withdrawal signs and symptoms. (Reprinted with permission. From Himmelsbach, 1942, *Archives of Internal Medicine* **69:** 764, copyright 1942, American Medical Association.)

sibility is that the disappointing success of behavioral treatments for smoking has made many reconsider their theories of why people smoke (Leventhal and Cleary, 1980). Second, nicotine gum has recently been shown to be a successful treatment for smoking. The success of nicotine gum is thought to be due to suppression of tobacco withdrawal (Hughes and Miller, 1984). Third, interest in the commonalities across different types of substance abuse has increased recently (Krasnegor, 1978; Levinson et al., 1983; Mule, 1981).

Several reviews on tobacco withdrawal have already appeared (Hatsukami and Hughes, 1985; Hatsukami, 1988; Larson and Silvette, 1961, 1968, 1971, 1975; Mangan and Golding, 1984; Murray and Lawrence, 1984; Shiffman, 1979; West, 1984). We believe another review is worthwhile because prior reviews have been less than comprehensive and because well-done research in the area has increased remarkably in the last few years.

This chapter first proposes five subtypes of abstinence effects: indefinite, offset, transient, rebound, and novel effects. Next, the methodology of our review, criteria for inclusion of studies and criteria for conclusions are outlined and defended.

The major sections of the chapter review the biochemical, physiological, behavioral, and subjective effects of abstinence. For these effects, the consistency across studies, validity, reliability, generalizability, magnitude, incidence, and time course are examined. Whether the effect is best classified as an indefinite, offset, transient, or rebound effect is discussed. Also, data on whether the effect appears to be due to nicotine deprivation are reviewed. This section is quite detailed, and the reader may wish to review only the summary statements and tables unless he/she has a particular interest in a certain abstinence effect.

The final sections review the determinants, clinical significance, and treatment of abstinence effects.

## 2. TYPES OF ABSTINENCE EFFECTS

As used in this chapter, *abstinence effect* is a generic term that simply indicates a change due to abstinence from tobacco. For this chapter we propose five subtypes of abstinence effects: indefinite, offset, transient, rebound, and novel effects. These subtypes are distinguished by the time patterns of abstinence effects and by the amount of data and follow-up necessary to define the subtype.

Noteworthy in this classification is the absence of the term *withdrawal*. In the past, *withdrawal* has been applied to all of these subtypes. In this chapter we purposely avoid the term *withdrawal* as use of it is often confusing and problematic.

### Indefinite Effects

Many studies of abstinence effects provide only a single postcessation measure (Fig. 2). Since such results give no indication of the time pattern of abstinence effects, they will be termed *indefinite effects*.

## Offset Effects

Studies that give at least two data points postcessation produce results that can be termed offset or transient effects. Studies in which the two data points indicate a *uniphasic* change in a direction opposite to the agonist effects of nicotine followed by a stabilization can be referred to as offset effects (Fig. 2). The simplest explanation of this pattern is that cessation of tobacco allowed the variable being measured to return to a tonic level; i.e., the effect is due to the "offset" of drug effects. Many investigators would not refer to these effects as withdrawal or even abstinence effects because then withdrawal or abstinence effects would have to be said to occur with almost all drugs, as the removal of most drugs produces a return to the predrug baseline. On the other hand, offset effects can be important as they can be aversive (e.g., increase in weight) and could lead to relapse.

In the past, we and others have incorrectly assumed such offset effects are *return-to-baseline* effects; i.e., the new level represents the pretobacco level (Hatsukami and Hughes, 1985; Hatsukami et al., 1984; Hughes and Hatsukami, 1986). However, this assumption may be incorrect because the level at which the measures stabilize could represent a new baseline produced by nonreversible effects of a drug.

## Transient Effects

Results in which the postcessation data points indicate a *biphasic,* finite time course can be referred to as transient effects (Fig. 2). Thus, offset and transient effects are mutually exclusive. Note that this effect cannot be explained as a simple offset of a drug effect. Transient effects are important as most clinical definitions of *withdrawal* require demonstration of transient effects because *withdrawal* implies a short-lived perturbation of behavioral and physiological systems.

## Rebound Effects

Rebound effects are a special subtype of transient effects. Although many use the term *rebound* to refer to transient effects, for most investigators rebound effects are a special type of transient effect. A rebound effect refers to a transient effect that is in the direction opposite to the agonist effect of a drug and exceeds the predrug baseline, i.e., an "overshoot" (Fig. 2). Such rebound effects are characteristic of withdrawal of the classical opiate/sedative type (Martin, 1977; see Section 14 for further explanation). Rebound effects actually require not only more postcessation data points, but also a measure of predrug functioning. Although such predrug values are easily obtained in animal studies, they are almost impossible to obtain in humans. Often, values from non-drug users (i.e., never-smokers) are used to substitute for the predrug baseline. However, there are some problems with using these control groups as outlined in Section 4.

## Novel Effects

Abstinence from drugs can produce new effects. For example, abstinence from alcohol can produce tremor and seizures. Although these effects can sometimes be

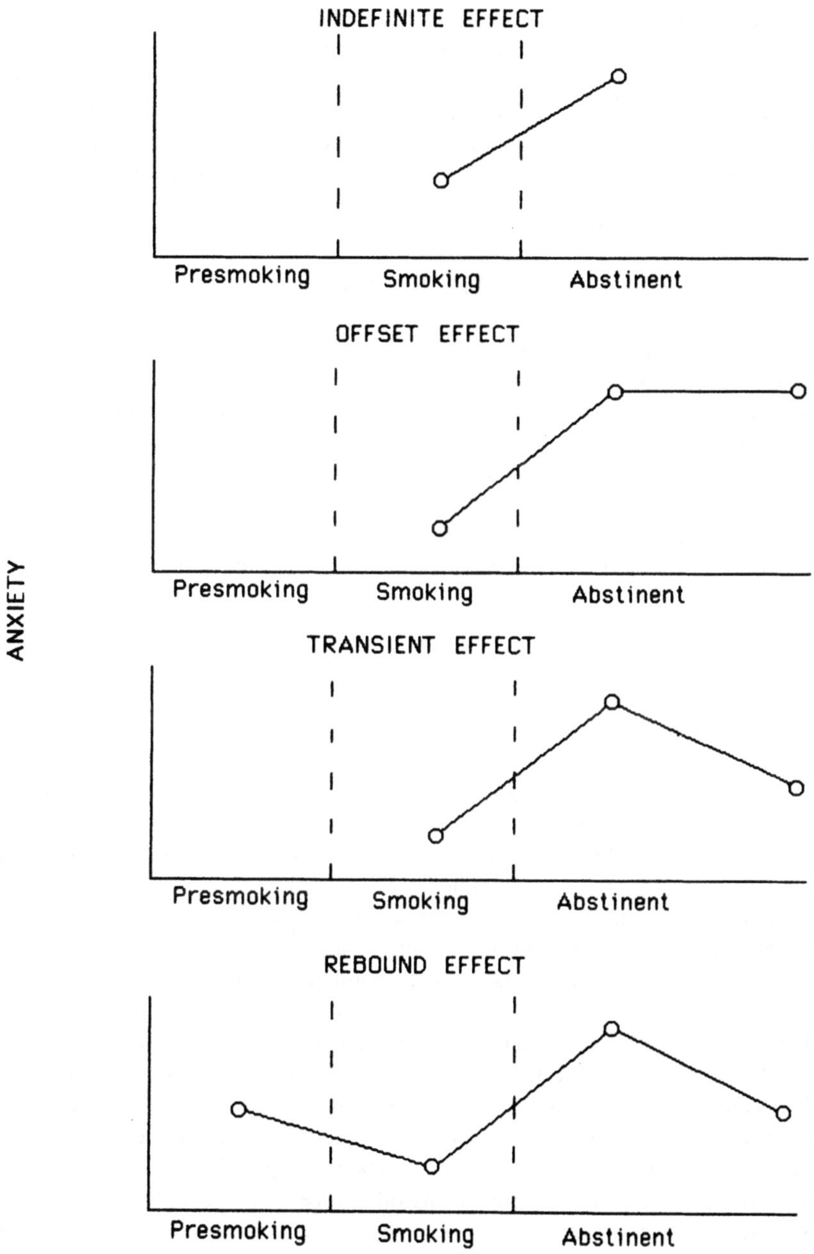


Figure 2. Subtypes of abstinence effects.

predicted by knowing the agonist effects of the drug (e.g., alcohol decreases tremor and increases the seizure threshold), these effects are so unusual they are best described as novel rather than transient effects. In our literature review we found no instances of novel effects from abstinence from tobacco or nicotine.

In summary, many investigators (ourselves included) have failed to distinguish indefinite, offset, transient, rebound, and novel effects and have thereby confused readers and sometimes implied a precision, a time course, or an etiology not justified by the data at hand. We hope this review will help clarify this confusion.

## 3. METHODOLOGY OF THIS REVIEW

Studies on the effects of abstinence from tobacco were located via five methods: (1) computer searches of *Index Medicus* and *Psychological Abstracts,* (2) *Bibliography on Smoking and Health,* (3) recent texts on smoking (e.g., Ashton and Stepney, 1982; Mangan and Golding, 1984), (4) reference lists of articles from 1–3, and (5) requests for in-press articles. The review was comprehensive through April 1988. Selected manuscripts were added after this time. Although we have tried to be inclusive, if we have missed some pertinent studies that fulfilled our inclusion criteria, we apologize to the investigators and would appreciate notification of such publications.

## 4. CRITERIA FOR INCLUSION OF STUDIES

### Baseline Values or Never-Smoker Control Groups Required

Our first criterion for inclusion in this review is that the study be a prospective study with either baseline values or a control group of never-smokers. It is important that the reader realize that this criterion eliminated all retrospective studies and many cross-sectional studies and prospective studies. Retrospective studies were excluded because they may be misleading not only because of memory problems, but also because of a "rationalization" bias. For example, unsuccessful quitters may overestimate the severity of abstinence effects to rationalize their inability to quit.

Cross-sectional studies (i.e., single-point comparisons of abstinent smokers and smoking smokers or relapsed smokers) without a control group of never-smokers were excluded for two reasons. First, differences between abstinent smokers and smoking smokers could be due, not to the effects of abstinence, but rather to the acute effects of smoking. Second, in cross-sectional studies subjects selected themselves into abstinent smoker, relapsed smoker, and continuing smoker groups. This self-selection bias may confuse abstinence effects with preexisting differences. For example, abstinent smokers and relapsed smokers appear to differ on many relevant characteristics *prior* to stopping smoking (Hughes, 1986*a*). For example, smokers who end up relapsing are more neurotic *a priori* than abstinent smokers (Eysenk and Eaves, 1980; Cherry and Kiernan, 1976). Thus, if a cross-sectional study finds that abstinent smokers are more anxious than relapsed smokers, it is unclear whether such a difference indicates the effects of abstinence or baseline differences.

Prospective studies that report only postcessation values were excluded, as baseline values are necessary to discriminate abstinence effects from trait effects. For example, if a smoker rates himself as anxious after smoking, without a baseline score it is impossible to know if this is due to abstinence or simply because the individual is chronically anxious.

Prospective and cross-sectional studies that lack baseline scores but do include scores not only for abstinent smokers but also for smoker and never-smoker control groups are included. For simplicity, we assume reports using "nonsmokers" are actually referring to never-smokers, i.e., not ex-smokers. However, this may not be true (Hughes and Valliere, 1988). In this design, the never-smoker group serves as a proxy for a predrug baseline value. If the scores of the abstinent smokers differ not only from smoking smokers but also from never-smokers (e.g., abstinent smokers are more anxious than smoking smokers *and* never-smokers; Fig. 3), then the result can be attributed to abstinence effects. On the other hand, if abstinent smokers differ from smoking

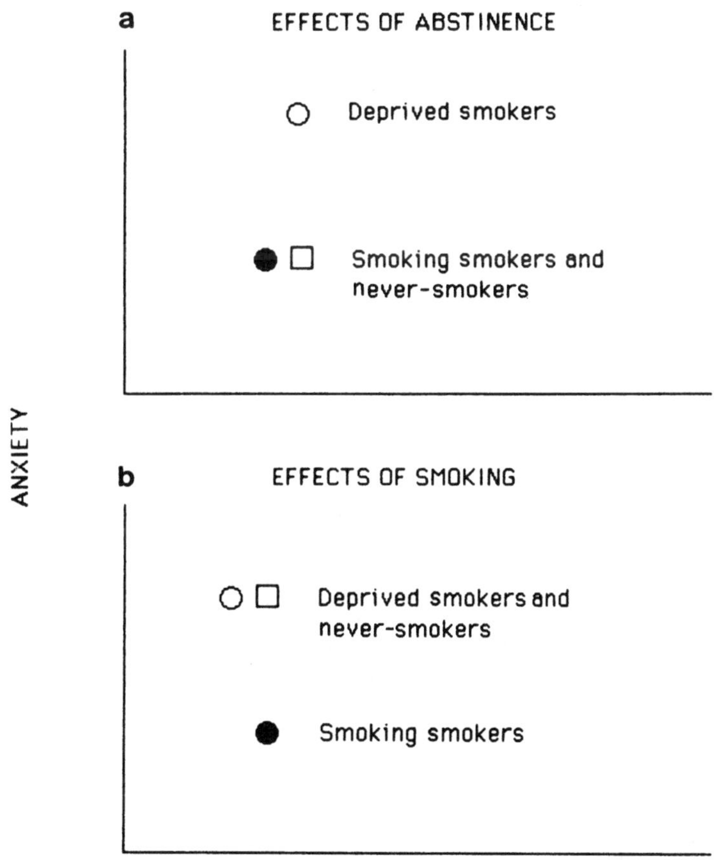


Figure 3. Possible outcomes of abstinence studies using deprived smokers (○), smoking smokers (●), and never-smokers (□). (a) Abstinence effects. (b) Acute effects of smoking.

smokers but are equivalent to never-smokers (e.g., abstinent smokers are more anxious than smoking smokers but equally anxious to nonsmokers; Fig. 3), then the result may be due to the acute effects of smoking.

Although results from this design that fit the first outcome (Fig. 3) are included in our review, the reader should be aware of an alternate interpretation of such results. This interpretation states that the differences between nonsmokers and abstinent smokers are due not to abstinence effects, but rather to *a priori* differences between nonsmokers and smokers. For example, individuals who become smokers (i.e., the abstinent smokers in Fig. 3) may be more anxious *a priori* than individuals who do not become smokers (i.e., the nonsmokers in Fig. 3; Cherry and Kiernan, 1976; Eysenk and Eaves, 1980; Hughes, 1986*a;* Seltzer and Oechsli, 1985).

To reiterate, our first inclusion criterion eliminates all retrospective studies, all cross-sectional studies, and all prospective studies that do not have either a baseline score or a score from a control group of smokers and nonsmokers. Some of the more comprehensive and widely cited studies that are eliminated by these criteria include Cummings et al., 1985*b;* Glassman et al., 1985; Guilford, 1966; Gunn, 1986; Manley and Boland, 1983; Pomerleau et al., 1978, 1983*a;* Shiffman and Jarvik, 1976; Stumpfe, 1984; Williams, 1979.

## Overnight Deprivation Excluded

Our second criterion is that studies of overnight abstinence are excluded. A common design in smoking research is to have smokers abstain overnight or for a brief period of time and then measure a dependent variable before smoking and then again after smoking. Usually the difference in the pre- and postsmoking scores is attributed to the acute effects of smoking. However, one could interpret the presmoking score as representing an abstinence score and the postsmoking score as a baseline score and attribute the difference to an abstinence effect. Without a preabstinence score it is debatable whether the prescores represent abstinence effects. Thus, we have not included studies of overnight or short-term deprivation (i.e., $\leq$12 hr) in this review.

## Craving Excluded

Our third inclusion criterion is that studies of craving or desire to smoke are excluded. This was done for several reasons. First, use of the term *craving* is problematic (Kozlowski and Wilkinson, 1987). For example, high craving ratings occur in the absence of abstinence (Hughes and Hatsukami, 1986) and craving is poorly correlated with other abstinence effects (Goldstein et al., 1988; Hughes et al., 1986*b;* West 1986). Craving or desire to smoke was eliminated for a second, more pragmatic, reason. Inclusion of all studies that reported craving or desire to smoke after cessation of smoking would be overwhelming.

For these reasons, "withdrawal" studies that focused only on desire to smoke (e.g., Finnegan et al., 1945; Gritz and Jarvik, 1973) were excluded. For those interested in the effects of abstinence on craving, a recent review by West and Schneider (1987) is recommended.

## Beneficial Effects of Abstinence Excluded

Our fourth criterion is that studies of the beneficial effects of cessation of smoking (e.g., improved cholesterol levels and pulmonary functions) are excluded. We did not consider these because the focus of this chapter is on abstinence effects that address the theory that smoking is a drug dependence or the theory that abstinence effects increase relapse to smoking.

## Critique of Our Inclusion Criteria

Some readers may believe our criteria are too stringent; however, these criteria provided a sufficient number of well-done studies to draw conclusions about most of the proposed effects of abstinence from smoking. Other readers may worry that the criteria are too lenient. These readers may believe that lumping indefinite and offset effects with rebound, transient or novel effects is unwarranted as the two classes of effects differ in their validity, etiologies, and so forth. We have intentionally included indefinite and offset effects. Our reason is that such effects are due to abstinence from tobacco, are often aversive, and could lead to relapse.

# 5. DESCRIPTION OF ABSTINENCE EFFECTS

In Sections 6–9, we review the evidence for physiological, behavioral, and subjective effects that have been attributed to tobacco abstinence. For each proposed effect, we first describe the agonist effects of smoking and, thus, the expected abstinence effects, i.e., opposite to the agonist effects. We then evaluate the validity of the effect by assessing its consistency across studies. We try to resolve any inconsistencies in the literature. Either in this section or a later section (Section 11) we describe the reliability, generalizability, magnitude, incidence, and time course of the effect. We also describe whether the effect appears to be an indefinite, offset, transient, or rebound effect. We review whether the effect appears to be due to nicotine deprivation. Finally, we state our conclusion about the literature on the effect of abstinence.

One important methodological issue (see Section 10 for others) is whether the studies are of smokers who are temporarily quitting for the purposes of the study or are of smokers who are making a serious attempt to stop smoking. Results from those two populations might vary substantially. *To help clarify this issue, we use "deprivation" to refer to abstinence induced by experimental manipulations and "cessation" to refer to abstinence induced by subjects trying to stop smoking.*

In the following sections, the reader will note three recurring patterns of results. First, there is a paucity of data in many areas. Second, many of the results are taken from book chapters, abstracts, brief reports, and so on, in which the quality of the study cannot be readily assessed. Third, even when many well-described results are available, they are often directly contradictory. Given this pattern of results, we were faced with two alternatives: (1) take an "educated guess" about the effects of abstinence using our experience and expertise or (2) present the results and eschew conclusions. In choosing between the two, we have leaned toward the latter, as we are afraid of premature closure in any one area in a field as unstudied as tobacco withdrawal. However, the result of this strategy is that, in many sections, the chapter reads as a compendium rather than an integrative text. It is difficult to integrate results that are either not available, not well described, or completely contradictory. Rather than an integrative chapter, we hope our chapter will help readers distinguish the abstinence effects in which there is a substantial consensus based on solid scientific evidence from those that are still speculative.

## 6. BIOCHEMICAL EFFECTS OF ABSTINENCE

The effects of abstinence on biochemical measures are outlined in Table 1.

### Acetycholine

Many of the effects of nicotine (e.g., improved performance) are thought to be due to increased cholinergic activity (Ashton and Stepney, 1982; Mangan and Golding, 1984). Based on this idea, abstinence would be expected to produce a *decrease* in cholinergic activity. Others have proposed that with chronic nicotine use, nicotine acts

Table 1. Biochemical Effects of Tobacco Abstinence[a]

| Type of abstinence effect[b] | Whether due to nicotine deprivation[c] |
|---|---|
| Rebound | Due to nicotine deprivation |
| ↑ Acetylcholine (nonhumans) | ↑ Acetylcholine (nonhumans) |
| Transient | Unclear evidence |
| ↓ Adrenaline | ↓ Adrenaline |
| Offset | |
| None | |
| Indefinite | |
| None | |
| Novel | |
| None | |
| Not an abstinence effect[d] | |
| ↓ Dopamine | |
| Unclear evidence[e] | |
| ↓ Acetylcholine (humans) | |
| ↓ Adrenocortical hormones | |
| ↓ Cortisol | |
| ↓ Endogenous opiates | |
| ↓ Noradrenaline | |
| ↓ Serotonin | |
| ↓ Sex hormones | |

[a]Only those effects tested by studies fulfilling the inclusion criteria were listed. At least two positive findings were required to classify effects.
[b]See Section 2 for definition of subtypes of abstinence effects.
[c]Among known abstinence effects.
[d]Not completely tested but weight of evidence is negative.
[e]Insufficient or contradictory evidence.

as a cholinergic blocker (Bachynsky, 1986) and, thus, have hypothesized abstinence will produce an *increase* in cholinergic activity (see Section 14). Studies of cholinergic activity are important because cholinergic mechanisms have been hypothesized to be operative in the performance-enhancing and other rewarding effects of smoking (Ashton and Stepney, 1982; Wesnes and Warburton, 1983; Mangan and Golding, 1984).

Direct assessment of the effect of abstinence on cholinergic activity in human smokers has not been reported. In nonhumans, deprivation appears to produce true rebound effects on acetycholine. Deprivation from chronic nicotine increases synthesis and release of acetycholine in autonomic ganglia and preganglionic and sciatic nerves that exceeds those of control (i.e., no-drug) nonhumans (Dahlstrom et al., 1980; Larsson et al., 1980). Whether similar effects occur in the central nervous system has not been reported.

*In summary, data on the effects of abstinence on acetycholine in humans are absent. In nonhumans, true rebound effects due to nicotine abstinence appear to occur, at least in the periphery.*

## Adrenaline/Noradrenaline

Smoking increases noradrenaline and adrenaline (Cryer et al., 1976); thus, one would expect that abstinence would *decrease* these neurotransmitters. On the other hand, some investigators have hypothesized that all drug withdrawal syndromes *increase* adrenergic activity as a common final pathway (Glassman et al., 1985). The study of adrenaline and noradrenaline is important, as they have been associated with changes in stress responsivity and task performance (Frankenhaeuser, 1971).

Abstinence produces a transient decrease in *adrenaline*. Urinary levels of adrenaline fall 30–50% on the first day of deprivation or cessation, remain decreased for up to 6 weeks, and are reversed by smoking (Elgerot, 1978; Hofstetter et al., 1986; Myrsten et al., 1977; Puddey et al., 1984; West et al., 1984*c*). One briefly reported study failed to replicate this result (Turnbull and Kelvin, 1971). A transient decrease and then increase over a 10-day period was found in one study (West et al., 1984*a*).

The evidence for the fall in adrenaline being due to nicotine deprivation is scant. Switching to a low-nicotine cigarette (West et al., 1984*b*) produces a nonsignificant decrease in adrenaline; however, nicotine gum does not reverse the decline in adrenaline levels (West et al., 1984*a*).

The effect of abstinence on *noradrenaline* is unclear. One to six weeks of deprivation has either no effect (West et al., 1984*c*), a small effect (Elgerot, 1976; Myrsten et al., 1977; Puddey et al., 1984), or a large effect (i.e., 45%; Hofstetter et al., 1986), and nicotine gum does not appear to affect noradrenaline (West et al., 1984*a*). Monoamine oxidase (MAO) is an enzyme that breaks down adrenaline, noradrenaline, and dopamine and thereby influences their levels. Deprivation from tobacco did not change platelet MAO in one small study (Littlewood et al., 1984), but cessation for 1 month dramatically decreased platelet MAO in all nine subjects in a better-designed study (Norman et al., 1987). Interestingly, a decrease in MAO should increase noradrenaline and adrenaline levels, which is *opposite* to the above-described findings.

*In summary, abstinence appears to produce a transient decrease in adrenaline. Whether this is due to nicotine deprivation is debatable, The effect of abstinence on noradrenaline is unclear.* This latter result may be because the effects of abstinence on noradrenaline may be limited to situations of high stress or high-performance demands. Abstinence may produce a decrease in MAO, but how this relates to changes in noradrenaline/adrenaline levels is unclear.

## Dopamine

Smoking appears to increase dopamine (Pomerleau and Pomerleau, 1984); thus, abstinence should decrease dopamine. The study of dopamine is important because dopamine is thought to mediate the reinforcing effects of stimulants (Wise, 1983).

As mentioned in the preceding section, cessation appears to decrease MAO, which should increase dopamine. However, cessation for 24 hr does not decrease and nicotine gum does not increase urinary dopamine in humans (West et al., 1984*a*) or prolactin, a hormone linked to dopamine (Puddey et al., 1984, 1985). Gradual reduction in smoking also does not change the dopamine metabolite dopamine B-hydroxylase (Zeidenberg et al., 1977).

*In summary, the few data available show abstinence does not affect dopamine.* Clearly, more research is needed before conclusions can be made.

## Serotonin

The effects of smoking on serotonin are unclear (Balfour, 1980; Hall, 1982). Research on serotonin is important as serotonin appears to be a major determinant of dysphoria and aggression (Feldman and Quenzer, 1984), both of which have been cited as abstinence effects.

The effects of abstinence on serotonin in humans have not been studied. An elegant and programmatic series of studies in rats has shown that following termination of chronic nicotine treatment, trytophan pyrrolase activity is increased approximately 150%. Since this enzyme controls serotonin degradation, the result is a decrease in brain serotonin by approximately 20% (Badawy and Evans, 1975*a;* Badawy et al., 1981*a,b*). These levels are significantly different from those in saline control nonhumans, indicating this is a rebound effect. Interestingly, similar effects occur during chronic treatment and discontinuation of other drugs (e.g., ethanol, morphine, and phentobarbitone) that are known to produce classic withdrawal syndromes (Badawy and Evans, 1973, 1974, 1975*a,b,* 1983; Badawy et al., 1980*a,b,* 1981*a*).

Another series of studies found dissimilar results. In rats, nicotine administration decreased and deprivation increased serotonin in the hippocampus (Balfour and Benwell, 1981; Benwell and Balfour, 1979, 1982). However, the effect of abstinence to increase serotonin was not replicated in two other studies by the same group (Benwell and Balfour, 1982; Vale and Balfour, 1987). In addition, the levels of serotonin and/or its metabolites in other brain areas were not changed by abstinence in this series of studies.

*In summary, the effect of abstinence on serotonin is quite unclear owing to contradictory results in nonhumans and the absence of studies in humans.* The reason for the contradictory results in the two series of studies cited is unclear, as neither of the two groups cites the other.

## Endogenous Opioids

Smoking high-nicotine cigarettes increases endogenous opiates (Pomerleau et al., 1983*b;* Seyler et al., 1986); thus, abstinence should decrease endogenous opiates. Study of endogenous opiates is important, as they are implicated in many of the presumed rewarding effects of tobacco (Pomerleau and Pomerleau, 1984).

The effect of abstinence on endogenous opiates in humans has not been studied directly. An indirect test of the role of opiates in tobacco abstinence effects is the effect of opiate antagonists. Such drugs do not precipitate tobacco abstinence effects, as would be expected (Gorelick et al., 1989; Karras and Kane, 1980; Nemeth-Coslett and Griffiths, 1986). In mice, discontinuation of chronic nicotine significantly reduces the endogenous opiate beta-endorphin 24 hr after the final drug injection. Beta-endorphin levels return to within control levels within 7 days postdrug and then, surprisingly, increase above control levels at 14 days postdrug (Rosecrans et al., 1985).

*In summary, there is a dearth of data on the effects of abstinence on endogenous opioids.*

## Hormonal Activity

Smoking increases adrenocortical hormones (Benowitz et al., 1984; Benwell and Balfour, 1979); thus, tobacco abstinence might be expected to *decrease* cortisol. On the other hand, cessation of several drugs *increases* cortisol (e.g., Kahn et al., 1984). Thus, the expected change in cortisol with abstinence is unclear. The study of adrenocortical hormones is important as these hormones have been linked to the effectiveness of coping with stress demands.

Deprivation for 24 hr increased cortisol but had no effect on sensitivity of cortisol to suppression by dexamethasone in one study (Hughes et al., 1988). Cessation decreased cortisol in two other studies (Puddey et al., 1984, 1985; R. J. West, personal communication; West et al., 1984*c*). Smokers deprived for 5 days on a research ward exhibited no change in cortisol (Benowitz et al., 1984).

Cessation of chronically administered nicotine increases the plasma corticosterone levels in nonstressed rats above control levels, i.e., a rebound effect (Badawy et al., 1981*b;* Benwell and Balfour, 1979). Similar increases occur following cessations of other drugs known to produce classic withdrawal syndromes (e.g., Pohorecky et al., 1978; Eisenberg and Sparber, 1979). However, in stressed rats (i.e., rats on an unsignaled avoidance schedule) neither nicotine nor its removal changed corticosterone (Balfour and Morrison, 1975). This result suggests abstinence does not potentiate stress-induced effects.

In terms of other hormones, smoking does not appear to affect sex hormones (Seyler et al., 1986) and neither does abstinence. No change in lutenizing hormone or testosterone at rest or in response to lutenizing hormone-releasing hormone (LHRH) was found after 3 weeks of deprivation in an all-male population (Burse et al., 1976). Resting follicular-stimulating hormone (FSH) was also not changed by deprivation, but the response of FSH to LHRH was higher during deprivation. However, this change did not reverse upon resumption of smoking.

Abstinence from tobacco affects several hormones involved in weight regulation. These are discussed in the section on weight and related effects (see Section 8).

*In summary, no conclusion can be reached about the effects of abstinence on adrenocortical and other hormones owing to the paucity of data and contradictory effects.*

## 7. PHYSIOLOGICAL EFFECTS OF ABSTINENCE

### Resting Electroencephalogram

Smoking is thought to increase alertness and improve information processing (Edwards and Warburton, 1983; Wesnes and Warburton, 1983); thus, abstinence has been hypothesized to induce changes in the resting and evoked electroencephalogram (EEG) to reflect drowsiness and poor concentration.

Deprivation reduces the dominant *alpha frequency* (Herning et al., 1983; Knott and Venables, 1977, 1979; Ulett and Itel, 1969). Two less well-described studies failed to find this effect (Brown, 1968; Sannita et al., 1984). More disturbing was the fact that one group was unable to replicate the decrease in alpha frequency in a study that was better designed than the original study (Itel et al., 1971).

Other evidence for the slowing of the EEG is that deprivation increases *slow-wave activity* (Ulett and Itel, 1969; Itel et al., 1971), *theta power* (Herning et al., 1983), and *sleeplike activity* (Itel et al., 1971). Consistent with this effect, high-frequency-wave activity shows little, if any, changes with deprivation (Itel et al., 1971; Ulett and Itel, 1969).

Changes in *alpha amplitude* have not been found (Knott and Venables, 1977, 1979; Szalai et al., 1986). *Alpha power* appears to increase with deprivation, but this has been attributed to the increase in theta power (Herning et al., 1983).

Another study examined the separate and combined effects of alcohol and overnight tobacco deprivation on alpha amplitude and frequency (Knott and Venables, 1979). Tobacco deprivation, with or without alcohol, did not change alpha amplitude. Tobacco deprivation did reduce alpha frequency, but only when subjects abstained from alcohol also.

The above-described EEG changes are reversed with smoking (Herning et al., 1983; Knott and Venables, 1977, 1979; Ulett and Itel, 1969). The single study with more than 24 hr of abstinence (i.e., 2 days) found that the EEG changes were restricted to the first 24 hr of cessation (Herning et al., 1983).

One study examined the effect of auditory stimuli (words and numbers) on alpha amplitude and the ability to regulate alpha amplitude using feedback in smoking and overnight deprivation conditions (Szalai et al., 1986). Abstinent smokers did not differ in reaction to stimuli or in ability to enhance alpha from smoking smokers or never-smokers; however, in terms of ability to suppress alpha amplitude with feedback, abstinent smokers did *better* than smoking smokers or never-smokers.

Nicotine gum appears to improve several EEG parameters during withdrawal (Herning and Pickworth, 1985), and mecamylamine, a nicotine antagonist, appears to produce withdrawal like EEG responses (Pickworth et al., 1988).

*In summary, it appears that abstinence "slows" the EEG, although contradictory results are available. Whether this is a transient or offset effect is unclear. A small amount of evidence suggests some EEG response changes are due to nicotine deprivation.* Although such EEG changes have been hypothesized to be associated with performance decrements (Edwards and Warburton, 1983; Wesnes and Warburton, 1983), this has not been directly tested; i.e., changes in EEG with abstinence have not been directly linked to performance decrements with tobacco abstinence.

## Evoked Responses

Smoking has been hypothesized to produce a "stimulus barrier" (Freidman et al., 1974; Wesnes and Warburton, 1983); thus, abstinence should increase the sensitivity to external stimuli. Evoked responses are EEG waveforms that result from auditory or visual stimuli. In one study, overnight deprivation from tobacco had no effect on the latency to any waveform but *decreased* the amplitude of the PIV-PV waveform in eight of nine subjects (Hall et al., 1973). Deprivation also dampened the responsivity of the PIV-PV waveform to increases in stimulus intensity. These effects occurred in the absence of subjective effects and were reversed by smoking.

A second study found opposite results. Overnight deprivation *increased* the latency to the PIV by 5–10% and increased amplitude of the PIV-PV waveform 30–50% (Knott and Venables, 1977). This effect also occurred at the lowest-intensity stimuli. The two studies did agree in that both reported deprivation *dampened* the sensitivity of PIV-PV to increases in stimulus intensity.

A third, small, and less well-described evoked-response study did not report on changes in the amplitude and sensitivity of the PIV-PV waveform but did report overnight deprivation increased latency to PIV-PV (Murphee, 1979). A fourth preliminary report did not state whether 36 hr of deprivation changed the PIV-PV waveform but did state that deprivation increased the amplitude of a "late positive" waveform (Sannita et al., 1984).

*In summary, the effects of abstinence on the EEG response to visual or auditory stimuli are unclear owing to completely contradictory results from different studies.* Unfortunately, none of the groups offer hypotheses to account for the discrepant results.

## Heart Rate

Smoking acutely increases heart rate (HR) (Ague, 1974; Benowitz et al., 1984; Cryer et al., 1976); thus, one would expect abstinence to decrease HR.

Many studies have shown that HR decreases in smokers trying to quit (e.g., Hughes and Hatsukami, 1986; Hughes et al., 1986*a;* Schneider et al., 1984; West et al., 1984*a*). A similar effect occurs in smokers temporarily abstaining and is reversed by smoking (e.g., Benowitz et al., 1984; Gilbert and Pope, 1982; Hatsukami et al., 1984; Hughes et al., 1984*c;* Karanci, 1985; Knapp et al., 1963; Nemeth-Coslett et al., 1986*b;* Nil et al., 1987). The few instances in which resting HR decrease has not been found have been in those temporarily deprived (e.g., Bojholm et al., 1980; Burse et al., 1975; Weybrew and Stark, 1967). The decrease in HR in those trying to quit is often large, e.g., mean of 12–14 bpm (Hughes and Hatsukami, 1986; West et al., 1984*a*).

The decline in HR appears to be an offset effect, but this is still somewhat unclear. Several studies have not found a transient pattern but examined only HR over short periods (5–8 days (Hughes and Hatsukami, 1986; Schneider et al., 1984). The single long-term study found that among a small sample of smokers able to remain abstinent for 5 weeks, there was no indication of a transient pattern of HR responses (West and Schneider, 1987). Contrary to this finding, one study reported HR declined and remained low for 8 days and appeared to return toward presmoking levels on the last 1–2 days; however, these last two data points may have been chance increases (Nemeth-Coslett et al., 1986*b*). Also, smokers who are more tolerant of the agonist effects of nicotine on HR appear to have greater decreases in HR upon smoking cessation (Hughes et al., 1984*b*). This should occur only if the HR decrease after cessation was a transient phenomenon.

To confuse the issue even more, two well-done studies have found that the HR of deprived smokers and smoking smokers did not differ in the morning but only after repeated smoking (Benowitz et al., 1984; Gilbert and Pope, 1982). This suggests the difference in abstinent smokers and smoking smokers is due, not to transient abstinence effects, but to the absence of the acute effects of smoking.

The decline in HR appears to be due to nicotine deprivation. First, nicotine replacement reverses the decline in HR (Schneider et al., 1984; West et al., 1984*a*) and deprivation from nicotine gum also decreases HR (West and Russell, 1985a). Some studies failed to find these effects (Hughes et al., 1984*a*, 1986*b*); however, these studies used the less-reliable manual palpation method to measure HR. Finally, long-term outpatient studies have found that switching to a low-nicotine cigarette decreases HR (Knapp et al., 1963; West et al., 1984*b*). A shorter inpatient study did not find this (Benowitz et al., 1984).

*In summary, abstinence produces a large decrease in HR, and this appears to be due to nicotine deprivation. The effect may be an offset effect, but this is unclear.*

## Blood Pressure

Smoking increases blood pressure (BP) (Ague, 1974; Cryer et al., 1976); however, over the long term, smokers' BP is either equal to or lower than that of nonsmokers (Higgins and Kjelsberg, 1967). Thus, it is unclear whether to expect abstinence to increase or decrease BP.

In humans, abstinence produces either a very small or no decrease in BP when followed for less than a year. Three to five days of deprivation slightly decreases systolic blood pressure (SBP) by 4–10 mm Hg and diastolic blood pressure (DBP) by 3–8 mm Hg, and this effect is reversed by smoking (Benowitz et al., 1984; Knapp et al., 1963). Other studies of smokers trying to quit (Hughes and Hatsukami, 1986; Puddey et al., 1984, 1985) and temporarily deprived (Glauser et al., 1970; Hatsukami et al., 1984; Nemeth-Coslett et al., 1986*b;* Weybrew and Stark, 1967) found no change in SBP or DBP. In one study, decreased BP occurred with switching to a low-nicotine cigarette (Benowitz et al., 1984), but this did not occur in another study (Knapp et al., 1963).

In nonhumans, administration of nicotine for 10 weeks decreases mean SBP and discontinuation of nicotine produces a large *increase* in SBP above predrug levels that does not return to control levels until 6 weeks of deprivation (Wenzel and Azmeh, 1970). Another study again found that chronic nicotine decreased and deprivation increased BP, but failed to find a rebound effect (Hutchinson and Emley, 1981). Although the latter study used the same dose of nicotine, it used a different species of nonhumans that were hypertensive and a shorter duration of nicotine treatment. Several cross-sectional studies indicate the blood pressure of ex-smokers does not differ from that of smokers or never-smokers (e.g., Schoenenberger, 1982).

*In summary, abstinence appears to have little effect on BP*. This is surprising as abstinence from tobacco has large effects on HR. However, covariance of HR and BP depends on several factors, e.g., internal vs. external stimuli. Surprisingly, more sophisticated studies using recent technological advances in cardiology have not been done. Such studies will be needed to determine whether BP changes with abstinence, and if not, what compensatory mechanisms stabilize BP in the face of a major decline in HR.

## Orthostasis

Smoking increases sympathetic activity (Ague, 1974; Cryer et al., 1976); thus abstinence should decrease sympathetic activity. One measure of sympathetic tone is the orthostatic response, i.e., the increase in HR and BP upon standing.

Consistent with the above prediction, abstinence diminishes orthostasis. One to four days of cessation or deprivation of cigarettes (Hatsukami et al., 1984; Hughes and Hatsukami, 1986; Hughes et al., 1984*c*) and deprivation from smokeless tobacco (Hatsukami et al., 1987) dampen the increase in HR on standing. Whether this effect is an offset, transient, or rebound effect is unclear. Nicotine replacement appears to reverse the effect (Hughes et al., 1984*a*).

*In summary, abstinence diminishes orthostasis. Whether this is an offset or transient effect or due to nicotine deprivation is unclear*. Although we have presented orthostasis as a measure of sympathetic activity, this is an oversimplistic approach. Again, much more sophisticated studies (e.g., simultaneous measurement of BP, HR, and catecholamines) are needed to relate changes in HR and BP on standing from abstinence from tobacco to changes in sympathetic activity.

## Respiratory Rate

Smoking increases respiratory rate (RR) (Hall, 1982); thus, short-term abstinence should cause a decline in RR.

Two well-designed studies found that deprivation did not change RR over 1–4 days of deprivation (Hatsukami et al., 1984; Karanci, 1985). Abstracts by Parsons and colleagues have reported deprivation decreased (Parsons et al., 1975*a;* Parsons and Hamme, 1975) and increased RR (Parsons et al., 1975*b*). *In summary, the better-described studies indicate abstinence does not change RR*.

## Body Temperature

Nicotine decreases body temperature in nonhumans: thus, one could hypothesize that abstinence would increase body temperature (Hall, 1982). From 1 to 21 days of deprivation does not change body temperature (Burse et al., 1976; Glauser et al., 1970; Hatsukami et al., 1984; Weybrew and Stark, 1967). However, one study found that those who scored high on a dependence scale had a decline in body temperature with deprivation (Fagerstrom, 1978). *In summary, abstinence does not appear to change body temperature.*

## Skin Temperature

Smoking decreases skin temperature owing to nicotine's action to constrict peripheral blood vessels (Ague, 1974). Thus, abstinence should increase skin temperature.

Finger temperature rises 2–4 degrees with 1–5 days of cessation or deprivation and is reversed with smoking (Gilbert and Pope, 1982; Myrsten et al., 1977; West et al., 1984*a*). One small study did not find this effect (Burse et al., 1975). Whether this is an offset, transient, or rebound effect is unclear. The effect does not appear to be due to nicotine deprivation. Switching to a low-nicotine cigarette (West et al., 1984*b*), chewing nicotine gum during cessation (West et al., 1984*a*), and stopping nicotine gum (West and Russell, 1985*a*) do not change skin temperature.

*In summary, cessation increases skin temperature, but whether this is an offset or transient effect is unclear. The effect has not been shown to be due to nicotine deprivation.*

## Tremor

Smoking produces a fine-grain tremor (Shiffman et al., 1983); thus abstinence should decrease tremor. Tremor significantly decreases for 1–4 days of cessation or deprivation (Gilbert and Pope, 1982; Hatsukami et al., 1984; Hughes and Hatsukami, 1986; Myrsten et al., 1977) and is reversed by smoking (Myrsten et al., 1977). The single study to examine the effect of nicotine on abstinence-induced tremor showed no effect of nicotine gum (Hughes et al., 1984*a*). *In summary, abstinence decreases tremor. Whether the effect is offset or transient or due to nicotine deprivation is unclear.*

## Pupillary Response

Nicotine produces an acute biphasic increase and then a decrease in pupil size (Henningfield et al., 1985). Thus, the expected effects of abstinence are unclear. The single study of pupillary diameter found no effect of 4 days of deprivation (Weybrew and Stark, 1967).

## Skin Conductance

One study reported that short-term deprivation decreased the level of skin conductance and the number of spontaneous skin conductance responses (Karanci, 1985).

## Drug Metabolism

Tobacco increases the biotransformation of several drugs (e.g., pentazocine, imipramine, warfarin) (Dawson and Vestal, 1982) and increases their clearance and half-life. Thus, cessation should increase the blood levels of such drugs. This section focuses on the effects of abstinence on three drugs of relevance to smokers: nicotine, caffeine, and theophylline.

Nicotine appears to influence its own metabolism. In fact, tobacco deprivation increases the clearance of nicotine itself (Lee et al., 1987*a*); i.e., nicotine is cleared from the body more quickly in abstinent smokers than in smoking smokers.

Caffeine intake is quite common among smokers (Istvan and Matarazzo, 1984). Three recent studies have documented increased caffeine levels postabstinence (Benowitz et al., 1988; Brown et al., 1988; Sachs and Benowitz, 1988). One study documented a transient 50% slower metabolism of caffeine during 4 days of deprivation (Brown et al., 1988), and another a 250% increase in plasma caffeine (Benowitz et al., 1988). This finding could be important in that it suggests the possibility that some of the symptoms of tobacco withdrawal (e.g., anxiety, restlessness, impatience) might be due to caffeine intoxication (Sachs and Benowitz, 1988).

Theophylline is a commonly used bronchodilator for chronic obstructive pulmonary disease, which is often present in smokers. Although two studies found no change in theophylline elimination immediately after abstinence (24–36 hr) (Eldon et al., 1987; Hunt et al., 1976), a larger, better-designed study with longer follow-up found that 1 week of deprivation increased theophylline levels by about one-third (Lee et al., 1987*b*). Nicotine gum does not appear to reverse this effect. How quickly and complete such reversals are for other drugs has not been well studied.

*In summary, abstinence appears to increase the elimination of nicotine and decrease the elimination of caffeine and theophylline. Similar effects probably occur with other drugs whose metabolism is affected by smoking. Although not completely tested, these are probably simple offset effects.* The effects may be due not to the absence of nicotine, but rather to the absence of the effects of hydrocarbons or other compounds on liver metabolism.

## 8. WEIGHT CHANGE AND RELATED EFFECTS

The effects of abstinence on weight change and related effects in both humans and nonhumans are outlined in Table 2.

Several recent articles have comprehensively reviewed the evidence for weight gain with smoking cessation and its possible causes (Bosse et al., 1980; Grunberg, 1985, 1986; Klesges et al., 1988*a;* Wack and Rodin, 1982). In this section we first review the effects of abstinence on weight and then review the possible causes of weight gain, e.g., increased eating, decreased activity, and decreased metabolic rate. Our review differs from prior reviews in that (1) it focuses only on the effects of abstinence and not on the effects of smoking *per se,* (2) it includes only studies that met our criteria (e.g., had baseline weights, etc.,) and (3) it is a critical rather than an integrative review.

### Weight Gain in Humans

Smoking decreases weight (Grunberg, 1985; Wack and Rodin, 1982) and weight gain is a commonly cited abstinence effect.

Table 2. Physiological Effects of Tobacco Abstinence[a]

| Type of abstinence effects | Whether due to nicotine deprivation |
|---|---|
| Rebound | Due to nicotine deprivation |
| None | ↓ Heart rate |
| Transient | Not due to nicotine deprivation[b] |
| None | ↓ Skin temperature |
| Offset | Unclear evidence |
| ↓ Drug metabolism | ↓ Drug metabolism |
| Indefinite | Slowing of EEG |
| ↓ Heart rate | ↓ Orthostasis |
| ↓ Orthostasis | ↓ Tremor |
| ↑ Skin temperature | |
| Slowing of EEG | |
| ↓ Tremor | |
| Novel | |
| None | |
| Not an abstinence effect[b] | |
| ↑ Blood pressure | |
| ↑ Body temperature | |
| ↓ Respiratory rate | |
| Unclear evidence | |
| ↑ Evoked response | |
| ↓ Pupillary diameter | |
| ↑ Skin conductance | |

[a]See Table 1 for footnotes.
[b]Not completely tested but weight of evidence is negative.

In studies that fulfill our criteria, cessation of smoking or temporary deprivation almost universally increases weight (Axelson and Brantmark, 1975; Bosse et al., 1980; Brozek and Keys, 1957; Brantmark et al., 1973; Hjalmarson, 1984; Cambien et al., 1981; Carney and Goldberg, 1984; Clearman and Jacobs, 1985; Comstock and Stone, 1972; Fehily et al., 1984; Freidman and Siegelaub, 1980; Garvey et al., 1974; Glauser et al., 1970; Gordon et al., 1975; Hatsukami et al., 1984; Hickey and Mulcahy, 1973; Hughes and Hatsukami, 1986; Klesges et al., 1988*a;* Lund-Larsen and Tretle, 1982; Melander et al., 1981; Malcolm et al., 1980; Nemeth-Coslett et al., 1986*b;* Powell and McCann, 1981; Puddey et al., 1984, 1985; Puska et al., 1979; Rabkin, 1984; Rodin, 1987; Schoenenberger, 1982; Stitzer and Gross, 1988; Tuomilehto et al., 1986). Since abstinence does not change height, abstinence increases measures of obesity such as relative weight (e.g., Rabkin, 1984) and skinfold thickness (e.g., Comstock and Stone, 1972; Rabkin, 1984).

The amount and incidence of the weight gain vary widely, depending on setting (research ward vs. natural environs), subject population (self-quitters vs. clinic attendees), duration of follow-up (4 days to 5 years), and inclusion of smoking and nonsmoking controls. The most valid and generalizable estimates suggest the mean weight gain attributable to abstinence is 0.5–0.9 kg after 4–8 days (Hatsukami et al., 1984; Hughes et al., 1986*b;* Melander et al., 1981), 1.2–2.9 kg after 1 month (Glauser et al., 1970; Malcolm et al., 1980), and 1–4 kg at 1–5 years (Bosse et al., 1980; Brozek and Keys, 1957; Comstock and Stone, 1972; Freidman and Siegelaub, 1980; Garvey et al., 1974;

Gordon et al., 1975). However, hidden in these mean values is the fact that a significant proportion of subjects either maintain their weight or lose weight with cessation (Rodin, 1987).

In several studies, examination of mean weight gain and the weights of smokers, nonsmokers, and ex-smokers suggests an offset pattern of effects such that abstinent smokers slowly gain weight until they weigh the same as never-smokers (Bosse et al., 1980; Comstock and Stone, 1972; Freidman and Siegelaub, 1980; Garvey et al., 1974; Gordon et al., 1975). However, one study found that long-term abstinent smokers exceed the weight of never-smokers (Lund-Larsen and Tretle, 1982). In addition, the most recent population-based study of weight suggests former smokers weigh more than never-smokers (0.6–1.5 kg) (Williamson et al., 1987).

Several studies have reported the prevalence of weight gain. However, since weight increases somewhat with time in all adults, to correctly estimate the prevalence of weight gain due to smoking cessation, one must compare the prevalence of weight gain in abstinent smoker groups with that in continuing smoker and never-smoker control groups. The single controlled study that did so reported 27–31% more abstinent smokers than smokers or never-smokers had gained weight 1–5 years postcessation (Bosse et al., 1980; Garvey et al., 1974).

Postcessation weight gain in humans appears to be due to nicotine deprivation, but this is still far from resolved. Subjects on nicotine gum show significant (Emont and Cummings, 1987; Stitzer and Gross, 1988) and nonsignificant (Axelsson and Brantmark, 1975; Brantmark et al., 1973; Malcolm et al., 1980) trends to gain less weight than those on placebo gum. On the other hand, other studies show essentially no difference in weight gain between nicotine and placebo groups (Hjalmarson, 1984; Puska et al., 1979; Tonneson et al., 1988). As another line of evidence, several trials reported that subjects who used more nicotine gum had less weight gain (Emont and Cummings, 1987; Fagerstrom, 1987; Stitzer and Gross, 1988), but another trial did not replicate this result (Tonneson et al., 1988). The single dose–response study showed no difference in weight gain between 2- and 4-mg doses of nicotine gum (Tonneson et al., 1988). One trial reported no weight gain when placebo was substituted for nicotine gum for 1 week (Hughes et al., 1986*b*).

*In summary, abstinence increases weight. The weight gain appears to be due to nicotine deprivation. Whether ex-smokers gain weight such that their weight exceeds that of never-smokers has not been clearly documented. Surprisingly, whether weight gain is a transient or offset effect has not been clearly outlined* (i.e., is weight gained only initially but then never lost, or is weight gain constant for many months postcessation?) Whether weight gain contributes to relapse is discussed in Section 16.

## Weight Gain in Nonhumans

The effect of deprivation of nicotine on weight and eating in nonhumans may vary by gender and dietary composition (Grunberg, 1986).

In *male* rats with *standard* chow available, four studies reported an increase in weight *gain* of 5–10% (Falkenborn et al, 1981; Grunberg and Bowen, 1985; Grunberg et al., 1987; McNair and Bryson, 1983). One other study reported deprivation had no effect on weight gain (Grunberg et al., 1984) (Table 3).

In *male* rats with *sweetened* substances available, two studies both found a similar increase in weight gain upon deprivation (Grunberg, 1982; Grunberg et al., 1985) and a third found a nonsignificant trend in the same direction (Grunberg et al., 1988*a*).

In *females* on *standard* chow, all five studies document 2–15% increases in weight gain after deprivation (Bowen et al., 1986; Grunberg et al., 1986, 1987; Levin et al., 1987; Morgan and Ellison, 1987). In the only study of females on *sweetened* chow there was a 2–6% increase in weight gain at 17 days after deprivation (Grunberg et al., 1988*a*).

When the *duration* of changes in weight gain following nicotine treatment is considered, again sex appears to be an important factor. Grunberg et al. (1987) found that *female* rats who had standard chow available achieved a normal absolute body weight by 1 month after discontinuation of nicotine treatment, whereas *males* remained 7% below controls for as long as 4 months postdrug. In a subsequent study with sweetened foodstuff available, average weight gain in females was 2–15% *above* controls 2 months after discontinuation of nicotine, whereas males averaged 4–12% *below* controls. Other studies in female rats report they rapidly regain normal absolute body weights when nicotine treatment is terminated (Levin et al., 1987; Morgan and Ellison, 1987; Schecter and Cook, 1976). One study reported that weights in male rats remained below controls at 3 months (Classen and Battig, 1976). In contrast, Falkenborn et al. (1981) found that male rats achieved a normal absolute body weight by 10–20 days after discontinuation of nicotine treatment. It is important to note that male rats are heavier than same-age females (cf. Grunberg et al., 1986); thus, the possibility that initial weight differences account for the gender differences needs to be tested in future studies.

Only one study has been conducted in nonhumans examining changes in percent body composition of fat and protein during chronic nicotine administration and after its discontinuation (Winders and Grunberg, 1987). Nicotine decreased fat and protein composition, and in male rats, discontinuation of nicotine increased them. This is an interesting finding that merits further study.

Whether weight gain after termination of chronic nicotine treatment is an offset, transient, or rebound effect is unclear. Three studies have reported slight increases in weight gain above control levels in female rats, suggestive of a rebound effect, but these effects generally were not statistically significant (Grunberg et al., 1988*a;* Levin et al., 1987; Morgan and Ellison, 1987). Other studies have found that, at least for female rats, they regain absolute weights equivalent to controls, which suggests an offset effect.

*In summary, nicotine deprivation increases weight gain in nonhumans. Several studies suggest weight gain is greater with sweet chow than bland chow. Some studies suggest gender (male vs. female) and food composition (bland vs. sweet chow) interact such that males may be less likely to gain weight on standard chow than females, but both genders gain weight on sweet chow.* Studies also suggest the effect of nicotine deprivation may cause the weight of females to exceed that of control females (i.e., a rebound effect), but this does not occur with males. However, these gender–food composition interactions are not completely consistent across studies.

## Taste

The effects of smoking on taste perception, preference, sensitivity, and threshold are unclear (Grunberg, 1985; Pangborn and Trabue, 1973; Wack and Rodin, 1982). In

Table 3. Effects of Nicotine Abstinence in Nonhumans in Weight by Foodstuff Available and Gender

| Standard food | | Sweetened food | |
|---|---|---|---|
| Males | Females | Males | Females |
| No effect | No effect | No effect | No effect |
| Grunberg et al., 1984 | No data | No data | No data |
| Increase | Increase | Increase | Increase |
| Falkenborn et al., 1981 | Bowen et al., 1986 | Grunberg, 1982 | Grunberg et al., 1988 |
| Grunberg and Bowen, 1985 | Grunberg et al., 1986 | Grunberg et al., 1985, 1988*a* | |
| Grunberg et al., 1987 | Grunberg et al., 1987 | | |
| McNair and Bryson, 1983 | Levin et al., 1987 | | |
| Winders and Grunberg, 1987 | Morgan and Ellison, 1987 | | |

one study smokers deprived overnight, smoking smokers and nonsmokers did not differ in sensitivity to a number of chemical, olfactory, and viscosity stimuli (Pangborn et al., 1967). The tactile stimuli included sucrose (sweet), sodium chloride (salty), and quinine and caffeine (bitter) solutions. A second study examined the intensity and pleasantness of sucrose (sweet), salt, and quinine (bitter) solutions in subjects deprived overnight, smoking smokers, and nonsmokers. These subjects were examined before and after a glucose load (Redington, 1984). There were no differences prior to the glucose load. After the glucose load, the group did not differ on salty and bitter ratings or in tasting of sweetness, but abstinent smokers did rate sweet solutions more pleasant than deprived smokers. However, deprived smokers were equivalent to nonsmokers, suggesting this was not due to deprivation in the deprived smokers but rather due to tobacco administration in the smoking smokers. The most recent study compared smokers who self-selected into smoking and cessation groups (Rodin, 1987). One week postcessation, the abstinent smokers and relapsed smokers did not differ in perceived intensity of salty or sweet taste. Abstinent smokers did rate sweet solutions as more pleasant (even without a glucose load). Whether sex differences were present was not reported.

*In summary, abstinence does not appear to influence taste threshold or sensitivity but may increase the perceived pleasantness of sweet commodities. The time pattern of this effect and whether it is due to nicotine are unknown.* Increased rating of sweets is commonly reported after cessation (but see Section 8.5). Thus further work on the relationship of changes in perceived pleasantness of sweets and changes in sweet consumption postcessation would be of interest.

## Appetite

Smoking appears to decrease self-reported appetite and hunger (Wack and Rodin, 1982) and abstinence consistently increases self-ratings of eating, hunger, or appetite (Burse et al., 1975; Hatsukami et al., 1987, 1988; Hughes et al., 1986*a;* Hughes and Hatsukami, 1986; Lawrence et al., 1982; Smith and Lombardo, 1986; West et al., 1984*a*, 1987). One study reported a specific increase in craving for sweets (Lawrence et al., 1982). Hunger persists longer than most abstinence symptoms but does appear to return toward baseline with time (Hughes et al., 1988; West et al., 1987).

It is unclear if the increased appetite or hunger is due to nicotine deprivation. Increased hunger was relieved by nicotine in two long-term studies (Hughes et al., 1986*a;* Stitzer and Gross, 1988), but not two shorter studies (Hughes et al., 1984*a;* West et al., 1984*a*). Hunger occurred on switching to a low-nicotine cigarette (West et al., 1984*b*) and with placebo substitution for nicotine gum in one study (Hughes et al., 1986 *b*) but not another (West and Russell, 1985*a*).

*In summary, abstinence transiently increases appetite, but whether this is due to nicotine deprivation is unclear.* Further tests of the nicotine deprivation hypotheses are important because increased eating can result from deprivation from nondrug reinforcers (Falk, 1981).

## Eating in Humans

Smoking appears to decrease caloric intake (Albanes et al., 1987; Jacobs and Gottenborg, 1981; Wack and Rodin, 1982); thus, abstinence should increase caloric intake. In addition, smoking appears to selectively decrease sweet intake (Grunberg, 1985); thus, abstinence should especially increase sweet intake.

Most studies, including several randomized trials, have found mean increases in caloric intake of 200–350 calories/day over periods of cessation or deprivation ranging from 1 day to 1 year (Clearman and Jacobs, 1985; Dalloso and James, 1983; Gilbert and Pope, 1982; Hughes et al., 1984*a,b;* Klesges et al., 1988*a;* Rodin, 1987; Stamford et al., 1986). Most studies that have examined specific changes in carbohydrate and sugar proportions of the diet have usually reported no specific changes (Dalloso and James, 1983; Klesges et al., 1988*a;* Rodin, 1987; Stamford et al., 1986). One study did report an increase in carbohydrates but did not indicate whether this was due to increase in sweets (Puddey et al., 1984, 1985). Surprisingly, the expected gender interaction such that females would especially eat more carbohydrates or sweets has not been found. Two studies have reported increases in "snacking" (Gilbert and Pope, 1982; Hughes et al., 1982*a*).

Studies of changes in alcohol and caffeine intake with abstinence are discussed in Section 9.

Longitudinal studies tracking changes in eating over time have not been done. Although studies have examined the effects of nicotine gum on postcessation weight, none have looked at the effect of gum use on actual eating behavior.

*In summary, abstinence typically increases caloric intake by 200–350 calories/day. This effect has not been shown to be due to any specific change in diet such as in sugar or carbohydrate. Whether the increased caloric intake is a transient effect or persists (i.e., is an offset effect) and whether the increased eating is due to nicotine deprivation is unclear.* Although studies suggest the entire weight gain cannot be attributed to increases in caloric intake, the relative contribution of caloric intake is unclear; i.e., does increased eating account for 20%, 50%, or 90% of the weight gain? Again, better studies of the effect of nicotine on increased caloric intake are needed to rule out the possibility that increased eating is a behavioral reaction to loss of a reinforcer (Falk, 1981).

## Food Intake in Nonhumans

The effect of termination of chronic nicotine on food consumption in rats appears to be affected by gender and dietary composition in a matter somewhat similar to that seen for weight.

In *male* rats on *standard* chow, three studies found that deprivation had no effect on food consumption (Clarke and Kumar, 1984; Grunberg et al., 1984, 1987); however, in one of these studies (Grunberg et al., 1987), there was a nonsignificant trend for increased food consumption with deprivation. On the other hand, four studies found an increase in food consumption under these conditions (Classen and Battig, 1976; Falkenborn et al., 1981; McNair and Bryson, 1983; Winders and Grunberg, 1987). (See Table 4.)

In *males* with *sweetened* lab chow or glucose solution available, two studies reported an increase in caloric intake (Grunberg, 1982; Grunberg et al., 1985) and a third study reported a nonsignificant trend in the same direction (Grunberg et al., 1988*a*).

In *females* on *standard* lab chow, both studies have reported increase in food consumption (Grunberg et al., 1987; McNair and Bryson, 1983). This pattern could suggest that females increase caloric consumption more reliably on standard chow than

Table 4. Effects of Nicotine Abstinence in Nonhumans in Eating by Foodstuff Available and Gender

| Standard food | | Sweetened food | |
|---|---|---|---|
| Males | Females | Males | Females |
| No effect | No effect | No effect | No effect |
| Clarke and Kumar, 1984 | No data | No data | No data |
| Grunberg et al., 1984 | Increase | Increase | Increase |
| Grunberg et al., 1987 | Grunberg et al., 1987 | Grunberg, 1982 | Grunberg et al., 1988 |
| Increase | Grunberg et al., 1986 | Grunberg et al., 1985 | |
| Classen and Battig, 1976 | Grunberg et al., 1988 | Grunberg et al., 1988*a* | |
| Falkenborn et al., 1981 | Bowen et al., 1986 | | |
| McNair and Bryson, 1983 | Levin et al., 1987 | | |
| Winders and Grunberg, 1987 | McNair and Bryson, 1983 | | |

males. However, as with the weight gain, direct comparisons of males and females on standard lab chow are contradictory. One study found that the increase in food consumption was statistically significant only for females but not males; however, the graphic display of the data suggests a clearly increasing trend for males (Grunberg et al., 1987). The other study reported that males exhibited significant increases in food consumption following discontinuation of treatment of 0.2, 0.4, and 0.6 mg/kg nicotine injections, while females exhibited increases only following discontinuation of the 0.6 mg/kg dose (McNair and Bryson, 1983).

There has only been one study in *females* on *sweetened* lab chow (Grunberg et al., 1988*a*). This study compared the effects of 6 and 12 mg/kg per day nicotine in male and female rats that had bland, salty, and sweetened food available. Males and females showed nonsignificant trends to increase consumption of the sweetened food. Females, but not males, also showed nonsignificant trends to increase consumption of the bland food. Consumption of salty foods was not reliably affected in males or females.

Food consumption levels sometimes significantly exceed control values following termination of chronic nicotine treatment, suggesting a true rebound effect (Bowen et al., 1986; Classen and Battig, 1976; Falkenborn et al., 1981; Grunberg et al., 1986; Levin et al., 1987). In three such reports, the investigators noted a transient pattern of increase (Classen and Battig, 1976; Falkenborn et al., 1981; Levin et al., 1987). In other reports, consumption levels either return to within control values (i.e., an offset pattern) or move in the direction of, but do not achieve, control levels (i.e., an indefinite pattern) (e.g., Grunberg et al., 1985, 1987; Grunberg and Bowen, 1985).

*In summary, nicotine deprivation increases caloric intake in nonhumans. Some studies suggest a specific increase in sweet food consumption.* Also, gender by food composition interactions similar to those proposed for weight gain have been discussed (e.g., males eat more sweet chow only, but females eat more sweet and bland chow). However, in our opinion, these interactions have not been conclusively shown.

## Fluid Intake and Output

Smoking releases antidiuretic hormone (Pomerleau et al., 1983*b;* Seyler et al., 1986); thus, one would predict that cessation could increase diuresis and, as a result, increase fluid intake. In addition, polydipsia is a common result of cessation of reinforcers, including drug reinforcers (Falk, 1981).

The single study to examine fluid intake in humans found a nonsignificant increase of 125 ml/day (Hatsukami et al., 1984). In terms of fluid output, deprivation does not appear to change urinary output or urinary creatinine (Hatsukami et al., 1984; West et al., 1984*c*).

In nonhumans, the effects of nicotine deprivation on fluid intake vary across studies. In male rats, most studies found that neither nicotine administration nor deprivation changed water intake, or if they did so, the changes were of small magnitude or transient (Clarke and Kumar, 1984; Grunberg et al., 1985, 1987, 1988*a;* Winders and Grunberg, 1987). However, Falkenborn et al. (1981) found a significant 20% decrease in water consumption in male rats treated with nicotine and this effect was still evident 28 days after discontinuation of nicotine treatment. Ingestion of sweetened fluids is significantly affected by nicotine (see the preceding section).

In female rats, nicotine administration decreases and nicotine deprivation increases water consumption. In two studies the effects appeared to be an offset effect (Grunberg et al., 1986, 1987), and in two others (Bowen et al., 1986; Levin et al., 1987) rebound effects (i.e., the increase intake exceeded that of a control group). In one study, nicotine deprivation increased fluid intake in female rats but not in male rats (Grunberg et al., 1987); however, a subsequent study in the same laboratory failed to find effects in either male or female rats (Grunberg et al., 1988*a*).

*In summary, changes in fluid intake or output have not been demonstrated in humans. The effect of nicotine deprivation on water consumption is variable in nonhumans, with increases, decreases, and no effect being reported.*

## Activity

Most studies report nicotine increases locomotor activity in rats or produces a biphasic effect consisting of an immediate decrease and a later increase in activity (Bowen et al., 1986; Clarke and Kumar, 1983; Grunberg, 1982; Grunberg and Bowen, 1985; Ksir et al., 1985; Morrison and Stephenson, 1972; Stolerman et al., 1973; Vale and Balfour, 1987). Tolerance to the initial decreases in activity develops rapidly, whereas the increases in activity become greater with repeated injections (Ksir et al., 1985; Morrison and Stephenson, 1972). With these complicated agonist and tolerance effects it is unclear what one would expect abstinence to do to motor activity.

Most well-described studies found no changes in self-reported activity or activity monitor scores during 1–7 days of deprivation (Hatsukami et al., 1984; Hofstetter et al., 1986; Klesges et al., 1988*a;* Puddey et al., 1984, 1985; Rodin, 1987). In humans, the single positive study was a brief abstract that reported pedometer scores were 14% lower on a deprivation day than a smoking day (Smith and Lombardo, 1986).

In nonhumans, cessation of chronic nicotine treatment produces inconsistent changes in locomotor activity across studies, with some reporting decreases (Clarke and Kumar, 1983; Grunberg and Bowen, 1985; Vale and Balfour, 1987), others reporting no change (Bowen et al., 1986; Grunberg et al., 1986; Grunberg, 1982; Stolerman et al., 1973), and still others reporting increases (Keenan and Johnson, 1972). The one common factor across the studies that reported no change after cessation of nicotine treatment was the absence of agonist effects of nicotine on activity (Bowen et al., 1986; Grunberg, 1982). For many psychoactive drugs, the nature of the behavioral effects observed depends on the baseline rates of responding (Dews and Wenger, 1977). Thus, perhaps rate of motor activity prior to cessation may determine the effects of abstinence. Also, if the agonist effects of nicotine on motor activity depend on the dose and duration of treatment, perhaps these variables also influence abstinence effects on motor activity. Since activity is an important variable in determining weight changes, understanding of postcessation weight gain requires some resolution of the effect of abstinence on motor activity.

*In summary, abstinence has not been shown to consistently change motor activity in humans or nonhumans.* Some smokers may voluntarily change activity levels to try to help them stop smoking. Future studies will have to try to eliminate such bias in order to assess the effect of abstinence *per se*. Also, better study of the types of activity (e.g., high- vs. low-intensity, etc.) is needed.

## Metabolic Rate/Energy Expenditure

Smoking appears to increase metabolic rate (Wack and Rodin, 1982); thus, cessation should decrease metabolic rate.

The first study on metabolic rate reported two results that suggest a decreased metabolic rate; i.e., after 3 months of cessation oxygen consumption decreased and respiratory quotient increased by 10% each (Glauser et al., 1970). However, oxygen consumption corrected for surface area was unchanged. In addition, this study did not control caloric intake, dietary composition, or activity level, all of which may change oxygen consumption and respiratory quotient. A second study examined resting metabolic rate after 48 days of deprivation and found no differences with deprivation (Stamford et al., 1986). A third study measured not only metabolic rate, but also energy expenditure by indirect calorimetry (Hofstetter et al., 1986). The study experimentally controlled diet and statistically controlled for physical activity. Deprivation for 24 hr did not change basal metabolic rate but did decrease total, diurnal, and nocturnal energy expenditure by 10%. Energy expenditure during exercise was not changed. A fourth study examined resting metabolic rate after 8 weeks of cessation and found a decrease of 4% (Dalloso and James, 1983). A fifth, small ($n = 3$), but intensive study was the only one that controlled diet and activity, both of which can effect metabolic rate (Burse et al., 1976). This study found that 3 weeks of deprivation produced no change in resting or walking oxygen consumption or in awakening, preprandial, or postprandial metabolic rates.

*In summary, despite popular belief, the effects of abstinence on metabolic rate are quite inconsistent across studies.* This may be due to inadequate controls for changes in diet, activity, other factors that alter metabolic rate, and change with cessation.

## Thyroid Function

The first study mentioned in the preceding section (Glauser et al., 1970) also found that 3 weeks of cessation decreased protein bound iodide, an index of thyroid function, by 10%. One study tested smokers before and 3–77 days ($x = 8$ days) after cessation (Melander et al., 1981) and found 5–10% decreases in thyroxine ($T_4$) and reverse triiodothyronine ($rT_3$), and a 5–10% increase in thyroid-stimulating hormone (TSH). No changes in triiodothyronine ($T_3$) or $T_3$ uptake were found. The authors interpreted these results to indicate cessation decreases secretion of thyroid hormone, but not by decreasing TSH secretion. They also noted that some of their findings may be the result of increased caloric intake rather than the cause of increased caloric intake. A second small study found a trend similar to these findings with 3 weeks of deprivation, but none of these reached statistical significance (Burse et al., 1976). In addition, this study found that deprivation potentiated the TSH response to thyroid-releasing hormone by 50%. The latter finding was interpreted to be a result of decreased thyroid activity.

*In summary, abstinence appears to decrease thyroid activity. Whether this is a transient or long-term effect or due to nicotine deprivation is unclear.* Whether this effect reflects thyroid gland, pituitary, or hypothalamic dysfunction is yet to be established. If these thyroid findings are corroborated, this would have a major impact on understanding the etiology of postcessation weight gain.

## Metabolic Substrates

Smoking appears to decrease serum insulin and increase serum glucose (Wack and Rodin, 1982); thus, cessation could cause a decreased glucose, which in turn could increase hunger and eating. In fact, hypoglycemia has been hypothesized to be a cause of abstinence effects (Bourne, 1985).

Two studies have examined serum glucose after 3–4 weeks of deprivation (Glauser et al., 1970; Burse et al., 1976). In both studies fasting glucose was unchanged. In one study the 30-min postingestion glucose level (in a glucose tolerance test) increased (Glauser et al., 1970), but the other study did not find this (Burse et al., 1976). In addition, in one small study, several hormones and substrates involved in metabolism—insulin, glucagon, growth hormone, and free fatty acids—did not change with cessation (Burse et al., unpublished). In one briefly described nonhuman study, nicotine deprivation appeared to increase serum insulin and produce a transient decrease in glucose (Grunberg et al., 1988*b*).

***In summary, the effect of abstinence on metabolic substrates has not been tested enough to make a conclusion.***

## Determinants of Weight Gain

In this section, we review several possible specific determinants of weight gain. The role of "generic" determinants, such as gender, number of cigarettes/day, and so on, is reviewed in Section 12.

Although many hypothesize weight gain to be greater in the more obese, prospective studies find no effect of absolute or relative weight (Carney and Goldberg, 1984; Emont and Cummings, 1987; Klesges et al., 1988*a;* Rabkin, 1984; Rodin, 1987) or that obese smokers gain *less* weight than lean smokers (Bosse et al., 1980). Whether maximum past weight predicts weight gain is debatable (Hall et al., 1986; Rodin, 1987). Surprisingly, weight gain on the last quit attempt does not appear to predict future weight gain (Hall et al., 1986).

In one study, smokers who scored high on an eating disinhibition scale and hunger scales gained more postcessation weight (Hall et al., 1986). Cognitive restraint on eating did not predict weight gain. Increased anxiety was unrelated to weight gain in one study (Rabkin, 1984), but decreased anxiety predicted weight gain in another study (Bosse et al., 1980).

One study examined lipoprotein lipase, an enzyme that helps form fat cells and appears to help maintain stable body weight (Carney and Goldberg, 1984). In this study smokers who had high levels of liprotein lipase gained more weight after 2–3 weeks of cessation.

One study tested whether several measures found to predict weight gain would also predict eating behavior (Duffy and Hall, in press). As mentioned earlier, in one study smokers who scored high on eating disinhibition and hunger scales gained more weight postcessation, but this effect was not true for scores in a restrained eating scale (Hall et al., 1986). In a follow-up eating study, smoking smokers and abstinent smokers (24 hr) were compared on eating in an ice cream taste test. Abstinent smokers who scored high on an eating disinhibition scale ate more ice cream than deprived smokers, but smokers who scored low on the scale did not differ in deprived and nondeprived conditions. Scores on hunger and eating restraint scales which had more weight fluctuation did not predict increased eating with cessation. Although the disinhibition scales differed between the two studies, the results suggest that the construct of disinhibition of eating predicts increases in both postcessation eating and weight.

*In summary, research on weight history and biological factors as determinants of postcessation weight gain has only begun; thus, until further replications are shown, no definitive conclusions can be drawn.*

### Summary of Weight and Related Effects

Abstinence from tobacco causes increases in weight, hunger, perceived pleasantness of sweets, caloric intake, and thyroid functioning. Whether these are offset, transient, or rebound effects is not known. The effects of abstinence on motor activity, fluid intake/output, and metabolic substrates are unclear.

Whether the increased weight and caloric expenditure *in humans* are due to nicotine deprivation is unclear. In nonhumans, nicotine deprivation does induce these effects. Whether the increase in hunger and decreased energy expenditure and thyroid activity are due to nicotine deprivation is also unclear. Gender and type of foodstuff appear to influence abstinence effects in nonhumans, but such interactions have not been demonstrated in humans.

## 9. BEHAVIORAL AND SUBJECTIVE EFFECTS OF ABSTINENCE

The effects of abstinence on behavioral and subjective variables are outlined in Table 5.

### Sleep

Smoking appears to interfere with sleep (Soldatos et al., 1980); thus, one might hypothesize sleep to improve with cessation. On the other hand, insomnia is a common symptom of many withdrawal syndromes (Martin, 1977). The data presented in this section suggest the effect of abstinence on sleep depends on the specific measure of sleep employed and whether self-report or EEG measures are used.

In terms of *sleep quality,* one group found a small decrease in self-reported sleep quality (Hughes and Hatsukami, 1986; Hughes et al., 1986*a*), but studies from this group and others have not replicated this finding (Hatsukami et al., 1984; Lawrence et al., 1982; Schneider and Jarvik, 1985; West et al., 1984*a*).

Studies of more specific self-reports indicate cessation and deprivation increase self-reported *number of awakenings* (Hatsukami et al., 1984, 1987, 1988; Hughes and Hatsukami, 1986; Weybrew and Stark, 1967). The effect appeared to be a transient one peaking at 2 days (Hatsukami et al., 1984; Hughes et al., 1984*b*). Nicotine gum does not reverse this effect (Hughes et al., 1984*a*) and deprivation from nicotine gum does not induce it (Hughes et al., 1986*b*).

Table 5. Weight and Related Effects of Tobacco Abstinence[a]

| Type of abstinence effect | Whether due to nicotine deprivation |
|---|---|
| Rebound | Due to nicotine deprivation |
| None | ↑ Caloric intake (nonhumans) |
| Transient | ↑ Weight (nonhumans) |
| ↑ Appetite | Unclear evidence |
| Offset | ↑ Caloric intake (humans) |
| None | ↑ Appetite |
| Indefinite | ↑ Pleasantness of sweets |
| ↑ Weight (humans and nonhumans) | ↓ Thyroid function |
| ↑ Caloric intake (human and nonhumans) | ↑ Weight (humans) |
| ↓ Thyroid function | |
| ↑ Rated pleasantness of sweet | |
| Novel | |
| None | |
| Not an abstinence effect | |
| ↑ Fluid intake | |
| ↓ Fluid output | |
| Unclear evidence | |
| ↑ Activity (humans and nonhumans) | |
| ↑ Hormones: e.g., free fatty acids, glucagon, glucose, growth hormone, insulin | |
| ↓ Metabolic rate | |
| ↑ Taste sensitivity or thresholds | |

[a]See Table 1 for footnotes.

Four days of cessation produces a significant decrease in self-reported *time asleep* in some studies (Hughes and Hatsukami, 1986; Hatsukami et al., 1984), but produces no change in smokers not trying to quit (Weybrew and Stark, 1967). In the positive studies cessation decreased sleep time by 30 min (Hughes and Hatsukami, 1986). The effect appeared to be of the offset pattern. Nicotine gum did not reverse the effect (Hughes et al., 1984*a*).

Cessation and deprivation increase *self-reported time awake* after asleep (Hatsukami et al., 1984; Hughes and Hatsukami, 1986), but decreases *EEG-measured time awake* (Kales et al., 1970; Soldatos et al., 1980).

Cessation and deprivation do not change *self-reported sleep latency* (Hughes and Hatsukami, 1986; Hatsukami et al., 1984; Weybrew and Stark, 1967) but do decrease *EEG-measured sleep latency* by 15–30 min (Soldatos et al., 1980; Parsons and Hamme, 1975).

Five to eleven days of deprivation slightly increases the absolute amount and percent of *REM sleep* (Kales et al., 1970; Soldatos et al., 1980) and *REM "bursts"* (Parsons et al., 1975*c*). Deprivation increased the intensity and amount of self-reported *dreaming* in one study (Kales et al., 1970) but not in another (Weybrew and Stark, 1967). We could not find a report on the effects of abstinence on *REM latency*. Two abstracts reported that deprivation increased *Stage III and IV sleep* (delta or "deep" sleep) (Parsons et al., 1975*c;* Parsons and Hamme, 1975), whereas a more well-described study found no change in sleep stages (Soldatos et al., 1980).

*In summary, abstinence appears to increase the number of awakenings and the amount of REM sleep. Neither of these effects has been shown to be due to nicotine deprivation. The effect of abstinence on other sleep parameters is unclear.* Since many of the proposed effects of abstinence vary between self-report and EEG measures, further research examining both measures would be especially helpful.

## Anger

In this section we have collated studies that measured behavioral aggression and observed or self-reported anger and irritability. Although these constructs are not identical, we felt them similar enough to review together. Smoking decreases aggression (Hutchinson and Emley, 1973; Cherek, 1981), and thus, abstinence would be expected to increase irritability and anger.

Spontaneous jaw contraction has been associated with aggression in nonhumans (Hutchinson and Emley, 1973). One briefly reported study found that 1–32 days of cessation increased spontaneous jaw contractions and the duration of high-force contraction (Hutchinson and Emley, 1973). Deprivation did not increase triceps contractions, indicating the effect was not due to a generalized increase in muscle tension. Another widely cited study reported deprivation caused subjects to deliver more shocks to a fictitious person (Schechter and Rand, 1974). However, the data indicated deprived subjects delivered more shocks than smoking subjects, but the same number as nonsmokers. Thus, in reality, the data do not indicate deprivation increases aggression, but rather that smoking decreases aggression.

Observer studies suggest abstinence increases anger and irritability. When spouses, friends, and others rated the irritability of smokers before and after cessation, cessation was found to increase observed irritability (Hughes et al., 1986*a;* Hughes and Hatsukami, 1986). On an inpatient ward (supposedly a less stressful environment), nurses did not note an increase in argumentativeness with cessation (Hatsukami et al., 1984).

Abstinence increased self-reported anger or irritability in many studies (Hatsukami et al., 1984, 1987, 1988; Hughes and Hatsukami, 1986; Hughes et al., 1984*c,* 1986*a;* Lawrence et al., 1982; Perlick, 1978; Schneider and Jarvik, 1985; Smith and Lombardo, 1986; Stitzer and Gross, 1988; West et al., 1984*a,* 1987). One study of smokers not trying to quit failed to find this effect (Weybrew and Stark, 1967). The effect appears to be transient (Hughes et al., 1986*a;* West et al., 1987).

Abstinence-induced anger and irritability appear to be due to nicotine deprivation. Both observer and self-reported increases in irritability are consistently decreased by nicotine gum (Brantmark et al., 1973; Hughes et al., 1984*a,* 1986*a;* Schneider and Jarvik, 1985; Stitzer and Gross, 1988; West et al., 1984*a*). Observed and self-reported irritability also occur upon placebo substitution for nicotine gum (Hughes et al., 1986*b;* West and Russell, 1985*a*). One study found that self-reported irritability did not increase on switching to a low-nicotine cigarette (West et al., 1984*b*). In addition, in nonhumans, large increases in aggressive behavior (postshock biting) occurred when chronically administered nicotine was discontinued (Hutchinson and Emley, 1973).

*In summary, abstinence transiently increases anger/aggression/irritability, and this appears to be due to nicotine deprivation.* Since there are several behavioral paradigms to measure aggression, further study using these objective measures could be illuminating.

## Performance

Smoking improves performance, especially on sustained attention tasks (Wesnes and Warburton, 1983); thus, abstinence should worsen performance.

Most of the data on the effects of abstinence come from two laboratories. The Addiction Research Center (ARC) laboratory has done three studies: a 9-day (Snyder et al., 1986), a 12-hr (Snyder and Henningfield, in press), and a 3-day deprivation study (Snyder et al., 1988). In the 9-day study, the effect of deprivation and of return to smoking was examined. In the 12-hr deprivation study, the effect of 0, 2, and 4 mg of nicotine was examined. In the 3-day study, the effect of chronic use of 2 mg of nicotine gum was examined. The other laboratory is that of Elgerot and colleagues in Sweden. They completed two studies that examined the effects of 15 hr (Elgerot, 1978) and 4 days of deprivation (Elgerot, 1976). As noted below, the ARC laboratory often found deprivation effects, whereas the Swedish laboratory did not. One obvious hypothesis to explain the discrepant results is that the laboratories used different tests of the same construct. However, it is not readily apparent why one task should show positive effects and another negative effects. Perhaps a more important explanation is that the ARC laboratory achieved stable baselines prior to testing, but the Swedish laboratory did not. *A priori* stable baselines are necessary to ensure that any effects of deprivation on the tasks are due to changes in performance, not due to changes in learning. Thus, the failure of the Swedish laboratory to find effects may be because it was studying learning not performance.

Arithmetic. The ARC group found that deprivation increased the number of errors by about 5% and increased the time to complete a rapid arithmetic task. The Swedish group found that deprivation either produced no change or improved arithmetic skills. Besides the performance/learning explanation mentioned above, the two sets of studies differed in that the ARC task was a *rapid* arithmetic task but the Swedish task was not.

Search Tasks. The ARC found that deprivation did not worsen the number of errors but did increase time to complete two letter search tasks. Another study from a different laboratory reported that 20 hr of deprivation decreased the detection of peripheral visual signals (Tarriere and Hartmann, 1964). Again, Elgerot (1976, 1978) found either no effect or an improvement. A third study from another Swedish laboratory also found no effects of 5 days of deprivation (Myrsten et al., 1977).

Logical Reasoning. The ARC found that deprivation did not increase the number of errors but increased the time to complete two logical tasks. Again, Elgerot (1976, 1978) found either no change or an improvement.

Memory. The ARC found deprivation caused a 10% increase in the number of errors and an increase in the time to complete a digit recall task. Another study examined the memory of high- and low-association nonsense syllables in smokers deprived for 24 hr, smokers allowed to smoke, and nonsmokers (Kleinman et al., 1973). Deprived smokers did worse than both smoking smokers and nonsmokers on memory of the more difficult low-association syllables, but deprived smokers did *better* than the two control groups on the easier high-association syllables.

Psychomotor Skills. In a study of driving skills (Heimstra et al., 1967), smokers deprived for 1–6 hr did worse than either smoking smokers or nonsmokers. In addition, two measures of visual vigilance were worse in deprived smokers than in the two control groups. Another study found that deprivation for 4 days did not change ability to copy geometrical patterns (Elgerot, 1978).

Reaction Time. Deprivation for 1 hr to 4 days does not worsen either simple or complex reaction time (Heimstra et al., 1967; Hatsukami et al., 1984; Hughes et al., in press-*b*). Deprivation does appear to increase the *variability* in reaction time responding (Hughes et al., in press-*b*).

Time Course. The 9-day ARC study (Snyder et al., 1986) found that the increases in errors in arithmetic peaked at 24 hr and then returned to normal, whereas the increased time to do arithmetic and the decrement in memory persisted for all 9 days of the study. The time course for the decrement in perceptual speed and logical reasoning was not described.

Nicotine Deprivation. The ARC (Snyder and Henningfield, in press) found nicotine reversed the effects of deprivation on arithmetic, perceptual speed, logical reasoning, and memory in a dose-dependent manner.

If nicotine deprivation causes performance deficits, then nicotine antagonists should produce similar effects; however, a central nicotine antagonist (mecamylamine) does not worsen performance on a perceptual speed task more than a peripheral nicotinic blocker (Stolerman et al., 1973).

*In summary, the effect of abstinence on performance differs across laboratories, but suggests that deprivation causes decreased memory, which is due to the offset of a nicotine effect. The data do not support that idea that abstinence increases reaction time. The effects of abstinence on arithmetic skills, perceptual speed, or psychomotor skills are unclear.*

## Self-Reported Difficulty Concentrating

Abstinence may have inconsistent effects on objective measures of concentration, but abstinence consistently decreases *self-reported* concentration (Hatsukami et al., 1984; Hughes and Hatsukami, 1986; Hughes et al., 1984*c*, 1986*a;* Schneider and Jarvik, 1985; Weybrew and Stark, 1967; West et al., 1984*a*, 1987). Only two small studies of smokers not trying to quit failed to find this effect (Hatsukami et al., 1988; Nemeth-Coslett et al., 1986*b*).

Whether decreases in self-reported concentration are due to nicotine deprivation is unclear. Studies have reported nicotine gum decreased difficulty concentrating (Hughes et al., 1984*a*, 1986*a;* Stitzer and Gross, 1988), yet others have not found this effect (Schneider et al., 1984; West et al., 1984*a*). One study reported placebo substitution for nicotine gum increased difficulty concentrating (Hughes et al., 1986*b*), but another did not (West and Russell, 1985*a*). Switching to low-nicotine cigarettes (West et al., 1984*b*) did not worsen concentration. The reason for these discordant results is unclear.

*In summary, abstinence transiently increases self-reported difficulty concentrating, but whether this is due to nicotine deprivation is unclear.* Future studies comparing abstinence-induced changes in performance and self-reported difficulty concentrating are needed to validate this self-reported effect.

## Pain

Smoking appears to decrease sensitivity to painful stimuli (Fertig et al., 1986); thus, abstinence should increase pain sensitivity.

Four studies have examined the effects of overnight deprivation on pain threshold and tolerance (Milgrom-Friedman et al., 1983; Nesbitt, 1973; Shiffman and Jarvik, 1984; Silverstein, 1982). In these studies, subjects were given a noxious stimulus (shock or ischemia via a tourniquet) and asked to indicate the point when they detect the stimulus (i.e., stimulus onset), the point it becomes painful (i.e., pain threshold), and the point it becomes intolerable (i.e., pain tolerance). The only study to report data on *stimulus onset* (i.e., measure of perceptibility of the stimulus) did not statistically analyze the results, but it appears that deprived smokers did not differ from nonsmokers (Silverstein, 1982). In terms of *pain threshold,* the data are quite varied. One study reported that deprived smokers had a *lower* threshold than smoking smokers and nonsmokers (Nesbitt, 1973). Two other studies found *no difference* in the pain threshold of deprived smokers and nonsmokers (Shiffman and Jarvik, 1984; Silverstein, 1982), and a fourth study found that deprived smokers had a *higher* threshold than smoking smokers and nonsmokers (Milgrom-Friedman et al., 1983). In terms of *pain tolerance,* again the data are contradictory, with some studies reporting that deprived smokers had a *lower* tolerance than smoking smokers and nonsmokers (Nesbitt, 1973; Silverstein, 1982) and others reporting a *higher* tolerance in deprived smokers (Milgrom-Freidman et al., 1983). In the latter study, administration of nicotine gum during deprivation did not affect the results. Since the studies reviewed are very similar in design, a readily apparent reason for the many discrepancies is not available. One study has noted some methodological differences that might account for the differences (Shiffman and Jarvik, 1984).

*In summary, the data on abstinence effects on pain are quite contradictory.* Future studies using within-subject designs, i.e., testing before and many times after cessation, might help clarify the issue.

## Impatience

Impatience can be operationally defined as the inability to inhibit responding and therefore can be measured by rates of false starts (i.e., errors of omission) on behavioral tasks. In such tasks, smoking improves the ability to inhibit responding (Mangan, 1982); thus, abstinence would be expected to worsen the ability to inhibit responding. Using this paradigm, a study compared the ability to inhibit responding in smokers before and after 24 hr of deprivation (Hughes et al., in press-*b*). Across the two tests, nonsmokers and smoking smokers decreased their false starts but deprived smokers did not. However, whether this represents an impairment in impatience or an impairment in learning due to abstinence is unclear.

Cessation increases observed and self-reported impatience in a transient manner (Hughes and Hatsukami, 1986; Hughes et al., 1986*a;* Rodin, 1987). Such increases in self-reported impatience appear to be due to nicotine deprivation, as impatience is decreased by nicotine gum and precipitated by placebo substitution for nicotine gum (Hughes et al., 1984*a,* 1986*a,b;* Stitzer and Gross, 1988). Finally, in nonhumans, false-positive errors on an attention task increase after cessation of chronic nicotine treatment (Nelson and Goldstein, 1972, 1973).

*In summary, impatience is a transient effect of abstinence from tobacco that appears to be due to nicotine deprivation.*

## Restlessness

Motor restlessness often co–occurs with impatience and is a common symptom of withdrawal syndromes (Martin, 1977).

Both observed and self-reported restlessness is consistently increased by cessation (Hughes and Hatsukami, 1986; Hughes et al., 1984*c*, 1986*a;* Lawrence et al., 1982; Schneider and Jarvik, 1985; West et al., 1984*a*, 1987). The effect appears to be transient (Hughes et al., 1986*a*).

Whether restlessness is due to nicotine deprivation is unclear. Most studies have found that nicotine gum decreased observed or self-reported restlessness (Hughes et al., 1984*a*, 1986*a;* Stitzer and Gross, 1988), but others have not (Schneider and Jarvik, 1985; West et al., 1984*a*). One study found observed and self-reported restlessness occurred with placebo substitution for nicotine gum (Hughes et al., 1986*b*), but another did not (West and Russell, 1985*a*). Self-reported restlessness did not occur with switching to low-nicotine cigarettes (West et al., 1984*b*).

*In summary, transient restlessness often occurs with abstinence. It appears to be due to nicotine deprivation, but this is debatable.*

## Anxiety

Smoking itself is said to improve anxiety (Gilbert, 1979), and anxiety is a common feature of withdrawal syndromes (Hughes, in press).

Cessation and deprivation increase self and observer ratings of anxiety (Hatsukami et al., 1984, 1987, 1988; Hughes and Hatsukami, 1986; Hughes et al., 1984*c*, 1986*a;* Puddey et al., 1984, 1985; Rodin, 1987; Schneider and Jarvik, 1985; Smith and Lombardo, 1986). The studies that have failed to find this effect (Nemeth-Coslett et al., 1986*b;* West et al., 1984*a;* Weybrew and Stark, 1967) either used smokers not trying to quit or had short cessation and deprivation periods (i.e., <48 hr). The effect appears to be transient (Hughes et al., 1986*a;* West et al., 1987).

One study found that women deprived for 3 days appeared to have an increased *sensitivity* in perceived muscle tension (Russell et al., 1984). In addition, this effect was decreased by nicotine gum. Deprivation did not affect the *accuracy* of perceived muscle tension. Unfortunately, whether deprivation actually increased muscle tension was not reported in this or other studies that fulfill our criteria. One study reported abstinence had no effect on prolactin (Puddey et al., 1984, 1985), which is said to be a marker for stress. As mentioned earlier, two studies interpreted a decrease in pain tolerance from deprivation as increased anxiety, but this effect was inconsistent across studies.

Anxiety effects of abstinence have been studied with a novel use of the animal drug-discrimination paradigm. In this paradigm, nonhumans are taught to press one lever when a drug is administered at the beginning of a session and to press an alternate lever when saline is administered (Overton, 1984; Griffiths and Balster, 1979). When this arrangement is used, the interoceptive stimulus effects that accompany cessation of chronic nicotine treatment appear to be similar to those produced by anxiogenic drugs. In three studies, rats were first trained to discriminate between pentylenetetrazol (PTZ) and saline. PTZ is thought to produce anxiety-like signs and symptoms. When chronic nicotine treatment was discontinued, approximately half of the deprived rats pressed the PTZ lever, whereas few (e.g., 12.5%) of the control rats did so (Harris et al., 1986*a,b*, 1988). The investigators also found that this effect was blocked by diazepam and enhanced by isoniazid, which suggests involvement of the GABA/benzodiazepine system in the anxiety associated with abstinence (Harris et al., 1986*a,b;* Lal et al., 1985).

Whether the increased anxiety is due to nicotine deprivation is unclear. Nicotine gum relieves observed and self-reported anxiety, and placebo substitution for nicotine gum increased observed and self-reported anxiety in several studies (Hughes et al., 1984*a*, 1986*a,b;* Schneider and Jarvik, 1985; Stitzer and Gross, 1988). However, other studies have failed to replicate these findings (Brantmark et al., 1973; West et al., 1984*a;* West and Russell, 1985*a*).

*In summary, abstinence transiently increases anxiety. Whether this is due to nicotine deprivation is unclear.* Anxiety can be estimated via several behavioral and physiological indices. Future research using such objective measures might be especially fruitful.

## Dysphoria

Whether smoking improves depression is debatable (Gilbert, 1979; Hughes, 1988). Smoking is more prevalent in clinically depressed patients (Hughes et al., 1986*c*), perhaps as a self-modification to improve mood (Goldstein, 1987; Hughes and Hatsukami, 1987). Thus, one might expect abstinence to increase depression. In addition, abstinence from prototypic stimulants (e.g., amphetamines and cocaine) can induce clinical depressions (American Psychiatric Association, 1987). For these reasons, abstinence would be expected to increase dysphoria.

Psychiatrists distinguish dysphoria and clinical depressions (Hughes et al., 1982*b*). Dysphoria is the mood state of being sad, blue, and so on. Clinical depression is dysphoria to the point it significantly impairs functioning (e.g., at work, with family, and so on). In addition, clinical depression is accompanied by changes in eating, sleeping, and so on (American Psychiatric Association, 1987). Although case reports suggest cessation of tobacco can induce such depressions (Flanagan and Maany, 1982), scientific studies of cessation-induced clinical depressions are unavailable.

In contrast to clinical depression, several studies have reported self-reported mood decreased (i.e., dysphoria) after 1–30 days of cessation or deprivation (Hatsukami et al., 1984; Schneider and Jarvik, 1985; West et al., 1984*a*, 1987; Weybrew and Stark, 1967), but others have not found this effect (Hatsukami et al., 1987, 1988; Hughes and Hatsukami, 1986; Lawrence et al., 1982; Rodin, 1987). One possible explanation of the contradictory results is that most of the negative studies used a multiitem standardized scale (POMS), whereas all of the positive studies used single-item scales. Thus, the later studies may have been tapping a broader construct, such as total mood disturbance. The time course of dysphoria appears to be transient (West et al., 1987).

A few studies suggest depression may be due to nicotine deprivation. Studies have reported that nicotine gum relieves postcessation depression (Schneider and Jarvik, 1985; West et al., 1984*a*), but others have not (Brantmark et al., 1973). Placebo substitution for nicotine gum increased depression (Hughes et al., 1986*b*) and switching to low-nicotine cigarettes did not increase depression (West et al., 1984*b*). Finally, a central nicotine antagonist did not induce more dysphoria than a control peripheral nicotine antagonist (Stolerman et al., 1973).

*In summary, abstinence appears to induce dysphoria but has not been shown to induce true depression.* Future studies more clearly documenting abstinence-induced clinical depressions in smokers with a history of depression would be of interest (Hughes, 1988), as would a clearer definition of the dysphoria produced by cessation.

## Alertness

The decreased performance and slowed EEG from abstinence (see earlier sections) have been interpreted to indicate decreased alertness (Edwards and Warburton, 1983; Wesnes and Warburton, 1983); thus, one would expect abstinence to decrease alertness.

One to thirty days of cessation or deprivation has been reported to increase drowsiness (Hatsukami et al., 1987, 1988; Hughes 1984*c*, 1986*a*; Smith and Lombardo, 1986), to have no effect (Hatsukami et al., 1984; West et al., 1984*a*; Weybrew and Stark, 1967), and to have different effects on different measures of alertness and drowsiness (Hughes and Hatsukami, 1986).

In terms of nicotine deprivation, one study reported nicotine gum improved self-reported drowsiness (Stitzer and Gross, 1988); however, another did not (Hughes et al., 1984*a*), and drowsiness did not occur upon placebo substitution for nicotine gum (Hughes et al., 1986*b*).

*In summary, the effect of abstinence on alertness cannot be stated owing to wide variance in study results.* Studies using objective measures may help clarify these inconsistent results.

## Fatigue

The worsening in performance with abstinence could be attributed to fatigue (Wesnes and Warburton, 1983).

One direct measurement of fatigue is decrement in performance during a long task, e.g., a worsening of reaction time, errors, and variability in responding in a sustained attention task. Deprivation does not appear to potentiate such fatigue effect (Hughes et al., in press-*b*). In addition, cessation or deprivation does not worsen either self-reported or observed daily fatigue (Hatsukami et al., 1984, 1987, 1988; Hughes and Hatsukami, 1986; Lawrence et al., 1982; Nemeth-Coslett et al., 1986*b*; Rodin, 1987; West et al., 1984*a*; West and Russell, 1987; Weybrew and Stark, 1967) or fatigue during an exercise test (Myrsten et al., 1977). Only one abstract reported an effect of cessation on fatigue (Smith and Lombardo, 1986). Fatigue also does not appear to be relieved by nicotine gum (Brantmark et al., 1983) or to occur with deprivation from nicotine gum (West and Russell, 1985*a*).

*In summary, abstinence does not appear to increase fatigue.* This is interesting as fatigue is a common symptom of abstinence from prototypic stimulants (American Psychiatric Association, 1987).

## Physical Symptoms

Many physical symptoms have been attributed to abstinence from tobacco but few have been tested prospectively in more than one trial.

Headache is one of the commonly cited physical symptoms (American Psychiatric Association, 1980); however, all of the studies of headache failed to find an effect of 1–30 days of cessation and deprivation (Hughes and Hatsukami, 1986; Hughes et al., 1986*a*; West et al., 1984*a*; Weybrew and Stark, 1967). Gastrointestinal complaints are also often cited (American Psychiatric Association, 1980). Again, most studies have not found an effect of cessation or deprivation (Hughes and Hatsukami, 1986; Hughes et al., 1986*a*; West et al., 1984*a*; Weybrew and Stark, 1967). Dizziness was reported in one study (West et al., 1984*a*) but not in others (Hughes et al., 1984*b*; Lawrence et al., 1982; West et al., 1984*b*). Nausea was reported in one study (Weybrew and Stark, 1967) but not in others (Hughes et al., 1984*b*; Lawrence et al., 1982). Constipation was reported in one study (Lawrence et al., 1982) but not in others (Hughes et al., 1984*b*; West et al., 1984*a*). Other symptoms that have been tested and not found to occur include hiccups (West et al., 1984*a*), shakiness/tremor (Hughes et al., 1984*b*; West et al., 1984*a*; Weybrew and Stark, 1967), diarrhea (West et al., 1984*a*), sore throat (Lawrence et al., 1982; West et al., 1984*a*), cramps (Lawrence et al., 1982), sweating (Hughes et al., 1984*b*; Lawrence et al., 1982), skin rash (Lawrence et al., 1982), and palpitations (Lawrence et al., 1982). Other commonly cited symptoms, such as mouth ulcers (Gunn, 1986; Scheider and Jarvik, 1985) and increased cough and dry mouth (Gunn, 1986), have not been tested.

Some studies have examined composite scores of physical symptoms. Ratings of "physically well" do not increase with cessation (West et al., 1987). The Shiffman–Jarvik Inventory includes a subscale on physical effects (Shiffman and Jarvik, 1976). This scale did not increase in the one study that fulfilled our criteria (Hatsukami et al., 1987). Second, our group has collated several physical symptoms into a summary scale. We have found that scores on this scale increased with cessation (Hughes and Hatsukami, 1986; Hughes et al., 1986*a*) and that this increase was reversed by nicotine gum in one study (Hughes et al., 1984*a*) but not another (Hughes et al., 1986*a*), nor did scores on the scale worsen with placebo substitution for nicotine gum (Hughes et al., 1986*b*).

*In summary, abstinence from tobacco has not been shown to cause specific physical symptoms as in other withdrawal syndromes.* Although some would argue that the absence of such symptoms indicates tobacco withdrawal is not a true physiological withdrawal state, others have argued that behavioral outcomes as a result of cessation are sufficient to indicate withdrawal (Balster, 1985).

## Sociability

Abstinence appears to decrease sociability and composure in company and is reversed by nicotine gum (West et al., 1984*a*). However, cessation of nicotine gum

(West and Russell, 1985*a*) or switching to low-nicotine cigarettes (West et al., 1984*b*) did not decrease sociability.

*In summary, the evidence of the effect of abstinence in sociability is limited.* Since abstinence increases irritability, anxiety, restlessness, and impatience, further studies might show significant decreases in sociability.

## Drug Use

Smoking has been associated with the intake of several drugs, especially alcohol and caffeine (Istvan and Matarazzo, 1874), and abstinence from tobacco has been hypothesized to increase alcohol and caffeine intake.

Two prospective studies found that alcohol use decreased (by about 3/4 of a drink per day in one study) (Hughes and Hatsukami, 1986; Puddey et al., 1984, 1985). A third study reported that subjects who had a greater decrease in the number of cigarettes postcessation had a greater decrease in alcohol use (Olbrisch and Oades-Souther, 1986). Among long-term studies, abstinent smokers appeared to decrease alcohol intake in one study (Stamford et al., 1986) but not in another (Dalloso and James, 1983). Nicotine gum did not change alcohol intake in one of these studies (Hughes et al., 1984*a*). In these studies, it is unclear whether the decrease in alcohol was a result of cessation or a behavioral strategy used by smokers to help with cessation.

Cessation and deprivation did not change caffeine intake in several prospective studies (Hughes and Hatsukami, 1986; Puddey et al., 1984, 1985; Rodin, 1987). However, one briefly described study found a greater increase in caffeine use among those with a greater decrease in smoking (Olbrisch and Oades-Souther, 1986), whereas another study suggested a greater decrease in caffeine intake in quitters than continuing smokers (Benowitz et al., 1988). As described in Section 7, cessation of tobacco may increase caffeine levels even while intake remains constant, presumably through a pharmacokinetic interaction (Sachs and Benowitz, in press).

*In summary, tobacco abstinence appears to decrease alcohol intake but have no effect on caffeine intake. However, this issue has been studied surprisingly little, and no consensus can be reached on the time pattern of changes in alcohol intake or whether it is due to nicotine deprivation.* Future clinical studies will have to somehow control for voluntary changes in alcohol and caffeine intake as methods to enhance cessation to determine the true effect of abstinence *per se*.

## Operant Behavior in Nonhumans

Abstinence appears to disrupt the ability to avoid unanticipated aversive stimuli. Nicotine administration increases signaled and unsignaled avoidance responding in rats (e.g., Morrison, 1974*a,b*). In a series of studies, rats were trained on an unsignaled shock avoidance schedule while being chronically treated with nicotine (Balfour and Morrison, 1975; Hall and Morrison, 1973; Morrison, 1974*a,b*). When saline was substituted, avoidance responses decreased and the nonhumans received greater numbers of shock. Shock rates increased significantly above control levels, suggesting that this was a rebound effect. Since the behavior of the rats that had been trained on saline was not disrupted when nicotine was substituted for saline, a state-dependency explanation for this effect was dismissed. Interestingly, this effect was not observed in the nicotine group if a warning signal precedes the delivery of shock (Morrison, 1974*b*).

*In summary, these results are quite important because they indicate abstinence can produce behavioral changes in nonhumans that fulfill the criteria for rebound effects and are due to nicotine deprivation.*

## 10. METHODOLOGICAL ISSUES

Our conclusions have been based on the consistency of results across studies and on what we believe are the most valid and generalizable results in studies of humans. In general, we required at least two consistent studies to make any conclusions on whether an abstinence effect was present, the type of abstinence effect, and so on. In choosing which studies to rely on most heavily, we had to weigh the different merits of each study. We review our criteria for making conclusions not only to make them public, but also to illustrate some of the methodological problems of the literature. (See Table 6.)

### Substance Used

Cigarettes are the most commonly used form of tobacco in North America. Results of studies of abstinence from other forms of tobacco (e.g., smokeless tobacco) or from nicotine products (e.g., nicotine gum) were of secondary interest.

### Quitters vs. Nonquitters

Both smokers who are trying to quit smoking (i.e., cessation) and smokers temporarily abstaining for the purposes of a study (i.e., deprivation) have been examined in prior studies. Across similar protocols and measures, smokers not trying to quit appear to have fewer and less severe abstinence effects than smokers trying to quit (e.g., compare Hughes and Hatsukami, 1986, and Hughes et al., 1986*a*). In making conclusions, we gave more weight to cessation studies as these are of greater clinical interest.

### Self-Quitters vs. Clinic Attendees

Self-quitters appear to have fewer and less severe abstinence symptoms than those attending a smoking cessation clinic when similar protocols and measures are used (see Table 7). Although clinic attendees have been studied more often, they are less desirable subjects for several reasons. For example, few (<6%) smokers who quit attend clinics or specialized programs (e.g., Hughes et al., 1986*a*; Jamrozik et al., 1984). In addition, such smokers appear to be more "dependent" than nonclinic attendees (Russell et al., 1974). Finally, clinic attendees receive a treatment, and this treatment (e.g., relaxation) may influence abstinence symptoms. Thus, we gave more weight to studies of self-quitters, as they are a larger, more representative, and untreated sample. Unfortunately, there were fewer studies of abstinence effects in self-quitters.

Table 6. Behavioral and Subjective Effects of Tobacco Abstinence[a]

| Type of abstinence effect | Whether due to nicotine deprivation |
|---|---|
| Rebound | Due to nicotine deprivation |
| ↓ Avoidance (nonhumans) | ↑ Anger |
| Transient | ↓ Avoidance (nonhumans) |
| ↑ Anger | ↑ Impatience |
| ↑ Anxiety | ↓ Memory |
| ↑ Awakening during sleep | Not due to nicotine deprivation |
| ↑ Difficulty concentrating | ↑ Awakening during sleep |
| ↑ Dysphoria | Unclear evidence |
| ↑ Impatience | ↓ Alcohol use |
| ↑ Restlessness | ↑ Anxiety |
| Offset | ↑ Difficulty concentrating |
| ↓ Memory | ↑ Dysphoria |
| Indefinite | ↑ REM sleep |
| ↓ Alcohol use | ↑ Restlessness |
| ↑ REM sleep | |
| Novel | |
| None | |
| Not an abstinence effect | |
| ↑ Caffeine use | |
| ↑ Reaction time | |
| ↑ Fatigue | |
| Unclear | |
| ↓ Alertness | |
| ↓ Arithmetic skills | |
| ↓ Deep sleep | |
| ↑ Dreaming | |
| ↑ Pain | |
| ↓ Perceptual speed | |
| ↑ Physical symptoms | |
| ↓ Psychomotor skills | |
| ↑ Sleep latency | |
| ↓ Sleep quality | |
| ↓ Sociability | |
| ↓ Time asleep | |

[a]See Table 1 for footnotes.

## Gender

Although abstinence effects do not appear to differ by gender (see Section 12), for generalizability we gave more weight to studies of both sexes.

## Control Groups

Our inclusion criteria (Section 4) made it clear we gave greater weight to within-subject analyses with multiple data points over time. However, even these types of studies can benefit from appropriate control groups. For example, within-subject studies have described in detail the weight gain accompanying abstinence. However, other

Table 7. Incidence of Abstinence Effects 1 Week after Cessation

| Abstinence effect (self-reported) | % with an increase[a] Clinic attendees (Hughes and Hatsukami, 1986) | % with an increase[a] Self-quitters (Hughes et al., 1986a) | % with high rating[b] Clinic attendees (West et al., 1987) |
|---|---|---|---|
| Anxiety | 87 | 59 | — |
| Depression | — | — | 8 |
| Difficulty concentrating | 73 | 55 | 13 |
| Drowsiness | 22 | 40 | — |
| Hunger | 53 | 67 | 16 |
| Impatience | 76 | 52 | — |
| Insomnia | 84 | 38 | — |
| Irritability | 80 | 52 | 21 |
| Restlessness | 71 | 55 | 12 |

[a]Percentage of subjects in whom the effect increased from baseline to abstinence.
[b]Percentage of subjects who rated the effect as "extremely or very" or "all the time, almost all the time, or a lot of the time" as compared to a typical day.

studies with smokers as a control group indicate smokers also gain weight over time and thus all of the weight gain cannot be attributed to abstinence. Other studies with never-smoker control groups indicate that the weight gain in abstinent smokers does not make them obese, but rather returns them to the weight of never-smokers. Thus, we gave more weight to studies that use smoking smokers and never-smokers as control groups. Unfortunately, most studies that include these groups are cross-sectional rather than longitudinal.

## Setting

Environmental cues may be necessary to elicit tobacco abstinence effects (see Section 15). Laboratory studies lack such environmental cues and abstinence effects may not be as readily elicited in this setting. For example, subjects report abstinence symptoms are less than expected when they are hospitalized but increase upon discharge into their natural environs (Hatsukami et al., 1984). Thus, we gave more weight to studies performed in the natural environments of smokers.

## Abrupt Cessation

Abrupt and gradual cessation produce different abstinence effects (see Section 17). Abrupt cessation is the most common method of cessation and the method most likely to produce abstinence effects; thus, we gave more weight to studies of abrupt cessation.

## Nonrandomized Designs

The ideal design to study abstinence effects is to randomly assign subjects to either stop or not stop smoking. Although this is almost universally done in laboratory studies, it is rarely done in studies of smokers trying to quit.

Most cessation studies are of two designs. In the first design, smokers who were able to remain abstinent are studied before and after cessation using a within-subject design. This design is problematic because exclusion of subjects who were unable to stop smoking in all likelihood produces a selection bias in that those who have had the most aversive abstinence effects are the very smokers excluded. Since some long-term studies of abstinence report relapse rates of 80–90%, such studies are really reporting on the small subset (i.e., 10–20%) of smokers who are able to stay quit. Such small selected subsets could produce underestimates of abstinence effects or false-negative results.

The second design is to compare abstinent smokers and relapsed smokers. The problem here again is that smokers self-selected into groups and thus selection bias is highly likely. "Third variable" explanations of results would be common. For example, suppose those who quit drink less alcohol than those who relapse. Is this because abstinence decreases drinking or is it because those who drink less are more likely to become abstinent than those who do not?

Because nonrandomized trials make up >70% of the literature reviewed, the reader must be cautious not to overinterpret such results. The solution is to completely prevent relapse. Of course, this is impossible, and the longer the follow-up, the more dropout. In summary, we preferred studies with little relapse; however, this criterion was liberalized for studies of longer duration.

## Longitudinal vs. Cross-Sectional Analyses

A related problem is that some studies use cross-sectional analyses to track abstinence symptoms by using all abstinent smokers at each follow-up. Of course, the individuals in each follow-up sample change with each follow-up. An alternative is to report longitudinal data only on those smokers who remained abstinent for a certain period of time (e.g., at 1, 3, *and* 6 months). Although one could argue that longitudinal analysis restricts the sample and thus invokes some selection bias, we believe the fact that the analysis follows a single sample of subjects over time gives a truer view of the time course of abstinence effects than a series of cross-sectional surveys of different samples. Thus, we believed longitudinal analyses were preferable to cross-sectional analyses and gave more weight to the latter.

## Biochemical Verification

Many subjects in treatment for smoking cessation report cessation but fail biochemical tests, suggesting they are falsifying their smoking status (Glynn et al., 1986). Thus, we gave more weight to studies examining abstinence effects only in biochemically verified abstinent smokers.

## Objective Measures

The high incidence of expectancies about abstinence effects of tobacco cessation makes objective measures especially desirable. In addition, self-reports of behaviors and internal states become less valid when subjects are asked to rate them over periods of time. This problem occurs when cessation studies ask subjects to retrospectively rate abstinence effects for long periods of time (i.e., 6–26 weeks) (Pertschuk et al., 1979). Thus, we gave more weight to studies that used objective measures of constructs, e.g., laboratory analogs or observer reports. In addition, if studies used self-report, we gave more weight to studies that asked subjects to rate abstinence effects over short periods of time (i.e., $<1$ day).

## 11. THE TOBACCO ABSTINENCE SYNDROME

This section deals with studies that collated several abstinence effects into one score. We also use this section to address issues that apply to all abstinence effects (e.g., reliability and generalizibility).

### Reliability

Many smokers state that abstinence effects differ from one cessation to another. Documenting that abstinence effects are reliable is important, as reliability is thought to be a prerequisite to validity. One small study ($n = 3$) found several abstinence effects to have test–retest consistency, i.e., heart rate, insomnia, caloric intake, irritability, restlessness, and drowsiness (Hughes et al., 1984*c*). That study also found that the total scores for mood disturbance on the Shiffman–Jarvik Withdrawal Scale and the Profile of Mood States were quite similar on two consecutive abstinence periods. The authors concluded that when method of cessation controlled tobacco abstinence, effects possess within-subject reliability. Obviously, larger studies of the reliability of abstinence effects are needed before a firm conclusion can be reached.

### Generalizability

Except for studies on weight, most all of the prospective data available are from smokers temporarily refraining from smoking for the purposes of the study or from clinic attendees. Temporary refraining may not produce the same degree of distress as trying to quit for good and may thereby underestimate abstinence effects. On the other hand, smokers attending a clinic appear to be more dependent on nicotine and thus studies of these subjects might overestimate abstinence effects (see Section 10). Surprisingly, we know of only one unpublished prospective study of abstinence effects in self-quitters (Hughes et al., 1986*a*). Encouragingly, this study found that the magnitude and evidence of abstinence effects are only slightly lower in self-quitters.

### Magnitude

Abstinence effects from tobacco have usually been described as mild (e.g., Hatsukami, 1988); however, some have described significant distress in certain individuals (Flanagan and Maany, 1982; Larson and Silvette, 1974). The only study that quantified the magnitude of distress from tobacco abstinence found that most subjects had four to six symptoms and, more important, that POMS scores (a mood checklist) during the first 4 days of abstinence were similar to the scores found in psychiatric outpatients (Hughes and Hatsukami, 1986). Empirical studies of how often abstinence effects cause dysfunction (e.g., decreased ability to work, marital discord, etc.) have not been reported.

Several investigators have stated that the variability in abstinence effects from nicotine is large and indicates that the syndrome is unreliable or not as pharmacologically determined as other drug withdrawal syndromes. However, comparison of the coefficient of variability in tobacco abstinence scores in our studies with those in studies of alcohol and opiate withdrawal suggests similar variability (Hughes, 1988).

## Incidence

The incidence of abstinence effects has been widely cited in studies using postcessation scores only; however, as discussed before, without baseline scores, these are misleading. Incidence scores can be more validly calculated as the percentage of smokers in whom postcessation scores are greater than baseline scores. The three studies that have used this procedure found the incidence of abstinence effects varies widely across effects (Table 5) (Hughes and Hatsukami, 1986; Hughes et al., 1986*a*; West et al., 1987). The most common effects are decreased heart rate (HR), anxiety, difficulty concentrating, impatience, irritability, and restlessness, all of which occurred in more than 70% of clinic attendees and more than 50% of self-quitters. The incidence of effects is usually 20–30% lower in self-quitters than clinic attendees, even with similar methods and scales. Incidence figures for observer ratings of anxiety, drowsiness, impatience, irritability, and restlessness among both clinic attendees and self-quitters are usually 0–10% less than those for self-reported effects (Hughes and Hatsukami, 1986; Hughes et al., 1986*a*).

## Time Course

Previous reviews have suggested that abstinence effects can occur within 2 hr and last several months (e.g., Shiffman, 1979); however, these statements were based on studies that did not fulfill our inclusion criteria. Studies have also reported abstinence effects to decrease and then increase again in the second week (Shiffman and Jarvik, 1976), but this has not been replicated.

Among studies that did fulfill our criteria, most transient effects (see Tables 2–5) occurred within 24 hr, peaked in the first 1–2 weeks, and were absent at 1 month (Hughes et al., 1986*a*; Lawrence et al., 1982; Stitzer and Gross, 1988; West et al., 1987). Increased hunger and weight gain were the exceptions and lasted at least 1–6 months, with some decline but no return to baseline (Hughes et al., 1986*a*; Stitzer and Gross, 1988; West et al., 1987).

With cessation of other drugs, a prolonged withdrawal syndrome has been postulated (e.g., Martin and Jasinski, 1969). With tobacco abstinence, total abstinence scores over longer periods of time return to baseline by 1 month and then decrease *below* baseline and remain there for 10–26 weeks (Fig. 4) (Hughes et al., 1986*a*; Stitzer and Gross, 1988). Thus, this evidence directly contradicts the notion of a prolonged tobacco abstinence syndrome. Unfortunately, these studies of long-term abstinence effects did

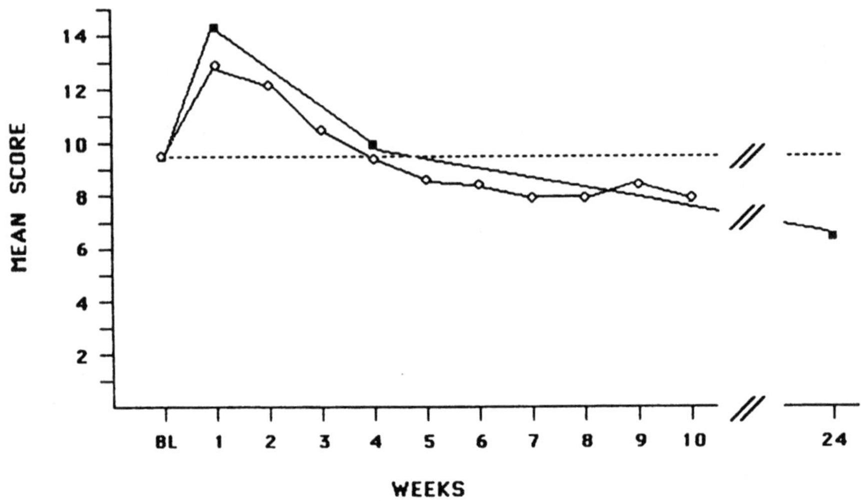


Figure 4. Long-term effects of abstinence on self-reported withdrawal. (From ■ Hughes et al., 1986*a*, and ◇ Stitzer and Gross, 1988. Reprinted with permission, National Institute on Drug Abuse.)

not include a control group of smoking smokers or nonsmokers to rule out the possibility that the decrease below baseline is simply due to repeated measurements or, more interestingly, occurs because nonsmokers and smokers have different before-smoking baselines.

Another time course variable that has been studied is time-of-day effects. According to two studies, abstinence symptoms are worse in the evening (Schneider and Jarvik, 1984; Shiffman and Jarvik, 1976). Unfortunately, neither study reported whether this same worsening of symptoms in the evening occurred in smoking smokers or nonsmokers.

## Nicotine Deprivation

In prior sections we have discussed whether individual effects could be due to nicotine deprivation. We now review the evidence in studies using total abstinence scores.

The most common line of evidence used to support the nicotine deprivation hypothesis is relief by nicotine gum (Hughes and Hatsukami, 1985). The majority of studies reported that nicotine gum decreases total abstinence scores (Fagerstrom, 1980; Hughes et al., 1984*a*, 1986*a*, in press; Killen et al., 1984; Schneider et al., 1984; Stitzer and Gross, 1988; West et al., 1984*a*; Westling, 1976), but a few did not (Gottlieb et al., 1987; Puska et al., 1979).

A second test of nicotine deprivation effects is to examine if nicotine via other routes of administration decreases abstinence effects. However, studies of nicotine nasal sprays and patches on abstinence effects did not take baseline data; thus, these results are not clearly interpretable (Jarvis et al., in press; Rose et al., 1985).

A third test of the nicotine deprivation hypothesis is whether abstinence is relieved by nicotine gum in a dose-related manner. One study found that the 2- and 4-mg-dose gums produced more relief from abstinence than the 0- and 1-mg doses of nicotine gum (Gust et al., 1985).

A fourth paradigm is to reduce the nicotine content of cigarettes as abstinence effects typically occur even with the simple reduction of drug intake (Martin, 1977). As discussed earlier, the results of the two studies of this paradigm differed in that one reported increased irritability (Perlick, 1978) whereas the other reported few effects (West et al., 1984*b*).

A fifth paradigm is to examine whether an abstinence effect occurs on placebo substitution for nicotine gum. Total observer and self-reported abstinence scores do appear to increase in such a paradigm (Hughes et al., 1986*b*).

A sixth paradigm is to change the pH of the urine, which should change the rate of elimination of nicotine and thereby change abstinence effects. Although studies have shown that administration of acidifying and alkanizing agents changes smoking behavior (Schachter, 1978), none of these studies measured abstinence effects.

A final paradigm to assess whether abstinence effects are due to nicotine deprivation is to see whether an antagonist precipitates abstinence effects (Stolerman, 1986*a*). Mecamylamine, a central nervous system (CNS) nicotine blocker, does induce dysphoria; however, this was not greater than that produced by pentolium, a peripheral nicotine blocker. Thus, the dysphoria appeared to be due to peripheral side effects of mecamylamine rather than to CNS antagonism of nicotine (Stolerman et al., 1973). Although one study suggested mecamylamine produced "withdrawal-like" changes in the EEG (Pickworth et al., 1988), other studies have mentioned that mecamylamine did not precipitate or worsen abstinence effects (Nemeth-Coslett et al., 1986*b*; Tennant et al., 1984). These data appear to contradict the nicotine deprivation hypothesis. However, it is important to note that none of these cited studies were set up specifically to test the ability of mecamylamine to precipitate abstinence effects. Interestingly, recent data indicate that although mecamylamine is a reliable blocker of nicotine's behavioral effects in nonhumans and humans, it is not a potent blocker of the recently discovered cholinergic nicotine receptor (Stolerman, 1986*b*). Thus, if abstinence effects are controlled by cholinergic nicotine receptors (see Section 14), then one would not expect mecamylamine to precipitate abstinence effects.

## 12. DETERMINANTS OF ABSTINENCE EFFECTS

### Age

Age was not associated with total abstinence discomfort in one study (Hughes and Hatsukami, 1986), and although younger quitters had more postcessation weight gain in some studies (Black et al., 1988; Bosse et al., 1980), this did not occur in other studies (Emont and Cummings, 1987; Klesges et al., 1988*a*; Rabkin, 1984).

### Gender

Whether women have more intense abstinence effects than men has been studied in several retrospective and prospective studies that do not fulfill our inclusion criteria. The results of these studies are unclear (Guilford, 1967; Gunn and Shapiro, 1979; Hall,

1984; Shiffman, 1979). The prospective studies that fulfill our criteria have found no sex differences in abstinence effects.

One article reviewed the data from two studies and found that of the 46 dependent variables, none differed significantly between men and women (Svikis et al., 1986). Women do not appear to have more total abstinence discomfort nor does such discomfort respond more to nicotine gum than in men (Hughes et al., 1984*b*; Hughes and Hatsukami, 1986; Schneider and Jarvik, 1985). Gender differences in specific physiological variables such as decline in HR (Gilbert and Pope, 1982) and catecholamines (Elgerot, 1978), as well as behavioral variables such as decreased performance (Elgerot, 1976), have been tested and not found.

Data from nonhumans could be interpreted to indicate greater postcessation weight gain and eating in females than males (see Section 8) but this effect is not reflected in the existing data in humans. Studies have reported that women gain more weight (Black et al., 1987; Klesges et al., 1988*a,b*), *less* weight (Freidman and Siegelaub, 1980; Rabkin, 1984), or a similar amount of weight (Emont and Cummings, 1987; Hall et al., 1986; Svikis et al., 1986) than men. Perhaps more women gain weight but gain less weight than men. This hypothesis would account for the clinical impression of weight gain or increase in women, yet data showing no differences in *mean* weight increases between men and women. Gender does not appear to influence the effect of nicotine on weight gain (Hall et al., 1986). The single study of caloric intake by gender found that women increased their snacking by 94% with deprivation, compared to 50% for men (Gilbert and Pope, 1982); this effect was not found in another study (Klesges et al., 1988*a*). The increase in overall caloric consumption does not appear to differ between men and women (Gilbert and Pope, 1982; Klesges et al., 1988*a*).

## Expectancy

Several studies that do not fit our inclusion criteria have been cited as evidence that expectancy influences abstinence effects (Gritz, 1980). In one study that did fit our criteria, subjects were asked if they believed they had received nicotine or placebo gum. Those who believed they had received placebo gum had more abstinence discomfort than those who could not tell what they had received, who in turn had more discomfort than those who thought they had received nicotine gum (Hughes and Krahn, 1985). Because this study used *post hoc* ratings, it is unclear whether belief in whether one received placebo or nicotine modified the level of abstinence effects, or vice versa, whether the level of abstinence effects modified the belief of whether one received nicotine or placebo.

Two trials have experimentally manipulated instructions and thereby directly tested whether expectancy influences abstinence effects. The first study randomly assigned smokers to a 2 × 2 design contrasting instructions (told received nicotine gum vs. told received placebo gum) and drug (received nicotine gum vs. received placebo gum) (Gottlieb et al., 1987). The majority of the measures of abstinence effects were unchanged by instructions or drugs. The physical symptoms and stimulation scores on the Shiffman-Jarvik Scale were less in the told nicotine group than in the told placebo group on some days but not on others. A second study used a similar design and found that abstinence symptoms were less in those who received nicotine than in those who received placebo group, but found no effect of instructions (Hughes et al., in press-*a*). In summary, the seemingly valid proposition that abstinence effects are highly influenced by expectancy has yet to be empirically verified.

## Biological Factors

Biological factors, such as the rate of elimination of a drug, should influence the severity of abstinence effects, as a faster decline in blood levels of a drug has been associated with greater abstinence effects (Martin, 1977). One study reported that smokers with shorter half-lives for nicotine (i.e., a quicker elimination) had more confusion and number of awakenings after abstinence than smokers with longer half-lives (Hatsukami et al., 1985). However, half-life was unrelated to several other abstinence effects.

In nonhumans, genetic factors can control the intensity of withdrawal from several drugs (Crabbe and Belknap, 1980). One preliminary study reported that abstinence effects and the degree of relief from nicotine gum were greatest in smokers who reported both parents smoked, less in those who reported one parent smoked, and least in those who reported neither parent smoked (Hughes, 1986*a*).

## Intensity of Smoking

Most withdrawal effects are dose-related to the intensity of drug self-administration throughout the entire dose range; i.e., even small amounts of a drug can induce some physical dependence (Katz and Valentino, 1986; Martin, 1977). Alternately, clinicians have often believed a certain amount of drug used for a certain duration is necessary for withdrawal to occur (Martin, 1977).

The results of retrospective and postcessation studies on whether abstinence effects are greater in those who smoke more *cigarettes per day* are inconclusive (Goldstein et al., 1988; Hatsukami, 1988; Pomerleau et al., 1983*a*; Shiffman, 1979, 1986; Williams, 1979). Studies that fulfill our criteria found either no relationship or a *negative* relationship between abstinence effects and the number of cigarettes per day (Hughes and Hatsukami, 1986; West and Russell, 1985*b*). Some studies have reported that weight gain is greater in heavier smokers (Clearman and Jacobs, 1985; Comstock and Stone, 1972; Emont and Cummings, 1987; Gordon et al., 1975; Hall et al., 1986); others have failed to find this relationship (Freidman and Siegelaub, 1980; Garvey et al., 1974; Rabkin, 1984). The reason for the contradictory results is unclear.

*Smoking topography* measured objectively or by self-report does not predict abstinence (Emont and Cummings, 1987; Hatsukami et al., 1985; Hughes and Hatsukami, 1986). *Strength* of the cigarette (i.e., nicotine yield) also does not appear to be related to overall discomfort (Hughes and Hatsukami, 1986). Strength of the cigarette was related to weight gain in one study (Bosse et al., 1980) but not in another (Emont and Cummings, 1987).

One possible reason that number of cigarettes, topography, and strength are poor predictors of abstinence effects may be because they are poor measures of tobacco or nicotine intake (Hatsukami et al., 1987). Thus, direct measurement of tobacco or nicotine in bodily fluids might better predict abstinence severity. Higher *serum nicotine* predicted more abstinence discomfort in one study (West and Russell, 1985*b*) but not in others (Hughes and Hatsukami, 1986; Hatsukami et al., 1985). Higher *serum cotinine* (a nicotine metabolite) appeared to predict greater abstinence effects in one study (Goldstein et al., 1988). But neither greater cotinine nor *thiocyanate* (a by-product of smoking) appear to be related to postcessation weight gain (Hall et al., 1986; Rabkin, 1984). Higher *breath carbon monoxide* did appear to be related to several abstinence effects (Nil et al., 1987; West and Russell, 1985*b*). Another possible reason that dose is a poor predictor of abstinence effects is that physical dependence is dose related only in the lower range (1–10 cigarettes) and not thereafter.

## Duration of Smoking

Duration of drug use typically increases the intensity of abstinence effects (Katz and Valentino, 1986; Martin, 1977) in experimental settings. However, some clinicians believe a minimal duration of use is necessary for the development of physical dependence. Contrary to this latter opinion is recent evidence that, at least with some drugs, physical dependence begins with the first dose of the drug (Bickel et al., 1988; Higgins et al., 1988).

Consistent with this notion is retrospective evidence that adolescents report abstinence effects even after only a few years of smoking (McNeill et. al., 1986). However, duration of smoking has not been found to be related to abstinence discomfort or weight gain (Carney and Goldberg, 1984; Hughes and Hatsukami, 1986; Rabkin, 1984). Thus, perhaps physical dependence develops rapidly after the onset of smoking and changes little thereafter.

## Route of Administration

The route that a drug is given (e.g., oral vs. intravenous) can influence the degree of abstinence effects (Katz and Valentino, 1986; Martin, 1977). The only study of a route of tobacco administration other than cigarettes compared abstinence effects from smokeless tobacco and cigarettes (Hatsukami et al., 1987). Abstinence from smokeless tobacco decreased heart rate and orthostasis and increased self-reported confusion, eating, number of awakenings, and observer-rated abstinence effects. Abstinence from cigarettes also caused these effects, but the effects of cigarette abstinence were consistently of greater magnitude. In addition, abstinence from cigarettes induced anger, anxiety, depression, drowsiness, and weight gain, none of which occurred with abstinence from smokeless tobacco.

## Dependence

Abstinence effects have been hypothesized to be greater in the more "dependent" smokers. Part of the problem with this hypothesis is that the scales for dependence vary in whether they are quantifying physical dependence (i.e., withdrawal) or behavioral dependence (i.e., desire for tobacco, tendency to relapse, etc.) or dependence on tobacco or on the nicotine in tobacco (Hughes, 1984). The Fagerstrom Tolerance Scale (TQ) consists mostly of items that refer to behavioral dependence on tobacco. The total TQ score predicted total abstinence discomfort in two briefly described papers (Fagerstrom,

1980; Goldstein et al., 1988) and weight gain in a well-done trial (Tonnesen et al., 1988). The single item from the TQ concerning time to first cigarette upon awakening appears to be the best predictor item (Hughes and Hatsukami, 1986; Emont and Cummings, 1987). On the other hand, two detailed studies have found negative results (Emont and Cummings, 1987; Hughes and Hatsukami, 1986).

The Reasons for Smoking Scale has two scales relevant to the dependence construct: the addiction scale and the negative affect scale (Ikard et al., 1969). Neither of these have been shown to predict abstinence effects or their relief by nicotine gum (Bosse et al., 1980; Hughes and Hatsukami, 1986).

Russell's Smoking Motivation Questionnaire has a subscale for dependence (Russell et al., 1974). In one study the scale predicted total abstinence discomfort and irritability but not restlessness, depression, hunger, or inability to concentrate (West and Russell, 1985*b*).

Other measures somewhat related to dependence include the severity of abstinence discomfort in the past, which appears to predict self-reported abstinence (Hughes and Hatsukami, 1986). One investigator hypothesized that some smokers are restrained smokers (i.e., voluntarily smoke less than they need to) and are chronically in withdrawal and found that even when smoking, such smokers are more irritable than nonsmokers (Schachter, 1978). Other generic scales, such as the MacAndrews Scale for Addiction (MacAndrews, 1979) and Eysenk Personality Questionnaire (Eysenk and Eysenk, 1975), do not predict abstinence discomfort and weight gain (Bosse et al., 1980; Hughes and Hatsukami, 1986). Finally, although one study found that self-reported smoking for stimulation predicted abstinence effects (Goldstein et al., 1988), a prior study had found no such relationship (West and Russell, 1985*b*).

A hypothesis related to the notion that highly dependent smokers will have more abstinence effects is that perhaps smokers with a history of drug or alcohol dependence will have greater abstinence effects. This hypothesis has not been tested.

In summary, the evidence that any dependence scale predicts abstinence effects is quite scanty. Further tests that use scales more specific for physical vs. behavioral dependence and dependence on nicotine vs. tobacco may find better results.

## 13. BEHAVIORAL THEORIES OF ABSTINENCE EFFECTS

### Extinction or Schedule Induction

When nonhumans are deprived of nonpharmacological reinforcers, several behaviors similar to abstinence effects occur, e.g., increased aggression, oral behaviors (e.g., paw licking), motor activity, polydipsia, and variability in responding (Falk, 1981). Interestingly, these effects are similar to the symptoms of abstinence from tobacco, i.e., irritability, eating more, restlessness, and impatience. These have been labeled extinction-induced behaviors (e.g., Azrin et al., 1966). Similar effects occur during periods of reinforcement schedules when reinforcement is prohibited or unlikely. These effects have been labeled scheduled-induced or adjunctive behaviors (Falk, 1981). Some of these effects have been shown to occur in humans as well (Falk, 1981). Demonstration that tobacco abstinence effects are due to extinction or scheduled-induced effects would require showing (1) smoking is serving as a reinforcer, (2) the abstinence effect is transient, and (3) changing the schedule of smoking changes the intensity of the abstinence effect.

## 14. PHARMACOLOGICAL THEORIES OF ABSTINENCE EFFECTS

### Nicotine Deprivation

As reviewed earlier, several lines of evidence indicate that the effects of abstinence from tobacco are due to nicotine deprivation: (1) abstinence effects are opposite to the agonist effects of nicotine, (2) abstinence effects are relieved by nicotine, and (3) abstinence effects from cessation of nicotine alone (e.g., from nicotine gum) are similar to those from tobacco. The weakest evidence for this hypothesis is that switching to low-nicotine cigarettes appears to produce few abstinence effects.

### Offset of Drug Effects

The simplest pharmacological theory to explain offset effects is that they represent the disappearance of the agonist effects of tobacco. Many believe that such effects should parallel the reduction in blood levels of the drug. If so, these effects should be quite short-lived, as five half-lives (when nicotine is almost totally eliminated) of nicotine would be 10 hr; i.e., withdrawal should occur almost every morning. However, some drug effects occur long after the disappearance of the drug, as the CNS effects of the drug (e.g., on receptors) may take longer to dissipate.

As mentioned earlier (Section 2), offset effects can represent not only a return to baseline, but irreversible effects of the drug. In other words, constant exposure to nicotine over 20–50 years may "reset" certain physiological effects at new levels.

Several abstinence effects do appear to be offset (see Tables 2–5). Other abstinence effects show a definite transient time course and thus cannot be explained by a simple offset of drug effects.

### Transient/Rebound Effects

Transient effects can be explained as behavioral reactions to the loss of reinforcer (as described in Section 13). However, they can also be explained as short-lived pharmacological perturbations prior to the body reaching a new homeostasis without the chronic agonist effects of nicotine. The most widely cited theory to explain such perturbations is that they represent withdrawal of the opiate/sedative type (e.g., Schachter, 1978; Solomon and Corbit, 1973).

Tolerance to Nicotine. Classical descriptions of withdrawal of the opiate/sedative type observe a strong relationship between the development and severity of tolerance and withdrawal effects (Martin, 1977). Several lines of evidence indicate tolerance to nicotine occurs in nonhumans (Balfour, 1982; Jarvik, 1979). In humans, tolerance occurs to the HR-increasing effects of nicotine (Jones et al., 1978; Benowitz et al., 1984; Jones, 1986). Tolerance to the HR-increasing and other effects of nicotine appears to be lost rapidly (Lee et al., 1987*a*; West et al., 1987). However, another study suggests that smokers abstinent for 1 year were more tolerant to the punishing effects of nicotine (Hughes et al., in press-*c*). Thus, tolerance in humans appears to be of both the acute (i.e., occurs and is lost each day) and chronic (i.e., persists from day to day) type.

Although experimental study of the development of tolerance in smokers is not available, it appears that adolescents develop a tolerance to the aversive effects of smoking quite rapidly and, according to a retrospective study, develop abstinence symptoms quite rapidly (McNeill et al., 1986). In addition, one study suggested tolerance to nicotine and abstinence effects are linked (Hughes and Hatsukami, 1986). This study found that on smoking a cigarette, smokers with a lower HR increase per unit increase in nicotine had greater abstinence symptoms. On the other hand, a more recent study found that on smoking a cigarette after abstinence, smokers with a lower HR per unit increase in carbon monoxide had *fewer* abstinence symptoms (West and Russell, 1987).

In the next sections we describe two generic theories of withdrawal of the opiate/sedative type: the dual action and homeostatic explanations. Then we describe more molecular theories, e.g., receptor induction and enzyme derepression. For each theory we discuss the evidence for and against applying the theory to tobacco. As will be seen, most theories have little empirical evidence.

## Dual Action

This general theory of withdrawal states that drugs have two actions—an excitatory and a depressant action. With depressant drugs, the depressant action is dominant, but the excitatory action cumulates with chronic dosing and accounts for tolerance. When the drug is withdrawn, the cumulative stimulant action persists as withdrawal (Martin, 1977). This theory is intriguing as nicotine is thought to have both depressant and stimulant effects (Hutchinson and Emley, 1986). However, we know of no direct applications of this theory to tobacco abstinence effects.

## Homeostasis Effects

This general theory of withdrawal states that drug exposure recruits a negative feedback process that opposes the drug effect (Martin, 1977). With repeated exposure this opposing effect becomes greater, thus decreasing the effect of the drug, i.e., tolerance. Cessation of the drug leaves the opposing effect unopposed, and this is withdrawal. The opponent process theory has elaborated this theory and applied it to cigarette smoking (Solomon and Corbit, 1973; Ternes, 1973).

Homeostasis theories require withdrawal effects to be opposite those of the agonist effects of the drug. Many would classify nicotine as a stimulant; thus, one could simply reverse the valence of effects and state nicotine withdrawal should be sedative in nature. This is clearly not the case. On the other hand, nicotine is not a prototypic stimulant. If one eschews the stimulant/depressant classification and simply looks at individual drug effects, many of the effects of cessation of tobacco are opposite to the agonist effects of the drug nicotine. For example, tobacco increases HR and adrenaline and abstinence causes a transient decrease in these. In addition, tobacco improves aggression, hunger and concentration, and, as already seen, abstinence worsens aggression, hunger, and concentration. On the other hand, effects opposite to the agonist effects of nicotine have not been documented for motor activity, pain, and alertness. In addition, some transient abstinence effects e.g., restlessness, insomnia, and depression, do not appear to be the opposite of the agonist effects of nicotine.

## Receptor Induction

Several theories to explain homeostasis have been proposed (Martin, 1977). The receptor induction theory states that drug exposure changes the number of receptor sites for the drug in the CNS and this causes tolerance. When drug is stopped, this change in receptor site activity causes withdrawal effects. This theory requires that receptors for the drug exist in the CNS. In nonhumans, several nicotinic receptors exist. At present the cholinergic/nicotinic receptor seems the most specific for the pharmacological effects of nicotine via tobacco (Schwartz et al., 1982; Stolerman, 1986*b*). Chronic nicotine increases the number, but not the affinity, of these receptors (Ksir et al., 1985; Marks et al., 1983, 1985; Schwartz and Kellar, 1983, 1985). In nonhumans this increase is related to tolerance (Marks et al., 1985). Postmortem studies of smokers and nonsmokers suggest the same effects occur in humans (Benwell et al., 1988). Although this evidence could support the receptor-induction theories, the functional significance of these up-regulated cholinergic nicotine receptors is unclear (Marks et al., 1985); i.e., whether changes in these receptors covary with abstinence effects is also unclear.

## Enzyme Derepression

This theory states that drug exposure inhibits the enzyme that converts a precursor to an active neurotransmitter (Martin, 1977). The resultant decrease in neurotransmitter causes more precursor to be made to overcome the enzyme inhibition and this accounts for tolerance. Cessation of the drug allows full activity of the enzyme to occur in the presence of a large amount of precursor and the resultant excessive activity accounts for withdrawal.

One investigator has applied this theory to tobacco (Bachynsky, 1986). He cited evidence that chronic use of nicotine inhibits the enzyme that converts choline precursor to acetycholine (choline acetyltransferase; CAT). According to this theory, upon cessation there is an abundance of the precursor choline in the presence of the now uninhibited CAT. This produces an excessive amount of acetycholine at CNS muscarinic–cholinergic sites, which accounts for tobacco abstinence effects (Bachynsky, 1986). Evidence for this application from the few data available suggests abstinence does increase acetycholine in the synaptic cleft *in peripheral ganglia* (see Section 6). In addition, abstinence causes decreased HR and gastrointestinal symptoms, both thought to be cholinergic effects. Finally, a briefly described, noncontrolled trial suggested antimuscarinic drugs (i.e., anticholinergics) help smokers quit (Bachynsky, 1986). On the other hand, studies have not found high levels of acetycholine *in the CNS* after cessation of chronic nicotine treatment (Edwards and Warburton, 1983).

## Disuse Supersensitivity

This theory states that drug exposure decreases neurotransmitters at the synaptic cleft, which causes the postsynaptic receptors to become hypersensitive to the drug in a manner similar to denervation supersensitivity (Martin, 1977). This model is intriguing as nicotine itself appears to be a CNS neurotransmitter. On the other hand, chronic nicotine appears to change the number, but *not* the affinity (i.e., sensitivity), of the CNS cholinergic/nicotinic receptor.

## Neuronal Redundancy

This theory states drug exposure depresses a neuronal pathway and, in response, a parallel pathway is recruited (Martin, 1977). Upon cessation, the unopposed action of the parallel pathway accounts for withdrawal. We are unaware of evidence that parallel pathways exist for nicotine. However, an interesting similarity exists on the level of receptors rather than pathways. Several nicotine receptors have tentatively been identified. Perhaps during chronic nicotine use, different receptor populations are recruited in a manner similar to that of different neuronal pathways.

## Sympathetic Overactivity

Three pharmacological theories have hypothesized specific neurohormonal changes involved in abstinence effects.

One theory states that craving is associated with sympathetic overactivity across many types of withdrawal (Glassman et al., 1985). Evidence supportive of this theory includes the fact that several abstinence effects, e.g., restlessness, anxiety, and irritability, could be due to increased sympathetic activity. In addition, alpha-2 agonist drugs, which block sympathetic activity, reduce withdrawal effects from opiates and alcohol (e.g., Cushman et al., 1985; Jasinski et al., 1985). Such effects have also been shown for tobacco abstinence (Glassman et al., 1985). Evidence against this theory includes the finding that many of the effects of tobacco abstinence are those of *decreased* sympathetic activity (e.g., decreased HR). Also, several critical pieces of evidence for this theory have not been reported; e.g., (1) abstinence from tobacco or nicotine increases sympathetic activity in the CNS, and (2) the severity of abstinence effects covaries with the degree of sympathetic arousal.

## Decreased Cholinergic Tone

This theory states that the symptoms of tobacco abstinence are due to *decreased* central cholinergic (i.e., adrenergic or catecholaminergic) tone (McCarty, 1982). Evidence for this theory includes findings that many of the abstinence effects can be attributed to decreased adrenergic activity: drowsiness, poor concentration, increased rapid eye movement sleep, fatigue, and weight gain. Evidence against this hypothesis includes the finding that many other effects of tobacco abstinence do not appear to be due to decreased adrenergic activity: e.g., restlessness, anxiety, impatience, and irritability. In addition, we know of few direct tests of the effect of abstinence on cholinergic or adrenergic function in humans. The little amount of nonhuman work suggests abstinence *increases* acetylcholine at the synaptic cleft (see Section 6).

### Hypoglycemia

A third theory states the symptoms of tobacco abstinence are due to hypoglycemia (Bourne, 1985). Evidence for this hypothesis includes findings that nicotine increases blood glucose, abstinence decreases serum glucose (see Section 8), and administration of ACTH, which increases blood glucose, relieves tobacco abstinence symptoms (Bourne, 1985). Evidence against the hypothesis includes the fact that the therapeutic efficacy of ACTH is small, inconsistent, and not fully replicated (West, 1985). Further critical tests of this hypothesis would include tests of (1) whether glucose reliably decreases with abstinence, and (2) whether any such decreases are related to the onset and severity of abstinence effects.

## 15. COMBINED BEHAVIORAL AND PHARMACOLOGICAL THEORIES

### Multicausality

Although we have presented the different theories of abstinence effects separately, it is possible that some abstinence changes are due to behavioral effects and some to pharmacological effects. For example, some abstinence effects could be due to extinction-induced behaviors, some to drug offset effects, and others to physical dependence of the opiate/sedative type (e.g., Schneider and Jarvik, 1985). Although Tables 2–4 might be used to develop such a classification, much of the classification in these tables may be inaccurate owing to inadequate information. For example, some of the effects we have labeled offset effects may in reality be transient or rebound effects when studied more intensively or for longer periods. In addition, effects classified as not due to nicotine deprivation may be shown to be nicotine deprivation effects when they are studied with routes of nicotine administration that better mimic smoking.

### Conditioned Withdrawal

When drug ingestion or deprivation from a drug is paired with a stimulus, this stimulus can come to evoke agonist or abstinence effects; e.g., conditioned withdrawal effects (Siegel, 1983; Stewart et al., 1984; Wikler, 1980). Cigarette smoking would appear likely to generate conditioned drug or withdrawal effects because smoking occurs frequently, there is a short delay between drug ingestion and psychopharmacological effects, and both smoking and not smoking often occur in the presence of distinctive cues. Studies of conditioning with cigarettes have typically compared physiological responses that occur with the presentation of smoking and with the presentation of a neutral cue (e.g., Sideroff et al., 1987). In some smokers, HR appears to decrease with the presentation of a smoking cue (Abrams et al., 1987; Niaura et al., in press). Although this result suggests a conditioned withdrawal effect, studies of these effects have failed to employ proper control groups of nonsmokers, ex-smokers, or smoking smokers. Thus, unambiguous interpretation of these findings is not possible. For example, alternate interpretations, such as the possibility that the decrease in HR is an orienting response to a reinforcer, cannot be excluded.

### Overgeneralization

Overgeneralization refers to the possibility that smokers who repeatedly have true abstinence effects begin to falsely report that aversive states due to environmental events are tobacco abstinence effects (Solomon and Corbit, 1973; Ternes, 1973). For example, suppose a smoker reliably becomes more irritable with tobacco abstinence. Then, suppose he/she stops smoking and during abstinence is punished by some environmental contingency. The smoker may then report that the irritability due to the punishment contingency is due to abstinence from smoking.

## 16. SIGNIFICANCE

### Smoking as a Drug Dependence

The debate whether smoking is a dependence disorder has become more salient owing to the development of dependence-based treatments (e.g., brand fading, nicotine gum), the debate on whether tobacco industries are liable for "addicting" smokers, and the emphasis on the commonalities across substance abuse.

The existence of a tobacco withdrawal syndrome is crucial to most definitions of dependence (American Psychiatric Association, 1987; Brady and Lukas, 1984; Edwards et al., 1981; Jaffe, 1977, 1980). Some of these definitions distinguish between *physical* (or physiological) dependence and *psychological* (or behavioral) dependence (e.g., Jaffe, 1980). The term "physical dependence" has been used in several ways but always indicates the presence of a withdrawal syndrome. To some, the term "physical" implies materialistic changes are necessary and the term "dependence" implies that withdrawal leads to drug seeking (Edwards et al., 1981). This interpretation of the term "physical dependence" has led to the proposal of another term—"neuroadaptation"—to replace the terms "withdrawal" and "physical dependence" (Edwards et al., 1981; WHO, 1981). The term "neuroadapation" is proposed to indicate withdrawal effects are an adaptive mechanism and can occur without leading to drug seeking.

In contrast to physical dependence, the term "psychological dependence" refers to regular self-administration of a drug. Physical dependence and psychological dependence often coexist, but also often occur independently; i.e., psychological dependence can occur without physical dependence, and physical dependence can occur without psychological dependence (Falk, 1983; Goldberg and Stolerman, 1986). In the following section we examine the hypothesis that physical dependence influences psychological dependence among tobacco users.

Although most clinicians believe withdrawal has a significant role in the maintenance and cessation of opiates and alcohol, this belief has been subjected to only a few direct tests (Cappell and Leblanc, 1971). Most investigators believe withdrawal is a sufficient, but not necessary, cause of alcohol/opiate use (Cappell and Leblanc, 1971).

## Maintenance of Smoking

Although many have hypothesized that the maintenance of smoking is due to the avoidance of abstinence effects (Schachter, 1978), a direct test of this hypothesis is not available. By a direct test, we mean a test that shows both that abstinence effects occur during daily smoking *and* that abstinence effects prompt smoking behavior.

## Smoking Cessation

One of the most widely cited hypotheses of the nicotine dependence theory is that abstinence effects from smoking prevent smokers from stopping (Schachter, 1978). Most accounts of this hypothesis refer to the onset of transient or rebound abstinence effects; however, as we have argued earlier (Section 2), offset effects can also be aversive and lead to relapse. Actually, the fact that offset effects are continuous, i.e., they do not abate like transient or rebound effects, could make them *more* likely to cause relapse.

Two lines of thought can be used to argue that offset effects could be potent causes of failures to stop smoking. The first line of thought is that smokers use cigarettes as a psychological tool to decrease aggression, anxiety, and hunger, and to improve concentration (Mangan and Golding, 1984; Ashton and Stepney, 1982). Over time smokers could lose their own abilities to cope with these problems. Then, upon cessation the day-to-day problems of frustration, anxiety, hunger, and concentration are unsolved and are, thus, more aversive than when they were smoking. Although pieces of evidence for this theory are available in individual studies (e.g., Abrams et al., 1987), a direct test is not available.

The second line of thought posits that those who choose to smoke have *a priori* psychological problems (Eysenk and Eaves, 1980; Goldstein, 1987; Hughes and Hatsukami, 1987). Such persons find that the pharmacological effects of nicotine from smoking relieve these problems, and therefore they continue to smoke. When such persons stop smoking, the old psychological problems recur, are aversive, and lead them back to smoking. In other forms of drug abuse, this theory has been labeled the self-medication theory.

Some evidence for the latter line of thought exists. Individuals who choose to smoke *and* who are unable to stop are more aggressive and anxious before ever smoking than those who do not choose to smoke or cannot stop (Cherry and Kiernan, 1976; Eysenk and Eaves, 1980; Hughes, 1986*a*; Seltzer and Oechsli, 1985). Although the increased aggression and anxiety that occur *a priori* to smoking may be due to genetic effects (Hughes, 1986*a*), it is also possible these states are due to early behavioral histories. Other pieces of evidence embracing this line of thought are missing. For example, this theory would require that long-term ex-smokers differ from nonsmokers. Although many studies have compared smokers and nonsmokers, few have compared ex-smokers and nonsmokers on relevant psychological characteristics (Matarazzo and Saslow, 1960).

Many believe abstinence effects cannot have a major role in cessation of tobacco because most relapse occurs long after abstinence effects. However, this argument is based on relapse data from clinics. Data based on self-quitters suggest much relapse (50–70%) occurs in the first 2 weeks (Eiser et al., 1985; Trends, 1985). Another argument against the role of abstinence effects in relapse cites studies that reported most self-quitters do not attribute relapse to abstinence effects (e.g., Shiffman, 1982). However, other studies have found that 33–35% of smokers report abstinence effects immediately prior to relapse (Cummings et al., 1985*a*).

In contrast to these indirect tests of the association of abstinence effects and relapse, some direct evidence is available. Several studies that did *not* fulfill our criteria found contradictory results (e.g., Eiser et al., 1985; Fagerstrom, 1980; Guilford, 1966; Killen et al., 1987; Puska et al., 1979). Surprisingly, we could only find four studies that fulfilled our criteria (Hughes and Hatsukami, 1986; Hughes et al., 1986*a*; Lawrence et al., 1982). One briefly reported study stated that those with more frequent abstinence symptoms were less likely to be abstinent at 6-week follow-up (Lawrence et al., 1982). A second, more detailed study reported that abstinence effects in the first 2 days did not predict the ability to refrain for the next 2 days (Hughes and Hatsukami, 1986). The third direct test of abstinence effects and relapse was a large study of whether smokers with high levels of abstinence discomfort in the first week or month after cessation would be more likely to have relapsed by 1-year follow-up (Hughes et al., 1986*a*). Analyses of the nine individual abstinence effects (craving, irritability, anxiety, difficulty concentrating, impatience, restlessness, insomnia, hunger, and physical symptoms) showed that *none* of these predicted relapse. Another study examined late relapse (i.e., relapse between 3 and 12 months postcessation). This study found that a past history of abstinence-induced anger predicted late relapse in men but not women (Swan et al., in press). Other psychological and physical symptoms in the past did not predict relapse. In summary, despite its face validity, abstinence effects have not consistently predicted relapse to smoking.

Postcessation weight gain has often been hypothesized to be a major cause of relapse, especially in women (Hall et al., 1986). Contrary to *a priori* hypotheses, the single prospective study found that more weight gain in the first 6 months prospectively predicted *less* relapse by 1 year (Hall et al., 1986). There was no difference in this prediction between men and women. Further support for this finding comes from one postcessation study that found women who reported eating more in the first 4 days were more likely to be abstinent at 6-month follow-up (Guilford, 1966). One explanation for this finding is that food deprivation increases the reinforcing effects of drugs (Carroll and Meisch, 1984). Cessation of smoking may decrease metabolic rate (see Section 7). If so, then to not gain weight, smokers may have to deprive themselves of food and thereby increase the reinforcing effects of cigarettes taken during minor slips.

In the context of these unexpected results, it is of interest that fear of weight gain appears to predict relapse (Klesges and Klesges, 1987).

## Abstinence Discomfort

If abstinence effects are not related to cessation, it may still be important to treat abstinence effects. As described earlier, abstinence effects do induce a significant amount of distress (Hughes and Hatsukami, 1986). Thus, treatment of abstinence effects may be important in itself. For example, for humanitarian reasons, physicians treat pain with injuries, even though the analgesic treatment may not improve outcome.

## 17. TREATMENT OF ABSTINENCE EFFECTS

### Psychological Treatments

Behavioral procedures, such as relaxation and social skills training, might relieve abstinence effects, such as anxiety, irritability, and impatience. Suprisingly, behavioral, group, and other therapies have not reported the effects of their treatments on abstinence effects. One dissertation reported that a behavioral program for postcessation weight gain was ineffective (Grinstead, 1981). Nicotine fading (i.e., reducing the nicotine yield of a cigarette) appears to induce few abstinence effects, despite a 60% decrease in nicotine blood levels (Hatsukami et al., 1988; West et al., 1984*b*).

Gradual reduction in number of cigarettes per day has been reported to produce *less* severe abstinence effects compared to complete abstinence (Hatsukami et al., 1988). This finding appears to contradict an earlier study that subjects who partially abstained from smoking reported *more* severe symptoms (Shiffman, 1979). These two studies vary widely in their methodology. The former *randomly* assigned subjects to *gradual* or abrupt cessation. The latter *post hoc* compared subjects who *self-selected* into *partial* and complete abstainers.

However, the real issue appears to be how one quantifies abstinence effects. In all likelihood, abrupt cessation causes greater symptoms over a shorter time, whereas gradual reduction produces less intense symptoms over a longer time. Whether the intensity of symptoms or their duration is more crucial to abstinence discomfort or the ability to remain abstinent is unclear.

### Pharmacological Treatments

As described earlier (Section 11), nicotine gum decreases abstinence discomfort, expecially anxiety, decreased memory, and irritability. On the other hand, nicotine gum does not reliably decrease hunger, restlessness, insomnia, difficulty concentrating, performance, or weight (Tables 2–4); (Hughes and Hatsukami, 1985; West, 1984). Whether similar results occur for other nicotine replacement therapies is unclear. Uncontrolled trials suggest nicotine nasal spray (Jarvis et al., in press), but not a nicotine patch (Rose et al., 1985), relieves abstinence effects.

Several well-done studies demonstrate alpha-2 agonists decrease abstinence effects. Oral clonidine (Glassman et al., 1985), and transdermal clonidine (Ornish et al., 1988), decreased postcessation anxiety, irritability, restlessness, and difficulty concentrating. Alprazolam, a benzodiazepine-like tranquilizer (Glassman et al., 1985), also decreases abstinence effects. Decreased sympathetic activity has been postulated to be the mechanism by which alpha-2 agonist drugs and benzodiazepines decrease abstinence effects. Although tobacco abstinence has some effects that could be attributed to sympathetic overactivity (e.g., anxiety, restlessness, and impatience), it lacks the typical signs and symptoms of sympathetic overactivity, such as tachycardia, diaphoresis, and hypertension. In addition, abstinence from other stimulant drugs does not produce syndromes characterized by sympathetic discharge. Thus, the mechanism by which alpha-2 agonists and benzodiazepines exert their effects is unclear. Elucidating this mechanism will be of special import (Hughes, 1988) now that clonidine has been shown to be an effective smoking cessation aid (Glassman et al., 1988).

Other pharmacological treatments for abstinence symptoms have been tested, but none of these studies reported baseline and postcessation values for abstinence symptoms. These treatments include doxepin (Edwards et al., 1988), anticholinergic drugs (Bachynsky, 1986), ACTH (Bourne, 1985), propranol (Dow and Fee, 1984), sodium bicarbonate (Fixx et al., in press), acupuncture (e.g., Fuller, 1982), meprobamate (Murphee and Shultz, 1968), and a nicotine antagonist (Tennant et al., 1984).

In summary, thus far only nicotine gum and clonidine have adequate empirical data to justify their use to treat the abstinence effects of smoking cessation.

## 18. TOBACCO VERSUS OTHER ABSTINENCE SYNDROMES

Abstinence from tobacco produces several symptoms that are common in almost all abstinence syndromes: anxiety, insomnia, irritability, impaired performance, impatience, and restlessness (American Psychiatric Association, 1987; Hughes, in press). Abstinence from tobacco is similar to that from prototypic stimulants (amphetamine and cocaine) in that both produce increased hunger and weight; however, abstinence from prototypic stimulants can produce clinical depressions and hypersomnia, which are not characteristic of tobacco abstinence. Abstinence from tobacco also differs from that from caffeine in that fatigue and headaches are prominent in the latter (Griffiths and Woodson, 1988).

Abstinence from tobacco differs from abstinence from sedatives and opiates mainly in its lack of physical signs, i.e., hyperthermia, increased tendon reflexes, lacrimation, nausea and vomiting, perspiration, pupillary dilatation, rhinnorhea, seizures, tremor, and yawning (American Psychiatric Association, 1987; Hughes, in press; Martin, 1977).

Clinical impression suggests the magnitude of discomfort due to abstinence from opiates, sedatives, and stimulants is much greater than that from tobacco. However, we are unaware of any direct comparisons of the magnitude of the syndromes. Such studies are needed as the perceived degree of difference in the syndromes is probably influenced by several factors, e.g., the samples being studied (e.g., outpatient problem drinkers vs. inpatients with histories of delirium tremens and self-quitters vs. those in clinics).

Studies suggest 25–50% of self-quitters and 75% of clinic attendees evidence tobacco abstinence effects (see Section 11). Although this appears similar to that seen with clinical samples of patients with alcohol, benzodiazepines, and opiate dependence, whether abstinence effects are more or less frequent than with cessation of other drugs is difficult to gauge from cross-study comparisons owing to differences in sample characteristics, differences in criteria for stating abstinence effects occur, and so on, across studies.

The onset of tobacco abstinence effects (i.e., in 6–24 hr) and the time of peak effects (2–3 days) are similar to acute abstinence syndromes for alcohol, sedative/

hypnotics, and stimulants. However, there does not appear to be a lag time between cessation of smoking and abstinence effects, as occurs with other drug withdrawal syndromes.

Withdrawal syndromes are usually associated with several features (Table 8) (Jaffe, 1980; Martin, 1977). Withdrawal and tolerance are typically associated as it is believed that they are manifestations of the same process. Tolerance to nicotine does occur among smokers and the degree of tolerance appears to be directly related to the degree of withdrawal (see Section 14).

Nonhuman models are available for most withdrawal states. Although some texts state that abstinence from nicotine produces no readily observable changes in nonhumans, as discussed earlier abstinence does have several effects in nonhumans, e.g., increased eating and weight (see Section 8) and disruption in avoidance responding (see Section 9).

Withdrawal syndromes often progress through stages (Mello and Mendelson, 1977). For example, tremor, sweating, and insomnia occur early in alcohol withdrawal, whereas seizures, disorientation, and hallucinations occur later. Whether progressions occur with tobacco abstinence has not been tested. Withdrawal syndromes are usually related to the intensity and duration of drug use, although this correlation may be rough and may include threshold effects (Kalant et al., 1971; Martin, 1977). Tobacco abstinence effects do not appear to be closely related to intensity or duration of smoking (see Section 12).

Withdrawal syndromes are typically relieved by drugs that are cross-tolerant with the drug discontinued (e.g., benzodiazepines relieve alcohol withdrawal). Whether nicotine-related compounds, such as cystine, lobeline, and cotinine, would suppress tobacco abstinence effects has not been tested.

Withdrawal syndromes are typically less with gradual reduction than with abrupt cessation. Although an early study suggested partial abstainers of cigarettes had *more* abstinence discomfort than complete abstainers, a more rigorous study reported abstinence effects were less with gradual reduction (see Section 17).

Table 8. Common Features of Withdrawal Syndromes

| | Tobacco | Alcohol/sedatives | Opioids |
|---|---|---|---|
| Associated with tolerance | Maybe | Yes | Yes |
| Animal models | Few | Yes | Yes |
| Symptom stages | ? | Yes | Yes |
| Cross-dependence | ? | Yes | Yes |
| Related to intensity and duration | ? | Yes | Yes |
| Reduced by gradual reduction | Probably | Yes | Yes |
| Precipitated by antagonists | No | Yes | Yes |
| Neonatal withdrawal | No | ? | Yes |
| Protracted abstinence | No | Yes | Yes |
| Conditioned withdrawal | ? | Yes | Yes |
| Associated with relapse | ? | Probably | Probably |

Withdrawal syndromes can often be precipitated by the antagonist (i.e., blocker) of a drug. The most widely known example is naloxone-precipitated opioid withdrawal. Mecamylamine is a CNS blocker of nicotine; however, it does not appear to precipitate withdrawal when given to smokers (see Section 11).

Neonates born to opioid-dependent mothers can have a characteristic withdrawal syndrome. Whether neonatal withdrawal occurs with other drugs, such as alcohol and cocaine, is debatable (Finnegan, 1981). Although neonates of smokers are underweight (Hasselmeyer et al., 1983), neonatal abstinence effects from tobacco have not been described.

Protracted withdrawal states have been described for both alcohol and opioids. With tobacco, the opposite appears to occur; i.e., abstinence symptoms are at baseline 1 month postcessation and below baseline 6 months postcessation (see Section 11).

Withdrawal signs and symptoms often become conditioned to environmental events. For example, the sight of opiate paraphenalia or of labeled alcohol beverage can produce physiological changes as in withdrawal (Siegel, 1983). Many investigators have hypothesized such changes occur in smokers because the high frequency of smoking produces numerous pairings between smoking and certain cues that should induce conditioning. However, at present there are only preliminary data to support such an effect (see Section 15).

Many clinicians and investigators believe the onset of withdrawal leads to relapse with alcohol and opioids among subjects who are physically dependent. Scientific demonstration of this belief is surprisingly not robust. The best that can be said is that withdrawal is sometimes a sufficient, but never a necessary, cause of relapse (Cappell and LeBlanc, 1971). Whether tobacco withdrawal leads to relapse is controversial. At present, prospective studies do not consistently support this contention (see Section 16).

In summary, as with other withdrawal syndromes, tobacco abstinence effects appear to occur in nonhumans, are related to the development of tolerance, are due to drug deprivation (nicotine), are time limited, and abate with drug replacement or gradual reduction. Unlike other withdrawal syndromes, tobacco abstinence effects are not clearly related to dose and duration, have not been precipitated by an antagonist, do not occur in neonates, are not clearly conditioned to environmental cues, and do not produce a protracted syndrome. The common notion that intense tobacco abstinence effects decrease the likelihood of stopping smoking has not been clearly shown.

## 19. CONCLUSIONS

The methodological issues listed in Sections 4 and 10 were used to compile the list that follows. We remind the reader that we required at least two studies with similar results to state a conclusion.

1. Abstinence from tobacco can induce offset, transient, and rebound effects. Unlike many other drugs of dependence, tobacco abstinence does not induce physical symptoms or novel effects (e.g., seizures).
2. Abstinence effects that are offset effects could still prevent smoking cessation.
3. For many of the proposed abstinence effects, there are few empirical data that

fit minimal scientific criteria (e.g., baseline values, randomization to abstinence or continued smoking, control groups of never-smokers).

4. Rebound effects of the opiate/sedative type are limited to nonhumans and include decreased avoidance responding and increased acetylcholine in peripheral nerves and ganglia.
5. Transient effects that occur with abstinence are decreased adrenaline and increased awakening, anger, anxiety, difficulty concentrating, hunger, impatience, and restlessness.
6. Offset effects that occur are decreased memory and tremor and increased levels of certain medications and weight.
7. Effects that occur but cannot be classified as transient, offset, or rebound (i.e., indefinite effects) are slowing of the EEG, decreased HR, orthostasis, thyroid function, and increased alcohol use, skin temperature, caloric intake, rapid eye movement sleep, and pleasantness of sweets.
8. Surprisingly, abstinence has not been clearly shown to influence alertness, caffeine use, dysphoria, fatigue, several hormones and neurotransmitters, blood pressure, evoked responses, taste sensitivity/thresholds, metabolic rate, or reaction time.
9. Among the valid abstinence effects listed (4–7), those found to be due to nicotine deprivation in humans are decreased HR and memory and increased anger, anxiety, and impatience. This evidence comes mostly from studies of the administration and cessation of nicotine gum. Further tests using more robust nicotine replacement strategies may show other abstinence effects are due to nicotine deprivation.
10. In nonhumans, nicotine deprivation decreases avoidance responding and increases acetycholine in the periphery, caloric intake, and weight.
11. Retrospective studies, cross-sectional studies, and prospective studies without baseline or control scores (i.e., from never-smokers) or without randomization to cessation and noncessation groups can produce results of doubtful validity. In addition, since abstinence cannot be induced in a blind manner, subjective measures are suspect. Studies of nonquitters or of clinic attendees can produce results of doubtful generalizability.
12. The validity of abstinence effects is indicated by the fact that the abstinence effects listed in 4–7 have been shown to possess inter- and intrarater reliability, to occur with abstinence from routes of administration other than smoking (e.g., nicotine gum and smokeless tobacco), and to reverse with smoking.
13. Abstinence effects occur in self-quitters but are less prevalent and severe than those that occur in clinic attendees.
14. Abstinence from tobacco typically produces four to six symptoms that are observable and of significant magnitude.
15. Most transient abstinence effects occur within the first 24 hr and dissipate by 1 month postabstinence. Offset effects, such as increased hunger, have been shown to last 1–6 months.
16. Individual differences in abstinence effects have not been consistently related to gender, smoking history, or even degree of dependence.

17. None of the behavioral or pharmacological theories of abstinence effects have been well tested. Theories that abstinence effects are due to extinction or schedule induction, offset of nicotine effects, or homeostasis via receptor induction have slighty more evidence than other theories.
18. Demonstration of abstinence effects supports the theory that smoking is a form of drug dependence.
19. Abstinence effects have yet to be clearly shown to be important in the maintenance or cessation of smoking.
20. Nicotine gum is the only treatment that has been consistently found to reduce abstinence effects. Alpha-2 agonists appear promising.
21. Many abstinence effects from tobacco cessation are similar to other drug withdrawal syndromes in that they occur in animals, are due to deprivation of a drug (i.e., nicotine), and abate with replacement therapy. Unlike other drug withdrawal syndromes, abstinence effects from tobacco are not clearly related to dose and duration of drug use, have not been shown to be precipitated by antagonists, do not appear to persist for prolonged periods, and have not been shown to be conditioned to environmental stimuli.

## 20. FUTURE RESEARCH

It is apparent from this review that many beliefs about abstinence effects from tobacco are either unexplored or marked by contradictory results. We believe research is especially needed in several areas. First, a prospective study in self-quitters is needed to assess the true incidence and magnitude of abstinence effects. Second, studies that quantify the magnitude of abstinence discomfort and the resultant dysfunction (e.g., at work), if any, are needed. Third, large studies testing whether abstinence effects prospectively predict the inability to quit are needed. Fourth, studies of abstinence effects that include baseline and several postcessation values, as well as never-smoker controls, are needed to determine whether any of the effects we have labeled indefinite, offset, or transient are true rebound effects. Fifth, studies of whether abstinence effects are conditioned to environmental stimuli are needed, as this is often hypothesized. Sixth, studies of whether abstinence occurs with forms and routes of tobacco administration other than cigarettes (e.g., cigars, low-nicotine cigarettes, pipes, wet and dry snuff) are needed, as some of these alternate forms of tobacco is increasing.

### ACKNOWLEDGMENTS

Preparation of this review was suppported by grant HL-39220 from the National Heart, Lung and Blood Institute and grants DA-03728 and DA-04066, a First Independent Research Scientist Transition DA-04545 (Dr. Higgins), and a Research Scientist Development Award DA-00109 (Dr. Hughes) from the National Institute on Drug

Abuse. The authors thank Neil Grunberg, Jack Henningfield, Lynn Kozlowski, and Robert West for their helpful comments on this manuscript.

## REFERENCES

Abrams, P., Monte, P., Pinto, R., Elder, J., and Brown, P., 1987, Psychosocial stress and coping in smokers who relapse or quit, *Health Psychol.* **6**:289–303.

Ague, C., 1974, Cardiovascular variables, skin conductance and time estimation: Changes after the administration of small doses of nicotine, *Psychopharmacology* **37**:109–125.

Albanes, D., Jones, Y., Micuzzi, M. S., and Mattson, M. E., 1987, Associations between smoking and and body weight in the U.S. population: Analysis of NHANES I, *Am. J. Public Health* **77**:439–444.

American Psychiatric Association, 1980, *Diagnostic and Statistical Manual,* 3rd ed., pp. 159–160, 176–178, American Psychiatric Association, Washington, DC.

American Psychiatric Association, 1987, *Diagnostic and Statistical Manual,* 3rd ed.—revised, pp. 150–151, 166–168, 181–182, American Psychiatric Association, Washington, DC.

Ashton, H., and Stepney, R., 1982, *Smoking: Psychology and Pharmacology,* Tavistock, New York.

Axelsson, A., and Brantmark, B., 1975, The anti-smoking effect of chewing gum with nicotine of high and low bioavailability, in: *Proceedings of the Third World Conference on Smoking and Health,* American Cancer Society, New York.

Azrin, H. H., Hutchinson, R. R., and Hake, D. F., 1966, Extinction-induced aggression, *J. Exp. Anal. Behav.* **9**:191–204.

Bachynsky, N., 1986, The case for anticholinergic drugs for smoking cessation: A pilot study, *Int. J. Addict.* **21**:789–805.

Badawy, A. A.-B., and Evans, M., 1973, The effects of chronic phenobarbitone administration and subsequent withdrawal on the activity of rat liver tryptophan pyrolase and their resemblance to those of ethanol, *Biochem. J.* **135**:555–557.

Badawy, A. A.-B., and Evans, M., 1974, The effects of ethanol on tryptophan pyrolase activity and their comparison with those of phenobarbitone and morphine, *Adv. Exp. Med. Biol.* **59**:229–251.

Badawy, A. A.-B., and Evans, M., 1975*a*, The effects of acute and chronic nicotine hydrogen (+)− tartrate administration and subsequent withdrawal on rat liver tryptophan pyrrolase activity and their comparison with those of morphine, phenobarbitone, and ethanol, *Biochem. J.* **148**:425–432.

Badawy, A. A.-B., and Evans, M., 1975*b*, The effects of ethanol on tryptophan pyrrolase activity and their comparison with those of phenobarbitone and morphine, *Adv. Exp. Med. Biol.* **59**:229–251.

Badawy, A. A.-B., and Evans, M., 1983, Opposite effects of chronic administration and subsequent withdrawal of drugs of dependence on the metabolism and disposition of endogenous and exogenous tryptophan in the rat, *Alcohol Alcoholism* **18**:369–382.

Badawy, A. A.-B., Punjani, N. F., and Evans, M., 1980*a*, The effects of ethanol on rat liver and brain tryptophan metabolism, *Substance Alcohol Actions/Misuse* **1**:507–515.

Badawy, A. A.-B., Punjani, N. F., Evans, C. M., and Evans, M., 1980*b*, Inhibition of rat brain tryptophan metabolism by ethanol withdrawal and possible involvement of the enhanced liver trypophan pyrrolase activity, *Biochem. J.* **192**:449–455.

Badawy, A. A.-B., Evans, M., and Punjani, N. F., 1981*a*, Reversal by naloxone of the effects of chronic administration of drugs of dependence on rat liver and brain tryptophan metabolism, *Br. J. Pharmacol.* **74**:489–494.

Badawy, A. A.-B., Punjani, N., and Evans, M., 1981*b*, The role of liver tryptophan pyrolase in the opposite effects of chronic administration and subsequent withdrawal of drugs of dependence on rat brain tryptophan metabolism, *Biochem. J.* **196**:161–170.

Balfour, D. J., 1980, Studies on biochemical and behavioral effects of oral nicotine, *Arch. Int. Pharmacodyn.* **245**:95–103.

Balfour, D. J., 1982, The pharmacology of nicotine dependence: A working hypothesis, *Pharmacol. Ther.* **15:**239–250.

Balfour, D. J., and Benwell, M. E., 1981, The effects of chronic nicotine administration and withdrawal on 5-hydroxtryptamine synthesis and uptake by rat brain synaptosomes, *Br. J. Pharmacol.* **72:**490.

Balfour, D. J., and Morrison, C. F., 1975, A possible role for the pituitary–adrenal system in the effects of nicotine on avoidance behavior, *Pharmacol. Biochem. Behav.* **3:**349–354.

Balster, R. L., 1985, Behavioral studies of tolerance and dependence, in: *Behavioral Pharmacology: The Current Status,* Neurology and Neurobiology, Volume 13 (L. Seiden, and R. L. Balster, eds.), pp. 403–418, Alan R. Liss, New York.

Benowitz, N. L., Kuyt, F., and Jacob, P., 1984, Influence of nicotine on cardiovascular and hormonal effects of cigarette smoking, *Clin. Pharmacol. Ther.* **36:**74–81.

Benowitz, N. L., Hall, S. M., and Moden, G. M., 1988, Caffeine levels and consumption following tobacco abstinence: Evidence for caffeine regulation, Unpublished manuscript.

Benwell, M. E., and Balfour, D. J., 1979, Effects of nicotine administration and its withdrawal on plasma corticosterone and brain 5-hydroxyindoles, *Psychopharmacology* **63:**7–11.

Benwell, M. E., and Balfour, D. J., 1982, Effects of chronic nicotine administration on the response and adaptation to stress, *Psychopharmacology* **76:**160–162.

Benwell, M. E., Balfour, D. J., and Anderson, J. M., 1988, Evidence that tobacco smoking increases the density of (−)[$^3$H] nicotine binding sites in human brain, *J. Neurochem.* **50:**1243–1247.

Bickel, W. K., Stitzer, M. L., Liebson, I. A., and Bigelow, G. E., 1988, Acute physical dependence in man: Effects of naloxone after acute morphine exposure, *J. Pharmacol. Exp. Ther.* **244:**126–132.

Black, P. M., Giovino, G. A., Ossip-Klein, D. J., Megahead, N., Reynolds, W., Lent, L., DeBole, N., Valenzuela, L., Leone, M. A., and Stiggins, J., November 1988. Weight gain following smoking cessation in a self-help population: An exploratory analysis, Presented at the Annual Meeting of the Association for the Advancement of Behavior Therapy, Boston.

Bojholm, S., Hansen, M., Meyer, J., Andersen, B. T., and Gyntelberg, F., 1980, Effect of smoking cessation on heart rate and blood pressure at rest and during exercise, *Danish Med. Bull.* **27:**96–98.

Bosse, R., Garvey, A. J., and Costa, P. T., 1980, Predictors of weight change following smoking cessation, *Int. J. Addict.* **15:**969–991.

Bourne, S., 1985, Treatment of cigarette smoking with short-term high-dosage corticotrophin therapy: Preliminary communication, *J. Roy. Soc. Med.* **78:**649–650.

Bowen, D. J., Evry, S. E., and Grunberg, N. E., 1986, Nicotine's effects on female rats' body weight: Caloric intake and physical activity, *Pharmacol. Biochem. Behav.* **25:**1131–1136.

Brady, J. V., and Lukas, S. E., eds., 1984, *Testing Drugs for Physical Dependence Potential and Abuse Liability,* NIDA Research Monograph 52, U.S. Govt. Printing Office, Washington, DC.

Brantmark, B., Ohlin, P., and Westling, H., 1973, Nicotine-containing chewing gum as an anti-smoking aid, *Psychopharmacology* **31:**191–200.

Brown, B. B., 1968, Some characteristic EEG differences between heavy smoker and non-smoker subjects, *Neuropsychiatry* **6:**381–388.

Brown, C. R., Jacob, P., Wilson, M., and Benowitz, N. L., 1988, Changes in rate and pattern of caffeine metabolism after cigarette abstinence, *Clin. Pharmacol. Ther.* **43:**488–491.

Brozek, J., and Keys, A., 1957, Changes of body weight in normal men who stop smoking cigarettes, *Science* **125:**1203.

Burse, R. L., Bynum, G. D., Pandolf, K. B., Goldman, R. F., Sims, E. A., and Danforth, E. R., 1975, Increased appetite and unchanged metabolism upon cessation of smoking with diet held constant, *Physiologist* **18:**157.

Burse, R. L., Goldman, R. F., Danforth, E., Horton, E. S., and Sims, E. A., 1976, Effects of cigarette smoking on body weight, energy expenditure, appetite, and endocrine function, Unpublished manuscript.

Cambien, F., Richard, J. L., Ducimetiere, P., Warnet, J. M., and Kahn, J., 1981. The Paris Cardiovascular Risk Factor Prevention Trial: Effects of two years of intervention in a population of young men, *J. Epidemiol. Comm. Health* **35:**91–97.

Cappell, H., and Leblanc, A. E., 1971, Tolerance and physical dependence. Do they play a role in alcohol and drug self-administration? in: *Research Advances in Alcohol and Drug Abuse,* Volume 6 (Y. Israel, F. B. Glaser, H. Kalant, R. E. Popham, W. Schmidt, and R. G. Smart, eds.), pp. 159–196, Plenum Press, New York.

Carney, R. M., and Goldberg, A. P., 1984, Weight gain after cessation of cigarette smoking, *N. Engl. J. Med.* **310:**614–616.

Carroll, M. E., and Meisch, R. A., 1984, Increased drug-reinforced behavior due to food deprivation, in: *Advances in Behavioral Pharmacology,* Volume 4 (T. Thompson, P. B. Dews, and J. E. Barrett, eds.), pp. 47–88, Academic Press, New York.

Cherek, D. R., 1981, Effects of smoking different doses of nicotine on human aggressive behavior, *Psychopharmacology* **75:**334–345.

Cherry, N., and Kiernan, K., 1976, Personality scores and smoking behavior: A longitudinal study, *Br. J. Prev. Soc. Med.* **30:**123–131.

Clarke, P. B., and Kumar, R., 1983, The effects of nicotine on locomotor activity in nontolerant and tolerant rats, *Br. J. Pharmacol.* **78:**329–337.

Clarke, P. B., and Kumar, R., 1984, Some effects of nicotine on food and water intake in undeprived rats, *Br. J. Pharmacol.* **82:**233–239.

Classen, W., and Battig, K., 1976, Nicotine induced changes in the regulation of body weight in growing rats, *Sozial-praventivmed., Med. Soc. E Prev.* **21:**142–143.

Clearman, D. R., and Jacobs, D. R., 1985, Relationships between weight and caloric intake of men who stop smoking, Unpublished manuscript.

Comstock, G. W., and Stone, R. W., 1972, Changes in body weight and subcutaneous fatness related to smoking habits, *Arch. Environ. Health* **24:**271–276.

Crabbe, J. C., and Belknap, J. K., 1980, Pharmacogenetic tools in the study of drug tolerance and dependence, *Substance Alcohol Actions/Misuse* **1:**385–413.

Cryer, P. E., Haymond, M. W., Santiago, J. V., and Shad, S. D., 1976, Norepinephrine and epinephrine release and adrenergic mechanism of smoking-associable hemodynamic and metabolic events, *N. Engl. J. Med.* **295:**573–577.

Cummings, K. M., Jaen, C. R., and Giovino, G., 1985*a*, Circumstances surrounding relapse in a group of recent ex-smokers, *Prev. Med.* **14:**195–202.

Cummings, K. M., Giovino, G., Jaen, C. R., and Emrich, L. J., 1985*b*, Reports of smoking withdrawal symptoms over a 21-day period of abstinence, *Addict. Behav.* **10:**373–381.

Cushman, P., Forbes, R., Lerner, W., and Stewart, M., 1985, Alcohol withdrawal syndromes: Chemical management with lofexidine, *Alcoholism Clin. Exp. Res.* **9:**103–108.

Dahlstrom, A., Booj, S., Heiwall, P. O., and Larsson, P. A., 1980, The effect of chronic nicotine and withdrawal on intra-neuronal dynamics of acetylcholine and related enzymes in a preganglionic neuron system of the rat, *Acta Physiol. Scand.* **110:**13–20.

Dalloso, H. M., and James, W. P. T., 1983, The role of smoking in the regulation of energy balance, *Int. J. Obesity* **8:**365–375.

Dawson, G. W., and Vestal, R. E., 1982, Smoking and drug metabolism, *Pharmacol. Ther.* **15:**207–221.

Dews, P. B., and Wenger, G. R., 1977, Rate dependency of the behavioral effects of amphetamine, in: *Advances in Behavioral Pharmacology,* Volume 1 (T. Thompson and P. B. Dews, eds.), pp. 167–227, Academic Press, New York.

Dow, R. J., and Fee, W. M., 1984, Use of beta-blocking agents with group therapy in a smoking withdrawal clinic, *J. Roy. Soc. Med.* **77:**648–651.

Duffy, J., and Hall, S. M., in press, Smoking abstinence, eating style, and food intake, *J. Consult. Clin. Psychol.*

Edwards, G., Arif, A., and Hodgson, R., 1981, Nomenclature and classification of drug and alcohol related problems: A WHO memorandum, *Bull. WHO* **59:**225–242.

Edwards, J., and Warburton, D., 1983, Smoking, nicotine and electrocortical activity, *Pharmacol. Ther.* **19:**147–164.

Edwards, N. B., Simmons, R. C., Rosenthal, T. L., Hoon, P. W., and Downs, J. M., 1988, Doxepin in the treatment of nicotine withdrawal, *Psychosomatics* **29:**203–206.

Eisenberg, R. M., and Sparber, S. B., 1979, Changes in plasma corticosterone level as a measure of acute dependence upon levorphenol in rats, *J. Pharmacol. Exp. Ther.* **211**:364–369.

Eiser, J., Van der Plight, J., Raw, M., and Sutton, S., 1985, Trying to stop smoking: Effects of perceived addiction, attributions for failure, and expectancy for success, *J. Behav. Med.* **8**:321–341.

Eldon, M. A., Lerecker, P. W., MacGee, J., and Ritschel, W. A., 1987, Lack of effect of withdrawal from cigarette smoking on theophylline pharmacokinetics, *J. Clin. Pharmacokin.* **27**:221–225.

Elgerot, A., 1976, Note on selective effects of short-term tobacco abstinence on complex versus simple mental tasks, *Percept. Motor Skills* **42**:413–414.

Elgerot, A., 1978, Psychological and physiological changes during tobacco: Abstinence in habitual smokers, *J. Clin. Psychol.* **34**:759–764.

Emont, S. L., and Cummings, K. M., 1987, Weight gain following smoking cessation: A possible role for nicotine replacement in weight management, *Addict. Behav.* **12**:151–155.

Eysenk, J. H., and Eaves, E. J., 1980, *The Causes and Effects of Smoking*, Maurice Temple Smith, London.

Eysenk, J. H., and Eysenk, S. B. G., 1975, *Manual of the Eysenk Personality Questionnaire*, Hodder and Stoughton, London.

Fagerstrom, K. O., 1978, Measuring degree of physical dependence to tobacco smoking with reference to individualization of treatment, *Addict. Behav.* **3**:235–241.

Fagerstrom, K. O., 1980, Physical dependence on nicotine as a determinant of success in smoking cessation, *World Smoking Health* **5**:22–23.

Fagerstrom, K. O., 1987, Reducing the weight gain after stopping smoking, *Addict. Behav.* **12**:91–93.

Falk, J. L., 1981, The environmental generation of excessive behavior, in: *Behavior in Excess: An Examination of the Volitional Disorders* (S. J. Mule, ed.), pp. 313–337, Free Press, London.

Falk, J. L., 1983, Drug dependence: Myth or motive? *Pharmacol. Biochem. Behav.* **19**:385–391.

Falkenborn, Y., Larsson, C., and Nordberg, A., 1981, Chronic nicotine exposure in the rat: A behavioral and biochemical study of tolerance, *Drug Alcohol Depend.* **8**:51–60.

Fehily, A. M., Phillips, K. M., and Yarnell, J. W. G., 1984, Diet, smoking, social class and body mass index in the Caerphilly Heart Disease Study, *Am. J. Clin. Nutr.* **40**:827–833.

Feldman, R. S., and Quenzer, L. F., 1984, *Fundamentals of Neuropsychopharmacology*, pp. 237–258, Sinauer, Sunderland, MA.

Fertig, J. B., Pomerleau, O. F., and Sanders, B., 1986, Nicotine-produced antinociception in minimally deprived smokers and ex-smokers, *Addict. Behav.* **11**:239–248.

Finnegan, J. K., Larson, P. S., and Haag, H. B., 1945, The role of nicotine in the cigarette habit, *Science* **10**:294–96.

Finnegan, L. P., 1981, Maternal and neonatal effects of drug dependence in pregnancy, in: *Substance Abuse: Clinical Problems and Perspectives* (J. H. Lowinson and P. Renz, eds.), pp. 545–581, Williams & Wilkins, Baltimore.

Fixx, A. J., Daughton, D., Kass, I., Smith, J. L., Wickiser, A., and Golden, C. J., in press, Urinary alkanization and smoking cessation, *J. Clin. Psychol.*

Flanagan, J., and Maany, I., 1982, Smoking and depression, *Am. J. Psychiatry* **139**:541.

Frankenhaeuser, M., 1971, Behavior and circulating catecholamines, *Brain Res.* **34**:241–262.

Freidman, G. D., and Siegelaub, A. B., 1980, Changes after quitting cigarette smoking, *Circulation* **61**: 716–723.

Freidman, J., Horvath, T., and Meares, R., 1974, Tobacco smoking and a "stimulus barrier," *Nature* **248**:455–456.

Fuller, J. A., 1982, Smoking withdrawal and acupuncture, *Med. J. Aust.* **1**:28–29.

Garvey, A., Bosse, R., and Seltzer, C., 1974, Smoking, weight change, and age, *Arch. Environ. Health* **28**:327–329.

Gilbert, D., 1979, Paradoxical tranquilizing and emotion reducing effects of nicotine, *Psychol. Bull.* **86**: 643–661.

Gilbert, R. M., and Pope, M. A., 1982, Early effects of quitting smoking, *Psychopharmacology* **78**: 121–127.

Glassman, A. H., Jackson, W. K., Walsh, B. T., and Roose, S. P., 1985, Cigarette craving, smoking withdrawal, and clonidine, *Science* **226**:864–866.

Glassman, A. H., Stetner, F., Walsh, B. T., Raizman, P. S., Fleess, I. L., Cooper, T. B., and Corey, L. S., 1988, Heavy smokers, smoking cessation and clonidine, *J. Am. Med. Ass.* **259**:2863–2866.

Glauser, S. C., Glauser, E. M., Reidenberg, M. M., Rusy, B. F., and Tallarida, R. J., 1970, Metabolic changes associated with the cessation of cigarette smoking, *Arch. Environ. Health* **20**:377–381.

Glynn, S. M., Gruder, C. L., and Jegerski, J. A., 1986, Effects of biochemical validation of self-reported cigarette smoking on treatment success and on misreporting abstinence, *Health Psychol.* **5**: 125–136.

Goldberg, S. R., and Stolerman, I. P., eds., 1986, *Behavioral Analysis of Drug Dependence*, Academic Press, New York.

Goldstein, A., 1987, Criteria of a pharmacologic withdrawal syndrome, *Arch. Gen. Psychiatry* **44**:392.

Goldstein, M. G., Ward, K., and Niaura, R., May 1988, Nicotine gum, tobacco dependence and withdrawal, Presented at the Annual Meeting of the American Psychiatric Association, Montreal.

Gordon, T., Kannel, W. B., Dawber, T. R., and McGee, D., 1975, Changes associated with quitting cigarette smoking: The Framingham study, *Am. Health J.* **90**:322–328.

Gorelick, D. A., Rose, J., and Jarvik, M. E., 1988, Effect of naloxone on cigarette smoking, *J. Substance Abuse* **1**:153–159.

Gottlieb, A. M., Killen, J. D., Marlatt, G. A., and Taylor, C. B., 1987, Psychological and pharmacological influences in cigarette smoking withdrawal: The effects of nicotine gum and expectancy on smoking withdrawal symptoms and relapse, *J. Consult. Clin. Psychol.* **55**:606–608.

Griffiths, R. R., and Balster, R. L., 1979, Opioids: Similarity between evaluations of subjective effects and animal self-administration results, *Clin. Pharmacol. Ther.* **25**:611–617.

Griffiths, R. R., and Woodson, P. P., 1988, Caffeine physical dependence: A review of human, laboratory and animal studies, *Psychopharmacology* **94**:437–451.

Grinstead, O. A., 1981, Preventing weight gain following smoking cessation: A comparison of behavioral treatment approaches, *Univ. Microfilms Int.* 82-06024:174.

Gritz, E. R., 1980, Smoking behavior and tobacco abuse, in: *Advances in Substance Abuse*, Volume 1 (N. Mello, ed.), pp. 91–158, JAI Press, Greenwich, CT.

Gritz, E. R., and Jarvik, M. E., 1973, Preliminary study: Forty-eight hours of abstinence from smoking, in: *Proceedings of the 81st Annual Convention, American Psychological Association*, pp. 1039–1040, American Psychological Association, Washington, DC.

Grunberg, N. E., 1982, The effects of nicotine and cigarette smoking on food consumption and taste preferences, *Addict. Behav.* **7**:317–331.

Grunberg, N. E., 1985, Nicotine, cigarette smoking and body weight, *Br. J. Addict.* **80**:369–377.

Grunberg, N. E., 1986, Behavioral and biological factors in the relationship between tobacco use and body weight, in: *Advances in Behavioral Medicine* (E. S. Katkin and S. B. Manich, eds.), pp. 97–129, JAI Press, Greenwich, CT.

Grunberg, N. E., and Bowen, D. J., 1985, The role of physical activity in nicotine's effects on body weight, *Pharmacol. Biochem. Behav.* **23**:851–854.

Grunberg, N. E., Bowen, D. J., and Morse, D. E., 1984, Effects of nicotine on body weight and food consumption in rats, *Psychopharmacology* **83**:93–98.

Grunberg, N. E., Bowen, D. J., Maycock, V. A., and Nespor, S. M., 1985, The importance of sweet taste and caloric content in the effects of nicotine on specific food consumption, *Psychopharmacology* **87**:198–203.

Grunberg, N. E., Bowen, D. J., and Winders, S. E., 1986, Effects of nicotine on body weight and food consumption in female rats, *Psychopharmacology* **90**:101–105.

Grunberg, N. E., Winders, S. E., and Popp, K. A., 1987, Sex differences in nicotine's effects on consumatory behavior and body weight in rats, *Psychopharmacology* **91**:221–225.

Grunberg, N. E., Popp, K. A., and Winders, S. E., 1988*a*, Effects of nicotine on body weight in rats with access to "junk" foods, *Psychopharmacology* **94**:536–539.

Grunberg, N. E., Nespor, S. M., Popp, K. A., Raygada, M., Sibolboro, E. C., Winders, S. E., August 1988*b*, Nicotine cessation affects plasma insulin and glucose levels in rats, Presented at the Annual Meeting of the American Psychological Association, New York.

Guilford, J. S., 1966, *Factors Related to Successful Abstinence from Smoking,* American Institute for Research, Pittsburgh.

Guilford, J. S., 1967, Sex differences between successful and unsuccessful abstainers from smoking, in: *Studies and Issues in Smoking Behavior* (S. V. Zagona, ed.), pp. 95–102, University of Arizona Press, Tucson.

Gunn, R. C., 1986, Reactions to withdrawal symptoms and success in smoking cessation clinics, *Addict. Behav.* **11**:49–53.

Gunn, R. C., and Shapiro, A., 1979, Life stress, weight gain and resuming smoking after success in a cessation clinic, *Psychol. Rep.* **57**:1035–1039.

Gust, S. W., Hughes, J. R., and Keenan, R., June 1985, A randomized, placebo-controlled study of the effects of dose on nicotine gum self-administration, Presented at the Annual Meeting of the International Study Group Investigating Drugs As Reinforcers, Baltimore.

Hall, G. H., 1982, Pharmacological responses to the intracerebral administration of nicotine, *Pharmacol. Ther.* **15**:223–238.

Hall, G. H., and Morrison, C. F., 1973, New evidence for a relationship between tobacco smoking, nicotine dependence and stress, *Nature* **243**:199–201.

Hall, R. A., Rappaport, M., Hopkins, H., and Griffin, R., 1973, Tobacco and evoked potential, *Science* **180**:212–214.

Hall, S. M., 1984, The abstinence phobias: Links between substance abuse and anxiety, *Int. J. Addict.* **19**:613–631.

Hall, S. M., Ginsberg, D., and Jones, R. T., 1986, Smoking cessation and weight gain, *J. Consult. Clin. Psychol.* **54**:342–346.

Harris, C. M., Emmett-Oglesby, M. W., Robinson, N. G., and Lal, H., 1986*a*, Withdrawal from chronic nicotine substitutes partially for the interoceptive stimulus produced by pentylenetetrazol, *Psychopharmacology* **90**:85–89.

Harris, C. M., Emmett-Oglesby, M. W., Robinson, N. G., and Lal, H., 1986*b*, Subjective effects of nicotine withdrawal: Evidence for role of GABAergic system, *J. Am. Osteopathic. Assoc.* **86**(689): 103–104.

Harris, C. M., Elkhayat, I. S., Bhadra, S., Wood, D., and Lal, H., June 1988, Comparison of pentylenetetrazol-like withdrawal stimulus after chronic treatment with amphetamine, nicotine and cocaine, Presented at the Internation Meeting of the Society for Stimulus Properties of Drugs, Falmouth, MA.

Hasselmeyer, E. G., Meyer, M. B., Longo, L. D., and Mattison, D. R., 1983, Pregnancy and infant health, in: *The Health Consequences of Smoking for Women: A Report of the Surgeon General,* pp. 189–250, U.S. Government Printing Office, Washington, DC.

Hatsukami, D. K., 1988, Nicotine: Withdrawal reactions (physical dependence) in: *The Health Consequences of Smoking: Nicotine Addiction* (N. L. Benowitz, N. E. Grunberg, J. E. Henningfield, and H. A. Lando, eds.), pp. 197–211, U.S. Government Printing Office, Washington, DC.

Hatsukami, D. K., and Hughes, J. R., 1985, Characterization of tobacco withdrawal: Physiological and subjective effects, in: *Pharmacological Adjuncts in Smoking Cessation,* NIDA Research Monograph No. 53 (J. Grabowski and S. M. Hall, eds.), pp. 56–67, U.S. Government Printing Office, Washington, DC.

Hatsukami, D. K., Hughes, J. R., Pickens, R. W., and Svikis, D. S., 1984, Tobacco withdrawal symptoms: An experimental analysis, *Psychopharmacology* **84**:231–236.

Hatsukami, D. K., Hughes, J. R., and Pickens, R. W., 1985, Blood nicotine, smoke exposure and tobacco withdrawal symptoms, *Addict. Behav.* **10**:413–417.

Hatsukami, D. K., Gust, S. W., and Keenan, R., 1987, Physiological and subjective changes from smokeless tobacco withdrawal, *Clin. Pharmacol. Ther.* **41**:103–107.

Hatsukami, D. K., Dalgren, L., and Hughes, J. R., 1988, Symptoms of tobacco withdrawal from abrupt cigarette cessation versus partial cigarette reduction, *Psychopharmacology* **94**:242–247.

Hatsukami, D., Morgan, S. F., Pickens, R. W., and Hughes, J. R., 1987, Smoking topography in a nonlaboratory environment, *Int. J. Addict.* **22**:719–725.

Heimstra, N. W., Bancroft, N. R., and DeKock, A. R., 1967, Effects of smoking upon sustained performance in a simulated driving task, *Ann. NY Acad. Sci.* **142**:295–307.

Henningfield, J. E., Miyasato, K., and Jasinski, D. R., 1985, Abuse liability and pharmacodynamic characteristics of intravenous and inhaled nicotine. *J. Pharmacol. Exp. Ther.* **234:**1–12.

Herning, R. I., and Pickworth, W. B., 1985, Nicotine gum improves stimulus processing during tobacco withdrawal, *Psychophysiology* **22:**595.

Herning, R. I., Jones, R. T., and Backman, J., 1983, EEG changes during tobacco withdrawal, *Psychophysiology* **20:**507–512.

Hickey, N., and Mulcahy, R., 1973, Effect of cessation of smoking on body weight after myocardial infarction, *Am. J. Clin. Nutr.* **26:**385–386.

Higgins, M. W., and Kjelsberg, M., 1967, Characteristics of smokers and nonsmokers in Tecumseh, Michigan, *Am. J. Epidemiol.* **86:**60–77.

Higgins, S. T., Preston, K., Cane, E., Henningfield, J., and Jaffee, J., 1988, Behavioral, physiological and hormonal effects of a naloxone challenge following acute morphine pre-treatment in humans, in: *Problems of Drug Dependence, 1987,* NIDA Research Monograph 81 (L. S. Harris, ed.), pp. 202–208, U.S. Government Printing Office, Washington, DC.

Hjalmarson, A. I., 1984, Effect of nicotine chewing gum in smoking cessation: A randomized, placebo-controlled, double-blind study, *JAMA* **252:**2835–2838.

Hofstetter, A., Schutz, Y., Jequier, E., and Wahren, J., 1986, Increased 24-hour energy expenditure in cigarette smokers, *N. Engl. J. Med.* **314:**79–82.

Hughes, J. R., 1984, Identification of the dependent smoker, Validity and clinical utility, *Behav. Med. Abstr.* **5:**202–204.

Hughes, J. R., 1986*a*, Genetics of smoking: A brief review, *Behav. Ther.* **17:**335–345.

Hughes, J. R., 1986*b*, Craving as a psychological construct, *Br. J. Addict.* **82:**38–39.

Hughes, J. R., 1988, Clonidine, depression and smoking cessation, *JAMA* **254:**2901–2902.

Hughes, J. R., in press, Similarities and differences in drug withdrawal syndromes in: *Addiction Counseling: The Role of the Family Physician,* The Medicine Group, Toronto.

Hughes, J. R., and Hatsukami, D. K., 1985, Short-term effects of nicotine gum, in: *Pharmacological Adjuncts in Smoking Cessation,* NIDA Research Monograph, No. 53 (J. Grabowski and S. M. Hall, eds.), pp. 68–82, U.S. Government Printing Office, Washington, DC.

Hughes, J. R., and Hatsukami, D. K., 1986, Signs and symptoms of tobacco withdrawal, *Arch. Gen. Psychiatry* **43:**289–294.

Hughes, J. R., and Hatsukami, D. K., 1987, Criteria of a pharmacologic withdrawal syndrome, *Arch. Gen. Psychiatry* **44:**393–394.

Hughes, J. R., and Krahn, D., 1985, Blindness and the validity of double-blind drug trials, *J. Clin. Psychopharmacol.* **5:**138–142.

Hughes, J. R., and Miller, S., 1984, Nicotine gum to help stop smoking, *JAMA* **252:**2855–2858.

Hughes, J. R., and Valliere, W., 1988, Are ex-smokers nonsmokers? Unpublished manuscript.

Hughes, J. R., Hatsukami, D., Carroll, K., and Pickens, R. W., August 1982*a*, Effects of smoking cessation on weight, eating and activity, Presented at Annual Meeting of the American Psychological Association, Washington, DC.

Hughes, J. R., O'Hara, M. W., and Rehm, L. P., 1982*b*, Measurement of depression in clinical trials: A critical overview, *J. Clin. Psychiatry* **43:**85–88.

Hughes, J. R., Hatsukami, D. K., Pickens, R. W., Krahn, D., Malin, S., and Luknic, A., 1984*a*, Effect of nicotine on the tobacco withdrawal syndrome, *Psychopharmacology* **83:**82–87.

Hughes, J. R., Hatsukami, D. K., and Pickens, R. W., 1984*b*, The effect of Nicorette on the signs and symptoms of the tobacco withdrawal syndrome, Project Report Y-84-07, Merrell Dow Research Institute, Indianapolis.

Hughes, J. R., Hatsukami, D. K., Pickens, R. W., and Svikis, D. S., 1984*c*, Consistency of the tobacco withdrawal syndrome, *Addict. Behav.* **9:**409–412.

Hughes, J. R., Gust, S. W., Keenan, R. M., Skoog, K. P., Pickens, R. W., Ramlet, D., and Healey, M., August 1986*a*, Efficacy of nicotine gum in general practice, Presented at the Annual Meeting of the American Psychological Association, Washington, DC.

Hughes, J. R., Hatsukami, D. K., and Skoog, K., 1986*b*, Physical dependence on nicotine gum: A placebo-substitution trial, *JAMA* **255:**3277–3279.

Hughes, J. R., Hatsukami, D. K., Mitchell, J. E., and Dahlgren, B. A., 1986*c*, Prevalence of smoking in psychiatric outpatients, *Am. J. Psychiatry* **143**:993–997.

Hughes, J. R., Arana, G., Amori, G., and Stewart, F., 1988, Effect of tobacco withdrawal on the dexamethasone suppression test, *Biol. Psychiatry* **23**:96–98.

Hughes, J. R., Gulliver, S., Amori, G., and Mireault, G., in press-*a*, Effects of instructions and nicotine gum on smoking cessation, withdrawal symptoms and self-administration of nicotine gum, *Psychopharmacology*.

Hughes, J. R., Keenan, R., and Yellin, A., in press-*b*, Effect of tobacco withdrawal on sustained attention, *Addict. Behav*.

Hughes, J. R., Strickler, G., King, D., Gulliver, S., Mireault, G., and Fenwick, J. W., Smoking history instructions and the effects of nicotine: Two pilot studies, *Pharm. Biochem. Behav*. (in press).

Hunt, S. N., Jusko, W. J., and Yurchak, A. M., 1976, Effect of smoking on theophylline distribution, *Clin. Pharmacol. Ther.* **9**:546–551.

Hutchinson, R. R., and Emley, G. S., 1973, Effects of nicotine on avoidance, conditioned suppression and aggression response measures in animals and man, in: *Smoking Behavior: Motives and Incentives* (W. L. Dunn, ed.), pp. 171–196, Holt, New York.

Hutchinson, R. R., and Emley, G. S., 1981, Nicotine ingestion reduces elevated blood pressures in rats and squirrel monkeys, *Life Sci.* **28**:801–809.

Hutchinson, R. R., and Emley, G. S., 1986, Behavioral effects of nicotine, in: *Advances in Behavioral Pharmacology*, Volume 4, (T. Thompson and J. Barrett, eds.) Academic Press, New York.

Ikard, F. F., Green, D. E., and Horn, D., 1969, A scale to differentiate between types of smoking as related to the management of affect, *Int. J. Addict.* **4**:649–659.

Istvan, J., and Matarazzo, J. D., 1984, Tobacco, alcohol and caffeine use: A review of their interrelationships, *Psychol. Bull.* **95**:301–326.

Itel, T. M., Ulett, G. A., Hsu, W., Klingenberg, H., and Ulett, J. A., 1971, The effects of smoking withdrawal on quantitatively analyzed EEG, *Clin. EEG* **2**:44–51.

Jacobs, D. R., and Gottenborg, S., 1981, Smoking and weight: The Minnesota Lipid Research Clinic, *Am. J. Public Health* **71**:391–396.

Jaffe, J. H., 1977, Tobacco use as a mental disorder: The rediscovery of a medical problem, in: Research in Smoking Behavior, NIDA Research Monograph No. 17 (N. Krasnegor, ed.), pp. 202–219, U.S. Government Printing Office, Washington, DC.

Jaffe, J. H., 1980, Drug addiction and drug abuse, in: *The Pharmacologic Basis of Therapeutics*, 6th ed. (A. G. Gilman, L. S. Goodman, and A. Gilman, eds.), pp. 535–584, Macmillan, New York.

Jamrozik, K., Vessey, M., and Wald, N., 1984, Placebo-controlled trial of nicotine chewing gum in general practice, *Br. Med. J.* **289**:794–797.

Jarvik, M. E., 1979, Biological influences on cigarette smoking, in: *Smoking and Health: A Report of the Surgeon General*, Chapter 15, U.S. Government Printing Office, Washington, DC.

Jarvis, M. J., Hajek, P., Russell, M. A. H., and West, R. J., in press, Nasal nicotine solution as an aid to cigarette withdrawal: A pilot clinical trial, *Br. J. Addict.*

Jasinski, D. R., Johnson, R. E., and Kocher, T. R., 1985, Clonidine in morphine withdrawal: Differential effects in signs and symptoms, *Arch. Gen. Psychiatry* **42**:1063–1066.

Jones, R. A., 1986, Individual differences in nicotine sensitivity, *Addict. Behav.* **11**:435–438.

Jones, R. T., Farrell, T. R., and Herning, R. I., 1978, Tobacco smoking and nicotine tolerance, in: *Self-administration of Abused Substances: Methods for Study*, NIDA Research Monograph, No. 20 (N. A. Krasnegor, ed.), pp. 202–208, U.S. Government Printing Office, Washington, DC.

Kahn, A., Ciraulo, D., Nelson, W. H., Becker, J. T., Nies, A., and Jaffe, J., 1984, Dexamethasone suppression test in recently detoxified alcoholics: Clinical implications, *J. Clin. Psychopharmacol.* **4**:94–97.

Kalant, H., LeBlanc, A. E., and Griffins, R. J., 1971, Tolerance to, and dependence on, some nonopiate psychotropic drugs, *Pharmacol. Rev.* **23**:135–191.

Kales, J., Allen, C., Preston, T., Tan, T., and Kales, A., 1970, Changes in REM sleep and dreaming with cigarette smoking and following withdrawal, *Psychophysiology* **7**:347–348.

Karanci, N. A., 1985, Individual nicotine requirements: The relationship between differences in nicotine intake and physiological response, *Biol. Psychol.* **21**:27–42.

Karras, A., Kane, J. M., 1980, Naloxone reduces cigarette smoking, *Life Sci.* **27**:1541–1543.

Katz, J. L., and Valentino, R. J., 1986, Pharmacological and behavioral factors in opioid dependence in animals, in: *Behavioral Analysis of Drug Dependence* (S. R. Goldberg and I. P. Stolerman, eds.), pp. 287–315, Academic Press, New York.

Keenan, A., and Johnson, F. N., 1972, Development of behavioral tolerance to nicotine in the rat, *Specialia* **5**:428–429.

Killen, J. C., Maccoby, N., and Taylor, C. B., 1984, Nicotine gum and self-regulation training in smoking relapse prevention, *Behav. Ther.* **15**:234–248.

Killen, J., Taylor, C., Maccoby, N., and Young, J., 1987, Investigating predictors of smoking relapse: An analysis of biochemical and self-report measures of tobacco dependence, Unpublished manuscript.

Kleinman, K., Vaughn, R., and Christ, T., 1973, Effects of cigarette smoking and smoking deprivation on paired-associate learning of high and low meaningful nonsense syllables, *Psychol. Rep.* **32**:963–966.

Klesges, R. C., and Klesges, L. M., 1987, Cigarette smoking as a dieting strategy in a young adult sample, Unpublished manuscript.

Klesges, R. C., Eck, L. H., Clark, E. M., Meyers, A. W., and Hanson, C. L., 1988*a*, The effects of smoking cessation and gender on dietary intake, physical activity and weight gain, Unpublished manuscript.

Klesges, R. C., Meyers, A. W., and LaVasque, M. E., 1988*b*, Smoking, body weight and their effects on smoking behavior: A comprehensive review of the literature, Unpublished manuscript.

Knapp, P. H., Bliss, C. M., and Wells, H., 1963, Addictive aspects in heavy cigarette smoking, *Am. J. Psychiatry* **119**:966–972.

Knott, V. J., and Venables, P. H., 1977, EEG alpha correlates of non-smokers, smokers smoking, and smoking deprivation, *Psychophysiology* **14**:150–156.

Knott, V. J., and Venables, P. H., 1978, Stimulus intensity control and the cortical evoked response in smokers and non-smokers, *Psychophysiology* **15**:186–192.

Knott, V. J., and Venables, P. H., 1979, EEG alpha correlates of alcohol consumption in smokers and nonsmokers: Effect of smoking and smoking deprivation, *J. Stud. Alcohol* **40**:247–257.

Kozlowski, L. T., and Wilkinson, D. A., 1987, Use and misuse of the concept of "craving" by alcohol, tobacco and drug researchers, *Br. J. Addict.* **82**:31–36.

Krasnegor, R. A., ed., 1978, *Self-Administration of Abused Substances: Methods for Study,* NIDA Research Monograph No. 20, U.S. Government Printing Office, Washington, DC.

Ksir, C., Hakan, P., Hall, D. P., Jr., and Kellar, K. J., 1985, Exposure to nicotine enhances the behavioral stimulant effect of nicotine and increases binding of [$^3$H] acetylcholine to nicotinic receptors, *Neuropharmacology* **24**:527–531.

Lal, H., Harris, C. M., and Emmett-Oglesby, M. W., May 1985, Nicotine withdrawal symptom is increased by a GABA synthesis inhibitor, Presented at Society for Neuroscience, Minneapolis, MN.

Larson, P. S., and Silvette, H., 1961, *Tobacco: Experimental and Clinical Studies,* Williams & Wilkins, Baltimore.

Larson, P. S., and Silvette, H., 1968, *Tobacco: Experimental and Clinical Studies,* Supplement I, Williams & Wilkins, Baltimore.

Larson, P. S., and Silvette, H., 1971, *Tobacco: Experimental and Clinical Studies,* Supplement II, Williams & Wilkins, Baltimore.

Larson, P. S., and Silvette, H., 1975, *Tobacco: Experimental and Clinical Studies,* Supplement III, Williams & Wilkins, Baltimore.

Larsson, P. A., Dahlstrom, A., Heiwaii, P-O., and Booj, S., 1980, The effect of chronic nicotine and withdrawal on intra-axonal transport of acetylcholine and related enzymes in sciatic nerve of the rat, *J. Neural. Transm.* **47**:243–251.

Lawrence, P. S., Amodei, N., and Murray, A., November 1982, Withdrawal symptoms associated with smoking cessation, Presented at the Annual Convention of the Association for the Advancement of Behavior Therapy.

Lee, B. L., Benowitz, N. L., and Jacob, P., 1987*a*, Influence of tobacco abstinence on the disposition kinetics and effects of nicotine, *Clin. Pharmacol. Ther.* **41**:474–478.

Lee, B. L., Benowitz, N. L., and Jacob, P., 1987*b*, Cigarette abstinence, nicotine gum and theophylline disposition, *Ann. Intern. Med.* **106**:553–555.

Leventhal, H., and Cleary, P. D., 1980, The smoking problem: A review of the research and theory in behavioral risk modification, *Psychol. Bull.* **88**:370–405.

Levin, E. D., Morgan, M. M., Galvez, C., and Ellison, G., 1987, Chronic nicotine and withdrawal effects on body weight and food and water consumption in female rats, *Physiol. Behav.* **39**:441–444.

Levinson, P. R., Gernstein, D. R., and Maloff, D. R., eds., 1983, *Commonalities in Substance Abuse and Habitual Behavior,* Lexington Books, Lexington, MA.

Littlewood, J., Glover, V., Sander, M., Peatfield, R., Petty, R., and Rose, F. C., 1984, Low platelet monoamine oxidase activity in headache: No correlation with phenolsulphastransferase, succinate dehydrogenose, platelet preparation method and smoking, *J. Neurol. Neurosurg. Psychiatry* **47**: 338–352.

Lund-Larsen, P. G., and Tretle, S., 1982, Changes in smoking habits and body weight after a three-year period—The Cardiovascular Disease Study in Finnmark, *J. Chronic Dis.* **35**:773–780.

MacAndrews, C., 1979, On the possibility of the psychometric detection of persons who are prone to the abuse of alcohol and other substances, *Addict. Behav.* **9**:11–20.

Malcolm, R. E., Sillett, R. W., Turner, J. A. McM., and Ball, K. P., 1980, The use of nicotine chewing gum as an aid to stopping smoking, *Psychopharmacology* **70**:295–296.

Mangan, G. L., 1982, The effects of cigarette smoking on vigilance performance, *J. Gen. Psychol.* **106**: 77–83.

Mangan, G. L., and Golding, J. F., 1984, *The Psychopharmacology of Smoking,* Cambridge University Press, Cambridge.

Manley, R., and Boland, F., 1983, Side-effects and weight gain following a smoking cessation program, *Addict. Behav.* **8**:375–380.

Marks, M. J., Burch, J. B., and Collins, A. C., 1983, Effects of chronic nicotine infusion on tolerance development and nicotine receptors, *J. Pharmacol. Exp. Ther.* **226**:817–825.

Marks, M. J., Stitzel, J., and Collins, A. C., 1985, Time course study of the effects of chronic nicotine infusion on drug response and brain receptors, *J. Pharmacol. Exp. Ther.* **235**:619–628.

Martin, W., ed., 1977, *Drug Addiction I and II: Handbook of Experimental Pharmacology,* Volume 45, Springer-Verlag, New York.

Martin, W. R., and Jasinski, D. R., 1969, Physiological parameters of morphine dependence in non-tolerance, early abstinence and protracted abstinence, *J. Psychiatr. Res.* **7**:9–17.

Matarazzo, J. D., and Saslow, G., 1960, Psychological and related characteristics of smokers and nonsmokers, *Psychol. Bull.* **57**:493–513.

McCarty, M. F., 1982, Nutritional support of central catecholaminergic tone may aid smoking withdrawal, *Med. Hypotheses* **8**:95–102.

McNair, E., and Bryson, R., 1983, Effects of nicotine on weight change and food consumption in rats, *Pharmacol. Biochem. Behav.* **18**:341–344.

McNeill, A. D., West, R. J., Jarvis, M., Jackson, P., and Bryant, A., 1986, Cigarette withdrawal symptoms in adolescent smokers, *Psychopharmacology* **90**:533–536.

Melander, A., Nordenskjold, E., Lundh, B., and Thorell, J., 1981, Influence of smoking on thyroid activity, *Acta Med. Scand.* **209**:41–43.

Mello, N. K., and Mendelson, J. H., 1977, Clinical aspects of alcohol dependence, in: *Drug Addiction, Handbook of Experimental Pharmacology,* Volume 45 (W. Martin, ed.), pp. 613–666, Springer-Verlag, New York.

Milgrom-Friedman, J., Penman, R., and Meares, R., 1983, A preliminary study on pain perception and tobacco smoking, *Clin. Exp. Pharmacol. Physiol.* **10**:161–169.

Morgan, M. M., and Ellison, G., 1987, Different effects of chronic nicotine treatment regimens on body weight and tolerance in the rat, *Psychopharmacology* **91**:236–238.

Morrison, C. F., 1974*a*, Effects of nicotine and its withdrawal on the performance of rats on signaled and unsignaled avoidance schedules, *Psychopharmacology* **38**:25–35.

Morrison, C. F., 1974*b*, Effects of nicotine on the observed behavior of rats during signalled and unsignalled avoidance experiments, *Psychopharmacology* **38:**37–46.

Morrison, C. F., and Stephenson, J. A., 1972, The occurrence of tolerance to a central depressant effect of nicotine, *Br. J. Pharmacol.* **45:**151–156.

Mule, S. J., 1981, *Behavior in Excess: An Examination of the Volitional Disorders,* Free Press, London.

Murphee, H. B., 1979, EEG effects in humans of nicotine, tobacco smoking, withdrawal from smoking and possible surrogates, in: *Electrophysiological Effects of Nicotine* (A. Remond and C. Izard, eds.), pp. 227–243, Elsevier/North Holland Biomedical Press, Amsterdam.

Murphee, H. B., and Schultz, R. E., 1968, Abstinence effects in smokers, *Fed. Proc.* **27:**220.

Murray, A. L., and Lawrence, P. S., 1984, Sequalae to smoking cessation: A review, *Clin. Psychol. Rev.* **4:**143–157.

Myrsten, A. L., Elgerot, A., and Edgren, B., 1977, Effects of abstinence from tobacco smoking on physiological and psychological arousal levels in habitual smokers, *Psychosom. Med.* **39:** 25–38.

National Institute on Drug Abuse, 1983, *Why People Smoke Cigarettes,* U.S. Government Printing Office, Washington, DC.

Nelson, J. M., and Goldstein, L., 1972, Improvement of performance on an attention task with chronic nicotine treatment in rats, *Psychopharmacology* **26:**347–360, 1972.

Nelson, J. M., and Goldstein, L., 1973, Chronic nicotine treatment in rats: 1. Acquisition and performance of an attention task, *Res. Commun. Chem. Pathol. Pharmacol.* **5:**681–693.

Nemeth-Coslett, R., and Griffiths, R. R., 1986, Naloxone does not affect cigarette smoking, *Psychopharmacology* **89:**261–264.

Nemeth-Coslett, R., Henningfield, J. E., O'Keefe, M. K., and Griffiths, R. R., 1986*a*, Effects of mecamylamine on human cigarette smoking and subjective ratings, *Psychopharmacology* **88:**420–425.

Nemeth-Coslett, R., Sampson, A., and Henningfield, J. E., August 1986*b*, Subjective and physiological correlates of cigarette deprivation, Presented at the Annual Meeting of the American Psychological Association, Washington, DC.

Nesbitt, P. D., 1973, Smoking, physiological arousal, and emotional response, *J. Person. Soc. Psychol.* **25:**137–144.

Niaura, R., Abrams, D., Demuth, B., Monti, P., and Pinto, R., in press, Response to smoking-related stimuli and early relapse, *Addict. Behav.*

Nil, R., Woodson, P. P., and Battig, K., 1987, Effects of smoking deprivation on smoking behavior and heart rate response in high- and low-CO absorbing smokers, *Psychopharm.* **92:**465–469.

Norman, T. R., Chamberlain, K. G., and French, M. A., 1987, Platelet monoamine oxidase: Low activity in cigarette smokers, *Psychiatry Res.* **20:**199–205.

Olbrisch, M., and Oades-Souther, D., August 1986, Smoking cessation and changes in food, alcohol, and caffeine intake, Presented at the Annual Meeting of the American Psychological Association, Washington, DC.

Ornish, S. A., Zisook, S., and McAdams, L. A., 1988, Effects of transdermal clonidine treatment on withdrawal symptoms associated with smoking cessation: A randomized, controlled trial, *Arch. Intern. Med.* **148:**2027–2031.

Overton, P. A., 1984, State dependent learning and drug discriminations, in: *Handbook of Psychopharmacology,* Vol. 18 (L. L. Iversen, S. D. Iversen, and S. H. Snyder, eds.), pp. 59–127, Plenum, New York.

Pangborn, R. M., and Trabue, I. M., 1973, Gustatory responses during periods of controlled and ad-lib smoking, *Percept. Psychophysics* **7:**139–144.

Pangborn, R. M., Trabue, I. M., and Barylko-Pikielna, N., 1967, Taste, odor, and tactile discrimination before and after smoking, *Percept. Psychophysics* **2:**529–532.

Parsons, L. C., and Hamme, S., 1975, The effects of nicotine withdrawal on the sleep awake cycle, *Va. J. Sci.* **27:**86.

Parsons, L. C., Avery, S., Christman, S., Hopkins, J., and Seal, M., 1975*a*, The effects of 48 hour nicotine withdrawal on heart rate and respiration through continuous monitoring of all night sleep patterns in adult females, *Va. J. Sci.* **26:**92.

Parsons, L. C., Bell, N., Comer, L., Swartz, A., and Weissenborn, C., 1975*b*, The effects of short-term nicotine withdrawal on day vigilance as measured electrophysiologically, *Va. J. Sci.* **27**:86.

Parsons, L. C., Luttrell, N., Mabe, J., and Pollock, P., 1975*c*, The effect of 48 hour nicotine withdrawal on all night sleep patterns in adult females, *Va. J. Sci.* **26**:92.

Perlick, D., 1978, The withdrawal syndrome: Nicotine addiction and the effects of stopping smoking in heavy and light smokers, cited in Schacter, 1978.

Pertschuk, M., Pomerleau, O., Adkins, D., and Hirsch, C., 1979, Smoking cessation: The psychological costs, *Addict. Behav.* **4**:345–348.

Pickworth, W. B., Herning, R. I., and Henningfield, J. E., 1988, Mecamylamine reduces some EEG effects of nicotine chewing gum in humans, *Pharmacol. Biochem. Behav.* **30**:149–153.

Pohorecky, L. A., Newman, B., Sun, J., and Bailey, W. H., 1978, Acute and chronic ethanol ingestion and serotonin metabolism in rat brain, *J. Pharmacol. Ther.* **204**:424–432.

Pomerleau, O. F., and Pomerleau, C. F., 1984, Neuroregulators and the reinforcement of smoking: Towards a biobehavioral explanation, *Neurosci. Biobehav. Rev.* **8**:503–513.

Pomerleau, O. F., Adkins, D., and Pertschuk, M., 1978, Predictors of outcome and recidivism in smoking cessation treatment, *Addict. Behav.* **3**:65–70.

Pomerleau, O. F., Fertig, J., and Shanhan, S., 1983*a*, Nicotine dependence in cigarette smoking: An empirically-based, multivariate model, *Pharmacol. Biochem. Behav.* **19**:291–299.

Pomerleau, O. F., Fertig, J. B., Seyler, L. E., and Jaffe, J., 1983*b*, Neuroendocrine reactivity to nicotine in smokers, *Psychopharmacology* **83**:61–67.

Powell, D. R., and McCann, B. S., 1981, The effects of a multiple treatment program and maintenance procedures on smoking cessation, *Prev. Med.* **10**:94–104.

Puddey, I. B., Vandongen, R., Berlen, L. J., and English, D., 1984, Haemodynmaic and neuroendocrine consequences of stopping smoking: A controlled study, *Clin. Exp. Pharmacol. Physiol.* **11**: 423–426.

Puddey, I. B., Vandongen, R., Berlen, L. J., English, D. R., and Ukich, A. W., 1985, The effect of stopping smoking on blood pressure: A controlled trial, *J. Chronic Dis.* **38**:483–493.

Puska, P., Bjorkqvist, S., and Koskela, K., 1979, Nicotine-containing chewing gum in smoking cessation: A double-blind trial with half year followup, *Addict. Behav.* **4**:141–146.

Rabkin, S., 1984, Relationship between weight change and the reduction or cessation of cigarette smoking, *Int. J. Obesity* **8**:665–673.

Redington, K., 1984, Taste differences between cigarette smokers and nonsmokers, *Pharmacol. Biochem. Behav.* **21**:203–208.

Rodin, J., 1987, Weight change following smoking cessation: The role of food intake and exercise, *Addict. Behav.* **12**:303–317.

Rose, J. E., Herskovic, J. E., Trelling, Y., and Jarvik, M. E., 1985, Transdermal nicotine reduces cigarette craving and nicotine preference, *Clin. Pharmacol. Ther.* **38**:450–456.

Rosecrans, J. A., Hendry, J. S., and Hong, J. S., 1985, Biphasic effects of chronic nicotine treatment on hypothalamic immunoreactive B-endorphin in the mouse, *Pharmacol. Biochem. Behav.* **23**:141–143.

Russell, M. A. H., Peto, J., and Patel, V. A., 1974, The classification of smoking by factorial structure of motives, *J. Roy. Statist. Soc. A.* **137**:313–333.

Russell, P., Epstein, L., Sittenfield, S., and Block, D., 1984, The effects of nicotine chewing gum and cessation on the perception of muscle tension, *Psychopharmacology* **89**:230–233.

Sachs, D. P. L., and Benowitz, N. L., in press, The nicotine withdrawal syndrome: Nicotine abstinence or caffeine excess? in: *Problems of Drug Dependence, 1988, NIDA Research Monograph* (L. S. Harris, ed.), U.S. Government Printing Office, Washington, DC.

Sannita, W., Crotti, N., Massa, T., Morasso, G., Rosadini, G., Timitilli, C., and Valerio, F., 1984, Electrophysiological concomitants of the long-term withdrawal from cigarette smoking: A pilot study, *Res. Commun. Psychol. Psychiatry Behav.* **9**:273–281.

Schachter, S., 1978, Pharmacological and psychological determinants of smoking, *Ann. Intern. Med.* **88**:104–114.

Schecter, M. S., and Cook, P. G., 1976, Nicotine-induced weight loss without an effect on appetite, *Eur. J. Pharmacol.* **38**:63–69.

Schecter, M., and Rand, M., 1974, Effect of acute deprivation of smoking on aggression and hostility, *Psychopharmacology* **35:**19–28.

Schneider, N. G., and Jarvik, M. E., 1984, Time course of smoking withdrawal symptoms as a function of nicotine replacement, *Psychopharmacology* **82:**143–144.

Schneider, N. G., and Jarvik, M. E., 1985, Nicotine gum vs. placebo gum: Comparisons of withdrawal symptoms and success rates, in: *Pharmacological Adjuncts in Smoking Cessation,* NIDA Research Monograph 53 (J. Grabowski and S. M. Hall, eds.), pp. 83–101, U.S. Government Printing Office, Washington, DC.

Schneider, N. G., Jarvik, M. E., and Forsythe, A. B., 1984, Nicotine vs placebo gum in the allievation of withdrawal during smoking cessation, *Addict. Behav.* **9:**149–156.

Schoenenberger, J. C., 1982, Smoking change in relation to changes in blood pressure, weight, and cholesterol, *Prev. Med.* **11:**441–453.

Schwartz, R. D., and Kellar, K. J., 1983, Nicotinic cholinergic receptor binding sites in brain: Regulation *in vivo, Science* **202:**214–216.

Schwartz, R. D., and Kellar, K. J., 1985, *In vivo* regulation of [$^3$H] acetylcholine recognition sites in brain by nicotinic cholinergic drugs, *J. Neurochem.* **45:**427–433.

Schwartz, R. D., McGee, R., and Kellar, K. J., 1982, Nicotine cholinergic receptors labeled by [$^3$H] acetycholine in rat brain, *Mol. Pharmacol.* **22:**56–62.

Seltzer, C. C., and Oechsli, F. W., 1985, Psychosocial characteristics of adolescent smokers before they start smoking: Evidence of self-selection, *J. Chronic Dis.* **38:**17–26.

Seyler, L. E., Pomerleau, O. F., Fertig, J. B., Hunt, D., and Parker, K., 1986, Pituitary hormone response to cigarette smoking, *Pharmacol. Biochem. Behav.* **24:**159–162.

Shiffman, S. M., 1979, The tobacco withdrawal syndrome, in: *Cigarette Smoking as a Dependence Process,* NIDA Research Monograph No. 23 (N. A. Krasnegor, ed.), pp. 158–185, U.S. Government Printing Office, Washington, DC.

Shiffman, S. M., 1982, Relapse following smoking cessation: A situational analysis, *J. Consult. Clin. Psychol.* **50:**71–86.

Shiffman, S. M., August 1986, Tobacco "chippers": A study of non-dependent cigarette smokers, Presented at the Annual Meeting of the American Psychological Association, Washington, DC.

Shiffman, S. M., and Jarvik, M. E., 1976, Smoking withdrawal symptoms in two weeks of abstinence, *Psychopharmacology* **50:**35–39.

Shiffman, S. M., and Jarvik, M. E., 1984, Cigarette smoking, physiological arousal, and emotional response: Nesbitt's paradox re-examined, *Addict. Behav.* **9:**95–98.

Shiffman, S. M., Gritz, E. R., Mallese, J., Lee, M. A., Schneider, N. G., and Jarvik, M. E., 1983, Effects of cigarette smoking and oral nicotine on hand tremor, *Clin. Pharmacol. Ther.* **33:**800–805.

Sideroff, S. I., Jarvik, M. E., and Mintz, J., 1987, Responses to stimuli associated with smoking: Comparison between ex-smokers and heavy smokers abstaining for 12 hours, Unpublished manuscript.

Siegel, S., 1983, Classical Conditioning, drug tolerance, and drug dependence, in: *Research Advances in Alcohol and Drug Problems,* Volume 7 (Y. Israel, F. B. Glaser, H. Kalant, R. E. Popham, W. Schmidt, and R. G. Smart, eds.), pp. 207–246, Plenum Press, New York.

Silverstein, B., 1982, Cigarette smoking, nicotine addiction, and relaxation, *J. Person. Soc. Psychol.* **42:**946–950.

Smith, P., and Lombardo, T., November 1986, Effect of abstinence from smoking on motor activity, Presented at the Annual Meeting for the Association for the Advancement of Behavior Therapy, Chicago.

Snyder, F., and Henningfield, J., in press, Effects of acute nicotine deprivation and administration: Assessment on computerized performance tasks, *Psychopharmacology.*

Snyder, F., Davis, F., and Henningfield, J., August 1986, Chronic tobacco abstinence reduces information processing capabilities in heavy smokers, Presented at the Annual Meeting of the American Psychological Association, Washington, DC.

Snyder, F. R., Davis, F. C., and Henningfield, J. E., 1988, Replacement of cigarette smoking with nicotine gum: Effects on information processing, in: *Problems of Drug Dependence, 1987,* NIDA

Research Monograph No. 81 (L. S. Harris, ed.), pp. 327–328, U.S. Government Printing Office, Washington, DC.

Soldatos, C., Kales, J., Scharf, M., Bixler, E., and Kales, A., 1980, Cigarette smoking associated with sleep difficulty, *Science* **207**:551–553.

Solomon, R. L., and Corbit, J. D., 1973, An opponent-process theory of motivation: Cigarette addiction, *J. Abnorm. Psychol.* **81**:158–171.

Stamford, B. A., Matter, S., Fell, R. D., and Papnek, P., 1986, Effects of smoking cessation on weight gain, metabolic rate, caloric consumption, and blood lipids, *Am. J. Clin. Nutr.* **43**:486–494.

Stewart, J., de Wit, H., and Eikelbom, R., 1984, The role of unconditioned and conditioned drug effects in the self-administration of opiates and stimulants, *Psychol. Rev.* **91**:251–268.

Stitzer, M. L., and Gross, J., 1988, Nicotine replacement: Effect on post-cessation withdrawal symptoms and weight gain, in: *Problems of Drug Dependence,* NIDA Research Monograph No. 81 (L. Harris, ed.), pp. 53–58, U.S. Government Printing Office, Washington, DC.

Stolerman, I. P., 1986*a*, Could nicotine antagonists be used in smoking cessation? *Br. J. Addict.* **81**:47–53.

Stolerman, I. P., 1986*b*, Psychopharmacology of nicotine: Stimulus effects and receptor mechanisms, in: *Handbook of Psychopharmacology,* Volume 19 (L. L. Iverson, S. D. Iverson, and S. H. Snyder, eds.), Plenum Press, New York.

Stolerman, I. P., Goldfarb, T., Fink, R., and Jarvik, M. E., 1973, Influencing cigarette smoking with nicotine antagonists, *Psychopharmacology* **28**:247–259.

Stumpfe, K. D., 1984, Tobacco withdrawal symptoms, *Munchen. Med. Wochenschr.* **126**:731–735.

Svikis, D. S., Hatsukami, D. K., Hughes, J. R., Carroll, K. M., and Pickens, R. W., 1986, Sex differences in the tobacco withdrawal syndrome, *Addict. Behav.* **11**:459–462.

Swan, G., Denk, C., Parker, S., Carmelli, D., Furze, C., and Rosenman, R., in press, Risk factors for late relapse in male and female ex-smokers, *Addict. Behav.*

Szalai, J., Allon, R., Doyle, J., and Zamel, N., 1986, EEG alpha-reactivity and self-regulation correlates of smoking and smoking deprivation, *Psychosom. Med.* **48**:67–72.

Tarriere, H. C., and Hartmann, F., 1964, Investigation into the effects of tobacco smoke on a visual vigilance task, in: *Proceedings of the Second International Congress of Ergonomics,* pp. 525–530, cited in Wesnes and Warburton, 1983.

Tennant, F. S., Tarver, A. L., and Rawson, R. A., 1984, Clinical evaluation of mecamylamine for withdrawal from nicotine dependence, in: *Problems of Drug Dependence, 1983,* NIDA Research Monograph No. 49 (L. S. Harris, ed.), pp. 239–246, U.S. Government Printing Office, Washington, DC.

Ternes, J. W., 1973, An opponent process theory of habitual behavior with special reference to smoking, in: *Research on Smoking Behavior,* NIDA Research Monograph No. 17 (M. E. Jarvik, J. W., Cullen, E. R. Gritz, T. M. Vogt, and L. J. West, eds.), U.S. Government Printing Office, Washington, DC.

Tonnesen, P., Fryd, V., Hansen, M., Helsted, J., Gunnersen, A., Forchammer, H., and Stockner, M., 1988, Effect of nicotine chewing gum in combination with group counseling on the cessation of smoking, *N. Engl. J. Med.* **318**:15–27.

Trends in US cigarette use, 1965 to 1980, 1985, in: *The Health Consequences of Smoking: Cardiovascular Disease,* Appendix B, U.S. Government Printing Office, Washington, DC.

Tuomilehto, J., Nissinen, A., Puska, P., Salonen, J. T., and Jalkanen, L., 1986, Long-term effects of cessation of smoking on body weight, blood pressure and serum cholesterol in the middle-aged population with high blood pressure, *Addict. Behav.* **11**:1–9.

Turnbull, M. J., and Kelvin, A. S., 1971, Cigarette dependence, *Br. Med. J.* **10**:115.

Ulett, J. A., and Itel, T. M., 1969, Quantitative electroencephalogram in smoking and smoking deprivation, *Science* **164**:969–70.

Vale, A. L., and Balfour, D. J. K., 1987, The role of hippocampal 5-HT in the effects of nicotine on habituation to an X-maze, *Eur. J. Pharmacol.* **141**:313–317.

Wack, J. T., and Rodin, J., 1982, Smoking and its effects on body weight and the systems of caloric regulation, *Am. J. Clin. Nutr.* **35**:366–380.

Wenzel, D. G., and Azmeh, N., 1970, Chronically administered nicotine and the blood pressure of normotensive and renal hypertensive rats, *Arch. Int. Pharmacodyn.* **187**:367–376.

Wesnes, K., and Warburton, D. M., 1983, Smoking, nicotine and human performance, *Pharmacol. Ther.* **21**:189–208.

West, R. J., 1984, Psychology and pharmacology in cigarette withdrawal, *J. Psychosom. Res.* **28**:379–386.

West, R. J., 1985, Corticotrophin injections to treat cigarette withdrawal symptoms, *J. Roy. Soc. Med.* **78**:1065–1066.

West, R. J., 1986, Use and misuse of craving, *Br. J. Addict.* **82**:39–40.

West, R. J., and Russell, M. A. H., 1985*a*, Effects of withdrawal from long-term nicotine gum use, *Psychol. Med.* **15**:891–893.

West, R. J., and Russell, M. A. H., 1985*b*, Pre-abstinence smoke intake and smoking motivation as predictors of severity of cigarette withdrawal symptoms, *Psychopharmacology* **87**:334–336.

West, R. J., and Russell, M. A. H., 1987, Cardiovascular and subjective effects of smoking before and after 24 hr of abstinence from cigarettes, *Psychopharmacology* **92**:118–121.

West, R. J., and Schneider, N., 1987, Craving for cigarettes, *Br. J. Addict.* **82**:407–415.

West, R. J., Jarvis, M. J., Russell, M. A. H., Carruthers, M. E., and Feyerabend, C., 1984*a*, Effect of nicotine replacement on the cigarette withdrawal syndrome, *Br. J. Addict.* **79**:215–219.

West, R. J., Russell, M. A. H., Jarvis, M. J., and Feyerabend, C., 1984*b*, Does switching to an ultra-low nicotine cigarette induce nicotine withdrawal effects? *Psychopharmacology* **84**:120–123.

West, R. J., Russell, M. A., Jarvis, M. J., Pizzey, T., and Kadam, B., 1984*c*, Urinary adrenaline concentrations during 10 days of smoking abstinence, *Psychopharmacology* **84**:141–142.

West, R. J., Hajek, P., and Belcher, M., 1987, Time course of cigarette withdrawal symptoms during four weeks of treatment with nicotine chewing gum, *Addict. Behav.* **12**:1–5.

Westling, H., 1976, Experience with nicotine-containing chewing gum in smoking cessation, *Lakartidningen* **73**:2549–2552.

Weybrew, B. B., and Stark, J. E., 1967, *Psychological and Physiological Changes Associated with Deprivation from Smoking,* U.S. Naval Submarine Medical Center Report No. 490, U.S. Navy, Washington, DC.

Wikler, A., 1953, Neurophysiological aspects of the opiate and barbiturate abstinence syndromes, in: *Metabolic and Toxic Diseases of the Nervous System,* Volume 32, *Proceedings of the Association for Research in Nervous and Mental Disease,* Williams & Wilkins, Baltimore.

Wikler, A., 1980, *Opioid Dependence: Mechanisms and Treatment,* Plenum Press, New York.

Williams, D., 1979, Different cigarette-smoker classification factors and subjective state in acute abstinence, *Psychopharmacology* **64**:231–235.

Williamson, D. F., Forman, M. R., Binken, N. J., Gentry, E. M., Remington, P. L., and Trowbridge, F. L., 1987, Alcohol and body weight in United States adults, *Am. J. Public Health* **77**:1324–1330.

Winders, S. E., and Grunberg, N. E., August 1987, Nicotine, body weight, food consumption and body composition in rats, Presented at the Annual Meeting of the American Psychological Association, New York.

Wise, R. A., 1983, Brain neuronal systems mediating reward processes, in: *Neurobiology of Opiate Reward Mechanisms* (J. E. Smith, and J. D. Lane, eds.), pp. 405–438, Elsevier Biomedical Press, New York.

Woods, J. H., Katz, J. L., and Winger, G., 1987, Abuse liability of benzodiazepines, *Pharmacol. Rev.* **39**:251–414.

World Health Organization, 1981, Nomenclature and classification of drug and alcohol-related problems: A WHO memorandum, *Bull. WHO* **59**:225–242.

Zeidenberg, P., Jaffee, J. H., Kazler, M., Levitt, M. D., Langone, J. J., and Van Vunakis, H., 1977, Nicotine: cotinine levels in blood during cessation of smoking, *Comp. Psychiatry* **18**:93–101.

# Index

MIX
Papier aus verantwortungsvollen Quellen
Paper from responsible sources
FSC® C105338

If you have any concerns about our products,
you can contact us on
**ProductSafety@springernature.com**

In case Publisher is established outside the EU,
the EU authorized representative is:
**Springer Nature Customer Service Center GmbH**
**Europaplatz 3, 69115 Heidelberg, Germany**

Printed by Libri Plureos GmbH
in Hamburg, Germany